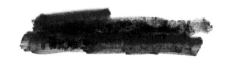

Respiratory Nursing

Author Bios

Michele Geiger-Bronsky, MSN, RN APNP, FNP-C has been an expert in the field of respiratory nursing for over two decades and was one of the first respiratory nurses to be recognized as a Fellow in the American Association of Cardiovascular and Pulmonary Rehabilitation. As the first Respiratory Clinical Nurse Specialist at Long Beach Memorial Medical Center in Long Beach, California, Michele developed a Respiratory Nursing Unit, an outpatient support group, and a comprehensive multidisciplinary Pulmonary Rehabilitation Program, all of which resulted in demonstrable differences in the lives of clients and staff and directly enhanced fiscal outcomes for the organization. Michele is a founding member of RNS, a past board member, and developed and served as the Editor of *Perspectives in Respiratory Nursing.* Following relocation to her home state of Wisconsin she now spends her time as the Executive Director and Nurse Practitioner of the Wellness Center of Door County and the Founder/President of the Door County Scottie Rally. She has been recognized as a 2008 champion of women's health by the Wisconsin Women's Health Foundation.

Donna J. Wilson, MSN, RN, RRT, is a clinical nurse specialist (CNS) and personal trainer who has been affiliated with the Integrative Medicine Service at Memorial Sloan-Kettering Cancer Center in New York City since 2000. During the past 30 years, she has gained extensive experience working with patients suffering from both acute and chronic respiratory diseases. Donna's post-graduate experience includes a MSN, awarded in 1991 from the Massachusetts General Hospital (MGH) Institute of Health Professions. The Aerobics and Fitness Association of America certified her as a personal trainer in May 2000 and, more recently, she was certified as a trainer for the T-Tapp Exercise Program. Her professional experience includes working at MGH for 17 years as a CNS, as the coordinator of the Respiratory Care Consultation Service in the Department of Anesthesia, and as the Lung Transplant Program nurse coordinator in the Thoracic Surgical Service.

In 1992, Donna joined the nursing staff at Memorial Sloan-Kettering Cancer Center as a pulmonary/thoracic CNS. Presently she creates and conducts exercise programs for a variety of individuals, many of whom are patients who are involved in ongoing cancer treatment programs. Activities include chair aerobics, step class, "Strong Bones for Osteoporosis," focused fitness classes for women, aerobics classes, and individual/group personal training. Her goals are to help patients rebuild strength, restore flexibility, achieve better balance, and decrease fatigue and breathlessness. To Donna, nursing is a means of giving of herself to the multiple roles serving as both a patient and family advocate. She also serves as collaborator, working with multiple health care teams and as a nursing care assessor to assist patients in coping with changes in their functional capacities in the course of daily activities. Donna has been involved in multiple national organizations focusing on respiratory diseases and is past president and board member of the Respiratory Nursing Society.

Respiratory Nursing

A Core Curriculum

Michele Geiger-Bronsky, MSN, RN APNP, FNP-C
Donna J. Wilson, MSN, RN, RRT
Editors

SPRINGER PUBLISHING COMPANY

New York

Springer Publishing Company, LLC
11 West 42nd Street
New York, NY 10036
www.springerpub.com

Acquisitions Editor: Allan Graubard
Production Editor: Rosanne Lugtu
Cover design: Joanne E. Honigman
Composition: Apex Publishing, LLC

08   09   10/   5   4   3   2   1

Library of Congress Cataloging-in-Publication Data

Respiratory nursing : a core curriculum / [edited by] Michele Geiger-Bronsky, Donna Wilson.
     p. ; cm.
 Includes bibliographical references and index.
 ISBN 978-0-8261-4444-7 (alk. paper)
 1. Respiratory organs—Diseases—Nursing.   I. Geiger-Bronsky, Michele.
II. Wilson, Donna, 1948–
 [DNLM: 1. Respiratory Tract Diseases—nursing. WY 163 R4344 2008]
RC735.5.R4697   2008
616.2'004231—dc22   2008005868

Printed in the United States of America by Bang Printing.

Contents

Contributors xi

Preface. xv

Acknowledgment. xvii

SECTION I   THE SPECIALTY OF RESPIRATORY NURSING

Chapter 1   Evolution of Respiratory Health Care 3
          Janet Larson and Suzanne C. Lareau

Chapter 2   Opportunities for Promoting Respiratory
          Health Across Clinical Settings 5
          Linda J. Schuyler

Chapter 3   Respiratory Nursing Research: Highlights
          and Future Directions 11
          Gerene S. Bauldoff and Leslie A. Hoffman

SECTION II   BASIC KNOWLEDGE

Chapter 4   Anatomy and Physiology of the Respiratory System 27
          Jacquenette Chambers-McBride and Rosalie O. Mainous

Chapter 5   Pathophysiology 51
          Janet Harris

Chapter 6   Respiratory Assessment. 61
          Lynn F. Reinke

Chapter 7   Pediatric Respiratory Assessment.....................71
             Pamela K. DeWitt

Chapter 8   Diagnostic Studies 75
             Deb Siela

Chapter 9   Provision of Patient Education......................97
             Susan Janson-Bjerklie

SECTION III   **NURSING CONCEPTS: HUMAN RESPONSE TO
               RESPIRATORY DYSFUNCTION**

Chapter 10   Dyspnea...109
             Audrey G. Gift and Anita Jablonski

Chapter 11   Impaired Sleep 123
             Terri E. Weaver

Chapter 12   Anxiety...135
             Mary Jones Gant and Judith Brown Sanders

Chapter 13   Depression..141
             Mary Jones Gant and Judith Brown Sanders

Chapter 14   Persistent Cough..................................151
             Cindy Balkstra and Sandy Truesdell

SECTION IV   **COMMON RESPIRATORY DISEASES AND DISORDERS**

Chapter 15   Emphysema and Chronic Bronchitis..................165
             Mary Beth Parr

Chapter 16   Asthma and Allergies..............................175
             Barbara Velsor-Friedrich and Susan Janson-Bjerklie

Chapter 17   Upper Respiratory Tract Infections 187
             Marianne Kwiatkowski, Enid Silverman,
             and Diane Dudas Sheenan

Chapter 18   Cystic Fibrosis...................................203
             Linda Tirabassi and Gwen McDonald

Chapter 19   Bronchiectasis....................................231
             Marilyn Borkgren and Cynthia Gronkiewicz

Chapter 20   Interstitial Lung Disease 243
Kathleen O. Lindell

Chapter 21   Pneumonias. 253
Janet Harris

Chapter 22   Lung Cancers. 275
Karen Leaton and Donna J. Wilson

Chapter 23   Pulmonary Thromboembolism 291
Christine Archer-Chicko

Chapter 24   Adult Obstructive Sleep Apnea. 311
Terri E. Weaver

Chapter 25   Respiratory Muscle Weakness. 317
Janet Crimlisk

Chapter 26   Respiratory Failure 353
Irene Grossbach

Chapter 27   Cor Pulmonale. 363
Elizabeth Burlew

Chapter 28   Pulmonary Complications of Human
Immunodeficiency Virus (HIV) 379
Ann Peterson

Chapter 29   Pulmonary Hypertension 393
Christine Archer-Chicko

Chapter 30   Tobacco and Other Substance Abuse. 417
Kathleen O. Lindell and Mary L. Wilby

SECTION V   **PEDIATRIC SPECIFIC DISORDERS**

Chapter 31   Newborn Respiratory Disorders 433
Rosalie O. Mainous

Chapter 32   Bronchiolitis. 447
Rebecca Tribby

Chapter 33   Respiratory Syncytial Virus 453
Pamela K. DeWitt

Chapter 34   Croup 459
Joyce J. LoChiatto and Mary Horn

SECTION VI   **THERAPEUTIC MODALITIES**

Chapter 35   Respiratory Pharmacology. 475
Christine V. Champagne and Richard Champagne

Chapter 36   Mechanical Ventilation 497
Irene Grossbach

Chapter 37   Tracheostomy 525
Jo Ann Frey

Chapter 38   Lung Transplantation 537
Christine Archer-Chicko

Chapter 39   Pulmonary Rehabilitation. 555
Bonnie Fahy, Paula Meek, and Jane Reardon

Chapter 40   Self-Care Management Strategies. 567
Cindy Kane

Chapter 41   Quality of Life and Functional Ability Issues 575
Georgia L. Narsavage

SECTION VII   **LEGAL AND ETHICAL ISSUES**

Chapter 42   Resource Utilization 589
Donna Smaha

Chapter 43   Patient Advocacy. 607
Anne H. Boyle and Dianne L. Locke

Chapter 44   Ethical Dilemmas 615
Sue Galanes

Chapter 45   End-of-Life Issues 621
Anne H. Boyle and Dianne L. Locke

Index 639

Contributors

Section Editors

Kathleen Ellstrom, PhD, RN, ACNS-BC
Pulmonary Clinical Nurse Specialist
Director, Pulmonary Rehabilitation
  Program
VA Loma Linda Healthcare System
Loma Linda, CA

Kathleen O. Lindell, PhD, RN
Clinical Nurse Specialist
Richard and Dorothy Simmons Center
  for Interstitial Lung Disease
Adjunct Assistant Professor
School of Nursing
University of Pittsburgh
Pittsburgh, PA

Anne Perry, EdD, RN
Professor
Co-Coordinator, Adult Health Nursing
  Specialty
Saint Louis University
St. Louis, MO

Contributors

**Christine Archer-Chicko,
  MSN, CRNP, CCRN**
Nurse Practitioner
Pulmonary Vascular Disease Program
University of Pennsylvania Medical
  Center/Presbyterian
Philadelphia, PA

Cindy Balkstra, MS, RN, CNS-BC
President, Georgia Nurses Association
Pulmonary Clinical Nurse Specialist
Dahlonega, GA

Gerene S. Bauldoff, RN, PhD
Assistant Professor
Ohio State University College of Nursing
Columbus, OH

Marilyn Borkgren, MS, RN, CCNS
Clinical Specialist
Suburban Lung Associates
Rolling Meadows, IL

Anne H. Boyle, RN, PhD
Clinical Assistant Professor
Department of Adult Health Nursing
Virginia Commonwealth University
  School of Nursing
Richmond, VA

Elizabeth Burlew, MSN, RN
Clinical Nurse Specialist
The Regional Medical Center
Memphis, TN

Christine V. Champagne, APRN,
  BC, CCRC
Nurse Practitioner
Midwest Chest Consultant, P.C.
St. Charles, MO

Richard Champagne, RPh, BCNSP,
  CCRC
Director of Research
Midwest Chest Consultant, P.C.
St. Charles, MO

Janet Crimlisk, MS, APRN-BC, NP
Clinical Nurse Educator
Adult Nurse Practitioner
Boston Medical Center
Boston, MA

Pamela K. DeWitt MN, RN
Clinical Specialist
Scottsdale, AZ

Bonnie Fahy, MS, RN
Pulmonary Clinical Nurse Specialist
Pulmonary Rehabilitation
St. Joseph's Hospital and Medical
  Center
Phoenix, AZ

Jo Ann Frey, MS, CNS, APRN, BC, CRRN
TriHealth Pulmonary Clinical Nurse
  Specialist
Good Samaritan Hospital/Trihealth
Cincinnati, OH

Sue Galanes, RN, ANP-BC, NP-C
Advanced Practice Nurse
Suburban Lung Associates
Winfield, IL

Mary Jones Gant, MSN, RN, RRT,
  APRN-BC, CM
Pulmonary Clinical Nurse Specialist
Christiana Care Health System
Wilmington, DE

Audrey G. Gift, PhD, RN, FAAN
Professor Emeritus
Michigan State University
College of Nursing
East Lansing, MI

Cynthia Gronkiewicz, MS, RN
Clinical Specialist
River Forest, IL

Irene Grossbach, MSN, RN
Pulmonary Clinical Nurse Specialist
Assistant Professor, Adjunct Faculty
Research Nurse
University of Minnesota, School of
  Nursing
Minneapolis, MN

Janet Harris, RN, PhD
Colonel Army Nurse Corps
Army Medical Department Center &
  School
Fort Sam Houston, TX

Leslie A. Hoffman, RN, PhD, FAAN
Professor and Chair
Department of Acute/Tertiary Care
University of Pittsburgh School of
  Nursing
Pittsburgh, PA

Mary Horn, MS, RN, RRT
Surgical Clinical Nurse Specialist
Children's Hospital
Boston, MA

Anita Jablonski, RN, PhD
Assistant Professor
College of Nursing
Seattle University
Seattle, WA

Susan Janson-Bjerklie, RN, ANP, MS, DNSc, FAAN
Professor and Mary Harms/Alumnae Chair
Department of Community Health Systems
Adjunct Professor, Department of Medicine
University of California, San Francisco
San Francisco, CA

Cindy Kane, RN, APRN-BC, MSN
Pulmonary Advanced Practice Nurse
Suburban Lung Associates
Elk Grove Village, IL
Clinical Educator
St. Alexius Medical Center
Hoffman Estates, IL

Marianne Kwiatkowski, MS, RN, GNP
Nurse Practitioner-Home Visit Program
Advocate Family Practice on Ravenwood
Chicago, IL

Suzanne C. Lareau, MS, RN, FAAN
Pulmonary Clinical Nurse Specialist
New Mexico VA Health Care System
Albuquerque, NM

Janet Larson, PhD, RN, FAAN
University of Michigan
School of Nursing
Division Director of Acute, Critical & Long term care programs
Ann Arbor, MI

Karen Leaton, RN, BSN, OCN
Research Coordinator
Kentuckiana Cancer Institute
Louisville, KY

Joyce J. LoChiatto, MS, RN, CPNP
Staff Development Specialist
Children's Hospital
Boston, MA

Dianne L. Locke, ANP-BC, RN
Adult Nurse Practitioner
Veterans Affairs Medical Center
Richmond, VA

Jacquenette Chambers-McBride, MSN, RN, CNS, CCRN
Respiratory Clinical Nurse Specialist
Long Beach Memorial Medical Center
Long Beach, CA

Gwen McDonald, MS, RN
(Retired-2004)
Respiratory Clinical Nurse Specialist
Salt Spring Island, BC, Canada

Rosalie Mainous, PhD, RN, C, NNP
Associate Professor and Coordinator
Neonatal Nurse Practitioner Graduate Program
School of Nursing
University of Louisville
Louisville, KY

Paula Meek, RN, PhD, FAAN
Professor and Senior Scholar
School of Nursing
University of Colorado
Denver, CO

Georgia L. Narsavage, PhD, APRN, BC, FAAN
Dean and Professor
School of Nursing
West Virginia University
Robert C. Byrd Health Sciences Center
Morgantown, WV

Mary Beth Parr, MSN, RN, CNS, CCRN
Coordinator of Sharp Health Care Human Patient Simulation Center
School of Nursing
San Diego State University
San Diego, CA

Ann Peterson, MSN, RN, CNS
Clinical Nurse Specialist
National Institutes of Health
Nursing Department
Bethesda, MD

**Jane Reardon, MSN, APRN, CS,
AE-C, FAACVPR**
Adult Care Nurse Practitioner
Hospitalist
Hartford Hospital Department of
Medicine
Hartford, CT

Lynn F. Reinke, PhD, ARNP
Nurse Investigator, Post Doctoral
Fellow
Department of Veterans Affairs,
Health Services
Seattle, WA

**Judith Brown Sanders, MSN,
APRN, CS**
Clinical Specialist of Psychiatry
Christiana Care Health System
Wilmington, DE

Linda J. Schuyler, MA, BSN, RN
Staff Nurse Pulmonary Department
Kaiser Permanente
Denver, CO

**Diane Dudas Sheenan, RN, MS,
FNP-C, CRRN**
Family Nurse Practitioner-Pediatric
Rehabilitation Program
Rehabilitation Institute of Chicago
Chicago, IL

**Deb Siela, PhD/DNSc, RRT,
APRN-BC, CCRN**
Assistant Professor of Nursing
School of Nursing
Ball State University
Muncie, IN

Enid Silverman, MS, RN
(Died - 2006)
Clinical Nurse Specialist

Rehabilitation Institute of Chicago
Chicago, IL

Donna Smaha, MSN, RN, CRNP
Clinical Director, Asthma Center of
Excellence
Nurse Practitioner, Brookwood
Seniors Health Center
Brookwood Medical Center
Birmingham, AL

Linda Tirabassi, MN, RN, CPNP
Clinical Nurse Specialist-Pediatrics
Long Beach Memorial Medical Center
Long Beach, CA

Rebecca Tribby, RN, MSN
Clinical Nurse Specialist/
Case Manager
Clinical Assistant Professor
Pediatric Pulmonary Center
UW American Family Children's
Hospital
Madison, WI

Sandy Truesdell, MSN, RN, CS
Pulmonary Rehabilitation Coordinator
Henry Ford Hospital
Detroit, MI

Barbara Velsor-Friedrich, PhD, RN
Associate Professor of Nursing
Loyola University
Chicago, IL

Terri E. Weaver, RN, PhD, CS, FAAN
Associate Professor and Chair
Biobehavioral and Health Sciences
Division
University of Pennsylvania School of
Nursing
Nursing Education Building
Philadelphia, PA

Mary L. Wilby, MSN, CRNP
Assistant Professor
La Salle University
Philadelphia, PA

Preface

It would not be odd if this introduction were to be started as "Once upon a Time" since it seems that is just how all great things begin—either a group or an individual comes up with an idea and things evolve from there. In the 1990s there was an intense interest in the concept of certification for Respiratory Nursing practice. It was clear to many of our respiratory nursing colleagues, who belonged to either the Respiratory Nursing Society (RNS) and/or the American Thoracic Society (ATS), that a CORE Curriculum needed to be established before certification could be considered.

After years of editing *Perspectives in Respiratory Nursing* for RNS, I agreed in 1999 to serve as the Editor of the *CORE Curriculum for Respiratory Nursing*. Following a tentative chapter outline including a framework for content, input from leaders in respiratory nursing and other disciplines was sought from across the United States. An assimilation of this feedback resulted in the framework for this 1st Edition of the *CORE Curriculum in Respiratory Nursing.*

Since the original plan called for nearly 50 chapters it was imperative that the CORE be divided into four Sections, each led by respiratory nursing experts who oversaw the editing and adherence to deadlines for purposes of the publication. At times the Section Editors became mentors and support lifelines for the authors. Every chapter was blindly peer reviewed by at least three persons; two of whom were content experts in the specific scope of the chapter. As time wore on additional revisions by authors were needed to ensure timeliness and accurate clinical content of the CORE.

Despite the time that has evolved, one thing has remained constant: Chapter after chapter continued to impress editorial staff; this is a work of which RNS deserves to be proud. In particular the authors deserve to be recognized and feel extremely proud of their contributions to the specialty of respiratory nursing.

No project can be completed independently and the *CORE Curriculum for Respiratory Nursing* is one that took an enormous amount of people, patience, and perseverance. Nearly a decade after its beginnings, this project has been brought to fruition with a total of 45 chapters. Many of our authors, as well as reviewers, have had life changing events—births of babies, job/career changes, relocations, completion of degrees and loss of family/friends that we've loved. It is important for readers to understand that the CORE Curriculum process has been a labor of love and *commitment* to the expertise that nurses need to possess and demonstrate when caring for persons with respiratory disease or compromised function. Every reviewer, editor and in particular author contributed countless volunteer hours in the creation of this resource. To each of you and your families, we say thank you.

When we began the CORE for Respiratory Nursing, its intent was to:

- Provide the basis and direction for clinicians who provide direct clinical care across all settings
- Create a foundation for development of staff education and curricula at the undergraduate and graduate level
- Serve as a resource by which respiratory nursing practice could be evaluated and
- Provide the basis for the development of a certification process for Respiratory Nursing

I believe that this CORE has met those objectives that RNS envisioned a decade ago.

For those readers who may find gaps in content or chapter inclusion—this is an opportunity for you to become involved in revisions of this important work. We encourage you to submit your ideas and willingness to contribute to the RNS office for future consideration!

Michele Geiger-Bronsky

Acknowledgment

On a personal note I want to extend a huge appreciation to the love of my life, Tom Bronsky, who always seems to understand and knows what support looks like, and to each of the section editors: Kathi Ellstrom, Donna Wilson, Anne Perry, and Kathleen Lindell. Each of these women have had multiple personal and professional demands on them during this process and deserve to be recognized for *their significant* contributions to the practice of respiratory nursing. And lastly, Donna Wilson deserves the highest recognition for bringing the CORE to fruition at a time when I could no longer lead the way. Donna took up the baton and finished the race. She will have my unending support and respect for ensuring the CORE's completion and publication.

Michele Geiger-Bronsky

I would like to thank my colleague, friend, and soulmate, my husband Dr. Roger S. Wilson, for his love and support.

Donna J. Wilson

The Specialty of Respiratory Nursing

I

1

Evolution of Respiratory Health Care

Janet Larson and Suzanne C. Lareau

I. Respiratory medicine/health care
   A. In the first half of the 20th century respiratory clinicians focused on the treatment and prevention of tuberculosis. This rather narrow focus was gradually broadened to include all types of respiratory-related conditions.
   B. In the last 25 years of the 20th century the respiratory specialization expanded to include a major focus on critical care and the care of people on mechanical ventilation.
   C. Respiratory specialization now spans a wide range of conditions that include the treatment and/or prevention of lung infections, restrictive and obstructive lung disease, respiratory and ventilatory failure, lung transplant, and pulmonary rehabilitation.
II. Specialty of respiratory nursing
   A. The specialty of respiratory nursing began to emerge in the 1940s when nurses received specialized education in the care of people with tuberculosis. The earliest education programs were funded by the American Lung Association (ALA) and its predecessors the National Tuberculosis Association (NTA) and the National Tuberculosis & Respiratory Disease Association (NTRDA) (Lareau et al, 1998).
   B. Growth of the specialty of respiratory nursing was fostered in the 1970s by the establishment of the American Thoracic Society (ATS) subsection on nursing and its educational programming at the annual ATS meeting.
      1. The current ATS Nursing Assembly is comprised of nursing researchers, clinicians, and educators who focus on advancing the science related to promoting the health and function of pulmonary patients.
   C. The advent of the clinical nurse specialist (CNS) role in master's programs in the 1970s contributed to developing the sub-specialty of respiratory nursing.

D. The organization structure for respiratory nursing matured in the 1990s with the founding of the Respiratory Nursing Society (RNS).
   1. The majority of RNS members focus on clinical practice promoting high quality nursing care to patients and families with pulmonary diseases. In addition, a major emphasis of RNS is delivering patient and professional education.
   2. Respiratory Nursing Society (RNS) standards and scope of practice
      a. The respiratory nurse collects comprehensive data pertinent to the patient's health or the situation, analyzes the assessment data to determine the diagnosis or issues of the respiratory patient, identifies expected outcomes for an individualized patient plan, develops and prescribes a plan, implements the plan, and coordinates the care delivery.
      b. The respiratory nurse employs strategies to promote respiratory health and a safe environment including clean air to breathe.
      c. The advanced practice registered nurse provides consultation to influence the identified plan and enhance the abilities of others to effect change. The advanced practice registered nurse also uses prescriptive authority, procedures, referrals, treatments. and therapies within state and federal laws and regulations.
      d. The Respiratory Nursing Society and American Nurses Association Standards of Care in its completed format are published on the RNS Web site: http://www.respiratorynursingsociety.org
III. Interdisciplinary approach to respiratory health care
   A. In the last half of the 20th century respiratory health care became very specialized in response to the growing body of knowledge about respiratory health and disease.
   B. The increasing complexity of clinical care required collaboration with professionals from multiple disciplines.
   C. Currently the care of people with actual or potential respiratory health problems is routinely administered by a multidisciplinary team.
      1. The multidisciplinary team includes physician, nurse, respiratory therapist, dietician, pharmacist, physical therapist, occupational therapist, and social worker.
      2. Each discipline brings a unique perspective and expertise to the team.

REFERENCE

Lareau, S., Breslin, E., Hansen, M., McDonald, G., Traver, G., & Wewers, M. E. (1998). *History of the American thoracic society assembly on nursing 1944 to 1998.* New York: American Lung Association.

Opportunities for Promoting Respiratory Health Across Clinical Settings

2

Linda J. Schuyler

INTRODUCTION

Prevention programs can be provided to individuals regardless of their state of health. Virtually all practice settings provide opportunities for educating individuals about respiratory health.

I. Primary, secondary, and tertiary prevention in respiratory nursing practice
   A. Levels of prevention
      1. "Health promotion is the science and art of helping people change their lifestyle to move toward a state of optimum health" (O'Donnell, 1989, p. 5).
      2. Pender defines two types of activities for improving and maintaining health status:
         a. Health promotion that is "motivated by the desire to increase well being and actualize human health potential" and
         b. Health protection that is "motivated by a desire to actively avoid illness, detect it early or maintain functioning within the constraints of illness" (Pender, 1996, p. 7).
      3. Leavell and Clark define three levels of prevention (1965).
         a. Primary prevention, which has two components: first, activities not directed at any specific disease or condition but at promoting general good health, and second, activities directed at the prevention of specific disorders.

      b. Primary prevention activities include
         i. Health education in the areas of nutrition, growth, and development, sex education, genetic, and environmental factors and preventive health evaluations.
        ii. Specific protection activities that include immunizations, protection from occupational and environmental exposures, i.e., carcinogens and allergens, and accident prevention.
      c. Secondary prevention involves early diagnosis and treatment of disease in order to prevent complications and limit disability.
      d. Secondary prevention activities include
         i. Case finding and screening of communities and individuals
        ii. Adequate treatment to prevent complications and limit disability
      e. Tertiary prevention is the prevention of complete disability after a disease process becomes stable.
      f. Tertiary prevention activities include provision of adequate rehabilitation programs enabling individuals to maximize the use of their remaining capabilities, and public education about individuals with disabilities.

B. Prevention programs: Tobacco avoidance (Centers for Disease Control [CDC], 1994; U.S. Department of Health and Human Services [HHS], 1994)
  1. Tobacco use is the chief preventable cause of premature death and disability in the United States. Tobacco use includes cigarettes, cigars, and smokeless tobacco.
  2. Almost all tobacco users start before they graduate from high school.
  3. Starting tobacco use at a younger age results in longer and heavier use of tobacco, with the attendant health risks: lung cancer, chronic obstructive pulmonary disease (COPD), and cardiovascular disease.
  4. Adolescents who use tobacco may reduce their rate of lung growth and impede the maximum level of lung function they can achieve.
  5. Adolescent tobacco users experience more of the following symptoms than their non-smoking peers: cough, shortness of breath, wheezing, and phlegm production.
  6. Adolescent tobacco use is associated with increased risk of alcohol and other drug abuse and other high-risk behaviors such as high-risk sexual practices, fighting, and use of weapons.
  7. Multiple risk factors influence tobacco use behavior in adolescents
    a. Low socioeconomic status
    b. Availability of tobacco products
    c. Peer pressure
    d. Lack of parental support
    e. Low academic achievement/involvement
    f. Low self esteem
    g. Lack of ability to refuse/resist offers to use tobacco
    h. Lack of understanding of the addiction potential and long term health effects of nicotine

8. Key elements of tobacco use prevention programs for adolescents include
   a. School-based prevention programs that are a part of a comprehensive school education program and that also involve parents, community, and the media.
   b. Enforcement of the ban on sale of tobacco products to minors.
   c. Increasing the price of tobacco products.
   d. Recognizing that nicotine addiction is as difficult to overcome for adolescents as it is for adults and that recruiting and retaining adolescents for smoking cessation programs is also difficult.
9. Recommendations from the CDC Guidelines for School Health Programs to Prevent Tobacco Use and Addiction (CDC, 1994, p. 7)
   a. "Develop and enforce a school policy on tobacco use"
   b. "Provide instruction about the short- and long-term negative physiologic and social consequences of tobacco use, social influences of tobacco use, peer norms regarding tobacco use and refusal skills"
   c. "Provide tobacco-use prevention education in kindergarten through 12th grade; this instruction should be especially intensive in junior high or middle school and should be reinforced in high school"
   d. "Provide program-specific training for teachers"
   e. "Involve parents or families in support of school-based programs to prevent tobacco use"
   f. "Support cessation efforts among students and all school staff who use tobacco"
   g. "Assess the tobacco-use prevention program at regular intervals"

C. Women and smoking (HHS, 2001)
1. Cigarette smoking became prevalent among men sooner than among women, but since the mid-1980s the prevalence has been about the same.
2. Increase in the quantity and duration of smoking among women had resulted in a corresponding increase in the number of smoking-related deaths in women.
3. Lung cancer has surpassed breast cancer as the leading cause of cancer-related deaths in women.
4. Cardiovascular disease risk is substantially increased for women who smoke. Cardiovascular disease includes: coronary heart disease, stroke, peripheral vascular disease, and abdominal aortic aneurysm. Oral contraceptives increase the risk of coronary heart disease.
5. Smoking during pregnancy increases the risk of
   a. Pregnancy complications such as premature rupture of membranes, placenta previa, abruptio placentae, and pre-term delivery
   b. Stillbirth, neonatal death, and SIDS
   c. Low birth weight
6. Postmenopausal women who smoke may have lower bone density than non-smokers and some increase risk for hip fracture.

7. In general, studies have not shown differences in the effectiveness of smoking cessation programs between men and women or between white women and non-white women.
8. Factors that influence women's decisions to smoke or not smoke include: pregnancy, fear of weight gain, depression, and social support needs.
9. More women stop smoking during pregnancy than at any other time. Two-thirds of those who quit will resume smoking within 1 year.

   D. Involuntary smoking (HHS, 1986)
1. Involuntary smoking (also termed *passive smoking* or *exposure to environmental tobacco smoke*) is a nonsmoker's unavoidable exposure to the tobacco smoke of others.
2. Environmental tobacco smoke comes from the end of a burning cigarette as well as from a smoker's exhalation.
3. The Report of the Surgeon General on the Health Consequences of Involuntary Smoking concludes
   a. "Involuntary smoking is a cause of disease, including lung cancer, in healthy non-smokers."
   b. "The children of parents who smoke, compared with the children on non-smoking parents have an increased frequency of respiratory infections, increased respiratory symptoms and slightly smaller rates of increase in lung function as the lung matures.
   c. "The simple separation of smokers and nonsmokers within the same air space may reduce, but does not eliminate, the exposure of nonsmokers to environmental tobacco smoke" (HHS 1986, p. 7).
4. Steps to reduce exposure to environmental tobacco smoke include (American Lung Association [ALA], 2007)
   a. Quit smoking
   b. Eliminate exposure by asking people not to smoke in your home or your car
   c. Make sure that your child's school and day care are smoke free
   d. Eat in a smoke-free environment
   e. Seek a smoke-free workplace
   f. Support legislation that promotes smoke-free environments
      i. Smoking cessation
      ii. Environmental exposures/air quality
      iii. Occupational exposures
      iv. Immunizations
      v. Rehabilitation

   E. Framework for prevention programs
1. Healthy People 2010
2. Models for health behavior change
3. Program development
4. Resources

II. Respiratory health care settings
   A. Factors driving prevention programs
1. Health care resources

  B. Practice settings
     1. Ambulatory/outpatient care
       a. Primary care
       b. Specialty care
       c. Community health care
         i. Home care
         ii. Hospice/palliative care
         iii. Occupational health
         iv. Parish nursing
         v. School nursing
     2. Acute/in-patient care
       a. Emergency department
       b. Acute care hospital
       c. Critical care units
       d. Skilled nursing facility/extended care
     3. Public and private education
       a. Child care
       b. Elementary education
       c. Secondary education

REFERENCES

American Lung Association. (2007, June). American lung association second-hand smoke fact sheet. Retrieved from http://www.lungusa.org

Centers for Disease Control and Prevention. (1994). Guidelines for school health programs to prevent tobacco use and addiction. MMWR 1994:43 (No. RR-2).

Leavell, H. R., & Clark, E. G. (1965). *Preventive medicine for the doctor in his community: An epidemiological approach* (3rd ed., pp. 19–28). New York: McGraw Hill.

O'Donnell, M. P. (1989). Definition of health promotion: Part III: Expanding the definition. *American Journal of Health Promotion, 3*(3), 5.

Pender, N. (1996). *Health promotion in nursing practice* (3rd ed.). Stamford, CT: Appleton & Lange.

U.S. Department of Health and Human Services (HHS). (1986). *The health consequences of involuntary smoking: A report of the surgeon general.* Rockville, MD: Public Health Service, Office on Smoking and Health.

U.S. Department of Health and Human Services (HHS). (1994). *Preventing tobacco use among young people: A report of the surgeon general.* Atlanta, GA: Public Health Service, Office on Smoking and Health.

U.S. Department of Health and Human Services (HHS). (2001). *Women and smoking: A report of the surgeon general: Executive summary.* Public Health Service, Office of the Surgeon General, Washington, DC: U.S. Government Printing Office.

Respiratory Nursing Research: Highlights and Future Directions

3

Gerene S. Bauldoff and Leslie A. Hoffman

INTRODUCTION

I. Definition, purpose, and importance of respiratory nursing research
Respiratory nursing focuses on reducing the impact of pulmonary disease and promoting respiratory wellness across the health care continuum and life span. State-of-the-art respiratory nursing is based on scientific evidence that has been derived from research, integrated into practice, and used to advance the health and well-being of pulmonary patients, families, and communities. By conducting research and disseminating research findings, nurses with expertise in respiratory nursing have had a major influence on multidisciplinary health care. Findings of respiratory nursing research have identified ways to enhance health promotion, improve the quality of care for individuals diagnosed with respiratory disease and for individuals at risk for developing pulmonary disease.

II. Priorities for research
A. Top five American nursing research priorities
A variety of nursing organizations and funding agencies have published research priorities that identify areas deemed most important for the generation of nursing knowledge in the 21st century. From a review of nursing literature published from 1994 to 1999, Hinshaw (2000) identified five research priorities most commonly cited by professional organizations or leading researchers in a clinical field. These priorities included: (a) quality of care outcomes and their measurement; (b) impact/effectiveness of nursing

interventions; (c) symptom assessment and management; (d) health care delivery systems; and (e) health promotion/risk reduction. While helpful, these statements are extremely broad and, thus, could encompass most, if not all, areas of nursing research.

B. National Institute of Nursing Research Priorities (NINR)
Research priorities have also been published by the NINR, a major funding agency for nursing research. In establishing priorities, the NINR attempts to identify areas for nursing research that meet four criteria: (a) the area represents a significant and costly current or future health care problem; (b) there are gaps in the state of the science underlying the problem or issue; (c) nursing can make a unique contribution in the area; and (d) there is potential for development of new knowledge. For the 5-year period of 2000–2004, NINR priorities were: (a) chronic illness experience; (b) cultural and ethnic considerations including interventions to decrease health disparities; (c) end of life/palliative care (NINR is the lead NIH institute in this area); (d) health promotion and disease prevention; (e) implications of genetic advances; (f) quality of life and quality of care; (g) symptom management; and (h) telehealth interventions and emerging technologies. NINR priorities include areas of general interest (chronic illness experience) and those with a more specific focus (telehealth). The NINR also addresses priorities by issuing a request for proposals (RFP). The RFP mechanism targets a specific problem (e.g., weaning from mechanical ventilation, the topic of a recent RFP), and the RFPs are then used to increase the number of proposals submitted in areas deemed highly promising for nursing research. The NINR Web site (www.nih.gov/ninr) lists current RFP and due dates.

C. American Thoracic Society (ATS) nursing assembly priorities
The ATS Nursing Assembly published *Research Priorities in Respiratory Nursing* in 1998 (Wewers et al., 1998). These priorities were organized into three broad categories—health promotion and disease prevention; therapeutic strategies: acute care; and therapeutic strategies: chronic care. Subsections within each category summarize accomplishments to date and research needed to further advance practice. These subsections address: tobacco use, prevention of pulmonary complications, weaning from long-term mechanical ventilation, high-tech home-care, oxygen delivery systems, end-of-life decision-making, pulmonary rehabilitation, cost-effectiveness research, and selected pulmonary conditions. This statement provides the most specific direction for respiratory nursing research.

D. American Association of Critical-Care Nurses (AACN) research priorities
The AACN Research Work Group selected five broad areas to guide future research activities (www.aacn.org/aacn/research). These priorities were developed from a review of over 3,000 practice questions received by the AACN Practice Resource Network and are designed to provide a framework to identify gaps in nursing knowledge. These priorities include: effective

and appropriate use of technology to achieve optimal patient assessment; management and/or outcomes; creating a healing, humane environment; processes and systems that foster the optimal contribution of critical care nurses; effective approaches to symptom management and prevention and management of complications. Priorities identified by AACN are practice-based but very general in scope.

III. Key respiratory nursing research

To highlight the vast contributions of pulmonary nurse researchers, the authors conducted a literature search using CINAHL (1982–February 2000) and Medline (1966–June 2000). The search included the names of all current Respiratory Nursing Society members (June 2000) and ATS Nursing Assembly members (1998 ATS Roster). From 1995 to 2000, a total of 155 articles were identified, 88 of which were databased. Using these 88 articles, findings published during the past 5 years were identified and summarized. It is recognized that seminal and substantial work was published before 1995. However, space limitations required a systematic decision for research inclusion. The research has been organized under headings used by the ATS Nursing Assembly and three additional areas: critical care, dyspnea, and instrumentation. Citations are at the end of the chapter.

A. Health promotion and disease prevention

1. Tobacco use

Nicotine dependence is a complex phenomena involving behavior, biological, and pharmacological components that influence smoking cessation rates. Pulmonary nursing research has focused on smoking behaviors specific to gender, race, cigarette composition, and stages of change.

2. Prevention of postoperative pulmonary complications (PPC)

PPC increase morbidity, mortality, and health care costs. Work in this area has focused on developing, testing and validating a model that predicts risk for PPC.

B. Therapeutic strategies: Acute care

1. Weaning from long-term mechanical ventilation (LTMV)

Research in this area has addressed varied topics, including developing a model of weaning from LTMV (the first to provide a framework for scientific inquiry in this area), testing ability of an outcomes-managed approach to speed weaning from LTMV (no significant effect was found), and testing use of patient-focused strategies during LTMV (reduced uncertainty and stress). In addition, researchers have used an animal model to explore the effect of various weaning modes on right heart hemodynamics. Findings suggested that weaning by pressure support was the preferred mode in the setting of cardiac dysfunction.

2. Critical care

Research in this area has addressed a broad variety of topics including daily inner cannula change (found not necessary), normal saline instillation (not recommended but used frequently), delay in initiating tube feedings (reduced by CNS practice), and tracheal gas insufflation (shown to increase CO_2 elimination efficiency). Additional topics include predicting risk for nosocomial infection (model development), efficacy of oscillation therapy (no difference compared to 2-hour turning), accuracy of pulse oximetry if cardiac function is impaired (SaO_2 overestimated), response to suctioning in head-injured patients, and performance of nursing interventions (core interventions defined).

3. High-technology home care

In a study that compared direct and indirect costs of home mechanical ventilation, the cost for adults was estimated at $7,642 per month using LPN rates and $8,596 using RN rates. No pediatric studies were identified in the designated time period.

4. End-of-life decision making

Work in this area supports that patients with chronic obstructive pulmonary disease (COPD) desire more information about end-of-life issues than is currently provided and regard pulmonary rehabilitation educators as a valuable source of this information. An educational intervention tested in a follow-up study was found to increase life-support discussions.

5. Oxygen delivery systems

Perceptions of the use of transtracheal oxygen delivery (TTOD) were explored using qualitative methodology. Patients with COPD feel isolated from their social worlds, but genuinely satisfied with the improvements offered by TTOD.

C. Therapeutic strategies: Chronic care

1. Asthma

Multiple nursing research studies have focused on how to most effectively promote optimal asthma self-management. Symptom perceptions have been explored. A number of studies have examined how to improve asthma self-management through education and factors that impact symptom severity, including the relationship between social support and immune function. Several studies examined issues in children with asthma using qualitative and quantitative methodology.

2. COPD

COPD has consistently been a strong focus area in pulmonary nursing research. Studies have focused on identifying factors influencing symptoms, fatigue, mood, and depression in these patients. Health-related quality of life and functional status were the focus of several studies involving patients with COPD, alpha-1 antitrypsin deficiency, and individuals undergoing lung volume reduction surgery. Additional research involved model testing (functional status, self-care capabilities), gender-based differences, and the impact of social support. A meta-analysis of 65 studies of the effect of education, exercise, and psychological support identified types of psychoeducational care shown to improve functioning and well-being in adults with COPD.

The experience of wives of persons with COPD was explored using qualitative methodology.

3. Lung cancer

   Work in this area was limited to one study that evaluated a nursing intervention for the management of breathlessness in patients with lung cancer.

4. Lung transplantation

   Effects of inhaled colistin were tested in lung transplant candidates with cystic fibrosis. All (100%) patients who used this therapy developed sensitive isolates, compared to 30% of patients who did not use inhaled colistin.

5. Sleep apnea

   Nursing research in patients with sleep apnea has focused on alternative positive airway pressure systems and adherence to therapy with emphasis on night-to-night variability, nightly duration of use, and the time nonadherent patterns develop.

6. Cystic fibrosis

   Factors with an adverse impact on adherence to treatment were found to include parent-child stress and lack of agreement between parents, leading to reduction in the health status and disease management of the child.

7. Pulmonary rehabilitation (PR)

   PR has been a focus for multiple nursing research studies. Studies have examined the short- and long-term impact of PR on health-related quality of life, functional status, 6- and 12-minute walk distance, respiratory muscle strength, and symptoms (e.g., dyspnea). Optimal training methods have been evaluated, for example, resistive inspiratory muscle training and systematic movement. Upper extremity training has been tested as a means to decrease symptoms in the laboratory and home setting. Studies have explored how self-efficacy and coping strategies impact response in patients with pulmonary dysfunction.

8. Dyspnea

   While dyspnea was not identified as a separate research priority by ATS, the wealth of nursing research in this area mandates its inclusion as a separate topic. The majority of research studies extend the definition and experience of dyspnea, progression, response to training, and impact on health-care utilization.

HEALTH DELIVERY

Few nursing studies have attempted to assess the cost-effectiveness of care. Only one study was identified that evaluated impact of a clinical pathway on length of stay, discharge disposition, and readmissions, including the impact of advanced practice nursing.

Instrument Development

Nurse researchers have been prominent in establishing the psychometrics of instruments used in pulmonary nursing research and the development of new instruments. Examples of new instruments include the Functional Performance Inventory (developed by Leidy), Pulmonary Functional Status Scale (developed by Weaver and Narsavage), and the Pulmonary Functional Status and Dyspnea Questionnaire (developed by Lareau). Other studies have established reliability and validity of varied physiologic and psychologic measures, for example, 6- or 12-minute walk distance, submaximal exercise, and tests of inspiratory muscle endurance.

No research was identified in the designated time period that related to the remaining topics listed in the ATS Nursing Assembly Research Priorities.

I. Performance improvement
    A. Definition and purpose
        Performance improvement (PI) is the process whereby problems are identified, a strategy is developed, change is instituted, and an outcome is assessed. It is similar to the nursing process with the addition of research to evaluate outcomes of practice; it provides a formal structure that can be used to critically evaluate research-based practice. Desired outcomes include improved patient health, cost reduction, and evidence supporting practice. PI promotes clinical research utilization by promoting the synthesis of research studies and their incorporation into clinical practice
    B. Joint Commission of Accreditation of Hospital Organizations (JCAHO) performance improvement
        In 1997, the JCAHO added a performance measurement component to the accreditation process called ORYX initiative. The goal of ORYX is integrating outcomes and other performance measures into the accreditation process. In May 2001, core measures for hospital-based settings were identified for acute myocardial infarction, heart failure, community-acquired pneumonia, and pregnancy and related conditions. These data will be collected in July 2002. While long-term care will adopt the Minimum Data Set (MDS), JCAHO performance improvement in home care will adopt the Outcome and Assessment Information Set (OASIS).
    C. Samples of PI systems
        Multiple tools and systems are available for process improvement. Two such tools include:
        1. STRAIGHT-A
            Select a process
            Team assignment
            Review process
            Analyze reasons for variance
            Implement improvement
            Gauge success by measuring against baseline
            Head back to step 4 if improvement not achieved

Test for stability for continued measurement

Assess whether continued improvement is possible or necessary

2. FOCUS-PDCA

Find a process that needs improvement

Organize a team that knows the process

Clarify current knowledge of the process

Understand the process and learn the causes of the variation

Select the improvement opportunities

Plan the changes

Do

Check the results

Act by implementing the change

D. Helpful hints for PI team leaders

1. Identify practice that does not demonstrate evidence basis.
2. Enlist assistance from persons of expertise, for example, use researchers to develop the problem analysis.
3. Utilize valid and reliable tools for data collection.
4. Promote multidisciplinary approach to PI, that is, use recommended practice guidelines from medical experts.
5. Develop timely, clear and concise communication tools (workshops, web sites, team meetings) to disseminate the findings and planned course of action.
6. With team input, select an innovation to be developed and tested.
7. Train all appropriate staff on the innovation to promote success of the process.
8. Provide open feedback lines for all staff to allow for adaptation of the innovation.

REFERENCES

Hinshaw, A. S. (2000). Nursing knowledge for the 21st century: Opportunities and challenges. *Journal of Nursing Scholarship 32*(2), 117–123. Retrieved from http://www.aacn.org/aacn/research.nsf/vwdoc/mainresearch?opendocument

Wewers, M. E., Brooks-Brunn, J. A., Hoffman, L. A., Janson, S., Kline-Leidy, N., Klijanowicz, A., Larson, J., et al. (1998). Research priorities in respiratory nursing. *American Journal of Respiratory and Critical Care Medicine*, 158, 2006–2015.

ADDITIONAL READING

U.S. Department of Health and Human Services Office of Disease Prevention and Health Promotion. (2000). *Healthy people 2010*. Rockville, MD: Author. Retrieved from www.healthypeople.gov

Tobacco Use

Ahijevych, K., & Gillespie, J. (1997). Nicotine dependence and smoking topography among black and white women. *Research in Nursing & Health, 20*(6), 505–514.

Ahijevych, K., Gillespie, J., Demirci, M., & Jagadeesh, J. (1996). Menthol and non-menthol cigarettes and smoke exposure in black and white women. *Pharmacology, Biochemistry & Behavior, 53*(2), 355–360.

Ahijevych, K., & Parsley, L. A. (1999). Smoke constituent exposure and stage of change in black and white women cigarette smokers. *Addictive Behaviors, 24*(1), 115–120.

Groner, J., Ahijevych, K., Grossman, L., & Rich, L. (1998). Smoking behaviors of women whose children attend an urban pediatric primary care clinic. *Women & Health, 28*(2), 19–32.

Postoperative Pulmonary Complications

Brooks-Brunn, J. A. (1997). Predictors of postoperative pulmonary complications following abdominal surgery. *Chest, 111*(3), 564–571.

Brooks-Brunn, J. A. (1998). Validation of a predictive model for postoperative pulmonary complications. *Heart & Lung, 27*(3), 151–158.

Weaning From Long-Term Mechanical Ventilation

Burns, S. M., Marshall, M., Burns, J. E., Ryan, B., Wilmoth, D., Carpenter, R., et al. (1998). Design, testing, and results of an outcomes-managed approach to patients requiring prolonged mechanical ventilation. *American Journal of Critical Care, 7*(1), 45–57.

Frazier, S. K. (1996). *Right heart hemodynamics during weaning from mechanical ventilation.* Unpublished doctoral dissertation, Ohio State University.

Knebel, A., Shekleton, M. E., Burns, S., Clochesy, J. M., & Hanneman, S. K. (1998). Weaning from mechanical ventilatory support: Refinement of model. *American Journal of Critical Care, 7*(2), 149–152.

Wunderlich, R. J., Perry, A., Lavin, M. A., & Katz, B. (1999). Patients' perceptions of uncertainty and stress during weaning from mechanical ventilation. *DCCN: Dimensions of Critical Care Nursing, 18*(1), 2–10.

Critical Care

Burns, S. M., Spilman, M., Wilmoth, D., Carpenter, R., Turrentine, B., Wiley, B., et al. (1998). Are frequent inner cannula changes necessary?: A pilot study. *Heart & Lung, 27*(1), 58–62.

Gowski, D. T., Delgado, E., Miro, A. M., Tasota, F. J., Hoffman, L. A., & Pinsky, M. R. (1997). Tracheal gas insufflation during pressure-control ventilation: Effect of using a pressure release valve. *Critical Care Medicine, 25*(1), 145–152.

Harris, J. R. (1996). *Predictors of nosocomial pneumonia in critically ill trauma patients.* Unpublished doctoral dissertation, University of Maryland at Baltimore.

Kerr, M. E., Rudy, E. B., Weber, B. B., Stone, K. S., Turner, B. S., Orndoff, P. A., et al. (1997). Effect of short-duration hyperventilation during endotracheal suctioning on intracranial pressure in severe head-injured adults. *Nursing Research, 46*(4), 195–201.

Kerr, M. E., Sereika, S. M., Orndoff, P., Weber, B., Rudy, E. B., Marion, D., et al. (1998). Effect of neuromuscular blockers and opiates of the cerebrovascular response to endotracheal suctioning in adults with severe head injuries. *American Journal of Critical Care, 7*(3), 205–217.

Miro, A. M., Hoffman, L. A., Tasota, F. J., Sigler, D. W., Gowski, D. T., Lutz, J., et al. (1997). Tracheal gas insufflation improves ventilatory efficiency during metacholine-induced bronchospasm. *Journal of Critical Care, 12*(1), 13–21.

Schwenker, D., Ferrin, M., & Gift, A. G. (1998). A survey of endotracheal suctioning with instillation of normal saline. *American Journal of Critical Care, 7*(4), 255–260.

Smatlak, P., & Knebel, A. R. (1998). Clinical evaluation of noninvasive monitoring of oxygen saturation in critically ill patients. *American Journal of Critical Care, 7*(5), 370–373.

Sulzbach-Hoke, L. M., & Gift, A. G. (1995). Use of quality management to provide nutrition to intubated patients. *Clinical Nurse Specialist, 9*(5), 248–251.

Titler, M. G., Bulechek, G. M., & McCloskey, J. C. (1996). Use of the nursing interventions classification by critical care nurses. *Critical Care Nurse, 16*(4), 38–40.

Traver, G. A., Tyler, M. L., Hudson, L. D., Sherrill, D. L., & Quan, S. F. (1995). Continuous oscillation: Outcome in critically ill patients. *Journal of Critical Care, 10*(3), 97–103.

High-Technology Home Care

Sevick, M. A., Kamlet, M. S., Hoffman, L. A., & Rawson, I. (1996). Economic cost of the home based care for ventilator-assisted individuals. *Chest, 109*(6), 1597–1606.

End-of-Life Decision Making

Heffner, J. E., Fahy, B., Hilling, L., & Barbieri, C. (1996). Attitudes regarding advance directives among patients win pulmonary rehabilitation. *American Journal of Respiratory and Critical Care Medicine, 154*(6 Pt 1), 1735–1740.

Heffner, J. E., Fahy, B., Hilling, L., & Barbieri, C. (1997). Outcomes of advance directive education of pulmonary rehabilitation patients. *American Journal of Respiratory and Critical Care Medicine, 155*(3), 1055–1059.

Oxygen Delivery Systems

Berg, J. (1996). Quality of life in COPD patients using transtracheal oxygen. *MED-SURG Nursing, 5*(1), 36–40.

Asthma

Berg, J. (1997). An evaluation of a self-management program for adults with asthma. *Clinical Nursing Research, 6*(3), 225–238.

French, C. L., Irwin, R. S., Curley, F. J., & Krikorian, C. J. (1998). Impact of chronic cough on quality of life. *Archives of Internal Medicine, 158*(15), 1657–1661.

George, M. R., O'Dowd, L. C., Martin, I., Lindell, K. O., Whitney, F., Jones, M., et al. (1999). A comprehensive educational program improves clinical outcome measures in inner-city patients with asthma. *Archives of Internal Medicine, 159*(15), 1710–1716.

Kang, D., Coe, C. L., Karaszewski, J., & McCarthy, D. O. (1998). Relationship of social support to stress responses and immune function in healthy and asthmatic adolescents. *Research in Nursing & Health, 21*(2), 117–128.

Kang, D., Coe, C. L., McCarthy, D. O., & Ershler, W. B. (1997). Immune responses to final exams in healthy and asthmatic adolescents. *Nursing Research, 46*(1), 12–19.

Smyrnios, N. A., Irwin, R. S., Curley, F. J., & French, C. L. (1998). From a prospective study of chronic cough: diagnostic and therapeutic aspects in older adults. *Archives of Internal Medicine, 158*(11), 1222–1228.

Yoos, H. L., & McMullen, A. (1996). Illness narratives of children with asthma. *Pediatric Nursing, 22*(4), 285–290.

Yoos, H. L., & McMullen, A. (1999). Symptom perception and evaluation in childhood asthma. *Nursing Research, 48*(1), 2–8.

COPD

Anderson, K. L. (1995). The effect of chronic obstructive pulmonary disease on quality of life. *Research in Nursing & Health, 18*(6), 547–556.

Anderson, K. L. (1999). Changes in quality of life after volume reduction surgery. *American Journal of Critical Care, 8*(6), 389–396.

Boyle, A. H. (1997). *Spouses of the chronically ill: The lived experience of wives of persons with chronic obstructive pulmonary disease.* Unpublished doctoral dissertation, University of Virginia.

Devine, E. C., & Pearcy, J. (1996). Meta-analysis of the effects of psychoeducational care in adults with chronic obstructive pulmonary disease. *Patient Education & Counseling, 29*(2), 167–178.

Gift, A. G., & Shepard, C. E. (1999). Fatigue and other symptoms in patients with chronic obstructive pulmonary disease: do women and men differ? *Journal of Obstetric, Gynecologic & Neonatal Nursing, 28*(2), 201–208.

Graydon, J. E., & Ross, E. (1995). Influence of symptoms, lung function, mood, and social support on level of functioning of patients with COPD. *Research in Nursing & Health, 18*(6), 525–533.

Graydon, J. E., Ross, E., Webster, P. M., Goldstein, R. S., & Avendano, M. (1995). Predictors of functioning of patients with chronic obstructive pulmonary disease. *Heart & Lung, 24*(5), 369–375.

Knebel, A. R., Leidy, N. K., & Sherman, S. (1999). Health related quality of life and disease severity in patients with alpha-1 antitrypsin deficiency. *Quality of Life Research, 8*(4), 385–391.

Metcalf, S. A. (1996). *Self-care actions as a function of therapeutic self-care demand and self-care agency in individuals with chronic obstructive pulmonary disease.* Unpublished doctoral dissertation, Wayne State University.

Narsavage, G. L. (1997). Promoting function in clients with chronic lung disease by increasing their perception of control. *Holistic Nursing Practice, 12*(1), 17–26.

Weaver, T. E., Richmond, T. S., & Narsavage, G. L. (1997). An explanatory model of functional status in chronic obstructive pulmonary disease. *Nursing Research, 467*(1), 26–31.

Yohannes, A. M., Roomi, J., Baldwin, R. C., & Connolly, M. J. (1998). Depression in elderly outpatients with disabling chronic obstructive pulmonary disease. *Age & Aging, 27*(2), 155–160.

Lung Cancer

Connolly, M., & O'Neill, J. (1999). Teaching a research-based approach to the management of breathlessness in patients with lung cancer. *European Journal of Cancer Care, 8*(1), 30–36.

Lung Transplantation

Bauldoff, G. S., Nunley, D. R., Manzetti, J. D., Dauber, J. H., & Keenan, R. J. (1997). Use of aerosolized colistin sodium in cystic fibrosis patients awaiting lung transplantation. *Transplantation, 64*(5), 748–752.

Sleep Apnea

Reeves-Hoche, M. K., Hudgel, D. W., Meck, R., Witteman, R., Ross, A., & Zwillich, C. W. (1995). Continuous versus bilevel positive airway pressure for obstructive sleep apnea. *American Journal of Respiratory and Critical Care Medicine, 151*(2 Pt 1), 443–449.

Weaver, T. E., Kribbs, N. B., Pack, A. I., Kline, L. R., Chugh, D. K., Maislin, G., et al. (1997). Night-to-night variability in CPAP use over the first three months of treatment. *Sleep, 20*(4), 278–283.

Cystic Fibrosis

Eddy, M. E., Carter, B. D., Kronenberger, W. G., Conradsen, S., Eid, N. S., Bourland, S. L., et al. (1998). Parent relationships and compliance in cystic fibrosis. *Journal of Pediatric Health Care, 12*(4), 196–202.

Pulmonary Rehabilitation

Bauldoff, G. S., Hoffman, L. A., Sciurba, F. C., & Zullo, T. G. (1996). Home-based upper arm exercise training for patients with chronic obstructive pulmonary disease. *Heart & Lung, 25*(4), 288–294.

Berry, J. K., Vitalo, C. A., Larson, J. L., Patel, M., & Kim, M. J. (1996). Respiratory muscle strength in older adults. *Nursing Research, 45*(3), 154–159.

Breslin, E. H., & Garoutte, B. C. (1995). Respiratory responses to unsupported arm lifts paced during expiration. *Western Journal of Nursing Research, 17*(1), 91–100.

Nield, M. A. (1999). Inspiratory muscle training protocol using a pressure threshold device: effect on dyspnea in chronic obstructive pulmonary disease. *Archives of Physical Medicine & Rehabilitation, 80*(1), 100–102.

Preusser, B. A., Winningham, M. L., & Clanton, T. L. (1994). High- vs. low-intensity inspiratory muscle interval training in patients with COPD. *Chest, 106*(1), 110–117.

Sassi-Dambron, D. E., Eakin, E. G., Ries, A. L., & Kaplan, R. M. (1995). Treatment of dyspnea in COPD. A controlled clinical trial of dyspnea management strategies. *Chest, 107*(3), 724–729.

Scherer, Y. K., & Schmieder, L. E. (1996). The role of self-efficacy in assisting patients with chronic obstructive pulmonary disease to manage breathing difficulty. *Clinical Nursing Research, 5*(3), 343–355.

Scherer, Y. K., & Schmieder, L. E. (1997). The effect of a pulmonary rehabilitation program on self-efficacy, perception of dyspnea and physical endurance. *Heart & Lung, 26(1),* 15–22.

Scherer, Y. K., Schmieder, L. E., & Shimmel, S. (1998). The effects of education alone and in combination with pulmonary rehabilitation on self-efficacy in patients with COPD. *Rehabilitation Nursing, 23*(2), 71–77.

Dyspnea

Carrieri-Kohlman, V., Gormley, J. M., Douglas, M. K., Paul, S. M., & Stulbarg, M. S. (1996). Exercise training decreases dyspnea and the distress and anxiety associated with it. Monitoring alone may be as effective as coaching. *Chest, 110*(6), 1526–1535.

Carrieri-Kohlman, V., Gormley, J. M., Douglas, M. K., Paul, S. M., & Stulbarg, M. S. (1996). Differentiation between dyspnea and its affective components. *Western Journal of Nursing Research, 18*(6), 626–642.

Lareau, S. C., Meek, P. M., Press, D., Anholm, J. D., & Poos, P. J. (1999). Dyspnea in patients with chronic obstructive pulmonary disease: does dyspnea worsens longitudinally in the presence of declining lung function? *Heart & Lung, 28*(1), 65–73.

Parshall, M. B. (1999). Adult emergency visits for chronic cardiorespiratory disease: Does dyspnea matter? *Nursing Research, 48*(2), 62–70.

Stulbarg, M. S., Carrieri-Kohlman, V., Gormley, J. M., Tsang, A., & Paul, S. (1999). Accuracy of recall of dyspnea after exercise training sessions. *Journal of Cardiopulmonary Rehabilitation, 19*(4), 242–248.

Cost-Effectiveness and Delivery of Health Care

George, E. L., & Large, A. A. (1995). Reducing length of stay in patients undergoing open heart surgery: The University of Pittsburgh Experience. *AACN Clinical Issues, 6*(3), 482–488.

Instruments

Covey, M. K., Larson, J. L., Alex, C. G., Wirtz, S., & Langbein, W. E. (1999). Test-retest reliability of symptom-limited cycle ergometer tests in patients with chronic obstructive pulmonary disease. *Nursing Research, 48*(1), 9–19.

Covey, M. K., Larson, J. L., & Wirtz, S. (1999). Reliability of submaximal exercise tests in patients with COPD. *Medicine & Science in Sports & Exercise, 31*(9), 1257–1264.

Hopp, L. J., Kim, M. J., Larson, J. L., & Sharp, J. T. (1996). Incremental threshold loading in patients with chronic obstructive pulmonary disease. *Nursing Research, 45*(4), 196–202.

Knebel, A., Leidy, N. K., & Sherman, S. (1998). When is the dyspnea worth it? Understanding functional performance in people with alpha-1 antitrypsin deficiency. *Image, 30*(4), 339–343.

Lareau, S. C., Breslin, E. H., & Meek, P. M. (1996). Functional status instruments: outcomes measure in the evaluation of patients with chronic obstructive pulmonary disease. *Heart & Lung, 25*(3), 212–214.

Lareau, S. C., Carrieri-Kohlman, V., Janson-Bjerklie, S., & Roos, P. J. (1994). Development and testing of the Pulmonary Functional Status and Dyspnea Questionnaire (PFSDQ). *Heart & Lung, 23*(2), 242–250.

Lareau, S. C., Meek, P. M., & Roos, P. J. (1998). Development and testing of the modified version of the pulmonary functional status and dyspnea questionnaire (PFSDQ-M). *Heart & Lung, 27*(3), 159–168.

Larson, J. L., Covey, M. K., Vitalo, C. A., Alex, A. G., Patel, M., & Kim, M. J. (1996). Reliability and validity of the 12-minute walk in patients with chronic obstructive pulmonary disease. *Nursing Research, 45*(4), 203–210.

Larson, J. L., Kapella, M. C., Wirtz, S., Covey, M. K., & Berry, J. (1998). Reliability and validity of the Functional Performance Inventory in patients with moderate to severe chronic obstructive pulmonary disease. *Journal of Nursing Measurement, 6*(1), 55–73.

Leidy, N. K. (1995). Functional performance in people with chronic obstructive pulmonary disease. *Image, 27*(1), 23–25.

Leidy, N. K. (1999). Psychometric properties of the Functional Performance Inventory in patients with chronic obstructive pulmonary disease. *Nursing Research, 48*(1), 20–28.

Leidy, N. K., Abbott, R. D., & Fedenko, K. M. (1997). Sensitivity and reproducibility of the dual-mode actigraph under controlled levels of activity intensity. *Nursing Research, 46*(1), 5–11.

Leidy, N. K., & Darling-Fisher, C. S. (1995). Reliability and validity of the Modified Erikson Psychosocial Stage Inventory in diverse samples. *Western Journal of Nursing Research, 17*(2), 168–187.

Leidy, N. K. & Haase, J. E. (1996). Functional performance in people with chronic obstructive pulmonary disease: A qualitative analysis. *Advances in Nursing Science, 18*(3), 77–89.

Leidy, N. K., & Haase, J. E. (1999). Functional status from the patient's perspective: the challenge of preserving personal integrity. *Research in Nursing & Health, 22*(1), 67–77.

Leidy, N. K., & Knebel, A. R. (1999). Clinical validation of the functional performance inventory in patients with chronic obstructive pulmonary disease. *Respiratory Care, 44*(8), 932–939.

Leidy, N. K., & Traver, G. A. (1995). Psychophysiologic factors contributing to functional performance in people with COPD: are there gender differences? *Research in Nursing & Health, 18*(6), 535–546.

Leidy, N. K., & Traver, G. A. (1996). Adjustment and social behavior in the older adults with chronic obstructive pulmonary disease: the family's perspective. *Journal of Advanced Nursing, 23*(2), 252–259.

Revicki, D. A., Leidy, N. K., Brennan-Diemer, F., Sorensen, S., & Togias, A. (1998). Integrating patient preferences into health outcomes assessment: The Multi-attribute Asthma Symptom Utility Index. *Chest, 114*(4), 998–1007.

Sevick, M. A., Sereika, S., Hoffman, L. A., Matthews, J. T., & Chen, G. J. (1997). A confirmatory factor analysis of the Caregiving Appraisal Scale for caregivers of home-based ventilator-assisted individuals. *Heart & Lung, 26*(6), 430–438.

Weaver, T. E., Laizner, A. M., Evans, L. K., Maislin, G., Chugh, D. K., Lyon, K., et al. (1997). An instrument to measure functional status outcomes for disorders of excessive sleepiness. *Sleep, 20*(1), 835–843.

Weaver, T. E., Narsavage, G. L., & Guilfoyle, M. J. (1998). The development and psychometric evaluation of the Pulmonary Functional Status Scale: An instrument to assess functional status in pulmonary disease. *Journal of Cardiopulmonary Rehabilitation, 18*(2), 105–111.

Yohannes, A. M., Roomi, J., Waters, K., & Connolly, M. J. (1998). A comparison of the Barthel Index and Nottingham extended activities of daily living scale in the assessment of disability in chronic airflow limitation in old age. *Age & Ageing, 27*(3), 369–374.

Process Improvement

Haase, R., & Miller, K. (1999). Performance improvement in everyday clinical practice. *American Journal of Nursing, 99*(5), 52–54.

Jones, J. (2000). Performance improvement through clinical research utilization: The linkage model. *Journal of Nursing Care Quality, 15*(1), 49–54.

Ramsey, C., Ormsby, S., & Marsh, T. (2001). Performance-improvement strategies can reduce costs. *Healthcare Financial Management,* 2001 HFM Resource Guide, 26.

Basic Knowledge

Anatomy and Physiology of the Respiratory System

4

Jacquenette Chambers-McBride and Rosalie O. Mainous

INTRODUCTION

1. Identify the major structures of the upper and lower respiratory tract and how they function.
2. Identify lung mechanics including heart-lung interrelationship, the differences between pulmonary and bronchial vascular circulation, and control of respiration.
3. State the basic principles of oxygenation.
4. Describe the ventilation/perfusion relationship of respiration.
5. Verbalize the physiological changes of the lungs during childhood, in pregnancy and with aging.

I. Function: The primary function of the respiratory system is to exchange oxygen and carbon dioxide between the atmosphere and the cells of the body. The lungs also perform metabolic and endocrine functions. It also is a site of hormone metabolism.
   A. Gas exchange
      1. *External respiration:* the exchange of gases between blood and the atmosphere by diffusion.
      2. *Internal respiration:* the exchange of gases between the capillary blood and the tissues.
      3. *Cellular respiration:* cannot be directly measured but is estimated by the amount of oxygen (O_2) consumed and carbon dioxide (CO_2) produced by the body. This ratio is called the *respiratory quotient (RQ)*. It is normally about 0.8 but can change based on nutritional substrate mix and metabolism, that is, the amount of carbohydrates, fats, and proteins consumed. Individuals with high blood glucose levels from

insufficient glucose metabolism or intravenous glucose infusion may have a higher RQ closer to 1.0 as a result of increased CO_2 production.

B. *Ventilation:* the movement of air in and out of the lungs (Scanlan, Wilkins, & Stoller, 1999).

C. *Blood reservoir:* The pulmonary circulation blood volume serves as a reservoir. Whenever cardiac output falls, it expands and increases capacity to compensate without significant changes in pulmonary vascular resistance.

D. *Systemic blood filter:* Pulmonary vessels trap fine particles that could enter the systemic circulation, that is, gas bubbles, blood clots, and white blood cells.

E. *Fluid exchange:* Alveoli are kept relatively free of fluid. Vessel and tissue pressure balances favor the retention of fluid within the vessels and pulls excess fluid from the alveoli into the blood (Goldstein, O'Connell, & Karlinsky, 1997).

F. Metabolic functions of the lungs

1. *Metabolism:* assists in protein and phospholipid synthesis. Enhances degradation and modification of circulating blood substances such as vasoactive substances.

2. *Surfactant synthesis:* produces a lipid protein that reduces pulmonary surface tension and aids in lung elastic recoil.

3. *Connective tissue synthesis:* collagen and elastin serve to support the lung and maintain its elasticity.

4. *Endocrine function:* assists in the regulation of hormonal levels in normal and pathologic circumstances.

5. *Defense mechanism:* provides air filtration, the removal of particles of foreign material, phagocytic defense, and participates in humoral and cell-mediated immunity.

6. *Acid-base balance:* assists in the regulation of the body's acid-base balance (McCance & Huether, 2002).

II. Basic structures

A. *Thorax:* cone-shaped and contains the rib cage, thoracic vertebrae, sternum, esophagus, trachea, lungs, heart and great vessels. It provides a bony structure to protect the vital organs. The thoracic bones and muscles interact to generate the pressures necessary to allow gas to flow in and out of the lungs (Bourke & Brewis, 1998).

1. *Rib cage:* consists of 12 pairs of ribs and cartilage, thoracic vertebrae, intervetebral discs, and the sternum. Ribs 1–7 are true or complete and 8–12 are false or incomplete.

2. *Sternum:* consists of the manubrium (body and process), suprasternal notch, and the sternal angle, also known as the *Angle of Louis.*

3. *Mediastinum:* divides the thorax vertically into the left and right pleural cavities, contains the lungs, is bound on either side by the parietal pleura and is divided into three subdivisions.

a. *Anterior compartment:* positioned between the sternum and the pericardium. It contains the thymus gland and anterior mediastinal lymph nodes.

b. *Middle compartment:* contains the pericardium, heart, great vessels, phrenic and upper portion of the vagus nerve, the trachea, main stem bronchi and associated lymph nodes.

c. *Posterior compartment:* positioned between the pericardium and the vertebral column. It contains the thoracic aorta, esophagus, thoracic duct, the lower portion of the vagus nerve, and the posterior mediastinal lymph nodes.

4. *Lungs:* two cone-shaped organs, pinkish in color at birth.

a. *Right lung:* thicker, wider and slightly shorter than the left lung to accommodate the higher right side of the diaphragm due to the position of the liver.

b. *Left lung:* thinner, longer, and narrower than the right lung to accommodate the heart.

c. *Fissures:* potential spaces that divide the lobes.

   i. *Minor:* lies at the fourth right rib and separates the middle and upper right lobes.

   ii. *Major (oblique):* extends from thoracic vertebrae 3 to 4 (T3–4) to the anterior level of the sixth rib. It separates the right upper and middle lobes and the left upper and lower lobes.

d. *Root of the lungs:* the lung's only attachment to other thoracic structures. It consists of the pulmonary veins, pulmonary artery, bronchus, nerves, and lymph nodes.

e. *Hilum:* a depression where structures enter and exit each lung root.

f. *Pleura:* The surface of the lungs and the chest walls are lined with two thin layers of pleura that have smooth shiny surfaces (Bourke & Brewis, 1998).

   i. *Visceral pleura:* the inner layer that covers the surfaces of the lungs and fissures.

   ii. *Parietal pleura:* the outer layer, named according to the regional area it comes into contact with (e.g. costal, diaphragmatic, or mediastinal pleura). It contains fibers for pain transmission. The acute angle where the costal pleura and the diaphragmatic pleura join is known as the *costophrenic angle.* Excess fluid tends to collect here when a person is upright and can be visibly seen on chest X-ray.

   iii. *Pleural cavity or space:* the potential space between the visceral and parietal pleura that is filled with 10 to 20 ml of serous fluid. It allows the pleura to slide past each other with minimal friction. This permits chest-wall forces to fluctuate during respiration.

III. Mechanics of breathing

  A. Breathing patterns

    1. *Quiet breathing:* the diaphragm performs 80% of the work of breathing (WOB) with the external and parasternal intercostal muscles doing the rest (Geiger-Bronsky, 1997).

2. *Active breathing:* the accessory, internal intercostal, scalene, sterno-cleidomastoid, abdominal, shoulder, and back muscles assist the diaphragm during deep breathing and with forced breathing.

B. Respiratory muscles

1. *Inspiration:* the active process of contracting the diaphragm downward to create a negative pressure within the thoracic cavity that draws gas into the lungs (Scanlan et al., 1999).

   a. *Diaphragm:* the major muscle of ventilation. It has a normal excursion of 1.5 cm during quiet inspiration that can increase to 6 to 10 cm with deep inspiration. Motor innervation of the diaphragm is at cervical vertebrae 3 to 5 (C3–5).

   b. *External intercostal muscles:* elevate the rib cage and increase the anterior-posterior (A-P) diameter of the thorax by 20% during inspiration. Motor innervation of the external intercostal muscles is at T1–11.

   c. *Abdominal muscles:* elevate the sternum and ribs and increase the A-P diameter.

   d. *Neck muscles (scalene and sternocleidomastoid):* elevate the sternum and ribs and increase the A-P diameter.

2. *Expiration:* the passive act of relaxing the respiratory muscles allowing a decrease in thoracic size and the elastic recoil of the lungs to deflate the lungs (Scanlan et al., 1999).

   a. *Intercostal and accessory muscles:* compress the ribs and decrease the A-P diameter. Motor innervation of the intercostal and accessory muscles is at T1–11.

   b. *Abdominal muscles:* force abdominal content upward to elevate the diaphragm.

3. *Respiratory muscle groups:* While the diaphragm contracts, other muscle groups work to stabilize the chest wall and convert the diaphragmatic contraction into intrathoracic pressure and volume changes.

C. Mechanical properties

1. *Lung elasticity:* Elastic recoil would occur if the lungs were removed from the chest. This is primarily due to elastin fibers within the alveolar walls, bronchioles, and capillaries (Dettenmeier, 1992).

2. *Compliance:* the ability of the lungs to be stretched or distended based on tissue pliability and intrathoracic pressures. If compliance is high, the lung is more easily distended. If compliance is low, the lung is stiff and difficult to expand (McCance & Huether, 2002).

3. *Pressure changes during breathing:* Alveolar pressure normally equals atmospheric pressure before a breath.

   a. *Inspiration:* When contraction of the inspiratory muscles occurs, intrapleural pressure drops from about -5 cm H_2O to -7 or -8 cm H_2O and air enters the lungs.

   b. *Expiration:* As alveoli are distended, the pressure inside them falls below atmospheric pressure, intrapleural pressure decreases, and the elastic recoil of the alveolar walls is increased. This compresses alveolar gas and raises alveolar pressure above atmospheric pressure, causing air to flow out of the lungs until alveolar pressure equals atmospheric pressure again. Airflow ceases until inspiration occurs again (Goldstein et al., 1997).

4. *Airway resistance (R_{aw}):* the difference between air pressure in the mouth and/or nose and the alveoli that causes a volumetric gas flow rate. Airway resistance must be overcome to generate flow through the airways. Airway caliber, airflow rate, pattern, and conditions that change the airway all effect airway resistance (Marino, 1998).

D. Control of breathing
   1. Neural
      a. *Medulla:* regulates respiratory rate and depth.
      b. *Pons:* is the pacemaker of respiration. It regulates the rhythm and assists in a smooth transition from inspiration to expiration.
      c. *Apneustic center:* initiates inspiration.
      d. *Pneumotaxic center:* inhibits inspiration by blocking apneustic center transmissions.
   2. Mechanical control
      a. *Stretch receptors:* nerve endings in the bronchial walls that sense lung inflation.
      b. *Irritant receptors:* nerve endings located in the lining of the airways that sense noxious stimuli, that is, bronchial irritants and inflammation.
      c. *Juxtacapillary receptors:* nerve endings in the alveoli and interstitial space that sense increases in interstitial volumes and pulmonary capillary pressure caused by inflammation or excessive blood volume in the right heart. Stimulation can cause bradycardia, hypotension, and constriction of the glottis.
      d. *Chest wall receptors:* nerve endings in the intercostal muscles that sense stretching of the chest wall. They assist in the regulation of action and timing of respiratory muscles.
   3. Chemical control
      a. *Central chemoreceptors:* located in the anterior medulla and sense changes in pH in the extracellular fluid (ECF).
      b. *Peripheral chemoreceptors:* located in the aortic and carotid bodies and sense changes in PO_2. They also play a minor role in sensing PCO_2.

E. Lung volumes
   1. *Total lung capacity (TLC):* the total volume of air contained in the lungs at maximal inhalation.
   2. *Tidal volume (V_t):* the volume of air inspired and expired with each normal breath at rest.
   3. *Inspiratory reserve volume (IRV):* the amount of air that can be inspired in addition to tidal volume.
   4. *Inspiratory capacity (IC):* amount of air that can be inspired after a passive expiration (from FRC); includes V_t and IRV.

5. *Functional residual capacity (FRC):* the amount of air that remains in the lungs at the end of a passive expiration (sum of RC & ERV); this is the point at which the lungs are at rest or mechanical equilibrium.

6. *Vital capacity (VC):* the volume of air exhaled after maximal inspiration.

7. *Residual volume (RV):* the volume of air left in the lungs after a maximal expiration.

8. *Expiratory reserve volume (ERV):* the amount of air that can be expired after a passive expiration.

9. *Negative inspiratory force (NIF):* the negative pressure created during a forced inspiration. It is an indicator of inspiratory muscle strength.

10. *Minute volume:* the ventilatory rate (breaths per minute) times the tidal volume (liters per minute) expressed in liters per minute (McCance & Huether, 2002).

IV. Functional anatomy

A. *Upper airway:* consists of the nasal and oral cavities, the pharynx, and the larynx. It conducts air into the lower airway and acts as a defense mechanism for the lungs by preventing foreign materials from entering (Scanlan et al., 1999).

1. *Nose:* possesses skeletal rigidity that prevents collapse during inspiration. It is shaped to produce airflow conducive to providing the lungs with maximum exposure to atmospheric gas. The nose humidifies and warms air to body temperature and filters inspired air by trapping particles >6 μm in diameter.

   a. *Alae:* the two flared openings of the external nose.

   b. *Vestibule:* posterior to the alae with hairs that filter particles.

   c. *Anterior nares:* the openings to the interior nose.

   d. *Septum:* the cartilage that separates the internal nasal passages into two.

   e. *Turbinates (superior, middle, and inferior conchae):* three bony shelf projections that divide the nasal cavities into superior, middle, and inferior passages.

   f. *Olfactory receptors:* smell receptors that are located above the superior turbinates.

   g. *Goblet cells:* mucous secreting cells located within the epithelium of the interior nasal passages that assist with particle trapping and the humidification of air.

2. *Paranasal sinuses:* the frontal, maxillary, ethmoid, and posterior sphenoid sinuses that provide temperature insulation, voice resonance enhancement, and additional strength to the skull.

3. *Oral cavity:* involved in digestion, speech, and respiration. It is considered a secondary respiratory passage.

   a. *Palate:* separates the oral and nasal cavities.

      i. *Hard palate:* the anterior two-thirds of the palate, which consists of bony skeleton.

  ii. *Soft palate:* the posterior third of the palate, consisting of soft tissue.
  b. *Uvula:* soft tissue protrusion that extends down, midline of the soft palate.
  c. *Vagal gag reflex:* a nerve root on the posterior surface of the tongue that when stimulated causes expulsion of foreign material up out of the upper airway and protects the lungs from aspiration.
  d. *Lingual tonsils:* lymphoidal tissues at the base of the tongue that are part of the immune system.
  e. *Palatine folds:* double webbed pockets located bilaterally at the end of the oral cavity that hold the palatine tonsils.
  f. *Palatine tonsils:* lymphoidal tissues that are part of the immune system.
4. *Pharynx:* posterior to the nasal cavity and mouth. It separates inspired air from food and water, opens the eustachian tubes to regulate middle ear pressure, and is a defense mechanism against infection.
  a. *Nasopharynx:* closes during swallowing and coughing.
  b. *Oropharynx:* contains lymphatic tissue that aids in controlling infection.
  c. *Laryngopharynx:* plays significant role in swallowing.
  d. *Pharyngeal musculature:* primary function is the act of swallowing and holds the sensory receptor for the glossophrayngeal nerve, the ninth cranial nerve.
5. *Larynx:* lies between the upper and lower airway at the level of C4–6. It consists of incomplete rings of cartilage, muscle, and ligaments.
  a. *Vocal cords:* When the larynx muscle contracts, it changes the shape of the vocal cords, producing vibrational sounds during respiration. Speech is a dynamic function of the vocal cords, lips, tongue, soft palate, and respiration. The temporal and parietal lobes of the cerebral cortex control speech.
  b. *Epiglottis:* the flat cartilage posterior at the base of the tongue that assists in establishing an airtight laryngeal closure during swallowing to prevent aspiration of foreign bodies into the lungs.
  c. *Glottis:* the opening between the vocal cords.
  d. *Cricoid cartilage:* the lower border of the larynx that is made up of a complete ridged ring. The inner diameter determines the size of endotracheal tube that can be passed through the larynx into the trachea.
B. *Lower airway:* consists of the tracheobronchial tree and lung parenchyma. It progressively subdivides into multiple branches. Its diameter narrows with each subdivision as the total cross-sectional area of the airway increases.
  1. Major airways
    a. *Trachea:* extends from the cricoid cartilage of the larynx to its bifurcation at T5. It is the beginning of the conducting airway. It warms and humidifies air. The posterior wall is free of cartilage and

consists of interlacing fibers, muscle (trachealis), and numerous mucous glands that provide support yet allows variation in diameter. The adult tracheal averages 2.0 to 2.5 cm in diameter and ranges from 10–15 cm long. Cilia along the tracheal wall propel secretions up and out of the airway (Scanlan et al., 1999).

b. *Carina:* the cartilage located at the bifurcation of the trachea and the right and left main stem bronchi.

c. Main stem bronchi

    i. *Right main stem bronchus:* is 2.5 cm in length, is wider than the left main stem bronchus and angles off at 20 to 30 degrees from midline. Objects aspirated in the upright position have a tendency to migrate to the right main stem bronchi. In supine patients, aspirates migrate toward the dependent lung.

    ii. *Left main stem bronchus:* is 5 cm in length and angles off more sharply than the right main stem bronchus at 40 to 60 degrees from midline.

d. Lobar and segmental bronchi

    i. *Right:* divides into the upper, middle, and lobar bronchi and 10 segmental bronchi branches (apical, posterior, anterior, lateral, medial, superior, medial basal, anterior basal, lateral basal, and posterior basal).

    ii. *Left:* divides into the upper and lower lobar bronchi and eight segmental bronchi branches (apical-posterior, anterior, superior lingula, inferior lingula, superior, anterior basal, lateral basal, and posterior basal).

e. *Subsegmental bronchi:* each branch bifurcates into two lower branches called *generations*. The bronchi continue to subdivide up to 14 generations until the diameter reaches 1 to 2 cm in size. These are referred to as the *small airways* (Geiger-Bronsky, 1997).

f. *Terminal bronchioles:* are smooth muscles without cartilage. Their cross-sectional area is 20 times greater than that of the trachea. They are sensitive to changes in CO_2 levels. When CO_2 levels increase, bronchiolar dilation occurs and conversely when CO_2 levels decrease, bronchiolar constriction occurs. Ciliated mucosal cells on the walls of the terminal bronchioles become progressively fewer toward the alveoli.

2. Conducting airway tissue

a. *Mucosa (epithelium):* is lined with ciliated columnar epithelium that consists of ciliated, goblet, and basal cells.

b. *Submucosa (lamina propria):* is loose fibrous tissue made of small blood and lymphatic vessels, nerves, and mast cells.

c. *Adventitia (cartilaginous layer):* is composed of cartilage and dense connective tissue. It serves as a protective fibrous covering around the airway. This layer thins through the progression of the generations until it disappears.

    d. Tracheobronchial surface lining
- i. *Cilia:* clears the respiratory tract of secretions and defends the airways from infection.
- ii. *Mucus (sol and gel layers):* bronchial glands produce 100 ml a day of secretions of which 95% is water. The *sol layer* is adjacent to the mucosal surface. The *gel layer* protects the sol layer and traps particles that are then carried out of the airway by the cilia (Scanlan et al., 1999).
- iii. *Mucociliary escalator:* Cilia beat in a rhythmic pattern about 20 times a second. This allows for continuous upward propulsion of secretions from the airways. In the nose, cilia move secretions back to the pharynx at 0.48 cm/min. In a healthy individual, particles inhaled are usually removed within 24 hours (Bourke & Brewis, 1998).

3. *Terminal respiratory unit (acinar):* considered the basic unit of the lung. It is composed of the respiratory bronchioles, alveolar ducts, and alveolar sacs. Its semipermeable membrane permits movement of gases according to pressure gradients. Laminar flow develops, which minimizes small airway resistance and decreases the WOB during inspiration. Low gas velocity assists with the rapid mixing of gases and provides a consistent and stable environment for gas exchange (Dettenmeier, 1992).
- a. *Lung lobule:* consists of 2 to 5 orders of respiratory bronchioles that are 1 to 2 cm in size. There are approximately 130,000 lobules with 2,200 alveoli in each lobule.
- b. *Respiratory bronchioles:* are the terminal branching of the airway involved with the distribution of air into the acinus.
- c. *Alveolar ducts:* are the entrances into the alveoli.
- d. *Alveolar buds:* are clusters of 10 to 16 alveoli. The alveoli are positioned back to back, separated by thin walls called *septa*.
- e. *Alveoli:* the primary site of gas exchange. The average adult has 300 to 500 million alveoli. Surface area for gas exchange ranges from 40 to 100 m^2 with an average of 70 m^2. The lungs have 35 times more surface area than that of the skin (Dale & Federman, 2000).
- f. *Alveolar space:* the air space of the alveolus.
- g. *Alveolar epithelium:* consists of Type I, II, and macrocytic cells.
  - i. *Type I:* squamous epithelium adapted for gas exchange. It covers approximately 90% of the alveolar surface and is extremely susceptible to injury by inhaled agents. It is structured to prevent fluid transudation into the alveoli.
  - ii. *Type II:* granular pneumocyte located within the distal portions of the alveoli. It produces and secretes surfactant.
  - iii. *Alveolar macrophage:* phagocytic cells that line the alveolar extracellular surface and remove bacteria and other foreign bodies that invade the alveoli.

h. *Pores of Kohn:* interalveolar openings or collateral channels that allow gas movement between contiguous alveoli.

i. *Surfactant:* lipoprotein that coats the inner surface of the alveoli and facilitates lung expansion during inspiration. It assists in maximizing gas exchange in the alveoli by lowering alveolar surface tension during exhalation and raises it during inspiration to prevent alveolar collapse. Surfactant decreases the WOB by allowing the alveoli to remain inflated at low pressures and reduces net forces in the alveoli that can cause tissue fluid accumulation. It also contributes to the compliance of lung tissue, detoxifies inhaled gases, and traps particles (McCance & Huether, 2002; Scanlan et al., 1999).

j. *Alveolar-capillary membrane:* consists of alveolar epithelium, the interstitial space, and capillary endothelium tissue. Located between the alveoli and capillary blood, it contains fluid, leukocytes, macrophages, and a dense capillary network, lining the respiratory bronchioles, alveolar ducts, and alveolar sacs. It forms the walls of the alveoli and is approximately 1 μm thick, which permits rapid diffusion of gases (Alspach, 1998).

k. *O_2 and CO_2 gas exchange pathway:* gas crosses to and from the alveolar epithelium, alveolar basement membrane, interstitial space, capillary basement membrane, capillary endothelium, blood plasma, the erythrocyte membrane, and erythrocyte cytoplasm.

l. *Interstitial space:* made up of connective tissue including elastin fibers, collagen fibers, and fibroblasts. It is drained by the lymphatic system.

V. Vascular supply: includes the pulmonary circulation, the bronchial circulation, and the lymphatic circulation.

A. *Pulmonary circulation:* carries mixed venous blood from the tissues to the lungs to be re-oxygenated. The pulmonary circulation pressure is lower and has less resistance than the systemic circulation, which is essential in maintaining fluid balance at the alveolar-capillary membrane. Mean pulmonary artery pressure normally ranges from 10–15 mm Hg; mean aortic pressure is normally 90 mm Hg. Because the pulmonary circulation is a low-pressure system, blood flow is partially dependent on gravity. The dispersion of pulmonary blood flow influences pulmonary gas exchange. Increased pressure in the pulmonary circulation, as in right heart failure or pulmonary hypertension, can cause fluid to leak into the interstitial space and alveoli, impairing gas exchange (Alspach, 1998). The pathway of blood flow from the heart to the lungs and back is:

1. *Right atrium:* collects mixed venous blood from the superior vena cava, inferior vena cava, and the coronary sinus. Blood passes through the *tricuspid valve* to the right ventricle.

2. *Right ventricle:* passes mixed venous blood through the *pulmonic valve* into the main pulmonary artery.

3. *Main pulmonary artery:* divides into right and left arteries just below the carina.

4. *Pulmonary arteries:* follow the right and left main stem bronchi and continue to divide as the bronchi into generations until they reach the pulmonary arterioles.

5. *Pulmonary arterioles:* pass into the acinar and subdivide into the alveolar capillary bed that lines the alveolar walls.

6. *Alveolar-capillary bed:* provides a large surface area for O_2 and CO_2 gas exchange. The diameter is large enough for only one red blood cell to pass through the bed at a time.

7. *Pulmonary venules:* collect oxygenated blood from the alveoli and carry it to 4 to 5 major pulmonary veins.

8. *Pulmonary veins:* return oxygenated blood to the left atrium for delivery to the systemic circulation. Normal mean pulmonary venous pressure is 4 to 12 mm Hg.

B. *Bronchial circulation:* supplies the lungs with an arterial blood supply. The lungs have a lower metabolic need than other tissues because of direct oxygen contact at the parenchyma (Scanlan et al., 1999).

1. *Right artery:* originates from the upper intercostal, right subclavian, or internal mammary artery.

2. *Bronchial arteries:* supply the left lung and branch from the upper thoracic aorta into 2 to 3 branches, following the subdivisions of the airways until they reach the alveolar-capillary bed.

3. *Bronchial-pulmonary circulation relationship:* compensatory in nature. A decrease in perfusion pressure in the pulmonary circulation causes an increase in bronchial artery circulation at the affected area. A decrease in bronchial circulation causes an increase in pulmonary arterial perfusion. This lung defense mechanism minimizes tissue ischemia and/or the size of infarct if blood flow is impeded, that is, pulmonary embolism (PE).

C. *Lymphatic circulation:* drains excess fluid and protein molecules that leak out of blood vessels from the interstitial space. It removes finer inhaled particles that have reached the alveolar surfaces. Lymph flow is 1–3 ml/hour but can increase 10 fold, if needed, as in the presence of increased pulmonary fluid or infection (Dale & Federman, 2000).

1. *Superficial vessels:* network of vessels that drain the pleura and the surface of the lungs.

2. *Deep vessels (peribronchovascular):* network of vessels that drain lung tissue around the acinar.

3. *Lymphatic channels:* merge in the pleura and carry lymph fluid to lymph nodes located near each hilum.

4. *Right lymphatic or thoracic duct:* carries lymphatic fluid from the hilum through the mediastinum to be drained into the systemic circulation.

D. *Metabolic activity:* as blood passes through the pulmonary circulation many humoral substances are regulated, for example, angiotension I is converted into the potent vasoconstrictor angiotensin II, and other vasoactive substances are completely or partially inactivated such as bradykinin, serotonin, prostaglandins, and norepinephrine.

VI. Gas exchange
  A. *Diffusion:* the process whereby alveolar gases move across the alveolar-capillary membrane to the pulmonary capillary bed and back, from an area of higher concentration to an area of lower concentration. Factors that affect diffusion include molecular weight, total surface area, gas solubility, the pressure gradient, alveolar-capillary membrane integrity, and blood flow rate (Alspach, 1998).
    1. *Lung diffusing capacity (D_L):* the number of milliliters of gas that can transfer from the lungs to the pulmonary blood in 1 minute for each torr of partial pressure difference between the alveoli and pulmonary capillary blood.
    2. *Lung diffusion capacity to alveolar volume ratio (D_{LCO}/V_A):* the ratio of the diffusing capacity for each liter of lung volume. It is an index that measures the total functional alveolar surface area available for diffusion.
    3. *Diffusion defects:* can occur when there is a thickening of the alveolar-capillary membrane due to disease, for example, pulmonary fibrosis. Thickening of the membrane increases the distance between the alveoli and the pulmonary capillaries.
  B. *Pressure gradients:* passively move from an area of higher pressure to lower pressure.
    1. *Oxygen pressure gradient:* the partial pressure of O_2 is 104 mm Hg at the alveolar spaces and 40 mm Hg at the pulmonary capillary bed.
    2. *Carbon dioxide pressure gradient:* the partial pressure of CO_2 is 45 mm Hg at the pulmonary capillary bed and 40 mm Hg at the alveoli.
  C. *A-a gradient:* the difference between the partial pressure of O_2 in the alveolar gas spaces (PAO_2) and the pressure in the systemic arterial blood (PaO_2). PaO_2 is dependent on multiple factors including age, lung function, altitude, and the presence of disease. Normal A-a gradient is less than 10 mm Hg on room air and no more than 65 mm Hg on 100% oxygen. It increases with age and with the percent of inspired O_2 (FIO_2). It can increase to as high as 20 mm Hg on room air in individuals over the age of 60 years. The A-a gradient is an index that measures how efficiently the lungs are able to equalize pulmonary capillary O_2 with alveolar O_2 and thus indicates whether gas transfer is normal. A high A-a gradient generally indicates a dysfunction in oxygen transfer from the lungs to the blood (Marino, 1998). A gradient >60 mm Hg represents a severe oxygenation deficiency. Causes include ventilation and perfusion problems, shunting, and diffusion abnormalities.

$$\text{A-a gradient} = PAO_2 - PaO_2$$

$$PAO_2 = PIO_2 - (PaCO_2/\text{RQ of } 0.8)$$

$$PIO_2 = (P_B - 47) \times FIO_2$$

PIO_2 = pressure of inspired air
P_B = barometric pressure (at sea level = 760 mm Hg)
47 = water vapor tension at 37° C.

$PACO_2$ = alveolar PCO_2

RQ = the respiratory exchange ratio, normally 0.8

Example: A-a gradient = FIO_2 (P_B – 47) – ($PaCO_2$/0.8) – PaO_2

0.21 (760 – 47) – (40/0.8) – 92 = 8

0.21 (713) – 50 – 92 = 8

D. Basic principles of oxygenation
1. *Oxygen transport:* the loading of O_2 onto hemoglobin (Hgb) and the unloading of O_2 at the tissue level. Blood carries O_2 two different ways:
   a. *Oxyhemoglobin (HbO$_2$):* Hgb carries the majority of O_2 inside the red blood cell. In whole blood each gram of Hgb can carry 1.34 ml of O_2. With an average Hgb of 15 g/dl, you can calculate the total oxygen-carrying capacity of the blood. Normal is 17 to 20 ml/dl in 100 cc of blood. Hgb is the major determinant of total amount of O_2.

HbO_2 = 1.34 ml × 15 g/dl = 20.1 ml/dl

   b. *Dissolved oxygen:* Some O_2 is dissolved in the plasma and the intracellular fluid of erythrocytes. Dissolved O_2 allows for relatively high O_2 tension to be maintained while significant amounts of O_2 carried by Hgb is released to the tissues.

PO_2 × 0.003.

100 mm Hg × 0.003 = 0.3 ml/dl

   c. *Factors that affect O_2 transportation:* pH, body temperature, organic phosphates (2,3-DPG), and abnormal Hgb (i.e. sickle cell, methemoglobin, carboxyhemoglobin, and fetal hemoglobin).
2. *Alveolar ventilation (V_A):* is the only part of ventilation that takes part in gas exchange at the alveolar-capillary membrane. It can not be directly measured; however, it can be inversely measured by using $PaCO_2$.

V_A = VCO_2 × 0.863

$PaCO_2$

VCO_2 = CO_2 production

0.863 = is the correction factor for unit measurement differences of 0°C and 760 torr pressure

3. *Minute ventilation (V$_E$):* the amount of air exchanged in 1 minute. Normal is around 6 L/minute.

$$V_E = V_T \times RR$$

$$500 \text{ ml} \times 12 \text{ bpm} = 6000 \text{ ml or } 6 \text{ L/min}$$

4. *Hemoglobin saturation (SaO$_2$):* the measure of the proportion of Hgb that is actually carrying oxygen.
5. *Oxygen transfer:* is normally 1,000 cc/min. It is calculated by taking the Hgb, times the O$_2$ carrying capacity, times the SaO$_2$, times cardiac output (CO).

$$\text{Hgb of } 15 \times 1.34 \times \text{SaO}_2 \text{ of } 0.99 \times \text{CO of } 5 = 1032.$$

6. *Hemoglobin-oxygen binding:* a reversible process that is sensitive to O$_2$ pressures (PO$_2$). When PO$_2$ is high as it is in the capillary membrane, O$_2$ binds readily to Hg. When PO$_2$ is low as in tissues of the body, O$_2$ is readily released.
7. *Oxyhemoglobin dissociation curve (ODC):* is a S-shaped curve (see Figure 4.1) that relates the percentage of hemoglobin saturation of O$_2$ and the partial pressure of oxygen (PO$_2$) in the blood (Alspach, 1998). When PO$_2$ is high (plateau portion) as in the lungs, oxygen readily binds with hemoglobin; when PO$_2$ is low as in the tissue (steep portion), oxygen is readily released.
   a. *Normal curve shape:* The upper flat portion of the curve represents arterial association. It shows how the body protects itself

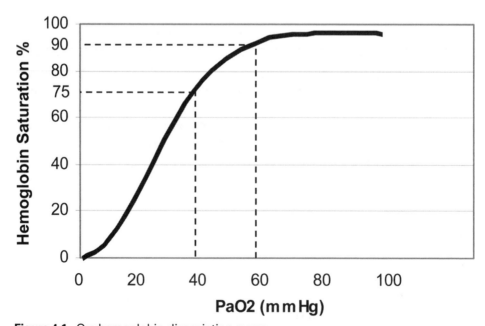

Figure 4.1. Oxyhemoglobin dissociation curve.

from hypoxemia by allowing O_2 uploading to Hgb despite large decreases in PaO_2. The lower, steep portion of the curve represents venous dissociation. It shows how the body protects itself from hypoxemia by allowing large amounts of O_2 to be unloaded to the tissues with small decreases in PaO_2 (Scanlan et al., 1999). An O_2 saturation of 75% correlates with a PaO_2 of 40 mm Hg and an O_2 saturation of 90% correlates with a PaO_2 of 60 mm Hg in a normal adult. Oxygen therapy is often instituted to maintain a PaO_2 of 60 minimally in a patient with compromised pulmonary functioning (Baldwin, Garza, Martin, Sheriff, & Hanssen, 1995).

   b. *Shift to the right:* indicates that more O_2 is being unloaded for a given PO_2. There is an increase in the amount of O_2 being delivered to the tissues. Causes for a right shift include:

      i. Decrease in pH
      ii. Increase in PCO_2
      iii. Increase in temperature
      iv. Increase in organic phosphates (2,3-DPG)

   c. *Shift to the left:* indicates that less O_2 is being released from the Hgb to the tissues because tissue and capillary O_2 is very low. Causes for a left shift include:

      i. Increase in pH
      ii. Decrease in PCO_2
      iii. Decrease in temperature
      iv. Decrease in organic phosphates (3,2-DPG)
      v. Carbon monoxide poisoning

E. *Carbon dioxide transport (CO₂):* the alveolar partial pressure of carbon dioxide ($PaCO_2$) varies based on the body's production of carbon dioxide (Vco_2) and inversely by alveolar ventilation (V_A). With a normal Vco_2 of 200 ml/min and a normal V_A of 4.2 L/min, the normal $PACO_2$ is 40 mm Hg. The $PACO_2$ will increase if there is an increase in Vco_2 production or a decrease in V_A.

$$PACO_2 = \frac{Vco_2}{0.863 \times V_A} \text{ so } \frac{200}{0.863 \times 4.2} = 40 \text{ mm Hg}$$

Carbon dioxide is carried in the blood in three forms:

1. 80% is carried as bicarbonate (HCO_3).
2. 12% is combined with Hgb as carbaminohemoglobin. The unloading of O_2 from Hgb potentates the loading of CO_2. This is called the *Haldane effect.*
3. 8% is dissolved in the blood ($PaCO_2$).

F. Ventilation and perfusion (V/Q)

   1. *Total lung ventilation:* the sum of alveolar ventilation and dead space ventilation.

     a. *Dead space ventilation:* the volume of inspired air that does not participate in gas exchange.

       i. *Anatomic:* the volume of air from the nose to the terminal bronchioles that does not participate in gas exchange, approximately a third of each inspired breath or 1 ml/lb.

      ii. *Alveolar:* the volume of gas in the acinus (excluding at the alveoli) that does not participate in gas exchange.

    iii. *Physiologic:* the total sum of the anatomic and alveolar dead space.

    iv. *Mechanical:* the dead space external to the patient on mechanical ventilation (ventilator circuit) that is inspired during the next breath.

2. Ventilation/perfusion relationships
   a. *V/Q ratio:* the alveoli receive air at the rate of 4 liters/min. The capillaries supply blood at a rate of 5 liters/min. The alveoli to capillary ratio is 4:5 or 0.8. Gravity affects the V/Q ratio based on lung location. It makes ventilation greater at the lung apex and perfusion greater at the lung bases. This widens the V/Q gap. The alveoli at the apex are under-perfused in relation to ventilation resulting in the V/Q of 3.0. This ratio gradually reverses itself downward, so the alveoli are over-perfused (Bourke & Brewis, 1998).
   b. Regional differences
      i. *Dependent areas:* have better perfusion than ventilation.
      ii. *Intrapleural pressure:* is more subatmospheric at the apex than at the base. Pressure is greater at the base to support the lung.
      iii. *Alveolar volumes:* are greater at the apex, decreases compliance, and directs the majority of inspired air down toward the bases where the volume per unit is greater.
   c. Positional changes
      i. *Upright:* basilar ventilation is greater than apex ventilation. Normally, a person receives more ventilation per lung unit due to the weight of the lungs. Alveolar ventilation is smaller in the apex and the change in volume per breath becomes progressively larger toward the bases of the lungs because of their capability to fully empty (Geiger-Bronsky, 1997).
      ii. *Supine:* apex ventilation is greater than basilar ventilation. When a person is supine, the lower lung airways become dependent. Increased lung volume and pressure are required to keep them open.
3. V/Q mismatches
   a. *Perfusion exceeds ventilation:* caused by poorly ventilated alveoli secondary to obstruction of the airways, for example, mucus plug, infectious process, atelectasis, or excessive rate of blood flow.
   b. *Ventilation exceeds perfusion:* caused by perfusion abnormality, for example, shunting, shock, hypovolemia, or embolism. Shunting

can occur for several reasons and is characterized by hypoxemia that is refractory to increasing FIO_2 (Grassi et al., 1999).

    i. *Anatomic shunting:* occurs when a portion of right ventricular blood does not pass through to the pulmonary capillaries, causing an uneven distribution of ventilation to perfusion.

    ii. *Normal physiologic shunting:* 2% to 5% of cardiac output is diverted into the bronchial and thebesian vein to supply the heart and lungs with an oxygenated blood supply.

    iii. *Other physiologic shunting:* occurs when all or part of a terminal unit does not come into contact with pulmonary capillary blood secondary to decreased lung compliance, hypoventilation, uneven distribution of ventilation, diffusion defects (e.g., pneumonia, pneumothorax, etc), intracardiac right to left shunting, and arteriovenous malformations.

VII. Life trajectory changes during the fetal and neonatal periods of development

  A. *Fetal circulation:* is different in three structural ways:

    1. *Ductus venous:* shunts blood from the umbilical vein through the liver and into the inferior vena cava.

    2. *Foramen ovale:* shunts blood between the right to left atrium.

    3. *Ductus arteriosus:* connects the pulmonary artery and the aorta, thereby allowing blood to by pass the lungs.

    4. *Placenta:* acts as the gas exchange organ during fetal life.

    5. *Fetal life means pulmonary hypertension.* Blood is shunted away from the lungs because the pressure in the lungs is higher than the pressure in the heart. A very small percentage of blood does flow to the lungs for the purpose of oxygenating pulmonary tissue itself. Fetal breathing is present in utero from about the 11th week and lung fluid is present from about the 13th week.

  B. *Neonatal (birth to 28 days of life):* As the infant passes through the birth canal, the chest is compressed and fluid is forced out of the conducting airways. After the cord is cut, PaO_2 and pH drops and $PaCO_2$ rises. This stimulates chemoreceptors, and the infant takes its first breath. During this first breath, a large negative intrathoracic pressure is created, which propels any remaining fluid from the lungs up and into the upper airway. As air displaces fluid in the lungs, the pressure decreases altering pressures in the heart, right heart pressure drops and left heart pressures rises, closing the foramen ovale (Loper, 1997). As the PaO_2 rises, it becomes the primary stimulus to close the ductus arteriosus and the prostaglandin level drops. Because there is no longer blood flow from the placenta to the umbilical vein, the ductus venosus ceases to function. The low resistance organ, the placenta, has been replaced and there is an increase in systemic pressure. Once the transition from fetal to neonatal circulation occurs, there is some increased WOB. The neonate overcomes pulmonary surface tension and lung compliance is established. Any remanding fluid in the lungs is absorbed by the lymphatic system (Zabloudil, 1999).

1. Congential anomalies
   a. *Diaphragmatic hernia:* This defect, where the abdominal organs are displaced in the chest, occurs with a frequency of 1 in 2,200 births (Miller, Fanaroff, & Martin, 1997). Usually the defect occurs on the left side due to the liver's anatomic placement on the right, and occurs about the 8th to 10th week of gestation. A significant problem for the neonate is the pulmonary hypoplasia on the ipsilateral side.
2. *Choanal atresia:* While this is rare, it still occurs with a frequency of 1 in 5,000 births, with two-thirds of those being unilateral (Miller, Fanaroff, & Martin, 1997). It is a disorder of the bony soft tissue obstructing the posterior nares. Because newborns are obligate nose breathers, this situation may become critical, particularily if the anomaly is bilateral.
3. *Pierre Robin:* This defect has a pronounced micrognathia due to mandibular undergrowth. The classic triad of micrognathia, glossoptosis, and cleft palate are known as Pierre Robin Sequence (Prows & Bender, 1999) because of the fact that a single defect, micrognathia, can cause a cascade of anomalies with an etiology of the primary defect. Often the tongue will fall back into the oropharynx, which will occlude the airway. They will present with varying degrees of respiratory distress. Pierre Robin may also occur as part of certain syndromes, such as cri-du-chat (Casey, 1999).
4. *Paralysis of the diaphragm:* This condition may result from a traumatic delivery with subsequent injury to the brachial plexus (seen as a unilateral affect) or a congential absence of the phrenic nerve(s) (possible bilateral). The chest movements will present as unequal. To determine diaphragmatic asymmetry in an infant on the ventilator, the practitioner must separate the infant's own breaths from those of the ventilator. X-ray will show an elevated diaphragm on the affected side.
5. *Neonatal pneumonia:* Pneumonia must be considered in every neonate that presents at birth with respiratory distress.
   a. Maternal history (Group B Strep positive mother)
   b. Rupture of membranes for more than 12 hours
   c. Maternal fever
   d. Maternal urinary tract infection
   e. Prolonged labor
   f. Congential infection: aspirates the infected amniotic fluid

C. Childhood periods
   1. *Infancy:* The respiratory system grows rapidly during the first 2 years of life with most of the growth concentrated in the lower airways of the lungs (Avery, Fletcher, & MacDonald, 1999).
      a. *Alveoli:* Rapid multiplication of alveoli occurs. Complications in utero or during infancy that decrease intrathoracic volume may affect the number of alveoli that will develop.

b. *Bronchi and bronchioles:* increase in diameter. However, the size of the respiratory system lends itself to small lumen obstruction and susceptibility to respiratory infections. The cricoid cartilage is located around C-4 with the bifurcation of the trachea at T-3.

c. *Diaphragm:* higher in the thorax in early childhood than in the adult. This is due to the abdominal organ to body proportion and organ pressure. Infants are diaphragmatic breathers; therefore, retraction of the intercostal, spinal extensor, and/or neck muscles with or without nasal flaring are signs of respiratory distress.

d. *Respiratory rate and rhythm:* rapid, ranging from 30 to 80 at birth, 30 to 60 at 6 months, and 22 to 40 by 1 year of age. Thus, normal respiratory rate of an infant is 30–40 times a minute.

2. *Toddler:* Growth of the respiratory system continues rapidly but begins to slow.

a. *Upper airway:* begins growing in width and length, particularly the larynx.

b. *Diaphragm:* pressure from the abdominal organs keeps the diaphragm higher in the chest than in older children.

c. *Alveoli:* continue to grow rapidly, increasing in both number and size with greatest emphasis on multiplication. Gas exchange qualitatively improves as expired CO_2 levels increase and expired O_2 levels decrease.

d. *Bronchi and bronchioles:* continue to increase in diameter. The cricoid cartilage and the trachea are still located at C-4 and T-3 respectively; however, supporting musculature and cartilage grow at the same rate as the alveoli. The lungs continue to be vulnerable to infection because the cartilage of the lungs remains soft and airway lumens remain small.

e. *Respiratory rate and rhythm:* varies with activity but is 20 to 28 times a minute.

3. *Preschool:* Growth of the respiratory system begins to slow.

a. *Thorax:* circumference of the thorax changes, becoming more cone-shaped. By school age the proportion of the transverse diameter to the anterioposterior diameter becomes 1:35, that of the normal adult.

b. *Upper airway:* continues to grow in length and width. Males typically have a larger larynx than females by age 3.

c. *Alveoli:* effectiveness of the terminal units steadily improves, giving the child greater lung functioning for strenuous activity.

d. *Bronchi and bronchioles:* diameter of the lumens continues to grow in size and the supporting musculature becomes stronger.

e. *Respiratory rate and rhythm:* varies with activity but decreases with age. Normal respiratory rate is 22 to 34 times a minute.

4. *School age:* Growth of the respiratory system continues to slow with little change during these years.

a. *Alveoli:* multiplication slows and growth is mainly that of widening.
b. *Bronchi and bronchioles:* lower airway continues to lengthen and expand with the bifurcation of the trachea at T-6 and the anterior margin of the lung at the fifth to sixth rib. Lung compliance gradually increases through childhood, as the lung tissue grows and matures.
c. *Respiratory rate and rhythm:* Respiratory effort changes at this time from primary diaphragmatic and includes costal muscles at approximately 7 to 8 years of age. Normal respiratory rate is 18 to 26 times a minute. The respiratory pattern normalizes to that of an adult.

5. *Adolescence:* The respiratory system grows during puberty.
a. *Upper airway:* increases in length, width, and thickness. The larynx is located at C-3 and the bifurcation of the trachea is located at T-5 to T-6.
b. *Alveoli:* number varies from person to person, but during puberty alveoli enlarge and total surface area increases. Differences in sex affect changes in gas exchange during puberty. Men inhale and retain more O_2 and exhale more CO_2 with each breath than women. The result is a greater alkali reserve. The oxygen dissociation curve also changes during adolescence, as the percentage of hemoglobin saturation of O_2 and the PO_2 of blood increases (Bowden, Dickey, & Greenburg, 1998).
c. *Bronchi and bronchioles:* increase proportionally in size and vital capacity. Sex differences become more apparent, as lung size and capacity are greater in males than in females. Respiratory infections decrease after puberty due to larger airway lumens, full development of the immune system, and completed lung growth.
d. *Respiratory rate and rhythm:* normal respiratory rate becomes the same as an adult at 12 to 20 times a minute.

D. *Pregnancy:* Changes between the first and third trimester
1. *Thorax:* changes early during pregnancy (Gabbe, Niebyl, & Simpson, 2001).
a. *Chest diameter:* increases 5 to 7 cm; however, there is no vital change in intrathoracic volume. The chest may not return to prepregnancy size after delivery.
b. *Subcostal angle:* of the rib cage increases from 68 to 103 degrees, causing a flaring of the rib cage and an increased A-P and transverse diameter of the chest.
c. *Diaphragm:* rises up to 4 cm as pregnancy progresses, decreasing the vertical diameter of the chest. Diaphragmatic excursion is not impeded by the enlarging uterus and actually increases 1 to 2 cm.
2. *Upper respiratory tract:* mucosa of the nasopharynx becomes hyperemic and edematous with increased production of mucus as a result of increased estrogen levels. This can lead to nasal congestion and

epistaxis. Polyposis of the nose and nasal sinuses sometimes occurs but usually reverses after delivery.

3. Lung volume and functioning
   a. *Total lung capacity:* decreases 5% because of diaphragm elevation, which decreases air volume in the lungs during the resting state.
   b. *Tidal volume (V_t):* increases by 30% to 40%.
   c. *Residual volume (RV):* decreases 20%.
   d. *Expiratory reserve volume (ERV):* decreases anywhere from 8% to 40% with an average of 20%.
   e. *Functional residual capacity:* decreases 20%.
   f. *Vital capacity* and *inspiratory reserve volume:* stay the same.
   g. *Airway resistance:* is reduced; however, the forced expiratory volume in 1 second (FEV_1) and the ratio of FEV_1 to forced vital capacity does not change.
   h. *Respiration:* no changes to a slight increase in depth and rate.
4. Gas exchange
   a. *Minute ventilation:* increases 30% to 40% by late pregnancy as a result of increased progesterone levels that enhance the respiratory center's sensitivity to CO_2.
   b. *Oxygen consumption:* increases 15% to 29%. Normal PaO_2 in late pregnancy is 104 to 108 mm Hg.
   c. *Carbon dioxide:* decreases 8% to 13%. Normal $PaCO_2$ in late pregnancy is 27 to 32 mm Hg. This change is significant, because it increases the CO_2 gradient, thereby facilitating transfer of CO_2 from the fetus to the mother.
   d. *Arterial acid/base balance:* by late pregnancy is compensated respiratory alkalosis. Arterial pH is maintained within normal limits (7.40 to 7.45) during pregnancy despite decreased CO_2 levels because the kidneys compensate by increasing bicarbonate excretion. Normal bicarbonate (HCO_3) concentration by late pregnancy is 18 to 31 mEq/L (VanderWal, 2000).
5. *Dyspnea:* occurs in approximately 60% to 70% of women during pregnancy, usually beginning late in the first trimester. The etiology has yet to be defined; however, it is thought to be due to respiratory alkalosis, reduced $PaCO_2$, and increased tidal volume that occurs with pregnancy.

E. *Normal changes with aging:* Changes are subtle and gradual in healthy, nonsmoking adults and vary greatly. Illness and disease increase O_2 demands and years of smoking can lead to decreased lung function. These factors are accumulative in nature. It is not until lung function is severely compromised that the effects are noticeable to the individual (Beers & Berkow, 2000).

1. *Thorax:* The ribs and vertebrae may become weakened by osteoporosis, particularly in women. The costal cartilage becomes calcified and the respiratory muscles diminish in size and strength. This can result in structural changes including kyphosis, shortening of the

thorax, chest wall stiffening, and an increased anterioposterior chest diameter, all of which diminish the effectiveness of respiration.

2. *Muscles of breathing:* Older adults compensate for structural changes in the thorax by increasing the use of accessory chest muscles during respiration. This requires more energy to be expended.

3. Upper respiratory airway

   a. *Nose:* Changes in connective tissue of the nose cause retraction of the columella, the lower part of the septum, and weakens the structural support, sloping the nose downward. This impairs airflow through the nasal cavity leading, to mouth breathing during sleep and increased incidence of snoring (Miller, 1999).

   b. *Oral cavity:* Decreased saliva production causes increased dry mouth, sore throat and frequent waking at night.

   c. *Trachea:* calcification of cartilage causes stiffening of the trachea.

   d. *Larynx:* There is a decline in cough and laryngeal reflexes that diminishes the efficiency of the gag reflex and increases the potential risk of aspiration.

4. *Control of breathing:* Heart rate and ventilatory responses to hypoxia and hypercapnia decrease with age, increasing the potential of hypoxic episodes from diseases that lower oxygen levels, for example, pneumonia, chronic obstructive pulmonary disease or congestive heart failure. The ability of central and peripheral chemoreceptors to sense hypoxia and hypercapnia decrease by 51% and 41% respectively by age 65 (Miller, 1999).

5. *Lungs:* The tissue loses firmness and structure and lung size decreases. The weight of the lung decreases by 20%.

6. *Terminal respiratory units:* Beginning around 30 years of age, the alveoli begin to enlarge and the walls thin. This process continues throughout adulthood at an average of 4% loss of alveolar surface area per decade, leading to a decrease in D_{LCO}.

7. *Pulmonary circulation:* The pulmonary artery thickens and the walls stiffen, increasing pulmonary artery pressure. There is a decrease in capillaries within the alveoli-capillary membrane, decreasing pulmonary capillary blood volume.

8. *Pulmonary compliance:* increases due to loss of elastin fibers in the alveoli and terminal bronchioles.

9. Lung volumes

   a. *Residual volume:* increases by 50%.

   b. *Vital capacity:* decreases by 25%.

   c. *FEV_1:* decreases approximately 20 ml each year after age 40.

   d. *Distribution of ventilation:* Loss of elastic recoil causes small airways to collapse during expiration, leading to air trapping in the terminal respiratory units, and increases physiologic dead space (Stone, Wyman, & Salisbury, 1999).

10. Gas exchange

a. *Arterial oxygen tension:* declines approximately 0.3% per year after the age of 40. Reciprocally, there is a gradual decline in PaO_2.
b. *Diffusion:* Thickening of the capillary-membrane and loss of surface area for gas exchange decreases diffusion capacity.
c. *Defense mechanisms:* The lungs decrease in their effectiveness to fight infection with age, due to decreased in macrophage activity.
d. *Airway clearance:* There is a decrease in the mobility of the mucociliary escalator with age.
e. *Humoral immunity:* the acute antibody response to extrinsic antigens such as those in pneumococcal and influenza vaccines reduces with age. The body's ability to sense changes in IgA and IgG levels and the lungs' ability to assist in the synthesizing of metabolic toxins decreases with age (Beers & Berkow, 2000).
f. *Cellular immunity:* Cell-mediated immunity decreases with age causing a delayed hypersensitivity to common antigens. The reliability of tuberculosis (TB) skin tests declines with age. There is also an increase of the reactivation of TB with aging (Stone et al., 1999).

REFERENCES

Alspach, J. G. (Ed.). (1998). *Core curriculum for critical care nursing* (5th ed.). Philadelphia: W. B. Saunders Company.

Avery, G. B., Fletcher, M. A., & MacDonald, M. G. (1999). *Neonatology pathophysiology & management of the newborn* (5th ed.). Philadelphia: Lippincott Williams & Wilkins Publishers.

Baldwin, K. M., Garza, C. S., Martin, R. N., Sheriff, S., & Hanssen, G. A. (1995). *Davis's manual of critical care therapeutics.* Philadelphia: F. A. Davis Company.

Beers, M. H., & Berkow, R. (Eds.). (2000). *The Merck manual of geriatrics* (3rd ed.). West Point, PA: Merck & Co.

Bourke, S. J., & Brewis, R. A. (1998). *Lecture notes on respiratory medicine* (5th ed.). Oxford: Blackwell Science Ltd.

Bowden, V. R., Dickey, S. B., & Greenberg, C. S. (1998). *Children and their families.* Philadelphia: W. B. Saunders Company.

Casey, P. M. (1999). Respiratory distress. In J. Deacon & P. O'Neill (Eds.), *Core curriculum for neonatal intensive care nursing* (2nd ed., pp. 118–150). Philadelphia: W. B. Saunders.

Dale, D. C., & Federman, D. D. (2000). *Scientific American medicine: Respiratory medicine.* New York: Healtheon/WebMD Corporation.

Dettenmeier, P. A. (1992). *Pulmonary nursing care.* St. Louis, MO: Mosby Year-Book, Inc.

Gabbe, S. G., Niebyl, J. R., & Simpson, J. L. (2001). *Obstetrics: Normal & problem pregnancies* (4th ed.). New York: Churchill Livingstone, Inc.

Geiger-Bronsky, M. (1997). *Respiratory nursing curriculum: Phase I.* Long Beach Memorial Medical Center. Long Beach, CA.

Goldstein, R. H., O'Connell, J. J., & Karlinsky, J. B. (1997). *A practical approach to pulmonary medicine.* Philadelphia: Lippincott-Raven Publishers.

Grassi, C., Brambilla, C., Costabel, U., Naeiji, R., Rodriguez-Roisin, R., Stockley, R., et al. (Eds.). (1999). *Pulmonary diseases.* Rome: McGraw-Hill International Ltd.

Loper, D. L. (1997). Physiologic principles of the respiratory system. In Askin, D. F. (Ed.). *Acute respiratory care of the neonate* (2nd ed., pp. 1–30). Petaluma, CA: NICU Ink.

Marino, P. L. (1998). *The ICU book* (2nd ed.). Philadelphia: Lippincott Williams & Wilkins.

McCance, K. L., & Huether, S. E. (2002). *Pathophysiology: The biologic basis for disease in adults and children* (4th ed.). St. Louis, MO: Mosby-Year Book, Inc.

Miller, C. A. (1999). *Nursing care of older adults: Theory & practice.* (3rd ed.) Philadelphia: Lippincott Williams & Wilkins.

Miller, M. J., Fanaroff, A. A., & Martin, R. J. (1997). Respiratory disorders in preterm and term infants. In A. A. Fanaroff & R. J. Martins (Eds.), *Neonatal-perinatal medicine* (6th ed., Vol. 2, pp. 1040–1065). St. Louis, MO: Mosby.

Prows, C. A., & Bender, P. L. (1999). Beyond Pierre Robin sequence. *Neonatal Network, 18*(5), 13–19.

Scanlan, C. L., Wilkins, R. L., & Stoller, J. K. (1999). *Egan's fundamentals of respiratory care* (7th ed.). St. Louis, MO: Mosby–Year Book.

Stone, J. T., Wyman, J. F., & Salisbury, S. A. (1999). *Clinical gerontological nursing: A guide to advanced practice* (2nd ed.). Philadelphia: W. B. Saunders Company.

VanderWal, B. (2000). *Physiologic changes in pregnancy.* Long Beach, CA: Long Beach Memorial Medical Center.

Zabloudil, C. (1999). Adaptation to extrauterine life. In M. T. Verklan & M. Walden (Eds.), *Core curriculum for neonatal intensive care nursing* (3rd ed., pp. 40–62). Philadelphia: W. B. Saunders.

Pathophysiology

5

Janet Harris

INTRODUCTION

Hypoxemia is a deficiency of oxygen in the blood, while hypoxia is a deficiency of oxygen in tissue. The causes of hypoxia include extrinsic causes, alveolar hypoventilation, diffusion defects, ventilation and perfusion mismatches, and inadequate transport and delivery of oxygen.

Hyperventilation-increased cardiac output, erythrocytosis, and right shift of the oxyhemoglobin dissociation curve are all physiologic adaptations to hypoxia.

Definitions

I. Hypoxemia: deficiency of oxygen in the blood (Table 5.1)
II. Hypercapnia: high $PaCO_2$ (above 50–55 mm Hg) with accompanying acidemia (pH < 7.30) and low PaO_2 (Alspach, 1998; Urden, Stacy, & Lough, 2002) (Table 5.2)
III. Hypoxia: a deficiency of oxygen at the tissue level; may have tissue hypoxia without hypoxemia

Causes of Hypoxia

I. Extrinsic
   A. Definition: low environmental oxygen
   B. Physiologic features: either the pressure or the concentration of inspired oxygen is decreased (Henneman, 1996)

The views of the authors are their own and do not reflect the official policy or position of the Department of the Army, the Department of Defense, or the United States Government.

Table 5.1	Causes of Hypoxemia

Diffusion Defect	V/Q Mismatch	Shunting
▓ Emphysema	▓ Asthma	▓ A/V Septal Defects
		▓ Pulmonary Edema
		▓ Atelectasis
▓ Fibrosis	▓ COPD	
▓ Pulmonary Edema	▓ Pulmonary Embolism	
▓ ARDS	▓ Mucus Plug	
	▓ Airway Obstruction	
▓ Aspiration		
▓ Near Drowning		
▓ Inhalation of Toxic Gas		
▓ Connective Tissues Diseases		

Table 5.2	Causes of Hypercapnia

Alveolar Hypoventilation

▓ Neurologic/Neuromuscular Disorder, e.g., polyneuritis disease, myasthenia graves
▓ CNS Depression, e.g., medications, anesthesia
▓ Spinal Cord Injuries
▓ Respiratory Muscle Diseases
▓ Obesity
▓ Upper Airway Structural Problems
▓ Lower Airway Structural Problems

C. Causes
1. High altitudes where atmospheric pressure is less than sea level
2. Conditions of diminished FiO_2 (fire in an enclosed space)
3. Discontinuation of delivered oxygen
D. Treatment: very responsive to oxygen therapy; by administering oxygen, you increase the pressure gradient and force more oxygen into the blood
II. Alveolar hypoventilation
A. Definition: The quantity, for example, the volume, of fresh gas entering the alveoli per unit time (alveolar ventilation) is reduced. If the alveolar ventilation is abnormally low, the alveolar PO_2 falls and Pco_2 rises (West, 2003).

B. Physiologic features
  1. Increased $PaCO_2$
  2. Decreased PaO_2
  3. PaO_2 does not fall to extremely low levels by hypoventilation alone; increased $PaCO_2$ is the dominant feature of hypoventilation
C. Causes (lungs often normal; commonly caused by diseases outside the lung parenchyma)
  1. Neurological (Farzan, 1997; West, 2003)
     a. Central nervous system (CNS) depression due to narcotics, sedatives, and anesthetic agents
     b. Central sleep apnea
     c. Diseases of the medulla
        i. Cerebral vascular accident (CVA)
        ii. Meningitis
        iii. Encephalitis
        iv. Head injury
        v. Neoplasm (rare)
  2. Disorders of the spinal cord (Farzan, 1997; West, 2003)
     a. Poliomyelitis
     b. Amyotrophic lateral sclerosis
     c. Spinal cord injuries
     d. Multiple Sclerosis
  3. Diseases involving nerves to the respiratory muscles
     a. Guillain-Barre
     b. Diphtheria
  4. Diseases of the myoneuronal junction
     a. Myasthenia Gravis
     b. Anticholinesterase poisoning
D. Structural causes
  1. Upper airways (Farzan, 1997; West, 2003)
     a. Obstruction
        i. Tongue/foreign body
        ii. Tracheal compression r/t thymoma
     b. Acute laryngitis or epiglottitis
     c. Anaphylaxis
     d. Obstructive sleep apnea (Not confined to the obese)
  2. Lower airways
     a. Thoracic cage abnormalities (West, 2003)
        i. Chest trauma
        ii. Kyphoscoliosis
     b. Obese patients (Pickwickian Syndrome)
     c. Severe lung disorders
        i. Emphysema
        ii. Bronchiolectasis
        iii. Hyaline membrane disease

E. Mixed causes
 1. Sudden Infant Death Syndrome (SIDS). Etiology not clear; CNS control of ventilation may not yet be fully developed and respiratory muscles lack coordination (West, 2003).
 F. Treatment for all causes of alveolar hypoventilation: Treat the underlying cause; support with supplemental O_2 to increase PaO_2 enough to overcome the problems caused by hypoventilation.

III. Diffusion defects
 A. Definition: "There is no equalization, for example, equilibration between the PO_2 in the pulmonary capillary blood and alveolar gas (West, 2003)." (Note: Diffusion defects do not normally effect CO_2 because with its higher solubility, CO_2 diffuses about 20 times faster than O_2.)
 B. Physiologic features
  1. $P(A-a)O_2$ (alveolar-arterial oxygen tension difference) rises
  2. PaO_2 decreases
  3. $PaCO_2$ unchanged
 C. Causes
  1. Lack of pressure gradient (without the driving pressure difference, O_2 will not diffuse into the blood)
  2. Decreased total surface area available for gas exchange, alveoli or capillaries
   a. Emphysema
   b. Trauma
   c. Emboli
  3. Increased diffusion distance produces incomplete equilibration (the alveolar lining or capillary endothelium may be thickened or the distance may be increased by fluid)
   a. Fibrosis
   b. Pulmonary Edema
   c. Pneumonia
   d. Acute Respiratory Distress Syndrome (ARDS)
   e. Smoking cocaine
   f. Asbestosis
   g. Sarcoidosis
   h. Connective tissue diseases affecting the lung (e.g., Scleroderma, Systemic Lupus Erythematosus)
 D. Treatment: Supplemental administration of oxygen helps to compensate for the increased diffusion resistance (West, 2003).

IV. Ventilation (V)/Perfusion (Q) {V/Q} Mismatch
 Extremely common mechanisms for hypoxemia (i.e., COPD, interstitial lung disease, and pulmonary embolus); the primary cause in critically ill patients (Wagner, 2002; West, 2004); generally identified by excluding other causes of hypoxemia.
 A. Definition: Adequate matching of ventilation and blood flow must occur in various regions of the lung, with the result that all gas transfer becomes inefficient (West, 2003). Compared to a lung having the

same total blood flow and alveolar ventilation, a lung that has a V/Q mismatch will exchange all gases in an inefficient manner (Wagner, 2002).

B. Physiologic features
1. Hypoxemia results when alveoli are underventilated relative to the amount of perfusion (i.e., blood flow) they receive. Unoxygenated blood passing by underventilated alveoli mixes with oxygenated blood and lowers the PaO_2 (Henneman, 1996; West, 2004).
2. Affects both gases, producing both hypoxemia and hypercapnia (Wagner, 2002).
    a. O_2 is affected more than CO_2 in very low V/Q regions
    b. CO_2 is affected more than O_2 in very high V/Q regions
    c. Creates alveolar-arterial differences for both O_2 and CO_2
3. Some regional V/Q inequality is normal due to the effects of gravity and gaseous properties. Both ventilation and perfusion increase from the apices (or nondependent regions depending on body position) to the bases (dependent regions). However perfusion increases at a faster rate producing a high V/Q ratio of about 3 in the apices (non-dependent regions) with a low V/Q ratio of about 0.6 in the bases (dependent region) (Wagner, 2002). For the normal lung, the average V/Q ratio is about 1 (Wagner, 2002).
4. Compensatory responses to V/Q inequalities.
    a. Pulmonary vasculature. Pulmonary arteriolar smooth muscle is very sensitive to the partial pressure of O_2 in the alveoli and hydrogen concentration in the blood (indirectly related to CO_2). This local control permits perfusion of well ventilated alveoli and the shunting of blood away from poorly ventilated alveoli (Stone, 1996).
        i. Increased alveolar O_2 results in vasodilation
        ii. Decreased alveolar O_2 results in vasoconstriction
        iii. Increased [H+] results in pulmonary vasoconstriction
        iv. Changes in total ventilation (see adaptation to hypoxemia)
        v. Changes in cardiac output (see adaptation to hypoxemia)
5. Systemic hypoxia also causes the pulmonary arterioles to constrict, resulting in an increase in pulmonary arterial pressure and pulmonary hypertension.
6. With certain disease processes the V/Q mismatch is exaggerated producing hypoxemia.
    a. Concomitant hypoventilation (overly sedated COPD patient)
    b. Reduction in cardiac output (causes fall of PO_2 of mixed venous blood leading to a fall of PaO_2 for the same degree of V/Q mismatch). May see in patients with myocardial infarction (MI) who develop mild pulmonary edema (West, 2003).

C. Causes of V/Q mismatch
1. Pulmonary diseases alter V/Q by increasing airway resistance, decreasing the diameter of airways, decreasing pulmonary compliance, or altering the caliber of pulmonary blood vessels (Stone, 1996).

   a. Asthma
   b. COPD
   c. Pulmonary edema
   d. Bronchospasm
   e. Mucus plug
   f. Atelectasis
2. Shunt (Most severe form of low ratio V/Q mismatch)
   a. Definition: "Some blood reaches the arterial system without passing through ventilated regions of the lung" (West, 2003).
   b. Causes
      i. Atrial or ventricular septal defects (often called right-to-left shunts)
      ii. "Mainstemming" an endotracheal tube (E-T tube inserted so that the end of tube is only in one mainstem [usually the right] producing ventilation to only 1 lung)
      iii. Pulmonary emboli
      iv. Alveoli completely collapsed from atelectasis
      v. Pneumonia
      vi. Pulmonary edema
      vii. Acute Respiratory Distress Syndrome (ARDS)
D. Treatment: Treat the underlying cause. O_2 therapy of minimal value. Differentiate shunt from low V/Q abnormalities by administering 100% O_2.
   1. Hypoxemia due to low V/Q ratio will respond to high FIO_2
   2. Hypoxemia due to shunting will not respond to high FIO_2
V. Inadequate transport and delivery of oxygen
   A. Definition: Inability to move adequate amounts of O_2 from the atmosphere to the tissues (West, 2003). Although the pulmonary system plays a vital role in preventing hypoxemia, other factors (hemoglobin concentration, position on the oxygen hemoglobin dissociation curve, cardiac output, and peripheral blood distribution) are important in oxygen delivery to the tissues.
   B. Physiological features (any or all of the following)
      1. Decreased hemoglobin
      2. Decreased cardiac output
      3. Decreased DO_2 (oxygen delivery)
      4. Decreased CaO_2
   C. Causes
      1. Decreased ability of the blood to carry oxygen
         a. Anemias—inadequate quantities of hemoglobin or abnormal hemoglobin (i.e., sickle cell anemia)
         b. Carbon monoxide poisoning—displaces O_2 on hemoglobin
         c. Left shift on oxygen-hemoglobin dissociation curve
      2. Decreased ability of the heart to deliver oxygenated blood to the tissue
         a. Decreased cardiac output

i. MI
ii. CHF
iii. Cardiac tamponade
b. Increased capacitance—Distributive shock states
3. Cellular defects—inability of tissue to use the oxygen provided
a. Sepsis
b. Cyanide poisoning
c. Tissue edema
D. Treatment: Treat the underlying cause; provide supplemental oxygen, however the responsiveness to oxygen may vary.
1. For anemia, abnormal hemoglobin, increasing the FIO_2 to 1.0 (100%) may provide up to a 30% increase in the amount of oxygen carried to the tissues.
2. For circulatory deficiency, oxygen is of slight value, since the problem is not due to lack of oxygen in blood but is due to inadequate pump function.
3. Oxygen may make a difference as a supportive measure when delivery is low as in the case of an acute MI with low cardiac output.
VI. Mixed causes of hypoxia
It is often impossible to accurately define the mechanism of hypoxia, especially in the acutely ill patient as the patient may exhibit more than one cause of hypoxia (West, 2003).
A. The patient requiring mechanical ventilation due to acute respiratory failure after an MVA may have a large shunt through unventilated lung in addition to severe V/Q mismatching.
B. The patient with interstitial lung disease may have some diffusion impairment that may be accompanied by V/Q mismatching and possibly a shunt.

Compensatory Mechanisms for Hypoxia

I. Hyperventilation
A. By increasing the depth of ventilation, more alveoli are recruited for gas exchange.
B. Hyperventilation is triggered by low levels of oxygen stimulating the carotid and aortic bodies (Cherniack & Pack, 2002).
C. The value of hyperventilation is limited in two ways.
1. It has no effect on anatomic or capillary shunt.
2. There is a point at which the demand for additional oxygen caused by the increased work of breathing matches or exceeds that available.
II. Cardiac output
A. This is the most important compensatory mechanism available to the body to correct hypoxia. In order to understand this, assume for a moment that the metabolic oxygen demand is constant.
1. Increasing the cardiac output moves the blood past the tissues faster.
2. The tissues do not have time to extract as much oxygen from a given amount of blood.

3. The venous saturation of the blood is higher as the blood leaves the tissue and returns to the right side of the heart, which means that it has less capacity for picking up more oxygen.
4. The diffusion gradient is therefore diminished.

B. Limitations of cardiac compensation
1. The heart beats faster and harder to try to meet the oxygen demand. This increases the heart's demand for oxygen and decreases the amount of time for blood to flow in the coronary arteries during diastole.
2. The heart muscle becomes hypoxic, which decreases its ability to pump.

III. Erythrocytosis
A. With chronic hypoxia (i.e., congenital defects, acclimatization to high altitudes, COPD) more RBCs will be produced to increase the oxygen carrying capacity of the blood.
B. However, the higher the hematocrit (more RBCs), the more viscous the blood. The more viscous the blood, the harder the heart has to work to pump it, resulting in an increased oxygen demand of the heart.

IV. Oxyhemoglobin dissociation curve shift (see Figure 4.1, chapter 4)
A. With chronic hypoxia and the resultant increase in anaerobic metabolism, the RBCs produce more 2, 3-diphosphoglycerate (DPG) (West, 2004).
B. An increase in 2, 3-DPG, shifts the oxyhemoglobin dissociation curve to the right and allows easier release of oxygen in a tissue capillary (West, 2004).
C. An increase in pCO_2, an increase in H+ concentration, and increased temperature also produce a right shift in the oxyhemoglobin dissociation curve (West, 2004).

REFERENCES

Alspach, A. G. (Ed.). 1998. *Core curriculum for critical care nursing*. Philadelphia: W. B. Saunders.

Cherniack, N. S., & Pack, A. I. (2002). Control of ventilation. In A. P. Fishman (Ed.), *Fishman's pulmonary diseases and disorders* (4th ed.). New York: McGraw-Hill.

Farzan, S. (1997). *A concise handbook of respiratory diseases*. Stamford, CT: Apple & Lange.

Henneman, E. A. (1996). Patients with acute respiratory failure. In J. M. Clochesy, C. Breu, S. Cardin, A. A. Whittaker, & E. B. Rudy (Eds.), *Critical care nursing* (2nd ed., pp. 630–655). Philadelphia: W. B. Saunders Company.

Stone, K. S. (1996). Respiratory physiology. In J. M. Clochesy, C. Breu, S. Cardin, A. A. Whittaker, & E. B. Rudy (Eds.), *Critical care nursing* (2nd ed., pp. 561–582). Philadelphia: W. B. Saunders Company.

Urden, L. D., Stacy, K. M., & Lough, M. E. (2002). *Critical care nursing: Diagnosis and management* (4th ed.). St. Louis: Mosby.

Wagner, P. D. (2002). Ventilation, pulmonary blood flow, and ventilation-perfusion relationships. In A. P. Fishman (Ed.), *Fishman's pulmonary diseases and disorders* (4th ed.). New York: McGraw-Hill.

West, J. B. (2003). *Pulmonary pathophysiology: The essential* (6th ed.). Baltimore: Williams & Wilkins.

West, J. B. (2004). *Respiratory physiology: The essential* (7th ed.). Baltimore: Williams & Wilkins.

Respiratory Assessment

Lynn F. Reinke

INTRODUCTION

Respiratory nursing involves the diagnosis and treatment of human responses to actual and potential pulmonary health problems (American Nurses Association & Respiratory Nursing Society, 1994). However, in order for the pulmonary nurse to develop a diagnosis, a thorough assessment of a patient's pulmonary history and health patterns, must be conducted, along with a full physical examination. The data obtained from the assessment of a physical examination will enable the nurse to implement the most appropriate pulmonary nursing interventions resulting in optimal health outcomes for the patient.

I. Completing the history
    A. Subjective data
        1. Inquire about the patient's past health history. This may include but is not limited to the following: frequency of upper respiratory infections (URIs), triggers, allergic reactions, history of asthma, chronic obstructive pulmonary disease (COPD), pneumonia, tuberculosis (TB), and so forth, and other medical conditions.
        2. Current medications. Prescribed, over-the-counters, herbal and complementary therapies, routes of administration (nebulizer, metered dose inhaler, oral, etc.), home O_2 therapy. Drug allergies? If yes, what drug and what type of reaction?
        3. Surgery or other treatments. Hospitalized for respiratory problem, surgical procedures, dates. Home treatments, for example, use of airway clearance devices, humidifier, peak flow meter monitoring device, and so forth.
        4. Occupational history. Includes length of exposure to chemicals, asbestos, fumes, and so forth. Farming? If yes, for how long and where?
        5. Pet exposure. For example, birds, pigeons, horses, cats, and so forth.

6. Recent travel, domestic or foreign.
7. Common cues to respiratory problems. When assessing the above chief complaints, the nurse may apply the PQRST framework to assure comprehensive evaluation:
   Precipitating factors/palliating factors
   Quality and characteristics of symptoms
   Radiation/related symptoms/systems
   Severity/impact on activities of daily living
   Timing of symptoms
   a. Dyspnea
   b. Wheezing
   c. Pleuritic chest pain
   d. Cough
   e. Sputum production
   f. Hemoptysis
   g. Voice change
   h. Fatigue

B. Functional health patterns
   1. Health perception—health management pattern
      a. Describe daily activities or recent changes
      b. Smoking status/history
      c. Health promotion activities, for example, Pneumovac, flu shot
      d. Ethanol (ETOH) consumption
      e. Illicit drugs
      f. Complementary therapies, for example, herbs, massage therapy, chiropractor sessions, and so forth
   2. Nutritional-metabolic pattern
      a. Recent weight loss or gain? quantity? intentional? early satiety? anorexia?
   3. Elimination pattern
      a. Independent toileting? Inactivity resulting in constipation?
   4. Activity-exercise pattern
      a. Assessment of exercise history. Type, frequency, tolerance, barriers?
      b. Dyspnea with exercise? at rest? stairs? distance ambulate, for example, one block.
      c. Does the patient implement dyspnea control techniques?
   5. Sleep-rest pattern
      a. Nocturnal dyspnea? Lie flat at night? how many pillows? sleep in chair? observed apnea episodes?
      b. Quality of sleep—does the patient feel rested upon awakening? frequency of awakenings? snoring? morning headaches? If yes, location of headaches, for example, occipital, temporal, and so forth.
   6. Cognitive-perceptual pattern
      a. Pain associated with breathing?
      b. Cognitive changes: restless, irritable, confused, depressed, anxiety? Difficulty remembering things?

7. Role-relationship pattern
    a. Respiratory problems causing difficulties with work, family, social relationships, self-image?
    b. Respiratory problems causing changes in social activities, for example, frequency, type, and so forth?
8. Sexuality-reproductive pattern
    a. Respiratory problems leading to change in sexual activity? Determine what dyspnea control techniques are used during sexual activities.
9. Coping-stress tolerance pattern
    a. How often does the patient leave home? Support group participation? Pulmonary rehab program? Does stress increase dyspnea? Does dyspnea alter emotions? Do emotions alter dyspnea?
10. Value-belief pattern
    a. Miss medications? Do prescribed treatments help? If not, why?
    b. Adherence to diet therapy, exercise therapy?
    c. Adherence to equipment maintenance, for example, tubing changes, spacers, MDIs, nebulizer, home oxygen equipment cleaning?
    d. Determine the value the patient places on health care plan (Dettemeier, 1992).

II. Objective data
    A. Physical examination includes vital signs
        1. Nose—assess inflammation, deformities, symmetry
        2. Mouth and pharynx—assess color, lesions, masses, gum retraction, bleeding, poor dentition, gag reflex
        3. Neck—assess symmetry, presence of tender/swollen area, assess lymph nodes
        4. Thorax and lungs—imaginary lines can be pictured on the chest to help identify abnormalities/location. For example, 2 cm from the right mid clavicular line.
    B. Inspection
        1. Patient should sit in upright position or lean on a bedside table with chest exposed. This position provides ease of the exam and is usually comfortable for the patient.
        2. Observe general appearance and work of breathing. Any evidence of respiratory disease? That is, tachypnea, use of accessory muscles, splinting, and so forth.
        3. Note shape and symmetry of chest. Chest movement should be equal on both sides and the anterior posterior (AP) diameter should be equal to the side to side diameter. Normal AP ratio is 1:2. An increase in diameter (barrel chest) may be a normal aging change or result from lung hyperinflation.
        4. Check sternum for abnormalities, such as, pectus carinatum or pectus excavatum.
        5. Respiratory rate, depth, rhythm. Normal rate 12–20 bpm, in elderly 16–25. Inspiration (I) should take half as long as expiration (E). I:E = 1:2.

63

Observe for abnormal breathing patterns such as, Kussmauls (rapid, deep), Cheyne-Stokes (a rhythmic increase and decrease in rate separated by apnea), or Biot's (irregular breathing with apnea every 4–5 cycles).

6. Skin color. Check for cyanosis, check conjunctivae, lips, palms, soles. Check for clubbing.

7. Inspect posterior chest. Note spinal curvature, may include kyphosis, scoliosis, or kyphoscoliosis.

C. Palpation

1. Check tracheal position. Normal is midline. Deviation occurs with tension pneumothorax, pneumonectomy and lobar atelectasis.

2. Check symmetry of chest expansion and extent of movement at the level of the diaphragm.

   a. Place hands over lower anterior chest wall along costal margins and move inward until the thumbs meet at midline.

   b. Ask the patient to breathe deeply and observe movement of thumbs away from each other. Normal expansion is 1 inch or 2.5 cm. Normal chest movement is equal.

   c. Abnormal findings: Unequal expansion occurs when air entry is limited by conditions involving the lung (atelectasis, pneumothorax), the chest wall (incisional pain), or pleura (effusion). Equal but diminished expansion occurs in conditions that produce a hyper-inflated or barrel chest or in neuromuscular disease.

3. Tactile fremitus. Vibration of the chest wall produced by vocalization.

   a. Place palms against the patient's chest and ask the patient to repeat "ninety-nine."

   b. Move hands from side to side and from top to bottom of the patient's chest. Compare vibrations from similar areas.

   c. Tactile fremitus is most intense in the first and second intercostal space lateral to the sternum and between the scapulae due to the proximity of the major bronchi.

   d. Abnormal findings: Increased fremitus occurs when the lung becomes filled with fluid or more dense (pneumonia, tumors, above a pleural effusion). Fremitus is decreased if the hand is further from the lung (pleural effusion or hyperinflation). Absent fremitus is noted with pneumothorax or atelectasis. Rhonchial fremitus is a palpable vibration caused by air traveling past thick bronchial mucus. It may change when the patient takes a deep inspiration and may change or clear with coughing.

D. Percussion—assesses density or aeration of the lungs

1. Directions

   a. Have patient in semi-sitting or supine position.

   b. Anteriorly start below clavicles and percuss downward, interspace by interspace. The area over lung tissue should be resonant.

   c. Posteriorly, have the patient sit leaning forward with arms folded. The posterior chest should be resonant over lung tissue to the level of the diaphragm.

2. Abnormal findings:
   a. Hyperresonance is a loud, lowered-pitched sound over areas that normally produce a resonant sound. This may indicate lung hyperinflation (COPD), lung collapse (pneumothorax), air trapping (asthma).
   b. Dullness is a medium-pitched sound over areas that normally produce a resonant sound. This may indicate an increased density (pneumonia, large atelectasis) or increased fluid in the pleural space (pleural effusion).

E. Auscultation
   1. Directions
      a. Instruct the patient to breathe slowly and deeply via mouth.
      b. Compare opposite sides of chest from the lung apices to the bases, including lateral fields.
      c. Place stethoscope over lung tissue vs. bony prominences. At each placement of stethoscope, listen to one cycle of inspiration and expiration.
      d. Note the pitch, duration of sound, presence of adventitious or abnormal sounds.
   2. Three normal breath sounds are vesicular, broncho-vesicular, and bronchial.
      a. Vesicular are soft, low pitched, gentle rustling sounds. Heard all over the lung areas except the major bronchi. Ratio 3:1 with inspiration, longer than expiration.
      b. Broncho-vesicular are medium pitch and intensity, heard anteriorly over mainstem bronchi on either side of sternum and posteriorly between scapulae. Ratio 1:1 with inspiration = expiration.
      c. Bronchial are louder and higher pitched and resemble air blowing through a hollow pipe. Ratio 2:3 with a gap between inspiration and expiration. Heard over manubrium.
   3. Normal auscultatory sounds are depicted in Figure 6.1.
   4. Abnormal breath sounds:
      a. Described bronchial or broncho-vesicular sounds heard in the peripheral lung fields.
      b. Adventitious sounds—crackles, rhonchi, wheezes, pleural friction rubs.
   5. Vocal auscultatory techniques
      a. Bronchophony, whispered pectoriloquy: spoken or whispered syllable more distinct than normal on auscultation. This may indicate pneumonia.
      b. Egophony: Spoken *e* similar to *a* on auscultation because of altered transmission of voice sounds. This may indicate pneumonia or pleural effusion (Reinke & Hoffman, 1999).
   6. Common assessment abnormalities of the thorax and lungs are presented in Table 6.1.

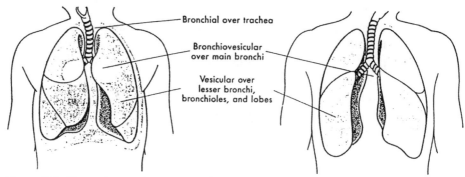

Figure 6.1. Normal ausculatory sounds.

Source: Beare, P. G. & Myers, J. L. (1994). In *Principles and practice of adult health nursing* (2nd ed., p. 529). St. Louis, MO: Mosby.

III. Normal findings related to aging
  A. Structural changes—decreased elastic recoil, decreased chest wall compliance, increased AP diameter, decreased functioning alveoli. These may lead to the following differences in assessment findings:
    1. Barrel chest appearance
    2. Decreased chest wall movement
    3. Decreased respiratory excursion
    4. Decreased vital capacity and increased functional residual capacity
    5. Decreased breath sounds, especially at bases
    6. Decreased PaO_2 and SaO_2, normal pH and $PaCO_2$
  B. Defense mechanisms—Decrease cell-mediated immunity, decrease specific antibodies, decrease cilia function, decrease cough force, decrease alveolar macrophage function. These changes may lead to the following differences in assessment findings:
    1. Decreased cough effectiveness
    2. Decreased secretion clearance
    3. Increased risk of URI, influenza, pneumonia
  C. Respiratory control—decreased response to hypoxemia, decreased response to hypercapnia. These may lead to the following differences in assessment findings.
    1. Greater decrease in PaO_2 and increase in $PaCO_2$ before respiratory rate changes.
    2. Significant hypoxemia or hypercapnia may develop from relatively small incidents.
    3. Retained secretions, pain, excessive sedation, or positioning that impairs chest expansion may substantially alter PaO_2 or SpO_2 values. (Cotes, 1997)
IV. Key assessment tips
  A. Begin with obtaining the past medical history, treatments, all medications (prescribed and over-the-counters) and any complementary therapies being used.

Table 6.1	Thorax and Lungs, Common Assessment Abnormalities

Finding	Description	Possible Etiology and Significance
Inspection		
Pursed-lip breathing	Exhalation through mouth with lips pursed together to slow exhalation.	COPD, asthma. Suggests ↑ breathlessness. Strategy taught to slow expiration, ↓ dyspnea.
Tripod position; inability to lie flat	Leaning forward with arms and elbows supported on overbed table.	COPD, asthma in exacerbation, pulmonary edema. Indicates moderate to severe respiratory distress.
Accessory muscle use; intercostal retractions	Neck and shoulder muscles used to assist breathing. Muscles between ribs pull in during inspiration.	COPD, asthma in exacerbation, secretion retention. Indicates severe respiratory distress, hypoxemia.
Splinting	Voluntary ↓ in tidal volume to ↓ pain on chest expansion.	Thoracic or abdominal incision. Chest trauma, pleurisy.
↑ AP diameter	AP chest diameter equal to lateral. Slope of ribs more horizontal (90°) to spine.	COPD, asthma, cystic fibrosis. Lung hyperinflation. Advanced age.
Tachypnea	Rate >20 breaths/min; >25 breaths/min in elderly.	Fever, anxiety, hypoxemia, restrictive lung disease. Magnitude of ↑ above normal rate reflects increased work of breathing.
Kussmaul's respirations	Regular, rapid, and deep respirations.	Metabolic acidosis. ↑ in rate aids body in ↑ CO_2 excretion.
Cyanosis	Bluish color of skin best seen in earlobes, under the eyelids, or nail beds.	↓ Oxygen transfer in lungs, ↓ cardiac output. Nonspecific, unreliable indicator.
Clubbing of fingers	↑ Depth, bulk, sponginess of distal digit of finger.	Chronic hypoxemia. Cystic fibrosis, lung cancer, bronchiectasis.
Abdominal paradox	Inward (rather than normal outward) movement of abdomen during inspiration.	Inefficient and ineffective breathing pattern. Nonspecific indicator of severe respiratory distress.
Palpation		
Tracheal deviation	Leftward or rightward movement of trachea from normal midline position.	Nonspecific indicator of change in position of mediastinal structures. Medical emergency if caused by tension pneumothorax.
Altered tactile fremitus	Increase or decrease in vibrations.	↑ in pneumonia, pulmonary edema; ↓ in pleural effusion, atelectatic area, lung hyperinflation; absent in pneumothorax, large atelectasis.

(continued)

Table 6.1 Thorax and Lungs, Common Assessment Abnormalities (*continued*)

Finding	Description	Possible Etiology and Significance
▪ Altered chest movement	Unequal or equal but diminished movement of two sides of chest with inspiration.	Unequal movement caused by atelectasis, pneumothorax, pleural effusion, splinting; equal but diminished movement caused by barrel chest, restrictive disease, neuromuscular disease.

Percussion

▪ Hyperresonance	Loud, lower-pitched sound over areas that normally produce a resonant sound.	Lung hyperinflation (COPD), lung collapse (pneumothorax), air trapping (asthma).
▪ Dullness	Medium-pitched sound over areas that normally produce a resonant sound.	↑ Density (pneumonia, large atelectasis), ↑ fluid pleural space (pleural effusion).

Auscultation

▪ Fine crackles	Series of short, explosive, high-pitched sounds heard just before the end of inspiration; result of rapid equalization of gas pressure when collapsed alveoli or terminal bronchioles suddenly snap open; similar sound to that made by rolling hair between fingers just behind ear	Interstitial fibrosis (asbestosis), interstitial edema (early pulmonary edema), alveolar filling (pneumonia), loss of lung volume (atelectasis), early phase of congestive heart failure
▪ Coarse crackles	Series of short, low-pitched sounds caused by air passing through airway intermittently occluded by mucus, unstable bronchial wall, or fold of mucosa; evident on inspiration and, at times, expiration; similar sound to blowing through straw under water; increase in bubbling quality with more fluid	Congestive heart failure, pulmonary edema, pneumonia with severe congestion, COPD
▪ Rhonchi	Continuous rumbling, snoring, or rattling sounds from obstruction of large airways with secretions; most prominent on expiration; change often evident after coughing or suctioning	COPD, cystic fibrosis, pneumonia, bronchiectasis

(*continued*)

Table 6.1	Thorax and Lungs, Common Assessment Abnormalities (*continued*)

Finding	Description	Possible Etiology and Significance
Wheezes	Continuous high-pitched squeaking sound caused by rapid vibration of bronchial walls; first evident on expiration but possibly evident on inspiration as obstruction of airway increases; possibly audible without stethoscope	Bronchospasm (caused by asthma), airway obstruction (caused by foreign body, tumor), COPD
Stridor	Continuous musical sound of constant pitch; result of partial obstruction of larynx or trachea	Croup, epiglottitis, vocal cord edema after extubation, foreign body
Absent breath sounds	No sound evident over entire lung or area of lung	Pleural effusion, main-stem bronchi obstruction, large atelectasis, pneumonectomy, lobectomy
Pleural friction rub	Creaking or grating sound from roughened, inflamed surfaces of the pleura rubbing together; evident during inspiration, expiration, or both and no change with/coughing; usually uncomfortable, especially on deep inspiration	Pleurisy, pneumonia, pulmonary infarct
Bronchophony, whispered pectoriloquy	Spoken or whispered syllable more distinct than normal on auscultation	Pneumonia
Egophony	Spoken "e" similar to "a" on auscultation because of altered transmission of voice sounds	Pneumonia, pleural effusion

Source: Lynn F. Reinke and Leslie A. Hoffman. As printed in Reinke, L. F., & Hoffman, L. A. (1999). Nursing assessment: Respiratory system. In S. M. Lewis, M. M. Heitkemper, & S. R. Dirksen, *Medical-surgical nursing, Assessment and management of clinical problems,* ed 5, (5th ed., pp. 561–570). St. Louis, MO: Mosby.

B. Obtain detailed occupational history, including exposure to chemicals, asbestos, fumes, and so forth.

C. Obtain smoking history (packs per day multiplied by number of years), quit date, if current smoker, number of quit attempts and techniques used to quit.

D. Obtain history of exposure to animals, including household pets, birds, pigeons, horses, and so forth.

E. Perform physical exam in a systematic approach from head to toe, beginning with inspection to palpation, percussion, and auscultation.

F. Other tips for the physical assessment:
    1. Instruct the patient to cough prior to the exam to establish a normal baseline and clear any potential atelectatic sounds.
    2. Minimize audible noises external to the exam setting.
    3. Manage of excessive thoracic hair which may interfere with accurate auscultation findings.
    4. Ensure appropriate length of stethoscope tubing and clear the stethoscope of articles, such as, stuffed animals or covers, bed linens or clothing.
    5. Ensure correct presence of *normal* breath sounds at the correct location.

REFERENCES

American Nurses Association & Respiratory Nursing Society. (1994). *Standard and scope of respiratory nursing practice.* Washington, DC: American Nurses Publishing.

Cotes, J. E. (1997). Physiology in the aging lung. In R. G. Crystal, J. B. West, E. R. Weibel, & P. J. Barnes (Eds.), *The lung: Scientific foundations* (2nd ed., pp. 2193–2201). Philadelphia: Lippincott-Raven.

Beare, P. G., & Myers, J. L. (1994). *Principles and practice of adult health nursing* (2nd ed., p. 529). St. Louis, MO: Mosby.

Dettemeier, P. A. (1992). *Pulmonary nursing care.* St. Louis, MO: Mosby.

Reinke, L. F., & Hoffman, L. A. (1999). Nursing assessment: Respiratory system. In S. M. Lewis, M. M. Heitkemper, & S. R. Dirksen (Eds.), *Medical-surgical nursing: Assessment and management of clinical problems* (5th ed., pp. 561–570). St. Louis, MO: Mosby.

Pediatric Respiratory Assessment

Pamela K. DeWitt

I. Completing the history
   A. A complete respiratory history is obtained through interview and discussion. Include the child in the discussion as appropriate.
   B. A review of the past medical history will give you information about the child's normal state of health and would include
      1. Previous illnesses
      2. Injuries
      3. Surgeries
      4. Birth history
      5. Growth and development
         a. Height and weight plotted on a growth chart
         b. Recent, unexplained weight loss or a drop in percentage of the growth curve
         c. Developmental milestones
         d. Sexual development
         e. Nutrition
   C. Ask about habits or episodes of
      1. Drinking alcohol
      2. Drug use or exposure to those who use drugs
      3. Use of inhalants
      4. Smoking or exposure to secondhand smoke
      5. Unprotected sexual intercourse
   D. Explore allergies including exposure to molds and mildew.
   E. Determine possible triggers or hazards in the home environment including
      1. Exposure to pets
      2. The type of heating and cooling system
      3. Recent flooding of the home or water damage

4. The type of flooring in the home, especially where the child spends most of their time

5. The type of bedding used for the child

F. Inquire about the usual sleep patterns and any changes.

G. Ask if the child has had any recent change in energy level or appetite.

H. A review of immunization status includes

1. Up-to-date with all recommended immunizations

2. Recent exposure to communicable diseases

3. Skin tests and results

I. A psychosocial history to include

1. Family composition

2. School performance

3. Activities

4. Sports

5. Friends

J. Have the family describe the current respiratory illness. Determine the onset, duration, and severity of the illness.

K. Have the family describe any episodes of cough to include

1. A description of the sound

2. Duration

3. Time of day the child coughs

4. If the cough is positional

5. Any secretions produced and their description

L. If dyspnea is present, ask when it occurs, how severe it is, and if activity or exercise affects it in any way.

M. Inquire about the occurrence of chest pains and the relationship to respirations.

N. Make a list of all medications taken by the child.

O. Inquire about any routine home respiratory therapy, such as airway clearance techniques.

II. Inspection

A. Inspection or observation of the child should be done with the child in a secure position. Make the child as comfortable as possible.

B. Note the general size and shape of the chest. Determine any asynchronous movement of the chest when the child breathes.

C. Skin color changes related to respiratory problems most often include cyanosis, mottling, or pallor. These changes are influenced by

1. Rate of blood flow/perfusion

2. Skin thickness

3. Normal skin color

4. Hemoglobin

5. Cardiac output

6. Perception of examiner

D. If the child is able to produce sputum, inquire if the production is related to the child's position. Examine the sputum for

      1. Character
      2. Volume
      3. Color
      4. Odor
  E. Determine the child's level of consciousness, comfort or anxiety.
  F. Observe respirations while the child is in a position of comfort. Respirations should be assessed for rate, pattern, or splinting. Describe the respiratory effort and use of accessory muscles.
  G. Clubbing, a symptom of hypoxia, may be noted in the fingertips, lips, or end of the nose.
  H. Listen to the child breath and describe any sounds such as grunting. Ask the family if the child snores and have them describe the pattern.
  I. Note the position of the trachea. It should be in the midline position.
III. Palpation
  A. While palpating the chest, note any enlarged lymph nodes or areas of tenderness.
IV. Percussion
  A. With the child supine or sitting, percuss each side and note any areas of dullness. Usually, dullness will be heard over the diaphragm, heart, liver and any areas of consolidation. Resonance is usually heard from the shoulder to the 8th or 10th rib posteriorly (Wong, 1995).
V. Auscultation
  A. When possible, have the child sit. Place your hands over the rib cage with thumbs together and midline. Assess the conduction of sound through the respiratory track by having the child repeat the words *ninety-nine*, or *one, two, three*, or *eee-eee*. While the child speaks, move your hands symmetrically over the chest. Vibrations can be felt when air is passing over fluid. Other vibrations may include a pleural friction rub or crepitations (Wong, 1995).
  B. Breath sounds should be assessed by listening from side to side, anterior and posterior and over the trachea. Determine the location of any adventitious breath sounds and whether they are cleared with a cough. Listen for a change in the breath sounds in various positions. Adventitious breath sounds include:
      1. Crackles
      2. Wheezing
      3. Pleural friction rubs
      4. Stridor
      5. Decrease or absence of sound
VI. Pediatric age-specific findings
  A. Due to the size of the tongue, infants are obligate nose breathers.
  B. Infants breathe by moving their diaphragm and abdomen.
  C. The larynx is funnel shaped above the cricoid cartilage which increases the airway resistance

   1. Tracheal changes
      a. The narrowest portion of a child's trachea is the cricoid cartilage until approximately 10 years of age.
      b. The trachea is easily occluded due to soft and incomplete tracheal cartilage.
      c. The trachea at birth is approximately one-third the size of an adult's.
      d. The number of alveolar sacs continues to increase until the child is 7–10 years old.
   D. Common pediatric anomalies affecting the respiratory system include:
      1. Hypoplastic lungs—markedly reduced lung volume.
      2. Tracheal stenosis—narrowing of the trachea.
      3. Tracheoesophageal fistula—opening between the trachea and esophagus, occurs in one out of every 300 to 4,500 live births, may be associated with tracheal atresia (Moore & Persaud, 1998).
      4. Osteogenesis Imperfecta—brittle bones and short thoracic cage (Porth, 1994).
VII. Key assessment tips
   A. Begin the assessment with discussion and observation and then proceed to more invasive techniques.
   B. Communicate with children according to their cognitive level and involve them in the exam as appropriate for their age.
   C. Allow small children to examine the assessment equipment to decrease fear and gain their cooperation (Wong, 1995).
   D. Be knowledgeable of normal pediatric age-specific findings.
   E. Know growth and developmental milestones for the pediatric population.

REFERENCES

Moore, K. L., & Persaud, T. V. N. (Eds.). (1998). *The developing human: Clinically oriented embryology* (6th ed.). Philadelphia: W. B. Saunders.

Porth, C. M. (Ed.). (1994). *Pathophysiology: Concepts of altered health states* (4th ed.). Philadelphia: J. B. Lippincott.

Wong, D. (Ed.). (1995). *Whaley and Wong's nursing care of infants and children* (5th ed.). St. Louis, MO: C. V. Mosby.

Diagnostic Studies

8

Deb Siela

INTRODUCTION

The purpose of this chapter is to review diagnostic studies that are used to detect pathology or deterioration in a patient's pulmonary status. The outline for each diagnostic study will present both normal and abnormal findings. Nursing and clinical implications are provided for each diagnostic study. When caring for patients with pulmonary diseases the nurse must be aware of the type of diagnostic studies as well as the impact of the results of these studies on the patients and their families. It is important for the nurse to understand the purpose of diagnostic study, diagnostic study procedure, indications of diagnostic study, clinical indications of diagnostic study, normal values of findings of diagnostic study, abnormal values of findings of diagnostic study, complications of diagnostic study, precautions of diagnostic study, and nursing implications of diagnostic study.

NONINVASIVE DIAGNOSTIC STUDIES

Pulse Oximetry

I. Purpose
   A. To monitor oxygen saturation to evaluate oxygen needs at rest, ambulation/activity, or long-term or home oxygen therapy
II. Clinical indications
   A. To detect oxygen desaturation in disorders that affect oxygenation
   B. To monitor effectiveness of oxygen therapy
   C. To monitor or detect oxygen desaturation with activity

III. Setting
  A. Acute care setting
  B. Ambulatory care setting
  C. Home setting
IV. Patient preparation
  A. Explain use of sensor and selection of body sites to patient. Include the need for patient to remove nail polish, as nail polish can negatively impact accurate monitoring of oxygen saturation.
 V. Normal values (Pagana & Pagana, 2003)
  A. 95%–100% at rest breathing room air
  B. SpO_2 is approximately 2%–3% below ABG O_2 saturation readings
VI. Clinical implications of abnormal values
  A. Values below 95% may require oxygen therapy; conditions resulting in values below 95% may include pneumonias.
  B. Values below 90% may require oxygen therapy and perhaps other treatment, such as the use of Albuterol administered via metered dose inhaler (MDI) with exacerbations of reactive airway disease.
  C. Values below 85% will require oxygen therapy and other treatment, such as the need to control ventilation through the use of mechanical ventilation.

End Tidal CO_2

 I. Purpose
  A. To measure alveolar CO_2 at the end of exhalation, when CO_2 concentration is at its peak
  B. To detect hyper- or hypoventilation states
 II. Clinical indications
  A. To identify problems with CO_2 exchange
  B. To measure end-tidal CO_2 (et CO_2) during anesthesia
  C. To measure et CO_2 during mechanical ventilation
  D. To measure et CO_2 during cardiopulmonary resuscitation
III. Setting
  A. Operating room
  B. Acute care settings
  C. Emergency transport
IV. Patient preparation
  A. Explain the non-invasive procedure to patient.
  B. Add the tubing to ventilator circuit, disposable CO_2 detector to endotracheal tube, or monitoring catheter in nose.
 V. Normal values (Carroll, 1999; Pierce, 1995)
  A. et CO_2 averages 2 to 5 mm Hg less than arterial pCO_2 or about 38 mm Hg
  B. et CO_2 averages 5%
VI. Clinical indications of abnormal values (Carroll, 1999; Pierce, 1995)
  A. Low et CO_2 could indicate hyperventilation.
  B. Abruptly decreasing et CO_2 could indicate ventilator malfunction, pulmonary embolism with lack of perfusion, cardiac arrest with no

pulmonary perfusion, or severe bleeding with pulmonary hypoperfusion.

C. Gradual decrease in et CO_2 could indicate increased minute ventilation or decrease in cardiac output resulting in decreased pulmonary perfusion.

D. Gradual increase in et CO_2 could indicate decreased minute ventilation, increase in production of CO_2, or accumulation of secretions in airway that impair ventilation.

Pulmonary Function Test (PFT)

I. Purpose (Ruppel, 2004)
   A. To measure lung ventilatory and diffusing capacities
   B. To determine ventilatory and diffusing capacity in response to therapy
II. Clinical indications
   A. Presence of acute respiratory disease or illness.
   B. Determine the presence of lung disease or an abnormality of lung function.
   C. Determine the degree of respiratory impairment and overall progression of disease.
   D. Determine a course of therapy in the treatment of disease.
   E. Determine risk for postoperative pulmonary complications.
III. Setting
   A. Pulmonary function lab
   B. Portable spirometry in any setting
   C. Hand-held spirometry (home setting)
IV. Patient preparation
   A. Explain purpose of diagnostic test.
   B. Explain withholding of bronchodilator medications and others as needed.
   C. Explain breathing component of the PFT or spirometry.
V. Normal values equal 80%–120% of the predicted value based on age, gender, and height for all values except FEV1/FVC and RV/TLC (Des Jardins & Burton, 1995; Ruppel, 2004; Shortall & Perkins, 1999)
   A. Spirometry
      1. Forced vital capacity (FVC)
      2. Forced expiratory volume in 1 second (FEV1) equals 65% or greater
      3. Forced expiratory volume in 1 second over forced vital capacity ratio (FEV1/FVC)
      4. Forced expiratory flow 25%–75% (FEF 25%–75%)
      5. Peak expiratory flow (PEF)
      6. Maximum voluntary ventilation (MVV)
      7. Airway conductance (Raw)
      8. Airway resistance (Gaw)
   B. Lung volumes
      1. Vital capacity (VC)
      2. Inspiratory capacity (IC)
      3. Total lung capacity (TLC)
      4. Residual volume (RV)

5. Residual volume over total lung capacity ratio (RV/TLC)
6. Functional residual capacity (FRC)
7. Expiratory reserve volume
8. Minute ventilation (VE)
9. Tidal volume (Vt)
   C. Diffusion tests
1. Carbon monoxide diffusing capacity (DLCO)
2. Alveolar lung volume (VA)
3. Carbon monoxide diffusing capacity per unit alveolar lung volume (DLCO/VA)
VI. Clinical indications of abnormal values (Des Jardins & Burton, 1995; Ruppel, 2004; Shortall & Perkins, 1999)
   A. Spirometry
1. Percent predicted values less than 80% indicate obstructive lung disease or chronic airflow disease increasing in severity as the percent predicted decreases.
2. Some restrictive disease will have low percent predicted values due to low lung volumes.
   B. Lung volumes
1. Percent predicted values greater than 120% indicate obstructive lung disease or chronic airflow disease.
2. Percent predicted values less than 80% indicate restrictive lung disease.

Spontaneous Respiratory Parameters

I. Purpose
   A. To measure strength and endurance of ventilatory muscles.
   B. May be used to predict patient's ability to maintain spontaneous breathing.
II. Clinical indications
   A. To assess ventilatory status of an acute or chronically ill person, for example, a person with chronic lung disease.
   B. To assess for readiness to wean from mechanical ventilation.
   C. To detect ventilatory changes in people with neuromuscular disease, such as ventilatory fatigue.
III. Setting
   A. Acute care setting
   B. Ambulatory setting
   C. Home care setting
IV. Patient preparation
   A. Explain precise breathing maneuvers to patient.
V. Normal values (Hanneman, 2004; Hanneman, Ingersoll, Knebel, Shekleton, Burns, & Clochsey, 1994; Pierce, 1995). These values must be assessed in conjunction with the patients arterial blood gases.
   A. Minute ventilation (VE) between 5 and 10 liters
   B. Maximum voluntary ventilation of 50 to 250 L/min and/or double the VE

C. Tidal volume (Vt) of greater than 300 ml and/or 5 to 8 ml/kg
D. Vital capacity (VC) of 10 to 15 ml/kg
E. Maximum inspiratory pressure (MIP), negative inspiratory pressure (NIP), maximum inspiratory force (MIF), peak negative pressure (PNP), and inspiratory force (IF) of more negative than -20 cm H_2O (normal is -115 cm H_2O)
F. Respiratory rate of less than 30/minute
G. Consider ABG values of pH, pCO_2, pO_2, and level of oxygenation.

VI. Clinical indications of abnormal values (Hanneman, 2004; Hanneman et al., 1994; Pierce, 1995)
A. VE greater than 10 L with increased respiratory rate may be associated with respiratory muscle fatigue
B. MVV less than 50 L/min may indicate an inability to maintain ventilation under stress
C. Vt less than 5 to 8 ml/kg may indicate a decreased respiratory muscle endurance.
D. VC of less than 10 ml/kg may indicate a lack of ventilatory reserve and strength
E. MIP, and so forth, of more positive than -20 cm H_2O indicates poor respiratory muscle strength
F. Respiratory rate of greater than 30 may indicate inadequate respiratory muscle strength and/or increased minute ventilation demands
G. ABG values
1. pO_2 values of less than 70 on 0.5 FIO_2 may indicate a reduced ability to meet the oxygen demands of the body.
2. pCO_2 values of greater than person's normal range may indicate a reduced ability to meet ventilatory needs of the body.
3. pH of less than 7.32 usually indicates an inability to ventilate if pCO_2 is also elevated especially in COPD.

Polysomnogram/Nocturnal Desaturation Study

I. Purpose
A. To measure respiratory rate, heart rate, oxygen saturation, and episodes of apnea during sleep.
II. Clinical indications
A. To document nocturnal oxygen desaturation.
B. To diagnose obstructive sleep apnea and other breathing related disorders, such as excessive snoring, excessive daytime sleeping/narcolepsy; mood changes, inability to concentrate, reported episodes of breathing cessation by bed/sleeping partner, early a.m. headaches.
III. Setting
A. Sleep laboratory, most common
IV. Patient preparation
A. Explain procedure to patient, that is, avoidance of caffeine, monitoring devices, and so forth.

V. Normal findings (Pagana & Pagana, 2003)
   A. Respiratory disturbance index: less than 5–10 apneic episodes per study
VI. Clinical indications of abnormal findings (Des Jardins & Burton, 1995; Pagana & Pagana, 2003)
   A. Diagnosis of obstructive sleep apnea, or indication of central sleep apnea or cardiac sleep apnea
   B. Treatment of obstructive sleep apnea by CPAP/BIPAP
   C. Document need for nocturnal oxygen therapy

Magnetic Resonance Imaging (MRI)

I. Purpose
   A. Use of magnetic resonance to view cross-sectional images of the body
II. Clinical indications
   A. Diagnosis of tumors or lesions in the chest wall, mediastinum, or hilar regions
III. Setting
   A. Site of MRI scanner
IV. Patient preparation
   A. Explain about contradictions to MRI and the MRI procedure including the need to remain still and no implanted metal objects.
   B. Explain risk of claustrophobia, noise levels, need to remain still, and procedure length.
V. Normal values
   A. Absence of pathology
VI. Clinical indications of abnormal values
   A. If tumor noted, could be indicative of pulmonary cancers or benign pulmonary tumors, thus appropriate medical and nursing care must be implemented.

Computerized Tomography (CT)

I. Purpose
   A. To view soft tissue/vascular techniques of the chest cavity using tomograms (cross-sectional radiographs).
II. Clinical indications
   A. To diagnose pathology such as tumors, nodules, cysts, abscesses, pleural effusion, fractures, enlarged lymph nodes, and some vascular abnormalities.
III. Setting
   A. Site of computerized tomography scanner
IV. Patient preparation
   A. Explain procedure to patient including the need to lie still during procedure, noise, and length of procedure.
V. Normal values
   A. Absence of pathology

VI. Clinical indications of abnormal findings
  A. If pathology noted, appropriate medical and nursing management are indicated for the specific pathology.

Chest X-ray Reading and Interpretation

  I. Purpose
    A. To view internal structures of the chest through the chest using X-ray
 II. Clinical indications
    A. To determine etiology of signs or symptoms of acute or chronic respiratory/cardiac dysfunction
    B. To view lungs of patients with suspected mycobacterial disease in known purified protein derivative (PPD) converters or anergic individuals
III. Setting
    A. Acute care setting with radiology facilities
    B. Ambulatory care setting with radiology facilities
 IV. Patient preparation
    A. Explain procedure to patient including exposure to radiation
  V. Normal findings (Siela, 2002; Dettenmeier, 1995; Kersten, 1989; Scheffer & Tobin, 1997)
    A. Normal lungs and surrounding tissues
      1. Soft tissues have both fat and water density
      2. Trachea
        a. Shows a column of radiolucency or air density above the clavicles in the midline
        b. Endotracheal tube placement should show the tube tip approximately 3 to 7 cm above the carina
      3. Bony thorax has symmetry
        a. Articulation of humerous with scapula
        b. Symmetry of clavicles
        c. Straight thoracic spine
        d. Presence of 9 to 10 posterior ribs for frontal inspiratory film
        e. Symmetry of intercostal spaces
        f. Dome shaped diaphragms with right hemidiaphragm 1 to 3 cm higher than left hemidiaphragm, air-fluid level below left hemidiaphragm, for example, gastric bubble
        g. Sharp right and left costophrenic angles, may be slightly hazy in women due to breast tissue
        h. Minor fissure sometimes seen on frontal films separating right upper lobe (RUL) from right middle lobe (RML), major fissures are only seen on lateral films between right and left upper lobes and right and left lower lobes
      4. Mediastinum shows varying degrees of water density
        a. Right artrium on the right heart border
        b. Ascending aorta into descending aorta forms aortic knob

        c. May observe main pulmonary artery

        d. Left atrium and left ventricle form the left heart border

    5. Heart spans the entire width of the mediastinum and has a ratio of less than 1:2 in its width compared to the chest diameter.

    6. Hila have varying densities with the pulmonary blood vessels on the right extending further out than the left pulmonary blood vessels. Left hilar region slightly higher than right hilar region.

    7. Lung fields most radiolucent or blackest are composed of air density.

VI. Clinical indications of abnormal findings (Dettenmeier, 1995; Kersten, 1989; Scheffer & Tobin, 1997; Siela, 2002)

    A. Soft tissues of the chest

        1. Increased densities may indicate tumors or lesions.

        2. Air density may indicate subcutanous emphysema.

    B. Trachea

        1. Tracheal deviation may indicate either a tumor or mediastinal shift due to a pneumothorax.

    C. Bony thorax

        1. Rib fractures commonly appear laterally

        2. Intercostal spaces

            a. Widened intercostal spaces may occur due to COPD, large pneumothorax, or large pleural effusion.

            b. Narrowed intercostal spaces may occur due to decreased lung volume of atelectasis and interstitial fibrosis.

        3. Diaphragm

            a. Diaphragm elevation with less than 9–10 ribs showing may indicate abdominal distension, phrenic nerve paralysis, or lung collapse.

            b. Diaphragm depression when 10–12 ribs show may indicate air.

            c. Trapping that occurs with COPD.

            d. Diaphragm flattening indicates hyperinflation and is a more reliable indicator of COPD than diaphragm depression.

            e. Diaphragmatic flattening indicates air trapping with acute exacerbations of asthma.

        4. Costophrenic angles

            a. Dull or obliterated angle suggests pleural thickening.

            b. Horizontal fluid level indicates pleural effusion; in heart failure a right pleural effusion is usually larger than the left.

    D. Mediastinum

        1. Widened mediastinum indicates a possible tumor, enlarged lymph nodes, cardiomegaly, inflammation, aortic disruptions, cardiac tamponade, or vascular aneurysms.

        2. Mediastinal shift from midline may indicate a tumor or pneumothorax.

    E. Heart

        1. If heart size has a ratio greater than 1:2 with the chest diameter cardiac enlargement or cardiomegaly is indicated.

2. Increased convexity of the right heart border indicates outward positioning of the right artrium that is indicative of right ventricular enlargement.
3. When the left heart border sags and becomes rounded and distended in the apical area, it indicates left ventricle enlargement.

F. Hila
   1. Hilar elevation may indicate lung collapse in the upper lobes.
   2. Hilar depression may indicated lung collapse in the lower lobes.
   3. Hilar enlargement may indicate heart failure and possible presence of cancer.

G. Lung fields
   1. Alveolar pattern or acinar pattern appears as fluffy clouds. Alveolar pattern is replacement of air in alveoli with edema, mucus, blood, tumor, or inflammatory materials making a water density.
      a. Alveolar pneumonia
      b. Alveolar pulmonary edema
      c. Pulmonary embolism with infarction
      d. Pulmonary hemorrhage
      e. Pneumocystis carini in late stages
      f. Aspiration pneumonia
      g. Adult respiratory distress syndrome
   2. Air bronchogram sign is visualization of air in an airway such as when a bronchus is surrounded by a water density as in pneumonia.
   3. Interstitial patterns include reticular, nodular, and granular patterns. A thickened alveolar interstitum is visualized and is usually caused by fibrosis, fluid, or inflammatory by-products in interstitial pneumonias. Identified as fine, medium, or coarse.
      a. Interstitial pneumonia
      b. Interstitial pulmonary edema
      c. Diffuse interstitial fibrosis
      d. Sarcoidosis
      e. Scleroderma
      f. Metastatic cancer
      g. Silicosis
      h. Asbestosis
      i. Fungus infections
      j. Advanced tuberculosis
   4. Peribronchial cuffing is a radiopaque ring around a bronchus that occurs when fluid from fibrosis extends around the interstitum of a bronchus.
   5. Kerley's A lines are oblique septal lines that are visible in the upper lobes, which indicates increased fluid or tissue in the interstitum.
   6. Kerley's B lines are horizontal septal lines that are visible in the lower lobes peripherally, which indicates increased tissue or fluid in the interstitum.

Digital Imaging Chest X-ray

I. Purpose
   A. To detect lung lesions in the chest without interference of bone images that are eliminated by computer
II. Clinical indications
   A. Signs/symptoms of infection, cancer, and so forth
III. Setting
   A. Site with digital imaging chest X-ray
IV. Patient preparation
   A. Explain procedure to patient
V. Normal values
   A. Absence of pathology
VI. Clinical indications of abnormal findings
   A. See chest X-ray for clinical indications

INVASIVE DIAGNOSTIC STUDIES

Arterial Blood Gases

I. Purpose
   A. To determine acid-base balance (pH)
   B. To determine adequacy of ventilation (p_aCO_2, HCO_3)
   C. To determine oxygenation status (p_aO_2, $O_{2\ sat}$)
II. Procedure
   A. Puncture of an arterial vessel with subsequent withdrawal of arterial blood
III. Indications
   A. Signs/symptoms of respiratory or metabolic dysfunction: dyspnea, tachypnea, hyperventilation, hypoventilation, accessory muscle use, buccal cyanosis, and so forth
IV. Nursing implications
   A. Explain procedure to patient
   B. Prepare artery site for puncture
   C. Perform Allen test (only with radial site)
   D. Normal values (Pagana & Pagana, 2003)
      1. pH: 7.35–7.45
      2. p_aCO_2: 35–45 mm Hg
      3. HCO_3: 21–28 meq
      4. p_aO_2: 80–100 mm Hg
      5. O_2 saturation: > 95%
V. Clinical indications of abnormal values (Des Jardins & Burton, 1995)
   A. Decreased pH and increased pCO_2 is respiratory acidosis
      1. May require metabolic compensation per kidney or through medical intervention
      2. May require ventilatory assistance

B. Increased pCO_2 indicates poor ventilation or hypoventilation
   1. Breathing exercises may improve ventilation.
   2. Mechanical ventilation may improve severe hypoventilation.
C. Decreased pO_2 and/or O_2 saturation
   1. May require oxygen therapy
   2. May require mechanical ventilation
VI. Complications
   A. Bleeding from arterial site and hematoma
   B. Occlusion of artery
VII. Contraindications
   A. A negative Allen's test indicating no ulnar artery circulation
   B. AV fistula proximal to draw site
   C. Severe coagulopathy

Ventilation Perfusion Scan

I. Definition/purpose
   A. To determine adequacy of ventilation/perfusion to all lung regions.
II. Procedure
   A. Peripheral IV injection of radionuclide-tagged MAA with subsequent perfusion scan
   B. Inhalation of a tracer through a face mask with subsequent image scan
III. Indications
   A. Primarily for diagnosis of perfusion defects, such as pulmonary embolism, but sometimes for ventilatory defects, such as parenchymal disease.
IV. Clinical indications of abnormal findings (Des Jardins & Burton, 1995; Pagana & Pagana, 2003)
   A. Ventilation scan
      1. Ventilation defect indicates parenchymal disease such as pneumonia, pleural fluid, emphysema.
   B. Perfusion scan
      1. Perfusion defect indicates probable pulmonary embolus.
   C. Ventilation and perfusion scan
      1. Both ventilation and perfusion defects indicates parenchymal disease (a match).
      2. Perfusion defect without a ventilation defect indicates pulmonary embolus.
   D. Clinical indications for an abnormal perfusion scan
      1. Thrombolytic drugs
      2. Embolectomy
      3. Anticoagulant therapy
   E. Clinical indications for an abnormal ventilation scan
      1. Treatment of parenchymal disease such as pneumonia or emphysema
V. Nursing implications
   A. Promote oxygenation
   B. Prevention of complications

C. Continue patient monitoring
D. Administer anticoagulant therapy
VI. Complications
    A. Usually none
VII. Precautions
    A. None

Pulmonary Angiography

I. Purpose
    A. To objectively detect and document perfusion defects following a positive lung scan
    B. To detect congenital and acquired lesions of the pulmonary vessels
II. Procedure
    A. Injection of dye through a central line to visualize pulmonary arterial circulation in a timed sequence
III. Indications
    A. Pulmonary embolism, congenital and acquired lesions of the pulmonary vessels
IV. Abnormal findings
    A. Pulmonary embolism, tumor, congenital or acquired lesions of pulmonary vessels
    B. Treat pulmonary embolism with thrombolytics, anticoagulants, or embolectomy
V. Nursing implications
    A. Explain procedure to patient
    B. Monitor catheter site for inflammation, bleeding, or hematoma
VI. Complications
    A. Allergic reaction to dye or contrast material
    B. Cardiac dysrhythmias
VII. Precautions
    A. Allergies to iodine or shellfish
    B. Pregnant patients
    C. Bleeding disorders

Bronchoscopy

I. Definition/purpose
    A. To examine the larynx, trachea, and bronchi by using either a flexible fiberoptic bronchoscope or a rigid bronchoscope.
    B. To obtain bronchial washings and/or transtracheal biopsies
    C. To clear excessive mucus
    D. To retrieve foreign bodies in the airway
II. Procedure
    A. The patient's nasopharnyx and oropharnyx are anesthetized topically.
    B. The tube is inserted through the nose or mouth into the pharynx.
    C. The tube is passed further into the bronchial tree.

D. Biopsy and washings are taken if pathology is suspected.

E. If removal of secretions is necessary, aspiration is performed.

III. Indications (Pagana & Pagana, 2003)

    A. Diagnostic

      1. Direct visualization of tracheobronchial tree for abnormalities

      2. Biopsy of lung tissue from lesions seen on X-ray or CT scan

      3. Aspiration of sputum for culture & sensitivity and cytology

      4. Direct visualization of the larynx

    B. Therapeutic

      1. Aspiration of retained secretions or sputum in patients with obstructed airways

      2. Control of bleeding in the bronchus

      3. Removal of foreign bodies in the bronchial tree

      4. Bradytherapy (radiation) for treatment of malignancies

      5. Palliative laser obliteration of bronchial obstruction caused by neoplasms

IV. Nursing implications

    A. Explain procedure to patient.

    B. Keep patient NPO (nothing by mouth) 8 hours before the bronchoscopy.

    C. Do not allow patient to eat or drink after the procedure until gag reflex and anesthesia has worn off.

    D. Watch for obstructed airway post bronchoscopy.

    E. Watch for blood in sputum post bronchoscopy.

V. Complications

    A. Hemorrhage

    B. Laryngospasm

    C. Sore throat

    D. Aspiration

VI. Precautions

    A. No eating or drinking for at least 8 hours prior to bronchoscopy to prevent aspiration.

    B. No eating or drinking for 2 hours post bronchoscopy to prevent aspiration. Check agency policy and post-procedure orders.

Lung Biopsy

I. Definition/purpose

    A. To obtain a specimen of lung tissue for a histologic examination by using either an open or closed technique.

II. Procedure (Pagana & Pagana, 2003)

    A. Transbronchial lung biopsy

      1. Use forceps through a flexible bronchoscope to obtain specimen of desired lung area.

    B. Transbronchial needle aspiration

      1. Needle is inserted through bronchoscope into desired lung area and a specimen is aspirated.

C. Transbronchial brushing
  1. A brush is inserted through the bronchoscope to move over a suspicious area in the bronchial tube.
D. Percutaneous needle biopsy
  1. During fluoroscopy or CT scan the desired site for biopsy is determined, then a needle is inserted through the patient's chest wall into the desired site and a specimen is aspirated.
E. Open lung biopsy
  1. During a thoracotomy, a lung specimen is obtained.

III. Indications
  A. Diagnosis of carcinomas, granulomas, infections, and sarcoidosis

IV. Nursing implications
  A. Explain procedure to the patient
  B. Keep patient NPO after midnight on the day of the test
  C. Monitor for signs/symptoms of pneumothorax post procedure
  D. Monitor pulmonary secretions for hemorrhage

V. Complications
  A. Pneumothorax
  B. Pulmonary hemorrhage
  C. Empyema

VI. Contraindications
  A. No bullae or lung cysts
  B. No suspected vascular lung abnormalities
  C. Bleeding abnormalities
  D. Pulmonary hypertension
  E. Respiratory insufficiency

Thoracentesis

I. Definition/purpose
  A. To aspirate pleural fluid or air from the pleural space for diagnosis or treatment.

II. Procedure
  A. Patient placed upright leaning on a bedside table or in a side-lying position on unaffected side.
  B. Needle with attached syringe and stopcock is inserted into pleural space site determined by percussion, auscultation, or radiologic techniques to aspirate fluid.
  C. A catheter may be placed in the pleural space to drain fluid or air.

III. Indications
  A. Signs/symptoms of cancer, empyema, pleurisy, tuberculosis, pleural effusion on X-ray or physical examination, dyspnea, and so forth
  B. Therapeutic
    1. Relieve pain, dyspnea, and other symptoms of pleural pressure
  C. Diagnostic
    1. Obtain fluid for the etiology of pleural effusion

IV. Abnormal findings (Pagana & Pagana, 2003)
   A. Exudates are indicated if total protein >3, albumin gradient <1.1, total protein ratio >0.5, elevated pleural fluid/serum LDH ratio >0.6, or WBC count >1000.
   B. Transudates are indicated if total protein <3, albumin gradient >1.1, total protein ratio <0.5.
   C. Exudates may be associated with empyema, pneumonia, tuberculosis, pancreatitis, ruptured esophagus, tumors, lymphoma, pulmonary infarction, collagen vascular disease, and drug hypersensitivity.
   D. Transudates may be associated with cirrhosis, heart failure, nephrotic syndrome, hypoproteinemia, and trauma.
   E. Treat patient for diagnosed problem.
 V. Nursing implications
   A. Explain procedure to patient.
   B. Monitor VS, signs/symptoms of diaphoresis or light-headedness during procedure.
   C. Monitor for hemoptysis post procedure.
   D. Monitor for signs/symptoms of pneumothorax post procedure.
   E. Keep patient on bed rest for about one hour post procedure, check agency policy and post-procedure orders.
VI. Complications
   A. Pneumothorax
   B. Interpleural bleeding
   C. Hemoptysis
   D. Bradycardia and hypotension
   E. Pulmonary edema
VII. Precautions
   A. Bleeding disorders
   B. Anticoagulant or antiplatelet therapy

Mediastinoscopy

  I. Definition/purpose
   A. To inspect mediastinal lymph nodes and to remove biopsy specimens from lesions in the mediastinum.
 II. Procedure
   A. A mediastinoscope is inserted through an incision in the suprasternal notch into the superior mediastinum.
   B. Lymph nodes may be biopsied.
III. Indications
   A. Signs and/or symptoms of lung cancer, granulomatous infections, sarcoidosis, Hodgkin's disease, other lymphomas, thymoma, or tuberculosis
IV. Abnormal findings
   A. Lung cancer, metastasis, sarcoidosis, thymoma, tuberculosis, Hodgkin's disease, lymphoma, and infection

V. Nursing implications
    A. Explain procedure to patient.
    B. Monitor for mediastinal crepitus post procedure.
    C. Monitor for signs/symptoms of mediastinal hematoma, that is, jugular venous distension (JVD) or pulsus paradoxus (see chapter 6, "Respiratory Assessment").
    D. Monitor for signs/symptoms of pneumothorax, that is, sudden dyspnea, increased respiratory rate, chest pain, anxiety, hypotension.
VI. Complications
    A. Puncture of the esophagus, trachea, or blood vessels
    B. Pneumothorax
    C. Laryngeal nerve damage
    D. Infection
VII. Precautions
    A. Bleeding disorders
    B. Anticoagulant or antiplatelet therapy

Thoracoscopy

I. Purpose
    A. To directly view the pleura, lung, and mediastinum, obtain tissue for examination, drain fluid, and perform lung resection (video-assisted thoracotomy)
II. Procedure
    A. Patient is in the operating room in lateral decubitus position.
    B. A blunt tipped needle is inserted through a small incision and the lung is collapsed.
    C. The thorascope is inserted through a trocar to examine the lung area, obtain tissue for examination, or allow lung resection.
    D. A chest tube is placed for lung re-inflation.
III. Indications
    A. Staging and dissection of lung cancers
IV. Abnormal findings
    A. Primary lung cancer, metastatic cancer to lung or pleura, empyema, pleural tumor, pleural infection, pleural inflammation, and pulmonary infection
V. Nursing implications
    A. Explain procedure to patient.
    B. Keep patient NPO after midnight the day of the thoracoscopy.
    C. Assess for signs of bleeding and pneumothorax post procedure.
    D. Provide analgesics post procedure.
VI. Complications
    A. Bleeding
    B. Infection or empyema
    C. Pneumothorax

VII. Precautions
   A. Patients with previous lung surgery

Complete Blood Count With Differential

   I. Purpose
   A. To assess oxygen carrying capacity of the blood (hemoglobin, hematocrit)
   B. To detect inflammatory or infectious processes in the body white blood count (WBC, differential)
   II. Procedure
   A. Venous blood is obtained.
   III. Indications
   A. Signs/symptoms of hypoxemia or anemia
   B. Signs/symptoms of inflammation or infection
   C. Acute onset of fevers, chills, or fatigue
   IV. Nursing implications
   A. Explain procedure to patient.
   B. Prepare venous puncture site.
   V. Normal values (Pagana & Pagana, 2003)
   A. Hemoglobin (Hgb): Male: 14–18 g/dl and Female: 12–16 g/dl
   B. Hematocrit (Hct): Male: 42%–52% and Female: 37%–47%
   C. Red blood cell count (RBC): Male: 4.7–6.1 mm^3 and Female: 4.2–5.4 mm^3
   D. White blood cell count (WBC): 5000–10,000
   E. Neutrophils: 55%–70%, 2500–8000 mm^3
   F. Lymphocytes 20%–40%, 1000–4000 mm^3
   G. Monocytes 2%–8%, 100–700 mm^3
   H. Eosinophils 1%–4%, 50–500 mm^3
   I. Basophils 0.5%–1%, 25–100 mm^3
   VI. Clinical indications of abnormal values (Des Jardins & Burton, 1995; Pagana & Pagana, 2003)
   A. Decreased Hgb, Hct, and RBC indicates decreased oxygen carrying capacity.
   B. Increased WBC indicates respiratory inflammation, infection, or stress.
   C. Increased neutrophils indicates respiratory inflammation, infection, or stress.
   D. Increased lymphocytes indicates chronic bacterial respiratory infection, or viral infection.
   E. Increased monocytes indicates chronic respiratory inflammation, respiratory viral infections, or tuberculosis infection.
   F. Increased eosinophils indicates allergic responses.
   VII. Complications
   A. Hematoma at venipuncture site
   B. Bleeding at venipuncture site

VIII. Precautions
   A. Patients with bleeding disorders or those on anticoagulant or antiplate-
      let therapy may have increased risk of bleeding/hematoma at venipunc-
      ture site.

**Sputum Diagnostics: Inspection of Physical Characteristics
of Sputum, Culture and Sensitivity (C & S), Gram and
Acid-Fast Stains, and Cytology**

   I. Purpose of sputum diagnostics
      A. Inspection
         1. Describe characteristics
            a. Color
            b. Consistency
            c. Volume
            d. Odor
      B. C & S
         1. To detect presence of pathogenic bacteria, mycobacterium, and fun-
            gus by culture
         2. To determine drug resistance of microorganism(s)
      C. Gram stain
         1. To detect and identify types of gram positive and negative bacteria
      D. Acid-fast stains
         1. To detect the presence of acid-fast bacilli
      E. Cytology
         1. To detect the presence of malignant cells
  II. Procedure
      A. Provide the appropriate specimen container.
      B. Collect sputum with or without assistance.
 III. Indications
      A. Physical appearance
         1. Color
            a. Yellow or green sputum may indicate infection or retained secre-
               tions.
            b. Bloody sputum may indicate irritation, infection, tuberculosis, or
               malignancy.
         2. Consistency
            a. Thick may indicate poor hydration or retention.
            b. Thin may indicate adequate hydration.
            c. Frothy may indicate saliva or pulmonary edema and not sputum.
         3. Odor
            a. Foul-smelling odor may indicate anaerobic infection.
            b. Musty odor may indicate pseudomonas infection.
         4. Volume: greater than 1/4 cup daily is a large amount, may indicate
            acute infectious process, chronic inflammation, or chronic lung
            disease.

   B. C & S, gram stain, and acid-fast stain
      1. Signs/symptoms of respiratory infection: colored sputum, fever, adventitious sounds, and so forth
   C. Cytology
      1. Signs/symptoms of lung malignancy: bloody sputum, hoarseness, abnormal chest X-ray, and so forth
IV. Nursing implications
   A. Sputum collection by voluntary coughing
      1. Provide sputum container, need for lung sputum, a.m. collection time, and so forth
   B. Sputum collection by suctioning, transtracheal aspiration, or bronchoscopy
      1. Explain suctioning, transtracheal aspiration, and bronchoscopy procedures.
      2. Perform sputum collection procedures by suctioning, transtracheal aspiration, or assist in bronchoscopy specimen collection.
V. Normal sputum values
   A. Appearance: clear or white
   B. C & S: negative
   C. Gram stain: negative
   D. Acid-fast stain: negative
   E. Cytology: negative (although does not exclude malignancy)
VI. Clinical indications of abnormal findings
   A. C & S: Presence of specific microorganisms and/or any drug sensitivity or resistance will determine antimicrobial drug therapy.
   B. Gram stain: Presence of gram positive or gram negative bacteria will determine initial antibiotic drug therapy until C & S results are available.
   C. Acid-fast stain: Presence indicates tuberculosis infection and/or disease, if disease respiratory isolation may be indicated.
   D. Cytology: Presence of malignant cells indicate a malignancy, further diagnostic studies and/or medical treatment may be indicated.
VII. Complications
   A. Hypoxemia if obtaining sputum by suctioning
VIII. Precautions
   A. Provide oxygenation, hyperinflation if patient is intubated.

Immunoglobulins

I. Purpose
   A. To detect and monitor hypersensitivity diseases, immune deficiencies, autoimmune diseases, and chronic infections measuring levels of IgA, IgE, IgG, and IgM
II. Procedure
   A. Explain procedure to patient.
   B. Obtain venous blood.

III. Indications
   A. Diseases that may affect level of immunoglobulins
IV. Nursing implications
   A. Explain procedure to patient.
V. Normal values (Pagana & Pagana, 2003)
   A. IgA 85–385 adults and 1–350 children
   B. IgE minimal
   C. IgG 565–1765 adults and 250–1,600 children
   D. IgM 55–375 adults and 20–200 children
VI. Clinical indications of abnormal values (Pagana & Pagana, 2003)
   A. IgA
      1. Increased: chronic liver disease, chronic infections, inflammatory bowel disease
      2. Decreased: telangiectasia, hypoproteinemia, immunosuppresive drugs
   B. IgE
      1. Increased: allergy reactions, allergic infections
      2. Decreased: agammaglobulinemia
   C. IgG
      1. Increased: chronic granulomatous infections, hyper immunization reactions, chronic liver disease, multiple myeloma, autoimmune diseases
      2. Decreased: Wiskott-Aldrich syndrome, agammaglobulinemia, AIDS, hypoproteinemia, drug immunosuppression, Non-IgG multiple myeloma, leukemia
   D. IgM
      1. Increased: Waldenstrom's macroglobulinemia, chronic infections, autoimmune diseases, acute infections, chronic liver disorders
      2. Decreased: agammaglobulinemia, AIDS, hypoproteinemia, drug immunosuppresion, IgG or IgA multiple myeloma, leukemia
VII. Complications
   A. Bleeding or hematoma at venipuncture site
VIII. Precautions
   A. Patients with bleeding disorders or anticoagulation or antiplatelet therapy may be at greater risk for puncture cite bleeding or hematoma formation.

Skin Tests

I. Purpose
   A. To determine previous exposure to a specific antigen usually mycobacterium (PPD)
   B. To detect anergy (no response) and immune status using antigens to which exposure is common including candida, mumps, or trichophyton
II. Procedure
   A. Explain procedure to patient.

B. Place antigen as an interdermal injection on the skin.

C. Observe for induration 48 to 72 hours later.

III. Indications

    A. Induration of PPD intradermal site of greater than 10 mm

        1. Indicates prior exposure to tuberculosis.

        2. Further diagnostic testing may be indicated to determine active tuberculosis disease.

    B. No reaction (anergy) to candida, mumps, or trichophyton antigens

        1. May indicate a poorly functioning immune system.

IV. Nursing implications

    A. Positive PPD and clinical signs of tuberculosis

        1. Airborne precautions may be necessary in an acute care setting.

        2. If drug therapy is indicated, encourage patient to follow drug regimen.

    B. No reaction to candida, mumps, or trichophyton antigens

        1. Plan for measures of preventing opportunistic infections.

V. Complications

    A. Severe hypersensitivity to the antigen

VI. Precautions

    A. Avoid administration of a PPD to a person with known active tuberculosis.

    B. Avoid administration of a PPD to a person who has received BCG immunization.

    C. Avoid administration of PPD, serial chest X-rays may be used.

REFERENCES

Carroll, P. (1999). Evolutions: Capnography. *RN, 62*(5), 69–71.

Des Jardins, T., & Burton, G. (1995). *Clinical manifestations and assessment of respiratory disease.* St. Louis, MO: Mosby.

Dettenmeier, P. (1995). Assessment of the patient: Chest radiology. In *Radiologic assessment for nurses.* St. Louis, MO: Mosby.

Hanneman, S. (2004). Weaning from short-term mechanical ventilation. *Critical Care Nurse, 24*(1), 70–73.

Hanneman, S., Ingersoll, G., Knebel, A., Shekleton, M., Burns, S., & Clochsey, J. (1994). Weaning from short-term mechanical ventilation: A review. *American Journal of Critical Care, 3*(6), 421–441.

Kersten, L. (1989). Chest roentgenology. In *Comprehensive respiratory nursing* (pp. 400–452). Philadelphia: W. B. Saunders.

Pagana, K., & Pagana, T. (2003). *Mosby's diagnostic and laboratory test reference* (6th ed.). St. Louis, MO: Mosby.

Pierce, L. (1995). Weaning from mechanical ventilation. In *Guide to mechanical ventilation and intensive respiratory care* (pp. 288–311). Philadelphia: W. B. Saunders

Ruppel, G. (2004). *Manual of pulmonary function testing.* St. Louis, MO: Mosby.

Scheffer, K., & Tobin, R. (1997). Respiratory system. In *Better X-ray interpretation* (pp. 25–46). Springhouse, PA: Springhouse Corporation.

Shortall, S., & Perkins, L. (1999). Interpreting the ins and outs of pulmonary function tests. *Nursing 99, 29*(12), 41–46.

Siela, D. (2002). Using chest radiography in the intensive care unit. *Critical Care Nurse, 22*(4), 18–29.

Provision of Patient Education

Susan Janson-Bjerklie

I. Determine what patients need to know
  A. Keep the following questions in mind to assess learning needs.
    1. What information does the patient need?
    2. What attitudes and beliefs about health and illness and its treatment should be explored?
    3. What skills are needed to perform health care behaviors?
    4. What factors pose barriers to the performance of desired behaviors?
  B. Assessment provides information about what the patient knows, believes, and is capable of at the beginning of the relationship with the educator.
    1. Determine what the patient already knows about a given health topic.
    2. Assess the accuracy of the patient's knowledge and determine what the patient believes to be true.
    3. Plan for correction of misinformation and inclusion of specific detail where knowledge is incomplete.
  C. Use a health assessment instrument to gather and organize data.
    1. Health history: chief complaint, history of present illness, review of systems, past history, family history, occupational/social/habits, history.
    2. Checklist form or assessment guide: include information about the patient's specific learning needs and preferred learning style.
  D. Prioritize needs and problems recognizing readiness to learn.
    1. Maslow's hierarchy is a guide to setting priorities.
      a. Physiological/survival needs
      b. Safety and security
      c. Love, affection, belongingness
      d. Esteem
      e. Self-actualization

    2. Patients cannot attain self-actualization in management of an illness until the basic needs are met. Unmet needs in the lower levels become barriers to learning and prevent attaining the highest level of self-actualization.

    3. Ability to participate in learning is affected by physical discomfort, denial, anxiety, grieving, dependency needs, cognitive and developmental factors.

E. Mutually develop goals for patient learning.

    1. Goal setting is an activity where the patient and the educator agree on what the patient wants to accomplish.

    2. Set goals in collaboration with the patient and family by sharing objectives.

F. Objectives are specific behavioral statements that will be performed to meet the goal. Goals are the desired outcomes of learning.

G. Adult learning is fostered by using Malcolm Knowles's adult learning theory

    1. Maturation leads from dependency to self-direction.

    2. Life experiences are a resource for learning.

    3. Readiness to learn is related to developmental tasks and roles.

    4. Learning is problem-centered rather than subject-centered and requires immediate application rather than delayed or postponed application.

    5. Motivation to learn in adults is triggered by recognition of a gap between what they know and what they want to know.

II. Patient education interventions

A. Content is focused on what individuals or target populations need to know to survive and make health-related decisions.

    1. Teach the patient survival skills: recognizing developing problems; what to do about problems; how to avoid problems.

    2. Teach decision making about rescue actions, treatment steps, and when to seek urgent medical care. Rehearse these skills at every opportunity.

    3. Teach, practice, and review the relevant skills needed to perform self-care behaviors.

B. Behavior change results from three types of learning behaviors: cognitive (knowledge and information), affective (attitudes, beliefs, and values), and psychomotor (skills and performance). Examples of desirable behaviors in each of these areas by a patient with asthma are shown in Table 9.1.

C. Teaching and learning formats

Individual and group formats have advantages and disadvantages as listed in Table 9.2. These features must be weighed when selecting an appropriate format.

D. Teaching/learning activities

    1. Lecture: Succinct messages are highly effective for teaching and learning cognitive behaviors but not effective for learning affective or psychomotor behaviors.

Table 9.1	Desirable Self-Management Behaviors in Patients with Asthma

Cognitive Behaviors for Asthmatic Patients
  Able to describe the role of airway inflammation and bronchoconstriction in chronic asthma.
  Able to state the warning signs of worsening asthma how to know when to seek urgent medical care.

Affective Behaviors for Asthmatic Patients
  Able to describe why it is important not to delay seeking urgently needed treatment.
  Able to describe why taking medication consistently is the healthiest approach to controlling asthma.

Psychomotor
  Able to demonstrate correct use of metered dose inhalers and spacers.
  Able to accurately and reliably perform measurement of peak expiratory flow on a portable peak flow meter.

2. Group discussion: active participation by group members with the educator in application of knowledge, shaping attitudes or dispelling myths. Requires at least two participants plus the educator.

3. Demonstration: most effective for teaching psychomotor skills. Allow observation of the skill, practice, and reinforcement of techniques.

4. Role play: Return demonstration in potential scenarios is often used in combination with demonstration to practice applying knowledge, attitudes, and skills in life-like situations under supervision.

5. Age-appropriate video/pictures/graphics/models: Learning enhancements that provide visual, auditory, and tactile cues to reinforce all three types of learning. Media should be used as adjuncts not substitutes for a live teacher. Learning skills still require return demonstration not provided by media.

6. Computer-assisted instruction attributes
   a. Drill and practice lessons to teach facts
   b. Tutorials to individualize lessons
   c. Problem solving, simulations, games help patient learn information and practice decision making
   d. Testing to assess knowledge, attitudes, provide feedback

7. Printed material attributes
   a. Most commonly used tool for patient education
   b. Can be language specific
   c. Emphasizes the most important points
   d. Reinforces learning but does not ensure learning

| Table 9.2 | Advantages and Disadvantages of Teaching and Learning Formats |

Individual Teaching Advantages

■ Allows tailoring of the intervention to the specific needs of the patient and capitalizes on teachable moments when the patient is more open to learning, e.g., after recovery from a life-threatening asthma exacerbation.
■ Allows ongoing assessment and reinforcement of technical skills.

Group Teaching Advantages

■ Economical in targeted populations within health centers/agencies.
■ Patients learn from one another and derive support/inspiration.
■ Family members can be present to hear the information and adapt it to their family and cultural functioning.

Individual Teaching Disadvantages

■ May be more costly than group formats if the educator is not the primary provider of care.
■ Lack of peer group support.
■ Family members and partners often not present.

Group Teaching Disadvantages

■ Group size affects the educator's ability to meet individual learning needs. Small group (2–5 patients) is best for teaching and learning skills.
■ Group dynamics may not be conducive to learning. Competition among group members may impede discussion.
■ Group teaching works best if members meet the target criteria for the group before enrollment. Diversity in age, language skills, or literacy may impede learning in groups.

8. Games and simulations
   a. Games of strategy give patients the opportunity to use problem-solving strategies in a parallel, entertaining, competitive situation. May work well with adolescents.
   b. Simulations provide the opportunity to apply new skills in life-like situations where coaching and encouragement are available from the educator.
III. Barriers to patient education
   A. Literacy: One in four people in the United States is illiterate.
      1. Using print materials with patients who do not read is the most common mistake. Screen for literacy by asking, "How many newspapers and magazines do you read in a typical week?"
      2. Videos are not the perfect answer. People who are illiterate may learn differently; they don't necessarily understand diagrams or pictures.
      3. All patients prefer simple instructions.
      4. If print materials are appropriate, determine the reading grade level of the materials and match to patient's reading ability.

B. Language: In communities of mixed cultures often the language of the patient and the health educator are not the same.

C. Beliefs and attitudes
   1. Beliefs and attitudes may prevent the patient from hearing and accepting what the educator is teaching.
   2. Cultural beliefs about health and illness should be explored before standardized educational approaches are attempted.
   3. Concerns about diagnosis and medications as well as culturally based beliefs about health care practices need to be explored carefully.

D. Psychiatric illness co-existing with health care needs may present a formidable barrier to health education.

E. Use of alternative and/or complementary therapy may interfere with recommended or prescribed therapies. It is important to ask patients to describe what other approaches they may be trying to promote or control health, but it is also important to avoid implying judgment. Assess the mechanisms and effects of the therapy in question. Many complementary therapies are not harmful and should not be discouraged if the patient finds them useful.

IV. Factors that influence patient education
   A. Age
      1. Teaching parents of infants, small children, adolescents, adults, and elderly patients all require different approaches in patient education and different supplemental educational materials.
      2. Although age is an obvious consideration in designing patient education approaches, it is often overlooked in the preparation of educational materials.
      3. Motivation to learn in adults is triggered by recognition of a gap between what they know and what they want to know.
         a. Adult learning using Malcolm Knowles's adult learning theory
            i. Maturation leads from dependency to self-direction.
            ii. Life experiences are a resource for learning.
            iii. Readiness to learn is related to developmental tasks and roles.
            iv. Learning is problem-centered rather than subject-centered and requires immediate application rather than delayed application.
      4. Patient education for children depends on age. Identify who needs training.
         a. Treatment decisions are made for infants and very young children by parents and caregivers. When there are multiple caregivers, include as many as possible in the education program.
         b. Children as young as 2 years can begin learning and participating.
         c. Adolescents should be taught all information themselves.
      5. Age-dependent learning styles in children
         a. Preschoolers: attracted to bright colors and pictures; interested in exploring and playing with dolls; look to parents when confronted with new situations. Attention span is 2–3 minutes.

   b. School-age children: like pictures, games, videos, cartoons, computers, books; respond well to group learning. Attention span is 10–15 minutes.

   c. Preadolescents: prefer interactive hands-on learning; like models and computers. Attention span is about 15 minutes.

   d. Adolescents: respond best to peers and peer-idols; may not respond to formal education styles (lectures); respond well to problem-solving scenarios; want and need technical information. Environments that are not dominated by adults work best. Attention span: 20–30 minutes.

  6. Learning needs in older adults

   a. Older adults may be particularly interested in the details and in understanding the rationale for health-related recommendations.

   b. They often require adaptation of learning materials when visual or auditory impairments interfere with learning.

   c. They are often more willing to attend and participate in groups than younger adults due to available time, interest, and need for socialization.

 B. Ethnicity

  1. Differences in language, culture, beliefs, health practices influence the way patient education is delivered and received.

  2. Ethnicity and culture influence the meaning of illness and therefore the response to proffered treatments.

 C. Family/significant others

  1. How a family functions influences the health of its members and how they react to illness.

  2. The family is a resource that can be used effectively to reinforce information and skills and encourage adherence.

  3. There are many nontraditional family units. It is important to identify who the patient defines as *family* or *support system* and develop these resources.

 D. Socioeconomic status (SES)

  1. Patients of lower SES are less likely to seek treatment and access health care later than those of higher SES.

  2. Patient education in self-management can help by focusing on health risks that can be modified with healthier lifestyles and practices.

 E. Chronicity of disease

  1. Acute self-limiting problems require brief and specific educational intervention.

  2. Chronic disease requires long-term educational approaches focused on self-management, surveillance of chronic symptoms, skills in taking daily and rescue medications, and communication with the health care provider.

V. Adherence

 A. Adherence in health care is the behavior of the patients in following recommended and prescribed actions to achieve health-related goals.

Adherence to medications, diet, exercise, and preventive health behaviors is the usual focus.

B. Prevention of nonadherence
   1. It is important to understand the patient's reasons for nonadherence.
   2. Adherence requires behavior change. Assess readiness for change and for learning self-management skills.
   3. Provide a simplified regimen, cues for actions, information on how and why the medication or recommended therapy works, cost-effective therapy, clearly written instructions, opportunity to practice, reinforcement of newly learned skills, and build confidence for self-management.

C. Detection of nonadherence
   1. Persistent symptoms/problems despite adequate prescribed therapy suggests nonadherence to treatment
   2. Differentiate nonadherence from persistent severe therapeutic problems.
   3. Missed appointments and infrequent refills suggest nonadherence.
   4. Methods of detection: interview, pill counts, pharmacy refill frequency, biological markers, and inhaler electronic counters.

D. Types of medication nonadherence and interventions
   1. Intermittent nonadherence: forgetting to take the medication or missing doses at times while taking medication correctly at other times.
      a. Reasons: busy work/life schedule, inconvenient dosing schedule, forgetfulness, fatigue, and depression.
      b. Interventions: cues, reminders, minimal daily dosing, integrate medication taking with daily activity pattern, treat depression.
   2. Unwitting nonadherence: taking the wrong dose, taking the medication incorrectly or at the wrong dosing intervals.
      a. Reasons: language barriers, communication problems, misunderstanding, lack of a written plan, inadequate demonstration and practice of skills
      b. Interventions: careful instruction, demonstration of skills, written instructions, pictures
   3. Purposeful nonadherence: not filling the prescription or purposefully not taking the medication even after filling the prescription.
      a. Reasons: beliefs, attitudes, concerns, cost
      b. Interventions: open communication and discussion of issues and concerns, contracting, planned evaluation of progress and benefit

E. Treatment of nonadherence
   1. Determine why the patient is nonadherent.
   2. Determine the type of nonadherence and select an appropriate intervention.
   3. Devise a plan with the patient as a partner to ensure success.

VI. Evaluation of education interventions
   A. Determine which interventions were effective.
      1. Format: How was the patient taught and was it compatible with the patient's learning style and needs?
      2. Content: Was the necessary information received and did it result in behavior change?
      3. Teaching-learning activities: Did the patient participate, ask questions, and practice skills? Was the learning problem-centered and immediately applied by the learner? Was the method of teaching/learning appropriate?
      4. Media: Were the media resources appropriate and understandable to the patient and family?
      5. Patient and family satisfaction: Which activities did they find most and least useful? Were their concerns addressed? Do they believe what they learned is useful?
      6. Time, cost, and resources used: Were the resources adequate? Were there unmet needs due to lack of resources? Did deficits in resources for patient education create barriers for patient learning?
   B. Four levels of evaluation of outcomes of interventions
      1. Patient's participation during intervention
         a. Does the patient ask questions, seem alert and interested?
         b. Participate actively in discussion and goal-setting?
      2. Patient's performance immediately following learning experience
         a. Were performance objectives met and to what extent?
         b. What modifications are needed for reinforcement of learning or improvement in performance?
      3. Patient's performance at home
         a. Does the patient perform the learned behaviors at home?
         b. Were difficulties encountered (misunderstanding, inability to perform skills, problems remembering)?
      4. Patient's overall self-care and health management
         a. Did the management and education approaches resolve and/or control the health problems?
         b. Did objective markers (e.g., blood pressure, peak flow, glucose level) reflect successful self-care?
         c. What are the long-term results of patient education for self-management? Is adherence or skill performance maintained?
   C. Method of evaluation
      1. Direct observation of patient behavior and skill performance
      2. Daily patient records of performance and progress
      3. Reports of patients, family, caregivers, and health care providers on patient performance and behavior
      4. Oral, written, or performance tests
         a. Scenarios can be used to evaluate judgment and decision-making ability.
         b. Written tests can be used to evaluate cognitive learning.

   c. Skill checklists are used to evaluate skills that require a number of steps, such as correct metered-dose inhaler technique.
5. Critical incident review
   a. Interview based review of an incident involving a health problem, including the patient's appraisal of risk, actions taken, and outcomes.
   b. Use to evaluate progress in understanding and managing an episode or exacerbation of a health problem.

SUGGESTED READINGS

Glanz, K., Lewis, F. M., & Rimer, B. K. (Eds.). (1990). *Health behavior and health education.* San Francisco: Jossey-Bass.

Janson, S. L., Fahy, J. V., Covington, J. K., Gold, W., & Boushey, H. A. (2003). Impact of individual self-management education on clinical, biological, and adherence outcomes in asthma. *American Journal of Medicine, 115,* 620–626.

Davis, T. C., Michielutte, R., & Askov, E. N. (1998). Practical assessment of adult literacy in health care. *Health Education Behavior, 25,* 613–624.

Meade, C. D., & Smith, C. F. (1991). Readability formulas: Cautions and criteria. *Patient Education Counseling, 17,* 153–158.

Muma, R. D., Lyons, B. A., Newman, T. A., & Carnes, B. A. (Eds.). (1996). *Patient education: A practical approach.* Stamford, CT: Appleton & Lange.

Rankin, S. H., & Stallings, K. D. (2001). *Patient education: Issues, principles, practices* (4th ed.). Philadelphia: J. B. Lippincott.

Redman, B. K. (1988). *The process of patient education* (6th ed.). St. Louis, MO: Mosby.

Shumaker, S. A. (Ed.). (1998). *The handbook of health behavior change.* New York: Springer Publishing.

Stoloff, S. W., & Janson, S. (1997). Providing asthma education in primary care practice. *American Family Practitioner, 56*(1), 117–126.

Taggart, V. (1995). Compliance in asthma: Implementation of the guidelines. *European Respiratory Review, 5*(26), 112–115.

Nursing Concepts: Human Response to Respiratory Dysfunction

Dyspnea

Audrey G. Gift and Anita Jablonski

INTRODUCTION

Dyspnea is a subjective experience which is inadequately related to physiological changes. Although dyspnea reduction techniques have not been adequately tested in research, many are invaluable strategies to increase comfort and lower anxiety. Dyspnea should be monitored in repiratory patients, cardiac patients, cancer patients and those at end-of-life.

Dyspnea is a term used to characterize the subjective experience of breathing discomfort that consists of qualitatively distinct sensations that vary in intensity. The experience derives from interactions among multiple physiological, psychological, social, and environmental factors, and may induce secondary physiological and behavioral responses (Meek et al., 1999, p. 322).

ETIOLOGY/PATHOPHYSIOLOGY/THEORIES

I. Physiologic mechanisms
    A. Neuro-mechanical or efferent-reafferent dissociation theory of dyspnea
        1. Dyspnea is caused by a dissociation or mismatch between central respiratory motor activity and incoming afferent information from receptors in airways, lungs, and chest wall. Therefore dyspnea is intensified when changes in airflow, respiratory pressure, or respiratory movement is not appropriate for the outgoing motor command (Meek et al., 1999, p. 323).
        2. First introduced by Campbell and Howell in the 1960s under the name of "length-tension inappropriateness" (Meek et al., 1999, p. 323).

3. Dyspnea results from a heightened ventilatory demand, respiratory muscle abnormalities, abnormal ventilatory impedance, and abnormal breathing patterns.

B. Neuro-chemical

1. Changes in blood gases resulting in hypoxemia and hypercapnia stimulates chemoreceptors and result in respiratory motor activity. Blood gases may also have a direct dyspneogenic effect since dyspnea can occur even without ventilatory changes.

C. Psychosocial factors

1. Cognitive

a. Dyspnea severity is influenced by perception. Nield, Kim, and Patel showed in 1989 that an adaptive response occurs with long-standing dyspnea.

2. Affective

a. Dyspnea and anxiety are closely related (Carrieri-Kohlman, Gormley, Douglas, Paul, & Stulbarg, 1996a; Gift, 1991; Gift, Plaut, & Jacox, 1986; Janson-Bjerklie, Carrieri, & Hudes, 1986; Smith et al., 2001).

b. Dyspnea and anxiety are separate dimensions (Carrieri-Kohlman et al., 2001).

c. Dyspnea is related to emotional status (Martinez-Moragon, Perpina, Belloch, deDiego, & Martinez-Frances, 2003).

D. Other symptoms

1. Cough, pain, psychological distress, and organic factors (such as tumor growth) predict 33% of dyspnea in patients with lung cancer (Tanaka, Akechi, Okuyama, Nishiwaki, & Uchitomi, 2002).

2. Dyspnea is related to pain in patients with lung cancer (Smith et al., 2001).

E. Attention and judgment

1. Dyspnea is influenced by prior exposure to the sensation (Meek, 2000).

II. Dimensions of dyspnea

A. Self-report of dyspnea is a separate dimension from exercise-induced dyspnea and from pulmonary function results.

B. Anxiety and dyspnea are separate dimensions (Carrieri-Kohlman, Gormley, Eiser, & Demir-Deviren, 2001).

C. Dyspnea and effort are different phenomenon.

RISK FACTORS AND INCIDENCE

The prevalence of dyspnea is related to the number of risk factors a patient has (Dudgeon, Kristjanson, Sloan, Lertzman, & Clement, 2001).

I. Related diseases/disorders

A. COPD (Dudgeon et al., 2001)

B. Asthma (Dudgeon et al., 2001; Janson-Bjerklie et al., 1987)

C. Congestive heart failure (CHF) (Mahler et al., 1996)

D. Restrictive lung disease. Exposure to asbestos, coal dust, cotton dust, or grain dust is related to the presence of dyspnea (Dudgeon et al., 2001)

E. Cancer
   1. Dyspnea is most commonly associated with breast, lung, and colorectal cancers (Acheson & MacCormack, 1997, p. 210).
   2. Direct causes of cancer-related dyspnea are those resulting directly from tumor effect (Acheson & MacCormack, 1997, p. 210)
      a. Bronchial/airway obstruction
      b. Superior vena cava syndrome obstruction
      c. Tumor invasion of lung tissue
      d. Lymphangitic spread
      e. Phrenic nerve paralysis
      f. Pleural effusion(s)
      g. Pericardial effusion
      h. Ascites
      i. Hepatomegaly
   3. Indirect causes of cancer-related dyspnea are those resulting from other disease effects/debilitation (Acheson & MacCormack, 1997, p. 210)
      a. Anemia
      b. Cachexia
      c. Pulmonary embolism
      d. Pulmonary aspiration
      e. Pneumonia
      f. Electrolyte imbalance
      g. Mucositis
      h. Infection

F. Obesity

G. Psychological (Acheson & MacCormack, 1997, p. 210)
   1. Anxiety. Higher levels of anxiety have been shown to occur with higher levels of dyspnea (Gift, 1989).
   2. Fear. Those with late-stage cancer report having significant, prolonged dyspnea lasting 3 months or more. Dyspnea is accompanied by feelings of fear, extreme fatigue, loss of memory, concentration, and appetite (Brown, Carrieri, Janson-Bjerklie, & Dodd, 1986). Others have hypothesized a relationship between panic and dyspnea (Smoller, Pollack, Otto, Rosenbaum, & Kradin, 1996).

H. Treatment-related dyspnea
   1. Chemotherapy-induced toxicity (Acheson & MacCormack, 1997, p. 210)
   2. Respiratory disease
   3. Cardiomyopathy
   4. Radiation-induced toxicity (Acheson, & MacCormack, 1997, p. 210)

I. Pulmonary fibrosis

J. Pneumonitis

K. Ventilator dyspnea. Patients often report they experience dyspnea while being mechanically ventilated, even when arterial blood gas levels are normal and the ventilator supplies a large portion of their minute ventilation requirement. This is believed to result from a mismatch between the patient's ventilatory drive and the ventilator settings, such as flow rate that is too slow, a respiratory rate that is too fast, and/or a V_t that is too large. This can lead to increased anxiety in the patient (Knebel, Strider, & Wood, 1994).

II. Incidence/prevalence
   A. The incidence of dyspnea is not determined directly. It is inferred from the incidence of the diseases in which it is found, such as COPD, lung cancer, terminal illness, etc.
   B. The prevalence of dyspnea in lung cancer patients has been reported as from 46% (Dudgeon et al., 2001) to 87% (Smith et al., 2001)

III. Considerations across the life span
   A. Elderly
      1. Elderly experience changes in lung function and respiratory muscle function that results in increased air trapping and enhanced likelihood of dyspnea.
      2. Older patients report more dyspnea than younger patients (Martinez-Moragon et al., 2003; Tanaka et al., 2002)
   B. End of life
      1. Those with late-stage cancer report having significant, prolonged dyspnea lasting 3 months or more. It is accompanied by feelings of fear, extreme fatigue, loss of memory, concentration, and appetite (Brown et al., 1986).
      2. A study of terminally ill cancer patients showed them to be troubled by dyspnea and pain, with the dyspnea increasing until the time of death (Higginson & McCarthy, 1989).
      3. Dyspnea in the patient at end of life needs to be assessed along with other symptoms (Tranmer et al., 2003).
      4. Use of a proxy, such as the caregiver in end of life, may not be an adequate assessment of a patient's dyspnea (Klingenberg et al., 2003).
   C. Pregnancy
      1. Pregnancy results in increased dyspnea that is only partially explained by diaphragmatic compression.
   D. Children
      1. Children at end of life experience symptoms, such as dyspnea, that require assessment and treatment (Wolfe et al., 2000).
      2. Children are able to rate the intensity of dyspnea using a four-point word-descriptor scale: "Rotten," "Just Okay," "Good," and "Great" (Kohlman-Carrieri, Kieckhofer, Janson-Bjerklie, & Souza, 1991).
      3. Colors have been used to have children rate dyspnea (Kohlman-Carrieri et al., 1991).
   E. Neonates—no data found

IV. Cultural considerations
   A. African Americans cope with dyspnea using traditional medical care, self-care wisdom, self-care action, and self-care resources (Nield, 2000).
V. Complications
   A. Unrelieved symptoms requiring emergency room treatment have been shown to be predictive of impending death (Escalante et al., 1996).
   B. Even without emergency room treatment the presence of dyspnea is of deep concern because it has been shown to be associated with loss of function and increased mortality (Reuben & Mor, 1988).
   C. Dyspnea results in a decrease in quality of life (Smith et al., 2001).

ASSESSMENT

I. General concepts in assessing and managing dyspnea
   A. Dyspnea is a subjective symptom and needs to be evaluated accordingly.
   B. Dyspnea is multidimensional having intensity/severity, distress, frequency, duration, and quality.
   C. Different descriptors used to characterize the dyspnea experience connote different types of dyspnea (Simon et al., 1990).
II. History
   A. History and physical
      1. Onset
         a. Acute dyspnea characterized by rapid onset
         b. Chronic dyspnea characterized by persistence over time with changing intensity (McCarley, 1999)
      2. Frequency of occurrence
      3. Duration
      4. Intensity/severity or range of experience
      5. Quality, description of dyspnea. Descriptors that have been shown to be specific to the underlying cause of dyspnea are repeatable and have been found to be different in different diseases (Mahler et al., 1996; Simon et al., 1990)
      6. Precipitating factors. Dyspnea is contextual. It is dependent on level of activity and needs to be rated in relation to activities performed and effort required for performance. Dyspnea is often exacerbated by anxiety or other emotions. Pollution or other respiratory irritants can also exacerbate dyspnea (Shim & Williams, 1986).
   B. History of respiratory illness (asthma/COPD)
   C. History of co-morbid conditions (cardiac/cancer)
   D. Presence of risk factors
   E. Prior exposure to dyspnea influences sensitivity to the sensation (Meek, 2000).
   F. Dyspnea found to occur with other symptoms such as fatigue (Graydon, Ross, Webster, Goldstein, & Avendano, 1995) and sleep difficulties (Baker & Scholz, 2002).

    G. Dyspnea management/coping strategies used by the patient in coping with the symptom, such as decreasing activities, pursed lip breathing, avoiding emotional conflict and the like, will influence patient report of dyspnea (Baker & Scholz, 2002).

III. Physical
    A. Respiratory system
      1. Airway patency
      2. Respiratory rate and pattern, use of abdominal/accessory muscle use
      3. Specific positioning for breathing comfort (unable to lie flat, needs support, etc.)
      4. Lung sounds
    B. Neuropsychosocial
      1. Emotional state/level of distress: presence of fear, anxiety, depression, agitation, nervousness, restlessness
      2. Alertness/orientation: loss of memory, poor concentration, home and friends as support system
    C. Cardiac
      1. Heart sounds/apical pulse
    D. Fever
    E. Weight/edema: If weight retards diaphragmatic excursion, it will result in dyspnea.

IV. Diagnostic testing
    A. Pulmonary function tests (PFTs). Dyspnea shows low correlation with pulmonary function ratings (Wolcove, Dajczman, Calacone, & Kreisman, 1989). Thus PFTs cannot be used to evaluate the extent of dyspnea experienced by the patient. Dyspnea can occur in a person with normal or near normal PFTs.
    B. ABG measurements. These correlate poorly with dyspnea in the COPD patient during rest. Hypoxemia and/or desaturation that are acute, result in the sensation of dyspnea and fatigue.
    C. Pulse oximetry (at rest and with exercise)
    D. Distance walking or exercise testing
    E. Radiologic tests (CXR, VQ scan)

V. Measurement tools (Meek et al., 1999). Dyspnea is contextual and needs to be rated along with activities or situations provoking it. Dyspnea occurs along with other symptoms and changes over time so it needs to be measured along with other symptoms and monitored over time (Gift, Stommel, Jablonski, & Given, 2003).
    A. Visual Analogue Scale (VAS). (Can be horizontal or vertical) Patient rates dyspnea intensity along a straight line 100 mm long (Gift, 1989; See Figure 10.1).
    B. Borg scale. Used during exercise. Patient asked to indicate effort. Dyspnea and effort are not identical concepts (Demediuk et al., 1992; Steele & Shaver, 1992). Borg scale is highly correlated with physiological measures of lung function (Kendrick, Baxi, & Smith, 2000).

How much shortness of breath have you had in the last week?

Please indicate by marking the height on the column.

Shortness of breath as bad as it can be

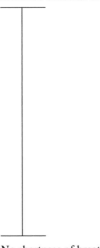

No shortness of breath

Figure 10.1. Visual analogue dyspnea scale.

C. Numeric Rating Scale (NRS). Dyspnea intensity rated on a scale from 1–10. Valid measure of dyspnea intensity that is easy for patients to use in a clinical setting (Gift & Narsavage, 1998) (See Figure 10.2).
D. Graphic/Verbal Rating Scale (GRS). Scores on a verbal rating scale with none, mild, moderate, severe and horrible as the ratings, correlate highly with dyspnea ratings using the visual analogue scale (Dudgeon et al., 2001).
E. Dyspnea intensity and distress (Carrieri-Kohlman et al., 1996a; Wilson & Jones, 1991).
F. Medical Research Council Scale (MRC)
   1. First developed by Fletcher in 1952
   2. Five-point scale requiring client to identify level of activity that results in dyspnea
   3. Lacks clear limits between grades
G. Baseline Dyspnea Index (BDI) (Mahler et al., 1992). Used in pulmonary rehabilitation to measure dyspnea at start of program. The Transitional Dyspnea Index is then used to quantify changes in dyspnea after rehabilitation.
H. Cancer dyspnoea scale is a 12-item scale that records a sense of effort, sense of anxiety and a sense of discomfort related to dyspnea. These factors were developed using a factor analysis. The scale has construct and convergent validity as well as internal consistency and test-retest reliability (Tanaka, Akechi, Okuyama, Nishiwaki, & Uchitomi, 2000).
I. Oxygen cost diagram—rarely used in a clinical setting.

On a scale of 1 to 10, indicate how much shortness of breath you have had in the past week.

0 = no shortness of breath

10 = shortness of breath as bad as it can be

Circle the number:

1   2   3   4   5   6   7   8   9   10

Figure 10.2. Numeric rating scale.

J. Breathlessness, cough and sputum scale—this is a new scale that evaluates two symptoms (dyspnea and cough) and one sign commonly seen in patients with respiratory disease (Leidy, Schmier, Jones, Lloyd, & Rocchiccioli, 2003).

COMMON THERAPEUTIC MODALITIES

I.   Pharmacologic (Acheson & McCormack, 1997)
   A. Opioids. Opiates have been recommended in the treatment of dyspnea because of their respiratory depressant effect on the central process of neural signals within the central nervous system. Some have found them to be effective in the relief of dyspnea (Bruera, Macmillian, Pither, & MacDonald, 1990). They have been shown to decrease expiratory volume (V_E) at rest and during submaximal levels of exercise. The danger with the use of these drugs is the concomitant increase in CO_2. Opioids have been described as alleviating dyspnea by blunting perceptual responses and decreasing the intensity of the respiratory sensation. They have been recommended for acute dyspnea but there is little research to recommend their use in long-term, progressive dyspnea such as in cancer (Meek et al., 1999).
   B. Benzodiazepines are recommended for use in the relief of dyspnea only when there is accompanying anxiety. The studies, however, involved large doses and much sedation of the patient (Greene, Pucino, Carlson, Storsved, & Strommen, 1989; Mitchell-Heggs et al., 1980; Woodcock, Gross, & Geddes, 1981)
   C. Corticosteroids and non-steroidal anti-inflammatories have been recommended to reduce the airway inflammation and create more patent airways. They are used in palliative care (Hardy, 1998). In addition to their anti-inflammatory effect is their effect on general well-being.
   D. Nebulized morphine. There is some evidence to indicate nebulized morphine to be effective in the relief of dyspnea (Zeppetella, 1997) but the evidence is minimal and this is not recommended for practice (Meek et al., 1999).
   E. Nebulized lidocaine. Some have recommended the use of nebulized lidocaine in the treatment of dyspnea in cancer patients. This, however, has not been found to be effective (Wilcox, Corcoran, & Tattersfield, 1994).

II. Non-pharmacologic
   A. Breathing patterns. Slowing the breathing to increase the expiratory phase has been shown to reduce dyspnea.
   B. Pursed lip breathing. Slows expiratory flow and maintain backpressure to avoid airway collapse during expiration. Also improves pattern of respiratory muscle recruitment (Breslin, 1992; Lareau & Larson, 1987).
   C. Position for comfort and adequate ventilation/perfusion: semi-Fowler's, tripod, leaning forward over table/chair. If lying in bed, position with good lung down.
   D. Anxiety reduction. Relaxation techniques have been shown to reduce dyspnea along with the anxiety (Gift, Moore, & Soeken 1992; Renfroe, 1988).
   E. Oxygen is frequently required to avoid desaturation and may offer placebo value when desaturation not present.
III. Radiotherapy. Palliative radiotherapy can reduce a cancer tumor and decrease dyspnea for a period of time. Radiation therapy can also result in dyspnea when it results in radiation pneumonitis.
IV. Respiratory function management
   A. Monitor patient's vital signs, respiratory pattern, lab values (esp. HGB/HCT, ABG/Pulse Ox), pulmonary function tests, peak flow results, and radiology results. Report to physician as necessary.
   B. Monitor for chronic signs: clubbing, barrel chest, pursed lip breathing, accessory muscle use
   C. Facilitate adequate ventilation
      1. Protect airway patency (suction, head tilt/chin lift, assist with intubation as necessary)
      2. Arrange for ventilator assistance and monitoring as necessary. Pattern of ventilation is as important as volume and oxygenation to reducing dyspnea
      3. Administer therapy as indicated: chest physiotherapy, humidified oxygen, medications
      4. Monitor response to therapy and report to physician as appropriate.
   D. Encourage adequate fluid intake (if no cardiac contradiction)
      1. Assists in thinning respiratory secretions for easier removal
      2. Encourage frequent sipping of water to keep oral mucosa moist
   E. Activity modification
      1. Slowing and/or pacing of activity to fit patient limitations
      2. Reduce the number or eliminate some steps necessary for task completion.
      3. Schedule tasks for peak energy periods.
      4. Reduce activities that require lifting unsupported arm activities (competes with respiratory accessory muscles and can produce dyspnea) (Lareau, Meek, Press, Anholm, & Roos, 1999).
      5. Encourage adequate sleep
         a. Limit environmental stimuli
         b. Keep sleep diary
         c. Encourage naps only if necessary

F. Exercise
   1. Encourage participation in exercise programs to provide graded exercises in a structured, safe, environment, desensitize patient to dyspnea (Carrieri-Kohlman, Douglas, Gormley & Stulbarg, 1993).
   2. Exercise training substantially improves the impact of a dyspnea self management program with a home walking prescription (Stulbarg et al., 2002).
   3. Exercise training improves aerobic capacity, increases neuromuscular coupling and improves tolerance to dyspnogenic stimuli (Gigliotti et al., 2003).
G. Patient education
   1. Teach pursed-lip breathing techniques (Breslin, 1992; Lareau & Larson, 1987).
   2. Teach relaxation techniques (Gift, Moore, & Soeken, 1992; Renfroe, 1988).
      a. Progressive muscle relaxation
      b. Guided imagery
      c. Biofeedback techniques
   3. Teach effective coping strategies and dyspnea self-management (Carrieri-Kohlman, Gormley, Douglas, Paul, & Stulbarg, 1996b; Kohlman-Carrieri & Janson-Bjerklie, 1986).
   4. Teach effective asepsis (hand washing, etc.) to prevent respiratory infections.
   5. Teach effective cough technique for airway clearance/removal of mucus plugs.
   6. Teach safe use and care of home medical equipment.
H. Acupuncture (Filshie, Penn, Ashley, & Davis, 1996)
V. Home care
   A. Equipment
      1. Oxygen
         a. Flow at the nose and across airway receptors may be more important than oxygen concentration.
      2. Ventilator
         a. Patients on a ventilator experience dyspnea. Alter flow rate if patient experiences dyspnea (Meek et al., 1999).
      3. Nebulizer
      4. ADL assistive devices (walkers)
   B. Caregiver and social support/psychosocial
      1. Encourage patient to build social support network
      2. Provide for respite care to relieve burden on caregiver

REFERENCES

Acheson, A., & MacCormack, D. (1997). Dyspnea and the cancer patient—an overview. *Canadian Oncology Nursing Journal, 7*(4), 209–213.

Baker, C. F., & Scholz, J. A. (2002). Coping with symptoms of dyspnea in chronic obstructive pulmonary disease. *Rehabilitation Nursing, 27*(2), 67–74.

Breslin, E. H. (1992). The pattern of respiratory muscle recruitment during pursed-lip breathing. *Chest, 101,* 75–78.

Brown, M. L., Carrieri, V., Janson-Bjerklie, S., & Dodd, M. J. (1986). Lung cancer and dyspnea: The patient's perception. *Oncology Nursing Forum, 13,* 19–24.

Bruera, E., Macmillian, K., Pither, J., & MacDonald, R. N. (1990). Effects of morphine on the dyspnea of terminal cancer patients. *Journal of Pain and Symptom Management, 5*(6), 341–344.

Carrieri-Kohlman, V., Douglas, M. K., Gormley, J. M., & Stulbarg, M. S. (1993). Desensitization and guided mastery: Treatment approaches for the management of dyspnea. *Heart & Lung, 22,* 226–234.

Carrieri-Kohlman, V., Gormley, J. M., Douglas, M. K., Paul, S. M., & Stulbarg, M. S. (1996a). Differentiation between dyspnea and its affective components. *Western Journal of Nursing Research, 18,* 626–642.

Carrieri-Kohlman, V., Gormley, J. M., Douglas, M. K., Paul, S. M., & Stulbarg, M. S. (1996b). Exercise training decreases dyspnea and the distress and anxiety associated with it: Monitoring alone may be as effective as coaching. *Chest, 110*(5), 1526–1535.

Carrieri-Kohlman, V., Gormley, J. M., Eiser, S., Demir-Deviren, S., Nguyen, H., Paul, S. M., et al. (2001). Dyspnea and the affective response during exercise training in obstructive pulmonary disease. *Nursing Research, 50*(3), 136–146.

Demediuk, B. H., Manning, H., Lilly, J., Fencl, V., Weinberger, S. E., Weiss, J. W., et al. (1992). Dissociation between dyspnea and respiratory effort. *American Review of Respiratory Disease, 146,* 1222–1225.

Dudgeon, D. J., Kristjanson, L., Sloan, J. A., Lertzman, M., & Clement, K. (2001). Dyspnea in cancer patients: Prevalence and associated factors. *Journal of Pain and Symptom Management, 21*(2), 95–102.

Escalante, C. P., Martin, C. G., Elting, Z. L. S., Cantor, S. B., Harle, T. S., Price, K. J., et al. (1996). Dyspnea in cancer patients: Etiology, resource utilization and survival. *Cancer, 78*(6), 1314–1319.

Filshie, J., Penn, K., Ashley, S., & Davis, C. L. (1996). Acupuncture for the relief of cancer-related breathlessness. *Palliative Medicine, 10,* 145–150.

Gift, A. G. (1989). Visual analogue scales: Measurement of subjective phenomena. *Nursing Research, 38*(5), 286–288.

Gift, A. G. (1991). Psychologic and physiologic aspects of acute dyspnea in asthmatics. *American Journal of Nursing Company, 40*(4), 196–199.

Gift, A. G. (1989). Validation of a vertical visual analogue scale as a measure of clinical dyspnea. *Rehabilitation Nursing, 14*(6), 323–325.

Gift, A. G., & Ausin, D. J. (1992). The effects of a program of systematic movement on COPD patients. *Rehabilitation Nursing, 17*(1), 6–10.

Gift, A. G., Moore, T., & Soeken, K. (1992). Relaxation to reduce dyspnea and anxiety in COPD patients. *Nursing Research, 41*(4), 242–246.

Gift, A. G., & Narsavage, G. (1998). Validation of the numeric rating scale as a measure of dyspnea. *American Journal of Critical Care, 7*(3), 200–204.

119

Gift, A. G., & Nield, M. (1991). Dyspnea: A case for nursing diagnosis status. *Nursing Diagnosis, 2*(2), 66–71.

Gift, A. G., Plaut, S. M., & Jacox, A. K. (1986). Psychologic factors related to dyspnea in subjects with chronic obstructive pulmonary disease. *Heart & Lung, 15,* 595–601.

Gift, A. G., Stommel, M., Jablonski, A., & Given, C. (2003). A cluster of symptoms over time in patients with lung cancer. *Nursing Research, 52,* 393–399.

Gigliotti, F., Coli, C., Bianchi, R., Romagnoli, I., Lanini, B., Binazzi, B., et al. (2003). Exercise training improves exertional dyspnea in patients with COPD. *Chest, 123,* 1794–1802.

Graydon, J. E., Ross, E., Webster, P. M., Goldstein, R. S., & Avendano, M. (1995). Predictors of functioning of patients with chronic obstructive pulmonary disease. *Heart & Lung, 24,* 369–375.

Greene, J. G., Pucino, F., Carlson, J. D., Storsved, M., & Strommen, G. L. (1989). Effects of aprazolam on respiratory drive, anxiety, and dyspnea in chronic airflow obstruction: A case study. *Pharmacotherapy, 9,* 34–38.

Hardy, J. (1998). Corticosteroids in palliative care. *European Journal of Palliative Care, 5,* 46–50.

Janson-Bjerklie, S., Carrieri, V. K., & Hudes, M. (1986). The sensations of pulmonary dyspnea. *Nursing Research, 35,* 154–159.

Kendrick, K., Baxi, S. C., & Smith, R. (2000). Usefulness of the modified 0–10 Borg scale in assessing the degree of dyspnea in patients with COPD and asthma. *Journal of Emergency Nursing, 26*(3), 216–222.

Klingenberg, M., Smit, J. H., Deeg, D. J., Willems, D. L., Onwuteaka-Philipsen, B. D., & van der Wal, G. (2003). Proxy reporting in after-death interviews: The use of proxy respondents in retrospective assessment of chronic diseases and symptom burden in the terminal phase of life. *Palliative Medicine, 17,* 191–201.

Knebel, A., Strider, V. C., & Wood, C. (1994). The art and science of caring for ventilator-assisted patients: Learning from our clinical experience. *Critical Care Nursing Clinics of North America, 6*(4), 819–829.

Kohlman-Carrieri, V., & Janson-Bjerklie, S. (1986). Strategies patients use to manage the sensation of dyspnea. *Western Journal of Nursing Research, 8*(3), 284–305.

Kohlman-Carrieri, V., Kieckhefer, G., Janson-Bjerklie, S., & Souza, J. (1991). The sensation of pulmonary dyspnea in school-age children. *Nursing Research, 40*(2), 81–85.

Lareau, S., & Larson, J. L. (1987). Ineffective breathing pattern related to airflow limitation. *Nursing Clinics of North America, 22,* 179–191.

Lareau, S. C., Meek, P. M., Press, D., Anholm, J. D., & Roos, P. J. (1999). Dyspnea in patients with chronic obstructive pulmonary disease: Does dyspnea worsen longitudinally in the presence of declining lung function. *Heart & Lung, 28*(1), 65–73.

Leidy, N. K., Schmier, J. K., Jones, M. K., Lloyd, J., & Rocchiccioli, K. (2003). Evaluating symptoms in chronic obstructive pulmonary disease: Validation of the Breathlessness, Cough and Sputum Scale. *Respiratory Medicine, 97*(Suppl. A), S59–S70.

Mahler, D. A., Faryniarz, K., Tomlinson, D., Colice, G. L., Robins, A. G., Olmstead, E. M., et al. (1992). Impact of dyspnea and physiologic function on general health status in patients with chronic obstructive pulmonary disease. *Chest, 102*(2), 395–401.

Mahler, D. A., Harver, A., Lentine, T., Scott, J. A., Beck, K., & Schwartzstein, R. M. (1996). Descriptors of breathlessness in cardiorespiratory diseases. *American Journal of Respiratory Critical Care Medicine, 154,* 1257–1363.

Martinez-Moragon, E., Perpina, M., Belloch, M., de Diego, A., & Martinez-Frances, M. (2003). Determinants of dypsnea in patients with different grades of stable asthma. *Journal of Asthma, 40*(4), 375–382.

McCarley, C. (1999). A model of chronic dyspnea. *Image: Journal of Nursing Scholarship, 31*(3), 231–236.

Meek, P. M. (2000). Influence of attention and judgment on perception of breathlessness in healthy individuals and patients with chronic obstructive pulmonary disease. *Nursing Research, 49*(1), 11–19.

Meek, P. M., Schwartzstein, R. M., Adams, L., Altose, M. D., Breslin, E. H., Carrieri-Kohlman, V., et al. (1999). Dyspnea: mechanisms, assessment, and management: A consensus statement. *American Journal of Respiratory and Critical Care Medicine, 159,* 321–340.

Mitchell-Heggs, P., Murphy, K., Minty, K., Guz, A., Patterson, S. C., Minty, P. S., et al. (1980). Diazepam in the treatment of dyspnoea in the "Pink Puffer" syndrome. *Quarterly Journal of Medicine, 49,* 9–20.

Nield, M. (2000). Dyspnea self-management in African Americans with chronic lung disease. *Heart & Lung, 29*(1), 50–55.

Nield, M., Kim, M. J., & Patel, M. (1989). Use of magnitude estimation for estimating the parameters of dyspnea. *Nursing Research, 38,* 77–80.

Renfroe, K. L. (1988). Effect of progressive relaxation on dyspnea and state anxiety in patients with chronic obstructive pulmonary disease. *Heart & Lung, 17,* 408–413.

Reuben, D. B., & Mor, V. (1988). Clinical symptoms and length of survival in patients with terminal cancer. *Archives of Internal Medicine, 148*(7), 1586–1591.

Shim, C., & Williams, M. H., (1986). Effects of odors in asthma. *The American Journal of Medicine, 80*(1), 18–22

Simon, P. M., Schwartzstein, R. M., Wwiss, J. W., Fencl, V., Teghtsoonian, M., & Weinberger, S. E. (1990). Distinguishable types of dyspnea in patients with shortness of breath. *American Review of Respiratory Disease, 142,* 1009–1014.

Smith, E. L., Hann, D. M., Ahles, T. A., Furstenbear, C. T., Mitchell, T. A., Meyer, L., et al. (2001). Dyspnea, anxiety, body consciousness and quality of life in patient with lung cancer. *Journal of Pain and Symptom Management, 21*(4), 323–329.

Smoller, J. W., Pollack, M. H., Otto, M. W., Rosenbaum, J. F., & Kradin, R. L. (1996). Panic anxiety, dyspnea, and respiratory disease. *American Journal of Respiratory and Critical Care Medicine, 154*(1), 6–17.

Steele, B., & Shaver, J. (1992). The dyspnea experience: Nocioceptive properties and a model for research and practice. *Advances in Nursing, 15,* 64–76.

Stulbarg, M. S., Carrieri-Kohlman, V., Demir-Deviren, S., Nguyen, H., Adams, L., Tsang, A., et al. (2002). Exercise training improves outcomes of a dyspnea self management program. *Journal of Cardiopulmonary Rehabilitation, 22,* 109–121.

Tanaka, K., Akechi, T., Okuyama, T., Nishiwaki, Y., & Uchitomi, Y. (2000). Development and validation of the cancer dyspnoea scale: A multidimensional, brief, self-rating scale. *British Journal of Cancer, 82*(4), 800–805.

Tanaka, K., Akechi, T., Okuyama, T., Nishiwaki, Y., & Uchitomi, Y. (2002). Factors correlated with dyspnea in advanced lung cancer patients: Organic causes and what else? *Journal of Pain and Symptom Management, 23*(6), 490–500.

Tranmer, J. E., Heyland, D., Dudgeon, D., Groll, D., Squires-Graham, M., & Coulson, K. (2003). Measuring the symptom experience of seriously ill cancer and noncancer hospitalized patients near the end of life with the Memorial Symptom Assessment Scale. *Journal of Pain and Symptom Management, 25,* 420–429.

Wilcox, A., Corcoran, R., & Tattersfield, A. E. (1994). Safety and efficiency of nebulized lidocaine in patients with cancer and breathlessness. *Palliative Medicine, 8*(1), 35–38.

Wilson, R. C., & Jones, P. W. (1991). Differentiation between the intensity of breathlessness and the distress it evokes in normal subjects during exercise. *Clinical Science, 80,* 65–70.

Wolcove, N., Dajczman, E., Calacone, A., & Kreisman, H. (1989). The relationship between pulmonary function and dyspnea in obstructive lung disease. *Chest, 96*(6), 1247–1251.

Wolfe, J., Grier, H. E., Klar, N., Levin, S. B., Ellenbogen, J. M., Salem-Schatz, S., et al. (2000). Symptoms and suffering at the end of life in children with cancer. *The New England Journal of Medicine, 342*(5), 326–333.

Woodcock, A. A., Gross, E. R., & Geddes, D. M. (1981). Drug treatment of breathlessness: Contrasting effects of diazepam and promethazine in pink puffers. *British Medical Journal, 283,* 343–346.

Zeppetella, G. (1997). Nebulized morphine in the palliation of dyspnoea. *Palliative Medicine, 11,* 267–275.

SUGGESTED READING

Mahler, D. A. (Ed.). (1990). *Dyspnea.* Mount Kisco, NY: Futura Publishing Company.

Impaired Sleep

Terri E. Weaver

INTRODUCTION

I. Although there is no generally accepted definition for impaired sleep, it is recognized as the perception of poor sleep quality and the inability to initiate or maintain sleep. Sleep is required for optimal physiological, neurobehavioral, and psychological functioning. Lack of sleep from poor sleep behaviors or sleep disorders produces deficits in cognitive processing, memory, mood, and functional performance. Sleep changes throughout the life cycle, although the clinical significance of this is still under not entirely understood. Sleep promotion is dependent upon the maintenance of good sleep hygiene that entails regular bedtime schedule and routine preparations for sleep.

   A. Definition

   Sleep is defined by the presence of several epochs of non-rapid eye movement (NREM) and/or rapid eye movement (REM) as documented during polysomnography or sleep study.

   1. NREM and REM sleep are differentiated by electroencephalogram (EEG), electroocculogram (EOG), and electromylogram (EMG) recordings.

   2. Non-REM sleep includes initial onset of sleep, progressing through very deep sleep, stages 1–4.

      a. Stage 1: Transitional stage to deeper stages of sleep occupying 1%–2% of adult total sleep time. At this stage, an individual is easily awakened and may experience fragmental thoughts. EEG shows waves that are of low voltage and mixed frequency.

      b. Stage 2: More stable stage of sleep that occurs for 50% of adult sleep time and characterized by slowing of the EEG waves.

      c. Stage 3 & 4: This stage of sleep, occupying 10%–15% of adult total sleep time, is a deeper restorative sleep. Known as *delta sleep* this stage is characterized by high voltage, low frequency, slow EEG waves and occurs in first third of night.

3. Active sleep (REM): rapid eye movement or dream sleep.
   a. This stage of sleep is identified by a desynchronized EEG that includes low voltage and mixed frequency waves.
   b. The EEG pattern is similar to that of being awake and is distinguished from that state by the presence of bilateral synchronous eye movements and muscle atonia.
   c. Autonomic nervous system activity fluctuates during REM sleep with changes in heart rate, BP, cerebral blood flow, metabolic rate, temperature regulation, and respiration.
   d. REM sleep occurs 4–6 times/night at 60–90 minute intervals. Periods can last from 40–60 minutes with greater duration toward morning. This stage of sleep occupies 20%–25% of the total sleep time.
   e. In children, sleep architecture completes its transition to a mature adult form with a 40% decrease in the amount of slow-wave sleep between the ages of 10 and 20 years and modest increases in light NREM sleep (Carskadon, 1982).

B. Etiology
   1. Physical factors
      a. Pain (Closs, 1992)
      b. Nocturnal exacerbation of such illnesses as asthma, GI distress, and cardiovascular conditions including angina and congestive heart failure
      c. Sleep disorders: obstructive sleep apnea (see below), periodic limb movements, narcolepsy, REM behavior disorder, insomnia, and parasomnias
      d. Medications that contain caffeine or other agents that alter sleep such as REM–suppressant drugs (narcotics, barbiturates, antidepressants) and NREM–suppressant drugs (benzodiazepines)
      e. Fever
      f. Age
      g. Perimenopause/menopause
      h. Prematurity
      i. Craniofacial or congenital anomalies in infants
      j. Low hematocrit with other airway issues
   2. Psychosocial factors
      a. Duration of prior wakefulness
      b. Alteration in sleep-promoting behaviors known as sleep hygiene such as alternating bedtimes and routines, extensive daytime napping
      c. Particularly in adolescence: bedtime resistance, poor sleep hygiene, and delayed sleep phase (DSPS—delayed sleep phase syndrome)
      d. Vigorous exercise and stimulating activity in evening hours
      e. Change in home environment including institutionalization

f. Environmental factors such as noise, temperature, exposure to daytime light (Redeker, 2000)

g. Loss of control (restraints, pharmacologic paralysis)

h. Fear, anxiety, depression, psychological stress

i. Factors related to institutionalization that can disrupt sleep such as diagnostic testing, physical assessment, nursing interventions, invasive procedures, and equipment noise

C. Risk factors

1. Sleep deprivation associated with ICU psychosis

a. Develops between 3rd and 7th day following admission and clears within 48 hours. More common in surgical patients (Schwab, 1994).

b. Contributing factors: illness severity, age, type of surgical procedure, medications, metabolic alterations (Redeker, 2000). Sleep deprivation primary cause.

2. Travel across time zones (altitude if oxygen saturation (O_2) baseline low)

D. Pathophysiology: dependent upon primary cause of sleep disruption

E. Relevant theories: none

F. Incidence

1. 67% of older adults experience one or more symptoms of a sleep problem at least a few nights a week; 71% of those aged 55–64; 65% of those aged 65–74; 64% of those 75–84 (National Sleep Foundation [NSF], 2003).

2. Sleep apnea, a common sleep disorder in middle aged individuals particularly among men, affects 4% men and 2% women (Young et al., 1993).

3. Insomnia is experienced by 20%–40% of the adult population (Kryger, Roth, & Dement, 2000; Mellinger, Balter, & Uhlenhut, 1985).

4. 48% of adults 55 and older experience the symptoms of insomnia—difficulty falling asleep, waking during the night, waking too early and being unable to fall back asleep, and waking feeling unrefreshed (NSF, 2003).

G. Considerations across the life span

1. Children

a. In children, the duration and distribution of normal sleep evolves with advancing age—from infancy (16–18 hours of sleep in 3–4 hour blocks), toddlers (11.4 hours), 13-year-olds (9 hours), to adolescence (7.9 hours) (Iglowstein, Jenni, Molinari, & Largo, 2003).

b. Infants spend 50% of their sleep time in REM (active sleep), recurring every 50–60 minutes alternating with periods of NREM sleep (quiet sleep). Sleep onset REM begins to subside by 3 months of age and overall REM declines to less than 30% of total sleep by 3 years. Sleep cycle length matures more gradually and by adolescents an adult cycle is attained of 90–100 minutes (Hoban, 2004).

c. Restless legs syndrome (RLS) and periodic limb movement disorder (PLMD) only recently identified in children (Hoban, 2004).

Emerging association between RLS/PLMD and daytime neurobehavioral symptoms. Survey of 138 adults with RLS identified onset at 20 years of age and 18% by 10 years of age suggesting that childhood onset may be more common than recognized earlier (Carroll, McColley, Marcus, Curtis, & Loughlin, 1995). One study found relationship between iron supplements and decrease in periodic limb movement in sleep (PLMS; Simakajornboon, 2003). In children, parasomnias, such as nocturnal enuresis, affect 15.7% of children 3–13 years of age (Laberge, Tremblay, Vitaro, & Montplaisir, 2000) and nightmares occur 57.6% in 5–7 years-olds (Smedje, Browman, & Hetta, 1999).

d. Delayed circadian phase more evident in adolescence.

e. Nasal congestion or obstruction can occur during first 3 months when most infants are obligatory nose breathers and tongue is larger proportionally.

f. Excessive daytime sleepiness not common sign of obstructive sleep apnea (OSA) in children like adults.

g. Central or obstructive apnea can occur in infancy due to any or all of the following: prematurity, GER, apparent life-threatening events (ALTE), shaken-baby syndrome, Munchausen by proxy, position in sleep/car seat or obstructing when held in arms, during feedings, low hematocrit levels, congenital anomalies, birth trauma, neurological damage at birth related to metabolic problems, asphyxia, complications, or rare life-threatening congenital central hypoventilation syndrome.

h. Craniofacial problems lead to obstructive sleep apnea in children and treatment may include surgical reconstruction and temporary tracheostomy due to narrow airways. There is evidence that infantile OSA, SIDS, and the adult OSA syndrome are related (McNamara & Sullivan, 2000; Rees et al., 1998).

i. Syndromes such as Down, Pickwickan, Prader–Willi, or Marfans can have an OSA component (Erler & Paditz, 2004).

j. Hypertrophy of the tonsils is a frequent cause of OSA in early childhood. If stridor is causing airway collapse, chin lift and jaw thrust while in the lateral position with adenotonsillar hypertrophy improves airway patency (Arai, Fukunaga, Hirota, & Fujimoto, 2004).

k. Vascular anomalies of the airway (venous, lymph malformations, hemmangiomas) at any age.

l. Airway tumors.

m. Chronic aspiration of saliva due to swallowing coordination.

n. Pertussis, croup, and epiglotitis can create apnea periods.

o. Suspect OSA if one of the following clinical symptoms are present: hyperactivity, poor concentration, nocturnal enuresis, deformities of the thorax, microsomia arterial or pulmonary hypertension; or sleep study identifies obstruction with desat, bradycardia or tachycardia, and/or arousals (Erler & Paditz, 2004).

        p. Features of sleep-related breathing disorders include peak age (3–6), gender (affected until adolescence), adenotonsillar hypertrophy (common), snoring (common, often continuous), pattern of obstruction (prolonged partial airway obstruction). Daytime symptoms include somnolence uncommon or intermittent, inattention, and behavioral disturbances (Hoban, 2004).

  2. Pregnancy

      a. Women report sleep problems throughout pregnancy (Mindell & Jacobson, 2000).

      b. Nocturnal awakenings reported by 97% of women by the end of pregnancy (Mindell & Jacobson, 2000).

      c. Frequent complaints are difficulty falling asleep and symptoms of sleep apnea (Mindell & Jacobson, 2000).

      d. By end of pregnancy, 23%–31% of women snored (Mindell & Jacobson, 2000).

      e. Little differences in sleep patterns across pregnancy, but women in late pregnancy sleep and nap more (Mindell & Jacobson, 2000).

      f. Potentially reduced oxygenation during sleep related to low functional residual capacity (FRC) and supine position (Kryger et al., 2000).

      g. Reduced sleep efficiency (Kryger et al., 2000).

      h. Increased amount of stage 1 sleep and decrease in REM sleep (Kryger et al., 2000).

      i. Development of periodic leg movement and restless leg syndrome common.

      j. Women with preeclampsia have reduced sleep quality, increased wakefulness, and periodic movements.

      k. Fetal growth retardation is more common in snorers and Apgar score <7.

  3. Elderly

      a. Greater sleep disruption with aging

      b. Increased nocturnal awakenings

      c. Increased latency to sleep and especially REM stage sleep

      d. Increased sleep fragmentation (Bliwise, King, Harris, & Haskell, 1992)

      e. Decreased slow-wave sleep (Bliwise et al., 1992)

      f. Changes in circadian patterns (Bliwise et al., 1992)

H. Cultural considerations

  1. Daytime napping or *siestas* are a common feature in some Latino cultures.

  2. Cobedding is utilized frequently in many cultures and sometimes associated with apnea in infants and/or apparent or acute life-threatening events (ALTE).

I. Complications/sequelae

  1. Excessive daytime sleepiness (EDS; Gottlieb et al., 1999) associated with:

a. Increased errors and accidents (Bedard, Montplaisir, Malo, Richer, & Rouleau, 1993; Findley, Smith, Hooper, Dineen, & Suratt, 2000; George & Smiley, 1999)

b. Decrements in neurobehavioral functioning, including difficulties with executive functioning, cognitive processing, sustaining attention, reaction time, and memory (Bedard et al., 1993; Engleman, Kingshott, Martin, & Douglas, 2000; Engleman et al., 1999)

c. Reduced functional status and quality of life (Engleman et al., 1999; Weaver et al., 1997)

2. Mental status changes associated with acute sleep disruption, especially related to ICU environment: hallucinations, disorientation, anxiety, depression, fear, paranoia, irritability, disorientation (Redeker, 2000; Schwab, 1994)

3. Depressed mood (Aikens, Caruana-Montaldo, Vanable, Tadimeti, & Mendelson, 1999; Millman, Fogel, McNamara, & Carlisle, 1989)

4. Respiratory system alterations—blunted chemosensitivity (Schwab, 1994)

a. 20%–24% decrease forced vital capacity, maximum voluntary ventilation, hypercapnic ventilatory response (Schwab, 1994)

b. 29% decrease in hypoxic ventilatory response (Schwab, 1994)

c. 24% decline in inspiratory muscle endurance (Schwab, 1994)

5. Immune system alterations—sleep deprivation may activate immune system (Dinges, Douglas, Hamarman, Zaugg, & Kapoor, 1995; Dinges et al., 1994)

a. Increase in WBC counts, granulocytes, monocytes, natural killer cell activity (Dinges et al., 1995)

II. Assessment

A. General concepts in assessing and managing impaired sleep
Frequent cause of impaired sleep in non-acute setting is poor sleep habits and sleep hygiene. Therefore, focus of assessment and management should be assessment of sleep habits and identification of potential risk factors and behavioral modification to restore sleep hygiene.

B. Identification of sleep disorder

C. History

1. General assessment

a. Usual time to bed and time of awakening

b. Quality and duration of sleep—number of and reason for awakenings

c. Behaviors prior to sleep (exercise and food, alcohol, caffeine, and nicotine intake)

d. Recent lifestyle or relationship changes or other sources of stress

e. Reports of awakening feeling unrefreshed

2. Assessment for sleep disorders

a. Presence of excessive daytime sleepiness including sleepiness-related accidents

      b. Symptoms of OSA including snoring, gasping, snorting, or apneic periods during sleep

      c. Reports of periodic limb movements prior to or during sleep (interfering with sleep) or sensation of "restless legs" or "crawling" feeling of the legs—indicative of periodic limb movement disorder

      d. Reports of cataplexy and daytime hallucinations along with excessive daytime sleepiness indicative of narcolepsy

      e. History of sleep walking, talking or eating during sleep

      f. Reports of difficulties initiating or maintaining sleep indicative of insomnia

      g. Difficulties with cognitive processes, concentration, memory, or disorientation.

   3. Physical exam/diagnostic tests

      a. Presence of small upper airway and other indications of OSA

      b. Body mass index >28 (males)

      c. Polysomnography (PSG) for detection of sleep disorder including EEG, EMG, EOG, and respiratory effort (inductive plethysmography), measurement of oronasal airflow

      d. Actigraphy—wristwatch-like device that contains a motion detector and memory bank that measures movement that can be used to evaluate sleep duration and quality. Correlates well with polysomnography for deep stages of sleep and wakefulness.

      e. In children: physical exam, endoscopic exam (ENT), exams and same exams as above in addition Ph Probe in reflux (24 hr), PFT's

III. Common therapeutic modalities (see chapter 24, "Adult Obstructive Sleep Apnea")

  A. Obstructive sleep apnea

   1. Weight loss

   2. Continuous Positive Airway Pressure (CPAP) produces a pneumatic splint that maintains airway patency during sleep. Required level of airway pressure determined during nocturnal PSG. Not impossible but difficult with younger children: mask uncomfortable, may cause midfacial hypoplasia (Erler & Paditz, 2004).

   3. Oral appliance: A device worn nocturnally that either holds the tongue in place and/or advances the mandible forward. In infancy, a nasal airway may be used to prevent tongue from falling back. To obstruct airway or in choanal atresia (small or no nasal opening) a tube within a nipple may be used temporarily to keep the mouth open prior to a tracheostomy.

   4. Surgery: Aim is to increase the pharyngeal space to increase the size of the airway.

      a. Uvulopalatopharyngoplasty

      b. Genial and hyoid advancement

      c. Retro-tongue-base-pharynx (RTBP) surgery including mandibular advancement, hyoid bone suspension, and tongue base reduction.

d. Lip-tongue adhesion for Pierre Robin

e. Preventing tracheostomy in select number of infants with OSA from tongue movement

5. Positional therapy: designed to keep patient from sleeping on their back, for example, tennis ball sewn into back of pajamas

B. Narcolepsy (Kryger et al., 2000)

1. Stimulants

a. Amphetamine

b. Methylphenidate

c. Mazindol

d. Pemoline

e. Modafinil

2. Adjunct effect drugs

a. Protriptyline

b. Viloxazine

3. Treatment of cataplexy, sleep paralysis, and hypnagogic hallucinations

a. Tricyclic antidepressant

b. Antidepressants

c. Gamma-hydroxybutyrate (experimental)

C. Insomnia (Ohayon, Caulet, & Lemoine, 1998)

1. Medications

a. Hypnotic agents

i. Benzodiazepines

ii. Clonazepam

iii. Diazepam

iv. Flurazepam

v. Zaleplon

vi. Zolpidem

b. Antidepressants

2. Psychological treatments

a. Cognitive therapy

b. Cognitive behavioral techniques

c. Relaxation

d. Sleep restriction

e. Stimulus control

IV. Interventions and outcomes

A. Treatment and intervention—Acute care setting

1. Schedule care to enable periods of sleep at least 2 hr in duration.

a. Decrease sensory stimulation in patient room including keeping equipment away from head of bed.

b. Entrain natural light in patient room.

c. Create routine prior to sleep to promote relaxation (back rubs, warm baths, use of white noise or ocean sounds).

d. Use hypnotic agents with short half-life judiciously such as benzo-diazepines or zolpidem.

     e. Provide cues to promote orientation to time of day such as clocks and calendars.

B. Treatment and intervention—Home setting

  1. Therapeutic modality appropriate for sleep disorder: Evaluation, promotion, and education regarding principles of sleep hygiene to nurture behavioral cues for sleep time.

    a. Regular sleep time, especially time of awakening

    b. Consistent and routine bedtime preparation

    c. Avoidance of caffeine, eating, alcohol, or smoking just prior to bedtime

    d. Decreased GI motility can cause GI distress during sleep if food intake prior to retiring

  2. Alcohol has same effect as caffeine on sleep. Mild sedation accompanies low blood concentration. With higher concentration, increased arousal occurs similar to cholinergic mechanism as blood alcohol levels decline. This disrupts sleep, preventing deeper restorative stages of sleep.

    a. Smoking prior to sleep period causes arousal. Effect is similar to caffeine producing alteration in sleep maintenance.

    b. Use of bed primarily for sleep and sexual activity. Avoid prolonged lounging in bed to read or watch TV as this will interfere with the development and maintenance of behavioral cues that the bed is for sleeping.

    c. Avoidance of exercise less than 3–4 hours prior to bedtime

    d. If awakening during the night, leave the bed. Avoid looking at the clock as it heightens anxiety increasing adrenaline interfering with sleep onset.

    e. Routine daytime naps >10–15 min should be avoided unless sleep deprived.

    f. Need for prolonged treatment with benzodiazepines should be consistently evaluated due to the potential for rebound effect and further sleep disruption.

  3. Home care considerations

    a. Equipment considerations: Patients should be taught how to care for their continuous positive airway pressure (CPAP) equipment (see OSA below; Oximeter for children with tracheostomies or CPAP)

  4. Caregiver considerations

    a. Bed partner may provide assessment of symptoms and treatment response

    b. Initiation of treatment at the urgency of the bed partner may affect patient adherence to CPAP treatment (Hoy, Vennelle, Kingshott, Engleman, & Douglas, 1999)

    c. Bed partners report improved sleep quality and fewer sleep disturbances when patients use their CPAP (McArdle, Kingshott, Engleman, Mackay, & Douglas, 2001)

5. Social supports
    a. Patient support organizations
        i. AWAKE—national support group for patients with obstructive sleep apnea
        ii. Narcolepsy Network
        iii. Sleep disorders organizations
        iv. National Sleep Foundation—provides information on sleep disorders for the professionals and the lay public
        v. Sleep Apnea Association
        vi. Restless Leg Syndrome Foundation
6. Web sites
    a. Sleep Net: http://www.sleepnet.com/
    b. NIH—National Center on Sleep Disorders Research
       http://www.nhlbi.nih.gov/health/public/sleep/index.htm
       http://www.nhlbi.nih.gov/health/prof/sleep/index.htm
    c. American Academy of Sleep Medicine: http://www.aasmnet.org/
    d. Children with tracheostomies: http://www.tracheostomy.com

REFERENCES

Aikens, J. E., Caruana-Montaldo, B., Vanable, P. A., Tadimeti, L., & Mendelson, W. B. (1999). MMPI correlates of sleep and respiratory disturbance in obstructive sleep apnea. *Sleep, 22*(3), 362–369.

Arai, Y. C., Fukunaga, K., Hirota, S., & Fujimoto, S. (2004). The effect of chin lift and jaw thrust while in the lateral position on stridor score in anesthetized children with adenotonsillar hypertrophy. *Anesthesia & Analgesia, 99*(4), 1631–1641.

Bedard, M. A., Montplaisir, J., Malo, J., Richer, F., & Rouleau, I. (1993). Persistent neuropsychological deficits and vigilance impairment in sleep apnea syndrome after treatment with continuous positive airways pressure (CPAP). *Journal of Clinical and Experimental Neuropsychology, 15*(2), 330–341.

Bliwise, D. L., King, A. C., Harris, R. B., & Haskell, W. L. (1992). Prevalence of self-reported poor sleep in a healthy population aged 50–65. *Social Science and Medicine, 34*(1), 49–55.

Carroll, J. L., McColley, S. A., Marcus, C. L., Curtis, S., & Loughlin, G. M. (1995). Inability of clinical history to distinguish primary snoring from obstructive sleep apnea syndrome in children. *Chest, 108,* 610–618.

Carskadon, M. A. (1982). The second decade. In C. Guilleminault (Ed.), *Sleeping and waking disorders: Indications and techniques* (pp. 99–125). Menlo Park, CA: Addison Wesley.

Closs, S. J. (1992). Patients' night-time pain, analgesic provision and sleep after surgery. *International Journal of Nursing Studies, 29*(4), 381–392.

Dinges, D. F., Douglas, S. D., Hamarman, S., Zaugg, L., & Kapoor, S. (1995). Sleep deprivation and human immune function. *Advanced Neuroimmunology, 5*(2), 97–110.

Dinges, D. F., Douglas, S. D., Zaugg, L., Campbell, D. E., McMann, J. M., Whitehouse, W. G., et al. (1994). Leukocytosis and natural killer cell function parallel neurobehavioral fatigue induced by 64 hours of sleep deprivation. *Journal of Clinical Investigation, 93*(5), 1930–1939.

Engleman, H. M., Kingshott, R. N., Martin, S. E., & Douglas, N. J. (2000). Cognitive function in the sleep apnea/hypopnea syndrome (SAHS). *Sleep, 23*(Suppl 4), S102–S108.

Engleman, H. M., Kingshott, R. N., Wraith, P. K., Mackay, T. W., Deary, I. J., & Douglas, N. J. (1999). Randomized placebo-controlled crossover trial of continuous positive airway pressure for mild sleep Apnea/Hypopnea syndrome. *American Journal of Respiratory and Clinical Care Medicine, 159*(2), 461–467.

Erler, T., & Paditz, E. (2004). Obstructive sleep apnea syndrome in children: A state of the art review. *Treatments in Respiratory Medicine, 3*(2), 107–122.

Findley, L., Smith, C., Hooper, J., Dineen, M., & Suratt, P. M. (2000). Treatment with nasal CPAP decreases automobile accidents in patients with sleep apnea. *American Journal of Respiratory and Clinical Care Medicine, 161*(3 Pt 1), 857–859.

George, C. F., & Smiley, A. (1999). Sleep apnea & automobile crashes. *Sleep, 22*(6), 790–795.

Gottlieb, D. J., Whitney, C. W., Bonekat, W. H., Iber, C., James, G. D., Lebowitz, M., et al. (1999). Relation of sleepiness to respiratory disturbance index: The Sleep Heart Health Study. *American Journal of Respiratory and Clinical Care Medicine, 159*(2), 502–507.

Hoban, T. F. (2004). Sleep and its disorders in children. *Seminars in Neurology, 24*(3), 327–340.

Hoy, C. J., Vennelle, M., Kingshott, R. N., Engleman, H. M., & Douglas, N. J. (1999). Can intensive support improve continuous positive airway pressure use in patients with the sleep apnea/hypopnea syndrome? *American Journal of Respiratory and Clinical Care Medicine, 159*(4 Pt 1), 1096–1100.

Iglowstein, I., Jenni, O., Molinari, L., & Largo, R. (2003). Sleep duration from infancy to adolescence: Reference values and generational trends. *Pediatrics, 111*(2), 302–307.

Kryger, M., Roth, T., & Dement, W. (2000). *Principles and practice of sleep medicine* (3rd ed.). Philadelphia: W. B. Saunders Co.

Laberge, L., Tremblay, R. E., Vitaro, F., & Montplaisir, J. (2000). Development of parasomnias from childhood to early adolescence. *Pediatrics, 106*(1), 67–74.

McArdle, N., Kingshott, R., Engleman, H. M., Mackay, T. W., & Douglas, N. J. (2001). Partners of patients with sleep apnoea/hypopnoea syndrome: Effect of CPAP treatment on sleep quality and quality of life. *Thorax, 56*(7), 513–518.

McNamara, F., & Sullivan, C. E. (2000). The genesis of adult sleep apnea in childhood. *Thorax, 55*, 964–969.

Mellinger, G., Balter, M., & Uhlenhut, E. (1985). Insomnia and its treatment: Prevalence and correlates. *Archives of General Psychiatry, 42*, 225–232.

Millman, R. P., Fogel, B. S., McNamara, M. E., & Carlisle, C. C. (1989). Depression as a manifestation of obstructive sleep apnea: reversal with nasal continuous positive airway pressure. *Journal of Clinical Psychiatry, 50*, 348–351.

Mindell, J. A., & Jacobson, B. J. (2000). Sleep disturbances during pregnancy. *Journal of Obstetric, Gynecologic, and Neonatal Nursing, 29*(6), 590–597.

National Sleep Foundation. (2003). *2003 Sleep in America poll.* Washington, DC: National Sleep Foundation.

Ohayon, M. M., Caulet, M., & Lemoine, P. (1998). Comorbidity of mental and insomnia disorders in the general population. *Comprehensive Psychiatry, 39*(4), 185–197.

Redeker, N. S. (2000). Sleep in acute care settings: An integrative review. *Journal of Nursing Scholarship, 32*(1), 31–38.

Rees, K., Wright, A., Keeling, J. W., & Douglas, N. J. (1998). Facial structure in the sudden infant death syndrome: Case-control study. *British Medical Journal, 317,* 179–180.

Schwab, R. J. (1994). Disturbances of sleep in the intensive care unit. *Critical Care Clinics, 10*(4), 681–694.

Simakajornboon, N., Gozal, D., Vlasic, V., Mack, C., Sharon, D., & McGinley, B. M. (2003). Periodic limb movements in sleep and iron status in children. *Sleep 26*(6), 735–738.

Smedje, H., Browman, J. E., & Hetta, J. (1999). Parents' reports of disturbed sleep in 5–7 year-old Swedish children. *Acta Paediatrica, 88*(8), 858–865.

Weaver, T. E., Laizner, A. M., Evans, L. K., Maislin, G., Chugh, D. K., Lyon, K., et al. (1997). An instrument to measure functional status outcomes for disorders of excessive sleepiness. *Sleep, 20*(10), 835–843.

Young, T., Palta, M., Dempsey, J., Skatrud, J., Weber, S., & Badr, S. (1993). The occurrence of sleep-disordered breathing among middle-aged adults. *New England Journal of Medicine, 328*(17), 1230–1235.

Anxiety

12

Mary Jones Gant and Judith Brown Sanders

INTRODUCTION

Anxiety is a pathologic state characterized by a feeling of dread and accompanied by somatic expressions of a hyper-alert autonomic nervous system. There are different classifications of anxiety, which include panic disorder, generalized anxiety disorder, phobic disorder, obsessive compulsive disorder, and posttraumatic stress disorder. Anxiety can be precipitated by a variety of medical illnesses including respiratory disease. Many of the pharmacologic interventions used to treat the precipitating medical conditions can also lend to symptoms of anxiety, including central nervous system stimulants, psychotropics, cardiovascular preparations, and respiratory medications. Anxiety affects approximately 2.4 million adult Americans and is twice as common in women often beginning in late adolescence. Psychotherapy is one of the common therapeutic modalities along with pharmacotherapy which include benzodiazepines, buspirone, tricyclics, Imipramine, and Trazodone. A variety of nursing interventions have been proven to be effective including providing a safe environment, relaxation techniques, and identification of coping mechanisms.

Anxiety is a human response to disease that is frequently seen in patients with lung disease. The most significant limiting symptom in patients with lung disease is shortness of breath. The feeling that one will not be able to perform this life sustaining act leads to feelings of anxiety for the future and how one will cope with difficult situations.

I. Definition

A pathologic state characterized by a feeling of dread and accompanied by somatic expressions of a hyper-alert autonomic nervous system

A. Panic disorder: spontaneous panic attacks and agoraphobia

1. Occurs 2–3 times a week
2. Course of remissions and exacerbations
3. Excellent prognosis with therapy

135

B. Generalized anxiety disorder: generalized anxiety for at least one month
   1. Symptoms may diminish with age
   2. Secondary depression may develop
C. Phobic disorder: irrational fear of a specific object or situation
   1. Fear is excessive or unreasonable
   2. Agoraphobia most resistant to treatment
D. Obsessive-compulsive disorder: intrusive ideas, impulses, thoughts, or patterned behavior that produce anxiety
   1. Insidious onset without clear precipitating stressors
   2. Fair prognosis with therapy and medication
E. Posttraumatic stress disorder: anxiety produced by extraordinary major life stress
   1. Trauma reexperienced periodically in thoughts and dreams
   2. Guarded prognosis with preexisting mental problems

II. Etiology
   A. Physical factors
      1. Cardiovascular excitation
      2. Superficial vasoconstriction
      3. Pupil dilation
      4. Insomnia
   B. Psychosocial factors
      1. Increased tension, apprehension
      2. Increased helplessness
      3. Decreased self-assurance
      4. Increased feelings of inadequacy
      5. Focus on perceived object of fear or unknown source of anxiety
   C. Risk factors
      1. Medical illnesses
         a. Endocrine and metabolic disorders: hyperthyroidism, hypoglycemia, Addison's disease, Cushing's disease, pheochromocytoma, electrolyte abnormalities
         b. Neurologic: seizure disorders, multiple sclerosis, chronic pain syndromes, traumatic brain injury, central nervous system (CNS), neoplasm, migraines, myasthenia gravis
         c. Parkinson's disease
         d. Cardiovascular: mitral valve prolapse, congestive heart failure (CHF), arrhythmias, post-myocardial infarction (MI), hyperdynamic beta adrenergic state, hypertension, angina pectoris, postcerebral infarction
         e. GI: PUD, Crohn's Disease, ulcerative colitis, irritable bowel syndrome
         f. Respiratory: COPD, asthma, pneumonia, pulmonary edema, cystic fibrosis, interstitial lung disease
      2. Psychiatric. Depression, mania, schizophrenia, adjustment disorder, personality disorders, delirium, dementia
      3. Drugs
         a. CNS stimulants: amphetamines, caffeine, cocaine, diethylproprion, ephedrine, PCP, phenylephrine, pseudoephedrine

      b. CNS depressant withdrawal: barbiturates, benzodiazepines, ethanol, opiates

      c. Psychotropics: antipsychotics, buproprion, buspirone, fluxetine, isocarboxazid

      d. Cardiovascular: captopril, enalapril, digitalis, disopyramide, hydralazine, Reserpine

      e. Others: albuterol, aminophylline, baclofen, theophylline, steroids, isoproteranol, NSAIDs

III. Pathophysiology

   A. Biological determinants (endogenous)

     1. Neurotransmitter

      a. gamma-aminobutyric acid (GABA)

     2. Catecholamine

     3. Metabolic

     4. Carbon dioxide

   B. Psychological determinants (exogenous)

     1. Behavioral

     2. Cognitive

IV. Relevant theories

   A. Theories related to biological etiology

     1. *Catecholamine:* massive β-adrenergic nervous system discharge

     2. *Locus Coeruleus:* increased discharge of central nervous system noradrenergic nuclei

     3. *Metabolic:* aberrant metabolic changes induced by lactate infusion

     4. *Carbon dioxide hypersensitivity:* hypersensitive brain stem dioxide receptors

     5. *GABA benzodiazepine:* abnormal receptor function leading to decreased inhibitory activity

   B. Theory related to behavioral etiology

     1. *Behavioral:* pairing of an unconditioned stimulus to a conditioned stimulus, leading to a conditioned response

     2. *Cognitive:* catastrophic cognitive misinterpretation of uncomfortable physical sensations and affects

V. Incidence

   A. General population: Affects approximately 2.4 million adult Americans and is twice as common in women as in men. It most often begins during late adolescence or early adulthood.

   B. Elderly: Prevalence of anxiety disorder in the general population of people over age 65 is 10% in women and 5% in men.

VI. Considerations across the life span

   A. Pediatric considerations (Kendall & Treadwell, 1996)

     1. History

      a. Vague somatic complaints

      b. School difficulties

      c. Behavioral regression

      d. Socially withdrawn

       e. Negative self-statements

       f. Alcohol/substance use or abuse

    2. Clinical manifestations

       a. Variable behavioral manifestations that may differentiate anxious from non-anxious children include having difficulty initiating conversations, trembling voice quality, and absence of eye contact.

       b. Children's self-reported anxiety was associated with their perception of greater parental control and less parental acceptance.

       c. Family characteristics such as maternal distress and family problem-solving abilities may be directly related to anxiety manifestations.

  B. Elderly (Waldinger, 1997)

    1. Physical illness is easily overlooked when an elderly person has symptoms of an anxiety disorder.

    2. If physical illness is detected, somatic issues may be treated but concurrent anxiety disorder may be overlooked.

VII. Cultural considerations (Purnell & Paulanka, 1998)

  A. Cultural responses to health and illness

    1. Sick role behaviors are culturally prescribed and vary among ethnic groups.

    2. How mental illness is perceived and expressed by a cultural group has a direct effect on how the patient will present to the health care provider and in turn how the health care provider will interact with these patients.

    3. Mental illness is culture bound. What may be perceived as a mental illness in one society may not be considered a mental illness in another.

    4. The health care provider must assess each patient and family individually and incorporate culturally congruent therapeutic intervention.

ASSESSMENT

  I. General concepts in assessing and managing

    A. Anxiety—The subjective symptom comprised of the moods of apprehension and worry, accompanied with physiological components of motor tension and autonomic hyperactivity.

      1. May present with some combination of the following

       a. Motor tension

       b. Apprehension and vigilance

       c. Palpitations, diaphoresis, tachycardia

       d. Nausea/diarrhea

       e. Dizziness/parathesia

       f. Dyspnea/tachypnea

  II. History

    A. Onset and duration of symptoms

    B. Specific events/situations that produce symptoms

C. Interference with daily activities
D. Associated somatic difficulties
E. Caffeine intake and medications
F. Previous treatments/results

III. Physical examination: Rule out medical conditions that may present as conditions.
A. Differential diagnosis
1. Angina, arrhythmias, congestive heart failure, myocardial infarction
2. Anticholinergic toxicity, digitalis toxicity, stimulants
3. Anemia
4   Hyperadrenalism, hyperthyroidism, menopause
5. Encephalopathies, seizure disorder
6. Asthma, chronic obstructive pulmonary disease, pneumonia, pulmonary embolism (Wingate & Hansen-Flaschen, 1997)

COMMON THERAPEUTIC MODALITIES

I. Psychotherapy (Hales, Yudofsky, & Talbott, 1999)
A. Insight-oriented: Self-understanding leads to cure.
B. Behavioral therapy: Change can occur through positive reinforcement.
C. Cognitive therapy: Correcting distorted belief system can effect cure.
D. Group therapy: Practice in social skills can relieve symptoms.
E. Meditation and biofeedback: utilizing the relaxation response.

II. Pharmacotherapy
A. Benzodiazepines: known efficacy; widely used; issues of dependence and withdrawal in certain patients; can depress respirations; should only be used short term
B. Buspirone: proven efficacy; generally well tolerated; a trial is generally indicated; compared with benzodiazepines, delayed action and not associated with a high; not associated with respiratory depression; may be used long term
C. Tricyclics: shown efficacy in few trials; delayed action compared with benzodiazepines; may be more effective for cognitive rather than physical symptoms of anxiety
D. Imipramine: shown efficacy; more side effects than benzodiazepines and buspirone
E. Trazodone: shown efficacy; more side effects than benzodiazepines and buspirone

III. Interventions and outcomes
A. Interventions
1. Avoid surprises; tell patient what to expect.
2. Include patient in planning of care.
3. Maintain calm and safe environment; decrease stimuli; reassure patient
4. Assist patient to identify those coping mechanisms that were successful in decreasing anxiety.

139

     5. Teach relaxation techniques.

     6. Involve family and/or significant other in patient's care.

  B. Expected outcomes

     1. Demonstrates decreased level of anxiety as evidenced by decreased tension, apprehension, and restlessness

     2. Ability to talk about fear/anxiety/concerns about symptoms that lead to anxiety

     3. Demonstrates effective coping skills as evidenced by increased ability to problem-solve and ability to meet self-care needs

     4. Verbalizes increased psychological comfort and coping skills

     5. Experiences a restful sleep

IV. Home care considerations (Carson, 1994)

  A. The home setting, surrounded by family and familiar environment create a sense of serenity, comfort, and peacefulness, which may lead to more holistic care and treatment.

  B. Aspects of the patient's condition when being cared for in the home include

     1. Support for the family and/or caregiver in assisting them to cope with the patient's behaviors

     2. An understanding of family dynamics and appropriate interventions

     3. Assisting the patient in selecting positive coping behaviors

REFERENCES

Carson, V. B. (1994). *Bay area health care psychiatric home care manual.* Baltimore, MD: Bay Area Health Care.

Hales, R. E., Yudofsky, S. C., & Talbott, J. A. (1999). *Textbook of psychiatry* (3rd ed.). Washington, DC: American Psychiatric Press.

Kendall, P. C., & Treadwell, K. R. H. (1996). Cognitive-behavioral treatment for childhood anxiety disorder. In E. D. Hibbs & P. S. Jensen (Eds.), *Psychosocial treatments for child and adolescent disorders* (pp. 23–41). Washington, DC: American Psychological Association.

Purnell, L. D., & Paulanka, B. J. (1998). *Transcultural health care: A culturally competent approach.* Philadelphia: F. A. Davis.

Waldinger, R. J. (1997). *Psychiatry for medical students* (3rd ed.). Washington, DC: American Psychiatric Press.

Wingate, B. J., & Hansen-Flaschen, J. (1997). Anxiety and depression in advanced lung disease. *Clinics in Chest Medicine, 18*(3), 495–505.

Depression

Mary Jones Gant and Judith Brown Sanders

INTRODUCTION

Depression is a mood disorder classified as Major Depressive Disorder, Bipolar Disorder, Cyclothymic Disorder, or Dysthymia. There are multiple medical disorders and medications that can lead to the development of depression. Approximately 9.5% of American adults suffer from a depressive illness with the incidence being twice as high for women than men. Common therapeutic modalities include medication, psychotherapy, or a combination of both.

Depression is a human response to disease that is frequently experienced by a patient with lung disease. The depression may range from mild dysthymia, adjustment disorder with depressed mood to a major depressive episode diagnosed as Major Depressive Disorder. Depression is a treatable condition that very frequently goes under-diagnosed and therefore under-treated in this population of patients. When practitioners screen and treat for this condition, patient's quality of life can be much improved.

I. Definition: Mood disorders are classified as Major Depressive Disorder, Bipolar Disorder, Cyclothymic Disorder, or Dysthymia.
   A. Major depression: At least five of the following symptoms must have been present during the same 2-week period.
      1. Depressed mood
      2. Loss of interest in usual activities (anhedonia)
      3. Weight loss or weight gain
      4. Insomnia or hypersomnia
      5. Psychomotor agitation or retardation
      6. Feelings of worthlessness
      7. Inability to concentrate
      8. Recurrent suicide ideation or thoughts of death
      9. Fatigue or loss of energy

B. Bipolar disorder: Presence of depression is identical to that of Major Depression Disorder. Crucial difference is presence of prior manic episode characterized by the following.
1. Elation, expansive mood
2. Increased energy
3. Inflated self-esteem
C. Cyclothymic: Similar to bipolar disorder but mood swings are less severe and occur with both depressive symptoms and hypomanic symptoms over a period of at least 2 years.
D. Dysthymia: Chronic, mild depressive disorder with depressive symptoms persisting ≥2 years. Symptoms are less severe than those of major depression and neurovegetative symptoms (disordered sleep and appetite) are minor or absent.

II. Etiology
A. Physical factors
1. Anhedonia
2. Somatic complaints
3. Fatigue
4. Weight change
5. Sleep disturbance
6. Slowed movement
7. Decreased libido
8. Decreased hygiene
9. Crying spells
B. Psychosocial factors
1. Worthlessness, guilt, or shame
2. Hopelessness, helplessness
3. Thoughts of death and suicide
4. Sadness
5. Pessimism
6. Irritability
7. Poor memory
C. Risk factors
1. Medical illnesses
a. *Central nervous system:* Alzheimer's disease, brain tumors, cerebrovascular accident, multiple sclerosis, Parkinson's disease, Huntington's disease, traumatic brain injury, dementias
b. *Pulmonary:* chronic bronchitis, emphysema, cystic fibrosis, interstitial lung disease, sleep apnea
c. *Cardiovascular:* congestive heart failure (CHF), myocardial infarction (MI), cerebral arteriosclerosis, angina, cardiomyopathies, coronary artery bypass surgery
d. *Endocrine:* Addison's disease, Cushing's disease, diabetes, hypothyroidism, hyperparathyroidism, parathyroid dysfunction
e. *Malignancies and hematologic disease:* pancreatic carcinoma, brain tumors, paraneoplastic effects of lung cancers, anemias

      f. *Metabolic disease:* electrolyte disturbances, renal failure, vitamin deficiencies or excess, acute intermittent porphyria, Wilson's disease, environmental toxins, heavy metals

      g. *Gastrointestinal disease:* irritable bowel syndrome, chronic pancreatitis, Crohn's disease, cirrhosis, hepatic encephalopathy

      h. *Autoimmune disease:* systemic lupus erythematosis, fibromyalgia, rheumatoid arthritis

  2. Drugs

      a. *CNS agents:* barbiturates, alcohol, amphetamines, benzodiazepines

      b. *Hormonal agents:* corticosteroids, estrogen, progesterone

      c. *Cardiovascular/antihypertensives:* digitalis, clonidine, reserpine, propranolol, procainamide

      d. *Anti-inflammatory and analgesic agents:* indomethacin, phenacetin, pentazocine

III. Pathophysiology

  A. Biological determinants (endogenous)

    1. Neurotransmitters

    2. Norepinephrine

    3. Dopamine

    4. Serotonin

    5. Hormonal levels

    6. Genetic factors

    7. Neurophysiological processes

  B. Psychological determinants (exogenous)

    1. Cultural influences

    2. Situational events

    3. Economic conditions

    4. Interpersonal relationships

    5. Social interactions

IV. Relevant theories

  A. Theories related to biological etiology

    1. Neuroendocrine abnormalities are a reflection of unknown biogenic amine input to hypothalamus.

    2. Biogenic amine activity is decreased in depression for unknown reasons.

    3. Both major depression and bipolar disorders appears to run in families.

  B. Theory related to psychological etiology

    1. Mourning of symbolic object loss with rigid superego that leads one to feel worthless.

    2. Cognitive triads of negative self-view, negative interpretation of experience, and negative view of the future.

V. Incidence

  A. General population

Approximately 9.5% of American adults suffer from a depressive illness. Women experience depression about twice as much as men. Although men are less likely to suffer from depression, 3 to 4 million men in the United States are affected.

B. Elderly

Prevalence is about 15% of the general population over age 65.

VI. Considerations across the life span

A. Pediatric (Milling & Martin, 1992)

1. History

   a. Developmental delays
   b. Disrupted attachments to others
   c. Social withdraw, boredom
   d. School difficulties
   e. Acting out in destructive ways
   f. Negative self-statements
   g. Alcohol/substance use or abuse
   h. Sexually acting out

2. Clinical manifestations

   a. Estimated prevalence is 2%–5% in school-aged children and teenagers. Depression may have detrimental effects on social and educational functioning.
   b. *DSM-IV-TR* criteria offer some age-related diagnosing criteria (APA, 2000). The Children's Depression Inventory is an age-appropriate self-report used to assess depression in children. Children may show significant weight change and/or skin abrasions/contusions/scars.

B. Elderly (Waldinger, 1997)

1. History

   a. Sadness
   b. Decreased appetite
   c. Insomnia
   d. Decreased energy
   e. Decreased libido
   f. Suicidal thoughts

2. Clinical manifestations

   a. Somatic complaints: may be only symptoms, the patient does not feel sad but develops a sense that they are physically unwell
   b. Pseudodementia: syndrome in which dementia is a result of the depression and not organic brain disease
   c. loneliness: need to distinguish between clinical depression and normal grief reactions

VII. Cultural considerations (Purnell & Paulanka, 1998)

A. Cultural responses to health and illness

1. Sick role behaviors are culturally prescribed and vary among ethnic groups.
2. How mental illness is perceived and expressed by a cultural group has a direct effect on how the patient will present to the health care provider and in turn how the health care provider will interact with these patients.

3. Mental illness is culture bound. What may be perceived as a mental illness in one society may not be considered a mental illness in another.
4. The health care provider must assess each patient and family individually and incorporate culturally congruent therapeutic intervention.

ASSESSMENT

I. General concepts in assessing and managing
   A. Depression in the elderly may be difficult to distinguish from dementia and delirium in the elderly as some symptoms of depression including disorientation, memory loss, and distractibility may suggest dementia.
   B. Three observations that may help distinguish between depression and dementia in the elderly
      a. Major depressive disorders occur over a period of days to weeks; dementia is slow and insidious.
      b. Depressed persons can answer questions correctly if given enough time, those with dementia cannot.
      c. A therapeutic trial of antidepressant medication produces improvement and/or recovery in the depressed patient and this does not occur in the patient with dementia.
II. History
   A. Onset, duration and description of symptoms
   B. Precipitating event
   C. Neurovegetative symptoms
      1. Loss of libido
      2. Weight loss/gain or anorexia
      3. Low energy level
      4. Insomnia/hypersomnia
      5. Constipation/dry mouth
      6. Decreased interest in usual activities
   D. Mood swings
   E. Personal and family history of depression
   F. Medication history
      1. Steroids
      2. Antihypertensives
      3. Estrogen
      4. NSAIDs
      5. Lanoxin
      6. Anti-Parkinson drugs
   G. Suicidal thoughts or attempts
III. Physical examination
   A. General appearance and behavior
      1. Tearful
      2. Downcast eyes
      3. Poor personal appearance

      4. Frustration

      5. Soft/low speech

      6. Psychomotor retardation or agitation

  B. Differential diagnosis

      1. Hypoxia or hypercapnia

      2. CNS Degenerative Disease

      3. Metabolic imbalance

      4. Medication side effects

      5. Other psychiatric disorders

      6. Insomnia or sleep depravation

      7. Depression related to chronic illness

      8. Isolation or lack of social support

  C. Diagnostic test

      1. Rule out organic cause

          a. CBC, sedimentation rate, chemistry profile, thyroid profile

          b. ECG

          c. Urinalysis

          d. Drug screen

  D. Self-administered depression tools

      1. Beck Depression Inventory (Beck, Ward, & Mendelson, 1961)

      2. Self-rating Depression Scale (Zung, 1965)

COMMON THERAPEUTIC MODALITIES

  I. Refer for treatment

    A. Bipolar and cyclothymic disorders

    B. Depression with psychotic symptoms

    C. High suicide risk

    D. Dysthymic disorder

    E. Neurovegetative signs

    F. Severe change in weight and/or sleep

    G. Major Depressive Disorder

  II. Treatment options include medication alone, psychotherapy alone, and combined treatment.

    A. 70% receiving medication experience marked improvement.

    B. Candidates for medication

      1. More severe symptoms

      2. Prior response to medical treatment

      3. Client preference

  III. Pharmacotherapy

    A. Depressed patients most likely to respond to antidepressant drug therapy are typified by the following

      1. Family history of depression, alcoholism, and/or response to somatic therapies

      2. Prominent vegetative signs

3. Mood congruent delusions (false beliefs that are congruent or consistent with the pervasive mood of the patient)

B. If patient not responsive to one drug class, change to an agent from another class of drugs (Salazar, 1996).

C. A trial of 4 to 8 weeks with a single agent should be pursued before changing to an alternate agent.

D. Drug classes

1. Selective serotonin reuptake inhibitors (SSRIs)

   Indications: Drug of choice due to effectiveness and safety as compared with the tricyclic antidepressants especially in the elderly

   Contraindications: These drugs should not be used in combination with MAO inhibitors or within 14 days of discontinuing MAO inhibitors. Use caution with other medications metabolized by cytochrome P450 liver enzymes. Patients may experience nervousness, insomnia, nausea, somnolence, ejaculatory disturbances, and hyponatremia.

   Medications: Fluoxetine (Prozac), sertraline (Zoloft), paroxetine (Paxil).

2. Monocyclic antidepressants

   Indications: May be useful for patients with mild bipolar disorder; useful for patients resistant to other agents and for those with atypical depression.

   Contraindications: Contraindicated in patients with a seizure disorder, current or prior diagnosis of bulimia or anorexia nervosa, or concurrent therapy with a MAO inhibitor. Fourteen days should elapse between discontinuing the MAOI and beginning this drug.

   Medication: Buproprion (Wellbutrin)

3. Selective serotonin-norepinephrine reuptake inhibitor

   Indications: This drug has a relatively short half-life and is successful in the treatment of depression. Rapid increases in dose may result in rapid response in patients with severe melancholic depression.

   Contraindications: Dose-dependent hypertension and other side effects similar to those of the SSRIs.

   Medication: Venlafaxine (Effexor)

4. Tricyclic antidepressants

   Indications: Have been replaced by the SSRIs. Use cautiously as they can cause cardiac complications.

   Contraindications: Use with caution in the elderly. Patient may experience dry mouth, constipation, tachycardia, postural hypotension, and sedation. Use only after other classes of medications have failed.

   Medications: Imipramine (Tofanil), amitriptyline (Elavil)

IV. Interventions and outcomes

A. Nursing interventions

1. Treat the patient as a person.
2. Give the patient as much control over the situation as possible.
3. Encourage patient to discuss feelings and concerns.
4. Use therapeutic touch.
5. Provide for diversional activities.

6. Initiate consultations with psychiatric liaison personnel as needed.
7. Provide opportunities for family/significant others to be with the patient, participate in the care, and so forth.
B. Expected outcomes
1. Uses effective coping mechanisms to manage the depression
2. Appears less depressed
3. Verbalizes feelings freely
4. States increased feelings of self-esteem and worth
5. Increased self-maintenance
6. Loss of suicidal ideation
V. Home care considerations (Carson, 1994)
A. The home setting, surrounded by family and familiar environment create a sense of serenity, comfort, and peacefulness, which may lead to more holistic care and treatment.
B. Aspects of the patient's condition when being cared for in the home include
1. Support for the family and/or caregiver in assisting them to cope with the patient's behaviors
2. An understanding of family dynamics and appropriate interventions
3. Assisting the patient in selecting positive coping behaviors

REFERENCES

American Psychiatric Association. (2000). *DSM-IV-TR. Diagnostic and statistical manual of mental disorders* (4th ed., text revision). Washington, DC: Author.

Beck, A. T., Ward, C., & Mendelson, M. (1961). An inventory of measuring depression. *Archives of General Psychiatry, 4,* 561–571.

Carson, V. B. (1994). *Bay area health care psychiatric home care manual.* Baltimore, MD: Bay Area Health Care.

Milling, L., & Martin, B. (1992). Depression and suicidal behavior in preadolescent children. *Handbook of clinical child psychology* (2nd ed.). New York: Wiley.

Purnell, L. D., & Paulanka, B. J. (1998). *Transcultural health care: A culturally competent approach.* Philadelphia: F. A. Davis.

Salazar, W. H. (1996). Management of depression in the outpatient office. *Medical Clinics of North America, 80,* 431–455.

Waldinger, R. J. (1997). *Psychiatry for medical students* (3rd ed.). Washington, DC: American Psychiatric Press.

Zung, W. W. K. (1965). A self-rating depression scale. *Archives of General Psychiatry, 12,* 63–70.

SUGGESTED READING

Depression Guideline Panel. (1993). *Depression in primary care: Volume 1, detection and diagnosis: Clinical practice guideline, No. 5.* (ACHPR Publication No. 93–0550). Rockville, MD: Author.

Hales, R. E., Yudofsky, S. C., & Talbott, J. A. (1999). *Textbook of psychiatry* (3rd ed.). Washington, DC: American Psychiatric Press.

Sarafolean, M. H. (2000). Depression in school-age children and adolescents. *A Pediatric Perspective, 9*(4), 1–4.

Shives, L. R., & Isaacs, A. (2002). *Basic concepts of psychiatric-mental health nursing* (5th ed.). Philadelphia: Lippincott.

Uphold, C. R., & Graham, M. V. (1994). *Clinical guidelines in family practice.* Gainesville, FL: Barmore Books.

Persistent Cough 14

Cindy Balkstra and Sandy Truesdell

INTRODUCTION

Though often trivialized by health care providers, persistent cough is a frequent cause of discomfort/disruption in people's lives. Although this process can take several months using a focused trial-and-error approach, persistent cough can be managed successfully in the majority of cases.

I. Definitions
   A. Acute and persistent (chronic) cough
      1. Acute cough lasts 3 to 4 weeks and usually follows a viral upper respiratory infection (i.e., common cold); only occasionally associated with life-threatening conditions such as pulmonary embolism
      2. Persistent (chronic) cough lasts for at least 8 weeks
   B. Cough as a reflex (See Table 14.1)
      1. Defense mechanism to help clear secretions and foreign material from the airways
      2. Components
         a. Cough or irritant receptors primarily found in the larynx, trachea, large bronchi; also present in the ear, sinuses, pharynx, diaphragm, pleura, stomach, pericardium.
         b. Receptors respond to both chemical and mechanical stimulation.
         c. Impulse travels to the brain via afferent neurons from the vagus, trigeminal, glossopharyngeal, and phrenic nerves.
         d. Cough center in the brain diffusely located in the medulla; not associated with the respiratory center. May be influenced by higher centers, which can cause cough to be voluntarily suppressed or initiated.

      e. Muscular activity achieved by stimulation of efferent neurons to the vagus, phrenic, intercostal, lumbar, trigeminal, facial, hypoglossal, and spinal motor nerves.

      f. Muscles involved include the diaphragm, intercostal, abdominal, bronchial, tracheal, accessory, and laryngeal.

3. Phases of an effective cough

      a. Inspiration of large volume of air (2.5 L) to increase intrathoracic pressure

      b. Closure of the glottis and vocal cords (entraps air in the lungs)

      c. Active contraction of the expiratory muscles (i.e., abdominal, intercostal) increases intrathoracic pressure

      d. Sudden opening of the glottis and vocal cords followed by extremely high expiratory flow rates (facilitates mucus removal) and narrowed central airways (dynamic compression of the airways increases the velocity of expiratory flow); essentially air under pressure in the lungs explodes outward

4. Factors of ineffective cough

      a. Altered cough mechanics, changes in the character of mucus, alterations in mucus clearance mechanism, medications, various medical diagnoses, such as neuromuscular conditions, cerebral vascular accident, and so forth

| Table 14.1 | Anatomy of a Cough Reflex | | | |

Receptors	Afferent Nerves	Cough Center	Efferent Nerves	Effector Organs
Larynx, trachea, bronchi, ear, canal, pleura, and stomach	Vagus	Diffusely located in medulla near the respiratory center: under control of higher centers	Vagus; phrenic; intercostals, and lumbar	Muscles of larynx and bronchi; diaphragm, intercostals, abdominal, and lumbar muscles
Nose and paranaseal sinuses	Trigeminal		Trigeminal, facial, hypoglossal, and accessory	Upper airways and accessory respiratory
Pharynx Pericardium, diaphragm	Glossopharyngeal Phrenic			

Corrao, W. M. (1996). Chronic persistent cough: diagnosis and treatment update. *Pediatric Annals, 25*(3), 162–168. Permission granted by Slack, Inc, Publisher.

II. Etiology
   A. Physical factors in persistent cough
      1. 85% of cases caused by postnasal drip syndrome (PNDS), asthma, and gastroesophageal reflux disease (GERD), or a combination of these problems
      2. Most frequent cause in adults is PNDS
      3. Second is asthma; third is GERD in adults <65 years of age
      4. Second is GERD; third is asthma in adults >65 years of age
      5. Asthma most frequent cause in children, followed by PNDS, then GERD
         a. Usually multicausal; thereby making treatment course difficult and prolonged
         b. Additional causes include nonasthmatic eosinophilic bronchitis, suppurative airway diseases (tracheitis, bronchitis, bronchiectasis, bronchiolitis), interstitial lung disease, cystic fibrosis, lung or throat cancer, sarcoidosis, chronic lung infections (i.e., post-viral, tuberculosis), fungal sinusitis, heart failure, aspiration, pertussis (especially adult recurrence), use of angiotensin-converting enzyme inhibitors (ACE-I) or other pharmaceutical agents
         c. In children other potential causes include recurrent viral or atypical infections, foreign body aspiration, congenital causes, dysmotile cilia syndrome, sequestration, bronchial cyst, compression of the airways by aberrant blood vessels, conditions altering the immune system
   B. Psychosocial factors
      1. Psychogenic cough
      2. Incidence greater in children, usually associated with underlying psychological problems
      3. No differentiating features
      4. All other causes should be excluded; 23% of referrals misdiagnosed
      5. Psychiatric therapy required
   C. Risk factors
      1. Smoking is most common risk factor, yet smokers rarely report the symptom.
      2. ACE-I causes onset of cough in 5%–20% of patients taking these drugs. Usually subsides within 1 week of discontinuing therapy.
      3. Lung infections due to malnutrition, poor social/financial supports, exposure to parasites/organisms or contagious diseases, lack of access to health care
      4. Often several risk factors involved
III. Pathophysiology
   A. Mechanical stimulation of the cough receptors in the upper airways such as with PNDS, bronchial tumors, inhaling irritants such as with smoking
   B. Inflammation of the airways such as in asthma, bronchitis, other respiratory infections and lung diseases, also with smoking, use of ACE-I

153

    C. Gross or microaspiration of gastric contents such as in GERD

    D. Afferent neural stimulation (most likely via the vagus nerve) as a result of gastric contents inciting a distal esophageal tracheobronchial reflex mechanism

  IV. Relevant theories (none known)

   V. Incidence

    A. Most common problem that causes patients to seek medical attention in the United States

    B. Accounts for 30 million office visits per year in the United States

    C. 14%–23% of nonsmokers report persistent cough

    D. 25% of 1/2 pack per day (ppd) smokers and 50% of 2 ppd smokers report persistent cough

    E. Cost estimated to exceed $1 billion (including over-the-counter and prescription medications)

    F. Contributes to the spread of infectious diseases

  VI. Considerations across the life span (see etiology)

 VII. Cultural considerations

    A. May significantly impact patient behavior in both seeking and following treatment

      1. Language or other cultural differences may limit the patient's access or willingness to seek treatment.

      2. Lifestyle changes such as dietary recommendations may not be culturally acceptable.

VIII. Complications/sequelae during vigorous coughing (see Table 14.2)

    A. Intrathoracic pressures reach up to 300 mm Hg

    B. Expiratory velocities go up to 28,000 cm/s or 500 miles/hour (85% of the speed of sound)

    C. Hemodynamic changes comparable to chest compressions

ASSESSMENT

   I. General concepts in assessing and managing persistent cough in immuno-competent adults

    A. Diagnostic algorithm

      1. Systematic evaluation of locations on the afferent limb of the cough reflex arc to determine etiology

      2. Includes history, physical exam, chest radiography, pulmonary function tests, and a variety of additional diagnostic studies

        a. Accurate diagnosis and effective treatment can occur in majority of cases

  II. History

    A. Symptom evaluation including character (barking, loose, productive, brassy, honking, single or repeated episodes), timing (onset, duration, associated activities), severity, aggravating and relieving factors, and complications (syncope, hemoptysis)

Table 14.2 | Complications of Cough

Cardiovascular

Arterial hypotension
Loss of consciousness
Rupture of subconjunctival, nasal, and anal veins
Dislodgement/malfunctioning of intravascular catheters
Bradyarrhythmias, tachyarrhythmias

Neurologic

Cough syncope
Headache
Cerebral air embolism CSF fluid rhinorrliea
Acute cervical radiculopathy
Malfunctioning ventriculoatial shunts
Seizures
Stroke due to vertebral artery dissection

GI

Gastroesophageal reflux events
1T.vdmthorax in peritoneal dialysis
Malfunction of gastrostomy button
Splenic rupture
Inguinal hernia

Genitourinary

Urinary incontinence
Inversion of bladder through urethra

Musculoskeletal

From asymptomatic elevations of serum creatine phosphokinase to rupture of rectus
    abdominis muscles
Rib fractures

Respiratory

Pulmonary interstitial emphysema, with potential risk of pocumalosis intestinalis,
    pneumomediastinum, pneumoperitoneum, pneumoretroperitoneum, pneumothorax,
    subcutaneous emphysema
Laryngeal trauma
Tracheobronchial trauma (e.g., bronchitis, bronchial rupture)
Exacerbation of asthma
Intercostal lung herniation

Miscellaneous

Petechiae and purpura
Disruption of surgical wounds
Constitutional symptoms
Lifestyle changes
Self-consciousness, hoarseness, dizziness
Fear of serious disease
Decrease in quality of life

The evidence from which this compilation has been derived consists of ease reports and descriptive
(Grade III) studies.

From: Irwin, R. S. et al. (1998). Managing cough as a defense mechanism and as a symptom: A
consensus panel report of the American College of Chest Physicians. *Chest, 114*(suppl. 2), 133–181.

B. Other associated factors
   1. Smoking behavior
   2. Exposure to irritants, smoke, or other allergens at home or work
   3. Known diagnosis of cardiopulmonary disease (see etiology)
   4. PNDS
      a. Mucus drainage, "runny nose"
      b. Throat clearing, mucus swallowing, dripping sensation in the back of the throat
      c. Allergies or sinus complaints
      d. Recent respiratory infection or flu-like symptoms
   5. Asthma
      a. Chest tightness, wheezing, or dyspnea
      b. Nocturnal cough
      c. Specific triggers for cough
      d. Family history of allergies, asthma, eczema
      e. Cough may be only symptom, especially in children
   6. GERD
      a. Heartburn, belching, sour taste in mouth, regurgitation; prominent in 6%–10% of patients with chronic cough
      b. Cough may be only symptom
      c. Symptoms may be clinically silent
   7. Underlying infection or malignancy
      a. Fever, chills, or night sweats
      b. Post-viral illness
      c. Bloody or foul-smelling green sputum
      d. Recent unintentional weight loss
   8. Medications
      a. ACE-I
      b. Beta-blockers (including eye drops)
      c. Miscellaneous: nitrofurantoin, amiodarone, others
      d. Improvement with use of decongestants and/or antihistamines
      e. Improvement with use of antacids or over-the-counter histamine 2 (H2) blockers
   9. Presence of additional symptoms such as chest pain, headaches, facial pain
      a. In patients greater than 50 years of age, investigate carefully for temporal arteritis
   10. Effect on patient's lifestyle
C. Pediatric history
   1. Neonatal
   2. Feeding
   3. Possibility of foreign body aspiration
   4. Allergies, eczema or presence of smoke, allergens or irritants in home/ daycare, including pets
   5. Sleep disorder
   6. Immunization record
   7. Medications

8. Family history of cystic fibrosis, tuberculosis, allergies, asthma, bronchitis, or chronic cough

II. Physical exam
   A. Evaluation of anatomic locations of receptors involved in cough reflex including nose, nasopharynx, and lungs
   B. Head and neck evaluation, including ear, nose, throat
      1. Pain on palpation over sinuses
      2. Watery, itchy eyes
      3. Drainage in posterior pharynx
      4. Nasal discharge
      5. Cobblestone appearance of oropharyngeal mucosa
      6. Mucus in oropharynx
   C. Chest evaluation
      1. Coarse crackles may indicate acute or chronic respiratory infection
      2. Fine crackles, especially at the bases, may indicate pulmonary edema
      3. Generalized wheezing may indicate asthma
      4. Isolated wheezing may indicate a tumor
      5. End-expiration wheezing may indicate airway obstruction
      6. Cardiac findings point to a need for more intensive cardiac work-up
   D. Skin and extremities evaluation
      1. Presence of clubbing may indicate chronic disease or carcinoma
      2. Rheumatic deformities may indicate interstitial lung disease
   E. Adenopathy at any site should trigger an evaluation for malignancy

III. Diagnostic tests
   A. Sputum analysis for microbiology and/or cytology
   B. Chest and/or sinus radiography
   C. Spirometry/pulmonary function tests
   D. Computerized tomography scan of chest and/or sinuses
   E. Blood work, such as complete blood count (CBC)
   F. Allergy testing
   G. Pulse oximetry or arterial blood gas
   H. Esophageal testing
      1. 24 hour pH probe
      2. Barium swallow (modified)
      3. Esophagoscopy
      4. Esophageal motility
   I. Flexible bronchoscopy
   J. Noninvasive cardiac studies

COMMON THERAPEUTIC MODALITIES

I. Antitussive therapy directed at causes
   A. Treatment of underlying infection, disease process, or malignancy
   B. Smoking cessation counseling

C. Environmental control measures

D. Medication review to exclude known triggers such as beta-blockers and ACE-Is

E. PNDS
   1. Nonallergic and postviral rhinitis best treated with older generation antihistamine/decongestant combinations.
      a. Ipratropium bromide (Atrovent) nasal spray reasonable alternative when above contraindicated
   2. Allergic rhinitis best treated with nasal steroids or cromolyn in combination with newer generation (nonsedating) antihistamines.
   3. Vasomotor rhinitis responds well to ipratropium bromide (Atrovent) and/or older generation antihistamine/decongestant combinations.
   4. Sinusitis requires antibiotics; nasal steroids and/or saline nasal irrigations may also be helpful.
   5. Older generation antihistamine/decongestant combinations can be added to the treatment as needed.
   6. Sinus surgery may be an option.
   7. Consider aspirin therapy for recurrent nonallergic sinusitis with nasal polyps.

F. Asthma (see chapter 16 "Asthma and Allergies")

G. GERD
   1. Treatment of cough may take months to be effective.
      a. Conservative measures—should not be ignored
         i. Weight reduction; increase activity
         ii. Low-fat (<30%), high-protein diet
         iii. Smaller meals
         iv. Avoid food/fluids that aggravate symptoms, that is, alcohol, caffeine, citrus, mint
         v. Remain in a vertical position (sitting or standing) after eating/drinking for at least 3 hours
         vi. Elevate head of bed on 4–6 inch blocks
         vii. Over-the-counter antacids, H2 blockers
         viii. Smoking cessation
   2. H2 blockers
   3. Proton-pump inhibitors
   4. Prokinetic agents
   5. Antireflux surgery (i.e., fundoplication, crural tightening, hiatal hernia repair)
   6. Consider empiric antireflux trial even without esophageal GERD symptoms in chronic persistent cough patients

II. General antitussive therapy
   A. Indicated while specific therapy is beginning to take effect, if the cause of cough cannot be determined, or if it is not treatable, such as late-stage lung cancer
   B. Pharmacologic agents found to be effective either alone or in combination; most often used as oral, inhaled, nebulized, or topical preparations

1. Anticholinergics such as ipratropium bromide (Atrovent) reduce smooth muscle spasms (i.e. bronchial) and suppress or decrease secretions.
2. Bronchodilators such as beta 2 agonists (Albuterol) relax bronchial smooth muscle by action on beta2-receptors.
3. Antihistamines such as diphenhydramine (Benadryl) and fexofenadine (Allegra) prevent or reduce increased capillary permeability (i.e., decrease edema, itching) and bronchospasm.
4. Decongestant sympathomimetic drugs such as pseudoephedrine (Sudafed) and phenylephrine (Neo-synephrine) work on the nasal mucosa by stimulating both alpha- and beta-adrenergic receptors or alpha-adrenergic receptors alone, as well as indirectly stimulating release of norepinephrine from storage sites. The end result is pronounced vasoconstriction in the nasal passages.
5. Corticosteroids reduce and control inflammation; inhaled such as fluticasone (Flovent) or intranasal (Flonase) preferred.
6. Non-narcotic antitussives containing dextromethorphan (Robitussin) selectively depress the cough center in the medulla.
7. Opiate agonists such as morphine, codeine, hydromorphone (Dilaudid), and oxycodone (Oxycontin) depress the cough center in the medulla. Antitussive effects occur at doses lower than those required for analgesia.
8. Topical anesthetizing agents such as benzonatate and viscous lidocaine act by numbing the stretch receptors of the vagal afferent fibers in the bronchi, alveoli, and pleura. Benzonatate also suppresses transmission of the cough reflex at the medulla.
9. Miscellaneous agents such as carbamazepine (Tegretol) and chlorpromazine (Thorazine) exert anti-cholinergic effects and serve to reduce irritation to the diaphragm.

C. Alternative therapies
   1. Herbal products such as slippery elm and plantain contain large amounts of mucilage that form a viscous solution able to coat the mucous membranes of the pharynx, larynx, and trachea. Protection from mechanical irritation of the cough receptors in these areas reduces the cough. The mucilage is not absorbed, so there are little or no side effects.

III. Protussive therapy
   A. Pharmacologic agents found to be effective either alone or in combination with other medications
      1. Expectorants such as guaifenesin (Humibid) and terpin hydrate act by increasing respiratory tract fluid, liquifying sputum, and facilitating expectoration by stimulating respiratory tract secretory glands.
   B. Non-pharmacologic therapies
      1. Chest physical therapy. A technique to enhance removal of secretions from the airways. This includes bronchial drainage, chest percussion, and vibration with deep breathing exercises.

INTERVENTIONS AND OUTCOMES

I. General measures
   A. Splinting of chest using a soft pillow
   B. Salt water gargle or nasal irrigation
   C. Hot beverages such as tea with lemon/honey
   D. Adequate fluid intake
   E. Cough drops or lozenges
   F. Over-the-counter analgesics
II. Patient/family education
   A. Possible causes of cough
   B. Medications
   C. Signs or symptoms to report
   D. Controlled coughing technique
   E. Treatment plan may include professional environmental evaluation of home and/or work setting
   F. Length of time needed for treatment plan to be effective
   G. Self-management methods and strategies
      1. Assessment of severity using a visual analog scale or other measuring tool
      2. Tobacco cessation (refer to chapter 30 "Tobacco and Other Substance Abuse")
   H. Environmental modifications/elimination of bronchial irritants
III. Patient outcomes
   A. Resolution of cough
   B. Improvement in quality of life
      1. Scores on survey tools, such as, Sickness Impact Profile, SF36, others
      2. Subjective responses
   C. Decrease in number of outpatient visits following resolution of cough
   D. Decreased amount of dollars spent on therapies once symptom resolved
   E. Improved understanding of symptom, cause, treatment and management
      1. Measured by results of various interventions such as weight reduction for GERD

HOME CARE CONSIDERATIONS

I. Equipment—specific to etiology
II. Caregiver considerations
   A. Recognition of patient's symptom and etiology
   B. Follow-through with treatment plan, management strategies such as dietary recommendations and environmental control measures
   C. Support and patience while waiting for the treatment(s) to take effect
      1. Asthma: 6–8 weeks
      2. GERD: 2–6 months or longer

3. Smoking cessation: at least 4 weeks
4. Use of angiotensin-converting enzyme inhibitor (ACE-I): 1–4 weeks is the amount of time off the drug. If the cough goes away then the ACE-I was the cause.

D. Close monitoring and gathering of information to assist with the diagnosis in children

E. Psychogenic cough (rare)
1. Psychological counseling

III. Social supports
A. Support groups for specific health disorders or issues
1. Tobacco cessation
2. Cancer
3. Asthma
4. Chronic obstructive pulmonary disease (COPD)
B. National organizations with local branches
1. American Lung Association
2. American Cancer Society

SUGGESTED READINGS

Corrao, W. M. (1996). Chronic persistent cough: diagnosis and treatment update. *Pediatric Annals, 25*(3), 162–168.

Daigle, K. L., & Cloutier, M. M. (2000). Evaluation and management of chronic cough in children. *Clinical Pulmonary Medicine, 7*(3), 134–139.

French, C. L., Irwin, R. S., Curley, F. J., & Krikorian, C. J. (1998). Impact of chronic cough on quality of life. *Archives of Internal Medicine, 158,* 1657–1661.

Gallagher, R. (1997). Use of herbal preparations for intractable cough. *Journal of Pain and Symptom Management, 14*(1), 1–2.

Harding, S. M. (2003). Chronic cough: practical considerations. *Chest, 123,* 659–660.

Hellmann, D. B. (2002). Temporal arteritis: A cough, toothache, and tongue infarction. *Journal of the American Medical Association, 287,* 2996–3000.

Irwin, R. S., Boulet, L., Cloutier, M. M., Fuller, R., Gold, P. M., Hoffstien, V., et al. (1998). Managing cough as a defense mechanism and as a symptom: A consensus panel report of the American College of Chest Physicians. *Chest, 114*(Suppl 2), 133–181.

Irwin, R. S., Corrao, W. M., & Pratter, M. R. (1981). Chronic persistent cough in the adult: The spectrum and frequency of causes and successful outcome of specific therapy. *American Review of Respiratory Diseases, 123,* 413–417.

Irwin, R. S., & Curley, F. J. (1991). The treatment of cough: A comprehensive review. *Chest, 99,* 1477–1484.

Irwin, R. S., Curley, F. J., & French, C. L. (1990). Chronic cough: The spectrum and frequency of causes, key components of the diagnostic evaluation, and outcome of specific therapy. *American Review of Respiratory Diseases, 141,* 640–647.

Irwin, R. S., French, C. L., Curley, F. J., Zawacki, J. K., & Bennett, F. (1993). Chronic cough due to gastroesophageal reflux: Clinical, diagnostic, and pathogenetic aspects. *Chest, 104,* 1511–1517.

Irwin, R. S., & Madison, J. M. (2000). The diagnosis and treatment of cough. *New England Journal of Medicine, 343,* 1715–1721.

Irwin, R. S., & Madison, J. M. (2002). The persistently troublesome cough. *American Journal of Respiratory and Critical Care Medicine, 165,* 1469–1474.

Mello, C. J., Irwin, R. S., & Curley, F. J. (1996). Predictive values of the character, timing, and complications of chronic cough in diagnosing its cause. *Archives of Internal Medicine, 156,* 997–1003.

Miller, M. M., McGrath, K. G., & Patterson, R. (1998). Malignant cough equivalent asthma: Definition and case reports. *Annals of Allergy, Asthma and Immunology, 80,* 345–351.

Murry, T. (1998). Chronic cough: In search of the etiology. *Seminars in Speech and Language, 19*(1), 83–91.

Poe, R. H., Harder, R. V., Israel, R. H., & Kallay, M. C. (1989). Chronic persistent cough: Experience in diagnosis and outcome using an anatomic diagnostic protocol. *Chest, 95,* 723–728.

Poe, R. H., & Israel, R. H. (1999). Evaluating chronic cough: Key points from the ACCP guidelines. *The Journal of Respiratory Diseases, 20*(5), 343–347.

Poe, R. H., & Kallay, M. C. (2003). Chronic cough and gastroesophageal reflux disease. *Chest, 123,* 679–684.

Pratter, M. R., Bartter, T., Akers, S., & DuBois, J. (1993). An algorithmic approach to chronic cough. *Annals of Internal Medicine, 119,* 977–983.

Schaefer, D. P., & Irwin, R. S. (2003). Unsuspected bacterial suppurative disease of the airways presenting as chronic cough. *The American Journal of Medicine, 114,* 602–606.

Smyrnios, N. A., Irwin, R. S., Curley, F. J., & French, C. L. (1998). From a prospective study of chronic cough: Diagnostic and therapeutic aspects in older adults. *Archives of Internal Medicine, 158,* 1222–1228.

Sullivan, N. C. (1997). Assessment and management of persistent cough in adults. *Clinical Excellence for Nurse Practitioners, 1,* 417–422.

Common Respiratory Diseases and Disorders

IV

Emphysema and Chronic Bronchitis

15

Mary Beth Parr

INTRODUCTION

Emphysema and chronic bronchitis belong to a category of diseases called obstructive disease. Cough, sputum production, dyspnea, airflow limitation that is not fully reversible, and impaired gas exchange characterize chronic obstructive pulmonary disease (COPD). The patient has difficulty getting air out of the lung, which leads to air trapping and hyperinflation. Emphysema is defined in terms of anatomic pathology and chronic bronchitis in clinical terms. The National Heart Lung and Blood Institute defines COPD as a disease state characterized by airflow limitation that is not fully reversible. The airflow limitation is usually both progressive and associated with an abnormal inflammatory response of the lungs to noxious particles or gases.

I. Emphysema
   A. Definition
      1. Abnormal permanent enlargement of the airspaces distal to terminal bronchioles
      2. Breakdown of alveolar interstitium due to alteration in the protease-antiprotease balance in the lower airways without obvious fibrosis
      3. Irreversible condition, which leads to poor gas exchange—low O_2 and increased CO_2
      4. Lungs damaged by emphysema gradually lose their elastic recoil
      5. Airways become floppy and collapse on exhalation
   B. Etiology of emphysema
      1. Exposure to tobacco smoke due to smoking—#1 preventable cause
      2. Secondhand smoke or passive smoking: nitric oxide, component of smoke, is a potent bronchodilator

3. Ambient air pollution
4. Alpha₁-antitrypsin deficiency: genetic abnormality accounts for less than 1% of COPD

C. Pathophysiology of emphysema

1. Formation of bullae: Destruction of acinar sacs produces 1–2 cm air-filled sacs called bullae. When a bullae ruptures it is called a *bleb*.
2. Loss of lung elasticity: Destruction of lung tissue causes loss of elastic recoil.
3. Lung hyperinflation: Lung does not recoil upon expiration so it remains inflated at the end of expiration. The residual volume (RV) is increased, which results in barrel chest deformity.
4. Air trapping and airway collapse: Airways are prone to collapse due to loss of elastic recoil.
5. These physiologic conditions lead to
   a. Dead space: with alveolar destruction and collapse, and bullae formation, the inspired air may not come in contact with the capillary blood flow with results in V/Q mismatch (ventilation/perfusion).
   b. Increased work of breathing: increased minute ventilation to compensate for lung destruction.

II. Chronic bronchitis

A. Definition

1. Inflammation of the bronchi, which leads to increased mucus production.
2. Presence of productive cough for 3 months for 2 consecutive years and other causes of chronic cough have been excluded.
3. American Thoracic Society defines bronchitis as non-neoplastic disorder of structure or function of the bronchi resulting from infectious or noninfectious irritation.

B. Etiology of chronic bronchitis

1. Exposure to tobacco smoke due to cigarette smoking
2. Secondhand smoke or passive smoking
3. Ambient air pollution and occupational irritants
4. Sex, race, and socioeconomic status: higher prevalence of respiratory symptoms in men, higher mortality rates in whites, and higher morbidity and mortality in blue-collar workers.
5. Occupational dusts and chemicals: vapors, irritants and fumes, particulate matter, organic dust

C. Pathophysiology

1. Mucus hypersecretion: increased size and number of submucous glands in the large bronchi. The increase of mucous leads to airway narrowing and airway obstruction.
2. In smaller airways, chronic inflammation leads to repeated cycles of injury and repair of airways and therefore scar tissue formation and narrowing airways
3. Reduction of alveolar ventilation due to increased secretions

    4. Expiratory airflow limitation

    5. Breathlessness due to airway narrowing and bronchoconstriction

D. Incidence: COPD is fourth leading cause of death in the United States and fourth leading cause of death in the world. Sources vary on the number of Americans affected, with a range of 5.4 to 15 million Americans. COPD is the most rapidly rising cause of death among Americans over 65 and this death rate has increased over 20% in the last decade. COPD is a major financial burden to society with costs upward of $15 million.

    1. Mortality rose 32.9% between 1979 and 1991. After the age of 45, COPD becomes the fourth or fifth leading cause of death in the United States.

    2. Morbidity increases with age and is greater in men than women. Morbidity is highest in countries where cigarette smoking has been or still is very common.

    3. Men and women have similar COPD mortality rates until age 55, then rate in men rises and at age 70, mortality more than doubles in men.

    4. Increases in mortality and morbidity are striking in older adults who continue to smoke.

    5. Sex, race, and socioeconomic status: Higher prevalence of respiratory symptoms in men; higher mortality rates in whites; and higher morbidity and mortality in blue-collar workers.

E. Considerations across the life span for COPD

    1. In nonsmokers the FEV_1 declines beginning at age 35. The rate of decline is steeper for smokers and steepest for heavier smokers. Those with COPD have frequent chest infections and added to decreased lung volume with age and smoking; older patients have increased difficulty breathing.

F. Complications/sequelae for COPD

    1. Acute exacerbation of chronic bronchitis (AECB): Infection— increased thick secretions increase the work of breathing. If the work of breathing becomes too high the patient may require mechanical ventilation.

        a. Dyspnea

        b. Cor pulmonale

        c. Respiratory failure

        d. Pneumothorax

        e. Bronchiectasis: recurrent bouts of bronchitis

        f. Decreased quality of life and functional status

        g. Decreased independence due to difficulty breathing and increased oxygen demands resulting in fatigue

        h. Assistance with activities of daily living (ADLs) as disease progresses

        i. Death

II. Assessment

A. History

    1. Exposure to risk factors

    2. Past medical history including asthma, allergy sinusitis, or nasal polyps

3. Family history of COPD or other chronic respiratory disease
4. Chronic cough: length of time, daily or intermittent, seldom nocturnal
5. Chronic sputum production: characteristics of sputum, change with the season, amount produced
6. Dyspnea that is progressive, persistent, worse with exercise, worse during respiratory infections
7. History of exposure to tobacco smoke, occupational dusts and chemicals, smoke from home cooking and heating fuels
8. Smoking history: pack years (number of packs per day multiplied by number of years smoking)
9. Age when first noticed symptoms
10. Current functional status and ability to perform ADLs
11. Limitation of activities
12. Pneumonia and other respiratory illnesses
13. Use of oxygen: liter flow and years of usage
14. Weight loss or weight gain
15. Sleep pattern and position during sleep: number of pillows used

B. Potential abnormal physical exam findings (will vary based on severity of illness)
1. Assessment of severity based on level of symptoms (see Table 15.1)
2. Severity of spirometric abnormalities
3. Characteristics of respiratory pattern: rate, depth, symmetry, and synchrony; breathlessness due to airway narrowing and broncho-constriction
4. Use of pursed lip breathing
5. Breath sounds: normal and adventitious: crackles, rhonchi and wheezes; hyperresonant lung fields; may be distant due to hyperinflation
6. Cough due to increased sputum production: usually worse in the morning
7. Sputum production: color, amount; usually increased with chronic bronchitis
8. Shortness of breath with speech: two or three words per breath
9. Dyspnea on exertion
10. Barrel chest as a result of increased RV
11. Use of accessory muscles
12. Resting pulse oximetry with potential drop with activity
13. Presence of complications such as respiratory failure and right heart failure
14. Cor pulmonale: right-sided heart failure to include edema, heart rate, blood pressure, jugular venous pressure (JVP)
15. Check for presence of murmurs, gallops, rubs, lifts, heaves, and/or thrills
16. Fluid retention and edema
17. Overall appearance: thin with muscle wasting and barrel chest *or* overweight with barrel chest

Table 15.1	Stages of COPD Based on The Global Initiative for Chronic Obstructive Lung Disease

Stage	Degree of COPD	Status of Airflow Postbronchodilator FEV_1 (forced expiratory volume in 1 second)
0	At Risk	normal spirometry chronic symptoms—cough and sputum production
I	Mild COPD	$FEV_1/FVC < 70\%$, $FEV_1 \geq 80\%$ predicted with or without chronic symptoms
II	Moderate COPD	$FEV_1/FVC < 70\%$, $50\% \leq FEV_1 < 80\%$ predicted with or without chronic symptoms
III	Severe COPD	$FEV_1/FVC < 70\%$, $30\% \leq FEV_1$ or $< 50\%$ predicted plus respiratory failure or right heart failure
IV	Very Severe COPD	$FEV_1/FVC < 70\%$ $FEV_1 < 30\%$ predicted or $FEV_1 < 50\%$ predicted plus chronic respiratory failure

The stages of COPD assist the clinician in a very general approach to management.

18. Enlarged abdominal girth or cachetic appearance
19. Enlarged liver with right-sided heart failure
20. Posture: hunched over with rolled shoulders
21. Pallor skin color
22. Generalized edema

B. Diagnostic tests
   1. Chest X-ray: air trapping; hyperinflation; increased A-P diameter; flattened diaphragms
   2. Postbronchodilator FEV_1
   3. Pulmonary function test: show decreased FEV_1 (up to 50% loss) and decreased FEF 25%–75%; increased functional residual capacity (FRC) due to air trapping and hyperinflation
   4. Arterial blood gases: may show increased CO_2 due to inability to expel all of the air (air trapping) and low O_2 levels due to ventilation/perfusion mismatch
   5. Assess dyspnea using a valid tool such as the Modified Borg scale or the Visual Analog Scale
   6. Oxygen saturation at rest and with activity
   7. Quality-of-life measure: baseline measurement
   8. Six-minute walk distance: baseline measurement

III. Therapeutic modalities (See chapter 35, respiratory pharmacology; chapter 39, pulmonary rehabilitation; chapter 30, tobacco and other substance abuse; and chapter 40, self-care management strategies for additional information)

A. Initial care and management

1. Effective management must include: assess and monitor disease, reduce risk factors, manage stable COPD, manage exacerbations.

2. Goals include improvement in gas exchange, airway clearance, improved breathing pattern, independent self care, improved activity tolerance.

3. Bronchodilators: central to symptomatic management of COPD. As needed or on regular basis. Inhaled is preferred and choice between Beta2 agonists, anticholinergic, theophylline, or combination therapy. Opens constricted airways, which helps to improve gas exchange and promote secretion removal. Current recommendations include long acting bronchodilators, which are more effective and convenient but more expensive.

4. Anticholingerics produce local, site-specific effects on the larger central airways. Also abolish vagally mediated reflex bronchospasm triggered by cigarette smoke, dusts, cold air, and range of inflammatory mediators.

5. Glucocorticosteroids: Regular treatment does not modify long-term decline of FEV_1 but they are appropriate for symptomatic COPD patients with $FEV_1 < 50\%$.

6. Oxygen: to maintain adequate oxygenation levels while not increasing CO_2 levels.

7. Airway clearance techniques such as: controlled cough and deep breathing, Flutter valve, Thairpy vest, and PEP therapy.

8. Hydration: to keep secretions thin and minimal, 6–8 glasses of water/day.

9. Nutrition: maintain physical condition with increased fats and decreased carbohydrates in order to decrease CO_2 production.

10. Patient teaching: metered dose inhaler use, turbohalers, panic control, relaxation techniques, cough control, pursed lip breathing, diaphragmatic breathing energy conservation, and environmental control to avoid irritants.

11. Dyspnea management strategies

12. Antibiotics: used when secretions become infected. COPD patients are encouraged to seek treatment early.

13. Smoking cessation

14. Relaxation techniques

15. Exercise conditioning

16. Mechanical ventilation in severe disease

17. Tracheostomy tube may be necessary if mechanical ventilation is long term or inadequate/ineffective cough for secretion removal.

B. Continued care and rehabilitation
   1. Smoking cessation: Addiction issues
      Smoking is addicting and this must be addressed in order to have success with smoking cessation.
   2. Pulmonary rehabilitation: educational and exercise program that trains and reconditions the patient along with the pulmonary muscles.
   3. Reinforce MDI correct use.
   4. Advance directives: Discuss wishes with family, physician and nurse practitioner and health care providers.
   5. Annual flu shot.
   6. Pneumonia vaccination: once every 6 years.
   7. Avoid others with cold and flu during high flu season. Stress importance of good hand washing.
   8. Consider referral for lung volume reduction surgery (LVRS) or lung transplant when appropriate. Still is unproven palliative surgical procedure. In LVRS, the size of the lungs is reduced and in theory, makes breathing easier.
   9. Bullectomy surgery: resection of bulla. In carefully selected patients, this procedure is effective in reducing dyspnea and improving lung function.
II. Home care considerations
   A. Oxygen
   B. Durable medical equipment
   C. Energy conservation
   D. Assistance with ADLs: family members and/or hired help
   E. Pulmonary rehabilitation and maintenance group
   F. Transportation
   G. Travel

WEB SITES

Agency on Healthcare Policy and Research (smoking cessation guidelines): http://www.ahcpr.gov
American Association of Cardiac and Pulmonary Rehabilitation: http://www.aacvpr.org
American Thoracic Society: http://www.thoracic.org
COPD Research Registry: http://www.COPDFoundation.org
Emphysema foundation (patient education): http://www.emphysema.net
European Respiratory Society: http://dev.ersnet.org
National Center for Tobacco Intervention: http://www.con.ohio-state.edu/tobacco
National Emphysema Treatment Trial: http://www.nhlbi.nih.gov/health/prof/lung/nett/lvrsweb.htm
National Heart Lung and Blood Institute: http://www.nhlbi.nih.gov
Respiratory Nursing Society: http://www.respiratorynursingsociety.org

SUGGESTED READINGS

American Thoracic Society Board of Directors. (1995). Standards for the diagnosis and care of patients with chronic obstructive pulmonary disease. *American Journal of Respiratory and Critical Care Medicine*, 152, S77–S120.

Barnes, P. J., Pedersen, S., & Busse, W. W. (1998). Efficacy and safety of inhaled corticosteriods. *American Journal of Respiratory and Critical Care Medicine*, 157, S1–S53.

Berry, M. J., & Walschlager, S. A. (1998). Exercise training and chronic obstructive pulmonary disease: past and future research directions. *Journal of Cardio-pulmonary Rehabilitation*, 18, 181–191.

Cole, T. K. (2001). Smoking cessation in the hospitalized patient using the transtheoretical model of behavior change. *Heart & Lung*, 30, 148–158.

Cook, D., Guyatt, G., Wong, E., Goldstein, R., Bedard, M., Austin, P., et al. (2001). Regular verses as-needed short acting inhaled B-Agonist therapy for chronic obstructive pulmonary disease. *American Journal of Respiratory and Critical Care Medicine*, 163, 85–90.

Dasgupta, A., & Mauer, J. (1999). Late-stage emphysema: When medical therapy fails. *Cleveland Clinic Journal of Medicine*, 66, 415–425.

Dean-Baar, S. L., Geiger-Bronsky, M., Gift, A., & Hagarty, E. (Eds.). (1994). *Standards and statement on the scope of respiratory nursing practice*. Washington, DC: American Nurses Publishing.

Ferguson, G. T. (1998). Management of COPD. *Postgraduate Medicine*, 103, 129–141.

GOLD. (2003). Global initiative for chronic obstructive pulmonary disease. NHL-BI/WHO, NIH. Retrieved from www.goldcopd.com

Grossman, R. F. (1998). The value of antibiotics and the outcomes of antibiotic therapy in exacerbations of COPD. *Chest*, 113, 249S–255S.

Kanner, R. E., Connett, J. E., Williams, D. E., & Buist, A. S. (1999). Effects of randomized assignment to a smoking cessation intervention and changes in smoking habits on respiratory symptoms in smokers with early chronic obstructive pulmonary disease: The Lung Health Study. *American Journal of Medicicne*, 106, 410–416.

Mahler, D. A. (1998). Pulmonary rehabilitation. *Chest*, 113, 263S–268S.

Man, S. F., McAlister, F. A., Anthonisen, N. R., & Sin, D. D. (2003). Contemporary management of chronic obstructive pulmonary disease. *Journal of American Medical Association*, 290, 2313–2316.

Matza, M. L., Balkstra, C. R., & Zugcic, M. (2001). Dyspnea near the end of life: An excerpt for the upcoming RNS 11th annual conference. *Heart & Lung*, 30, 164–165.

McFarland, G. K., & McFarlane, E. A. (1997). *Nursing diagnosis and intervention: Planning for patient care*. St. Louis, MO: Mosby.

O'Brien, G. M., & Criner, G. J. (1998). Surgery for severe COPD. *Postgraduate Medicine*, 103, 179–202.

Perry, T. L. (1998). Supportive therapy in COPD. *Chest*, 113, 256S–262S.

Rennard, S. I. (1998). COPD: Overview of definitions, epidemiology and factors influencing its development. *Chest, 113,* 235S–241S.

Senior, R. M., & Anthonisen, N. R. (1998). Chronic obstructive pulmonary disease. *American Journal of Respiratory and Critical Care Medicine, 157,* S139–S147.

Sin, D. D., McAlister, F. A., Man, S. F., & Anthonisen, N. R. (2003). Contemporary management of chronic obstructive pulmonary disease. *Journal of the American Medical Association, 290,* 2301–2312.

Wilson, B. A., Shannon, M. T., & Stang, S. L. (2002). *Nurse's drug guide.* Upper Saddle River, NJ: Prentice Hall.

Wilson, R. (1998). The role of infection in COPD. *Chest, 113,* 242S–248S.

Asthma and Allergies

16

Barbara Velsor-Friedrich and Susan Janson-Bjerklie

INTRODUCTION

Asthma is an extremely common chronic inflammatory disorder of the airways. Asthma sometimes coexists with allergies but not all people with allergies have asthma nor is the reverse true. With diligent management, asthma can be a well-controlled chronic disorder.

I. Definitions
   A. Asthma
      1. Asthma is a chronic inflammatory disorder of the airways in which many cells and cellular elements play a role.
      2. In susceptible individuals, inflammation causes recurrent episodes of wheezing, breathlessness, chest tightness, and coughing particularly at night, early morning, or with exercise. These symptom episodes are associated with widespread but variable airflow obstruction and are often reversible spontaneously or with treatment.
   B. Atopy
      1. The genetic predisposition for the development of an IgE-mediated response to common aeroallergens. It is the strongest identifiable predisposing factor for development of asthma.
      2. Atopy is found in 30%–50% of the general population worldwide and frequently found in the absence of asthma.
II. Etiology
   A. Asthma often begins in childhood, frequently in association with atopy. IgE antibodies and airway cells are sensitized and become activated when exposed to certain antigens.
   B. Family history of allergy in young children with wheezing is strongly associated with continuing asthma.

175

C. Approximately 70%–90% of children with asthma over the age of 5 years have some allergy (eczema, chronic rhinitis, and positive allergy; American Academy of Allergy, Asthma, and Immunology [AAAAI], 1999).

D. Asthma can occur at any time in life.

E. In some adults, no family history of allergy or IgE antibodies are detected but these adults with asthma often have coexisting sinusitis, nasal polyps, and sensitivity to aspirin or nonsteroidal anti-inflammatory drugs. The inflammatory process in this type of adult-onset asthma is similar to atopic asthma.

III. Pathophysiology

   A. Airflow obstruction in asthma is caused by
      1. Acute bronchoconstriction resulting from smooth muscle contraction
      2. Airway mucosal edema caused by increased microvascular permeability secondary to released mediators
      3. Chronic mucus plug formation
      4. Airway remodeling apparently related to structural changes in the airway matrix

   B. Airways are hyperresponsive, developing an exaggerated bronchoconstrictor response to a wide variety of stimuli.

   C. Acute and late phase responses to allergen
      1. Acute bronchoconstriction induced by allergen results from IgE-dependent release of mediators (histamine, tryptase, leukotrienes, and prostaglandins) from the airway mast cell. Aspirin and nonsteroidal anti-inflammatory drugs can also cause a non-IgE mediated acute bronchoconstriction. Other stimuli causing a similar acute bronchoconstriction include exercise, cold air, and irritants.
      2. A late response sometimes occurs several hours later characterized by a reoccurrence of bronchoconstriction, airway swelling, and inflammation marked by the presence of eosinophils and release of inflammatory cytokines. These cytokines cause airway inflammation with mucosal swelling, resulting airflow obstruction. The late response may result in chronic inflammation.

IV. Prevalence of asthma and allergies

   A. In the United States, asthma affects nearly 20 million people; 18 million are adults (Mannino et al., 2001).

   B. Age: 10.8 million asthmatic persons are under the age of 45; 8 million are 34 years or younger; 1.5 million are 65 years and older.

   C. Gender: Prevalence is higher among females after puberty. Women constitute 60% of the 18 million adults with asthma.

   D. Minority status: Prevalence is higher among ethnic minority populations. Puerto Rican Hispanics have the highest prevalence followed by African Americans.

   E. Socioeconomic status: Asthma prevalence is higher among low-income groups.

F. Global: Prevalence worldwide in children varies from zero in some countries to 30% in others. However, most verified prevalence information is from Western developed countries.

V. Considerations across the life span

A. Pediatric

1. Asthma in infants and children is very common and is often misdiagnosed and undertreated. It is the most common chronic illness in childhood and is often under diagnosed in preschool children.

2. Diagnosis of asthma in infants may be confirmed by evaluation of response to a trial of inhaled bronchodilators and anti-inflammatory medications.

3. 50%–80% of children with asthma develop symptoms before the fifth birthday. The most common cause of asthma symptoms in children under 5 years is viral respiratory infection.

4. Infants and young children who require treatment with bronchodilators more than two times per week should be given anti-inflammatory therapy, preferably inhaled corticosteroid, because over time, changes in the airway may become incompletely reversible due to airway remodeling (Child Asthma Management Program [CAMP], 2000). Sustained release theophylline is not recommended as an alternative long-term control medication for young children with mild persistent asthma.

5. Higher rates of asthma-related ER visits, hospitalizations, and mortality are associated with children who live in poverty and/or inner cities (AAAAI, 1999).

6. Poorly controlled asthma is the most frequent cause of school absences and can lead to negative effects on grades, academic achievement, self-esteem, and future success (AAAAI, 1999).

7. Active participation in sports, physical activities, exercise should be encouraged.

8. A written asthma management plan should be sent to the student's school and discussed with key school personnel.

B. Pregnancy

1. Poorly controlled asthma during pregnancy can result in increased perinatal mortality, prematurity, and low birth weight.

2. It is essential to maintain adequate lung function and oxygenation of the mother by maintaining asthma control to ensure adequate oxygen supply to the fetus.

3. Maternal smoking significantly increases the likelihood of wheezing in childhood.

4. Many asthma drugs are safe except brompheniramine, epinephrine, and alpha-adrenergic agents. Other drugs that pose a potential risk to the fetus are decongestants (except pseudoephedrine), antibiotics (tetracycline, sulfonamides, and ciprofloxacin), live virus vaccines, immunotherapy, and iodides. Always check the risk classification of medications for teratogenicity.

C. Elderly
1. Chronic bronchitis/emphysema may coexist with asthma. A trial of corticosteroids will determine the reversibility of airflow obstruction.
2. Some asthma medications may aggravate coexisting cardiac disease or osteoporosis.
3. There is increased risk of potential adverse drug/disease interaction, for example, aspirin, beta-blockers.
4. Treatment with inhaled corticosteroids may be essential to control asthma but concurrent treatment with calcium supplements and vitamin D and estrogen replacement (when appropriate) are recommended.

VI. Complications/sequelae
A. Undertreated and uncontrolled asthma results in increased morbidity and mortality. There are approximately 5,000 deaths per year, hundreds of thousands of hospitalizations annually, and millions of school absences and days of restricted activity due to asthma each year.
B. 85% of all asthma deaths occur in those 35 years and younger.
C. Annually there are nearly 2 million emergency department visits for asthma with African Americans having consistently greater numbers of visits than whites.
D. Continued exposure to irritants and allergens to which asthmatic patients are sensitive will increase asthma symptoms and continue to precipitate asthma exacerbations.
1. Allergens (factors that cause an IgE-mediated response) include animal dander, house dust mite, cockroach, mold, pollens, fungi.
2. Irritants include environmental tobacco smoke, wood smoke, bleach and household cleaners, perfumes, paint fumes, air pollution, and so forth.
E. Adult patients with severe persistent asthma, nasal polyps, or sensitivity to aspirin are at risk for severe or fatal exacerbations if exposed to aspirin or nonsteroidal anti-inflammatory drugs.
F. Chronic rhinitis, sinusitis, and gastroesophageal reflux may worsen asthma, making it more difficult to control. Therefore, these conditions should be treated.
G. Chronic persistent airway inflammation that is undertreated may result in airway remodeling and fixed airflow obstruction in susceptible individuals.

ASSESSMENT

I. History
A. History of present illness: Presence of symptoms of cough (coughing may be the only symptom that a child exhibits), wheeze, chest tightness, shortness of breath, sputum production.
B. Pattern of symptoms: episodic or continual, perennial or seasonal or both, onset duration, frequency, diurnal variations, nighttime awakenings.

C. Precipitating and/or aggravating factors: viral respiratory infections, allergens, exercise occupation exposures, environmental exposures such as irritants and environmental tobacco smoke, emotional expressions, medications, food additives, exposure to cold air, endocrine factors.

D. Disease development: age at onset, disease progress, present management and level of control, need for systemic corticosteroid bursts, comorbid conditions, need for hospitalization, intubation, emergency room visits, work/school asthma-related absenteeism, alteration in work/school performance, decreased exercise tolerance.

E. Profile of typical exacerbation and response to treatment
   1. Family history
      a. Asthma
      b. Sinusitis
      c. Rhinitis
      d. Nasal polyps in close relatives
      e. Allergies
      f. Skin conditions (atopic dermatitis)
   2. Social history
      a. Living situation and home exposures
      b. Tobacco use
      c. Substance abuse
      d. Education
      e. Occupation and employment
      f. Impact of asthma on family
      g. Work/school performance
      h. Economic impact
      i. Environmental tobacco exposure in home, work, social environment
      j. Functional status
      k. Quality of life
   3. Patient and family's knowledge of asthma, treatment, cultural beliefs, resources

II. Physical examination: Key findings
   A. Skin: check for presence of atopic dermatitis/eczema.
   B. Ear nose and throat (ENT): check tympanic membranes for signs of fluid, condition of nasal mucosa, presence of sinus tenderness, lymphadenopathy, nasal secretions/polyps.
   C. Chest: hyperexpansion of thorax, use of accessory muscles, sounds of wheezing, tachypnea.
   D. Cardiac: check normal heart sounds, absence of gallop, clicks, murmurs.

III. Diagnostic tests
   Measures of pulmonary function confirm asthma indicators obtained from the history and physical exam.
   A. Spirometry (FVC, FEV_1, FEV_1/FVC). Spirometry is recommended at initial assessment, after treatment has stabilized and at least every 1 to 2 years

B. Usually children under the age of 4 years cannot adequately complete spirometery testing, therefore, clinical judgement and/or response to treatment may be the best indicator for diagnosing asthma. Pulse oximetry may be useful in small children.

C. Assessment of diurnal variation by home peak flow monitoring.

D. Bronchoprovocation tests with methacholine.

E. Other tests that may be useful in selected patients: chest X-ray, allergy testing, rhinoscopy, gastroesophageal pH monitoring.

COMMON THERAPEUTIC MODALITIES

I. Goals of therapy
   A. Prevent chronic asthma symptom day and night.
   B. Prevent exacerbations.
   C. Maintain normal activity levels.
   D. Achieve and maintain normal or near-normal lung function.
   E. Increase patient and family's satisfaction with asthma care received.
   F. Optimize pharmacotherapy while minimizing side effects.

II. Pharmacological therapy
   A. Long-term control medications
      1. Inhaled corticosteroids are the most effective long-term control medication.
      2. Inhaled nonsteroidal anti-inflammatory medications (cromolyn, nedocromil).
      3. Long-acting inhaled beta$_2$ agonists. (Note: Theophylline is no longer recommended as a first-line long-term control agent. Patients should not be taking both long-acting inhaled beta$_2$ agonist and theophylline at the same time.)
      4. Leukotriene modifiers may be useful especially in patients with atopy and allergic rhinnitis.
      5. Note: Long-term use of oral corticosteroid is not recommended due to the devastating side-effects of this therapy when taken for long periods. However, some adults with very severe asthma may need longer treatment. Every attempt must be made to wean patients off long-term systemic corticosteroid medications. Consider every other day dosing if long-term oral corticosteroid is required.
   B. Quick relief medications
      1. Short-acting inhaled beta$_2$ agonists
      2. Oral corticosteroids: should be used in short-term bursts only

III. Step-therapy approach
   Start treatment at step appropriate to asthma severity at the time of presentation. Start with the level of therapy necessary to gain asthma control, then step down treatment to maintain control. (*Note:* Severity classifications are dynamic, not fixed, and can change quickly in response to exposures or treatment.)

A. Step 1: mild intermittent asthma

No daily medications, short-acting beta$_2$ agonist may be used to treat occasional symptoms.

B. Step 2: mild persistent asthma

Daily anti-inflammatory therapy + short-acting beta$_2$ agonist. Leukotriene modifiers may be tried.

C. Step 3: moderate persistent asthma

Daily anti-inflammatory therapy + long-acting beta$_2$ agonist + short-acting beta$_2$ agonist. Leukotriene modifiers may be tried.

D. Step 4: severe persistent asthma

Daily anti-inflammatory therapy + long-acting beta$_2$ agonist + short-acting beta$_2$ agonist + oral corticosteroid

E. Specific guidelines for the step-wise management approach for infants and children can be found in the document, "Pediatric Asthma, Promoting Best Practice" (AAAAI, 1999).

F. Consultation with an asthma specialist is recommended for infants and young children who require daily medications and are not meeting the goals of therapy within a 3–6 month period.

IV. Control of factors contributing to asthma severity

A. Allergens

Reduce exposure to allergens to which the patient is sensitive, especially indoor allergens, such as cats, dust mites, cockroach, mold. It is generally not possible to avoid exposure to outdoor allergens (pollens) but air conditioning may help reduce the concentration of pollens indoors.

B. Irritants

Avoid tobacco smoking; avoid exposure to secondhand smoke, wood smoke, household cleaners containing bleach, and other triggers.

C. Allergic rhinitis

Treat with intranasal steroids and antihistamines.

D. Sinusitis

Antibiotic therapy only if bacterial sinusitis is suspected; decongestants are sometimes necessary to promote drainage. Nasal lavage with salt water may be a useful adjunct therapy used prior to installation on intranasal steroids.

E. Gastroesophageal reflux

No eating within 3 hours of bedtime, elevate head of bed, use appropriate mediations to control chronic reflux.

F. Sulfite sensitivity

Avoid shrimp, dried fruit, processed potatoes, beer, and wine.

G. Medication interactions

Avoid nonselective beta-blockers; avoid aspirin and nonsteroid anti-inflammatory mediations if nasal polyps or severe persistent asthma is present.

H. Occupational exposures

Promote ventilation, respiratory protection, and a tobacco-free environment.

I. Viral respiratory infections
Annual influenza vaccinations and pneumovax for all patients, including children.

V. Patient self-monitoring
A. Monitor symptoms including frequency, duration, alleviating and aggravating factors.
B. Peak flow monitoring short term to evaluate exposures, response to treatment.
C. Long-term peak flow monitoring is recommended for patients with moderate or severe persistent asthma to detect exacerbations and need for early treatment.
D. Link monitoring to interpretation of symptoms and peak flow trends and to actions necessary to gain and maintain asthma control.

NURSING INTERVENTIONS

I. Asthma patient education
A. Teach basic information about asthma to patient, family members, and other caregivers emphasizing two components.
1. Airway inflammation
2. Bronchoconstriction
B. Describe the role of two classes of medications.
1. Long-term control medications
a. Inhaled corticosteroids
b. Inhaled nonsteroidal anti-inflammatories
c. Long-acting inhaled bronchodilators
d. Leukotriene modifiers
2. Quick relief medications
a. Short-acting inhaled beta$_2$ agonists
b. Systemic corticosteroids
C. Teach, demonstrate, and practice correct inhaler technique.
1. Metered dose inhaler closed-mouth technique
2. Metered dose inhaler open-mouth technique
3. Metered dose inhaler with a spacer/holding chamber
4. Dry powder inhaler technique
D. Teach self-monitoring of disease status.
1. Symptoms: chest tightness, cough, wheeze, dyspnea
2. Peak expiratory flow (PEF) monitoring
a. Determine personal best or predicted PEF.
b. Teach correct technique including deep inspiration followed by maximal expiration.
c. Teach patient to record the best of three tries every morning before taking medications to track peak flow trends.
3. Teach the warning signs of worsening asthma.
a. Waking at night with asthma symptoms

        b. Increased need for inhaled rescue beta$_2$ agonist

        c. Inability to engage in usual activity

        d. Falling or low PEF

    E. Teach when to seek urgent care by following an Asthma Action Plan.

      1. Write an action plan based on symptoms and/or PEF.

        a. Peak flow >80% of personal best and symptom-free, no action required. Follow usual daily plan.

        b. Peak flow <80% but >50% of personal best (symptoms may be present), self-treat with 2 puffs of short-acting inhaled beta$_2$ agonist. May repeat 3 times every 20 minutes if needed.

        c. Peak flow <50% of personal best, getting harder to breathe, take 2–4 puffs of short-acting inhaled beta$_2$ agonist and seek urgent care.

      2. Teach to self-treat when symptomatic or PEF <80% of personal best or predicted

      3. Teach to seek urgent care when it is becoming harder and harder to breathe or when PEF is <50% of personal best or predicted.

    F. Reinforce teaching at all patient encounters.

    G. Teach children with asthma, parents, siblings, any other caregivers and appropriate school personnel the components of the Asthma Action Plan.

    H. All patient education should be developmentally and culturally appropriate.

II. Home care considerations

    A. When to refill medications to ensure an adequate supply

      1. Divide total number of puffs on canister by number of puffs per day prescribed, result equals the number of days the medication will last. Put sticker with date of refill on vial.

      2. Ensure access to asthma medications at school.

      3. Rescue inhaler must be carried with the patient at all times.

    B. How to clean and care for dispensers, spacers, and home nebulizers.

    C. Environmental control measures

      1. Decrease home exposure to relevant allergens.

        a. Remove pets from home or keep out of bedroom.

        b. Cover mattress, box springs, and pillows with dust mite impermeable covers.

        c. Remove carpets from the bedroom.

        d. Decrease indoor humidity to <50%.

        e. Minimize number of stuffed toys and wash weekly.

      2. Decrease exposure to aerosolized irritants.

        a. Asthma patients should not smoke or be exposed to tobacco smoke.

        b. Avoid exposure to fumes, fireplaces, wood-burning stoves, sprays, perfumes, household cleaners containing bleach.

        c. Assess workplace or school environmental exposures.

    D. Refer patient and family to asthma resource organizations/support groups.

      1. American Lung Association

      2. National Asthma Education and Prevention Program

3. Allergy and Asthma Network/Mothers of Asthmatics, Inc.
4. Asthma and Allergy Foundation of America
5. American Academy of Allergy, Asthma, and Immunology

WEB SITES

National Asthma Education and Prevention Program: http://www.nhlbi.nih.gov
Allergy and Asthma Network/Mothers of Asthmatics, Inc.: http://www.aanma.org
American Academy of Allergy, Asthma, and Immunology: http://www.aaaai.org
American Academy of Pediatrics: http://www.aap.org
American College of Allergy, Asthma, and Immunology: http://acaai.org
The American Lung Association: http://www.lungusa.org
Asthma and Allergy Foundation of America: http://www.aafa.org

REFERENCES

American Academy of Allergy, Asthma, and Immunology. (1999). *Pediatric asthma: Promoting best practice: Guide for managing asthma in children.* Rochester, NY: Academic Service Consortium University of Rochester.

Child Asthma Management Program. (2000). Research Group. Long-term effects of budesonide or nedocromil in children with asthma. *New England Journal of Medicine, 343,* 1054–1063.

Mannino, D. M., Homa, D. M., Akinbami, L. J., Moorman, J. E., Gwynn, C., & Redd, S. C. (2002). Surveillance for asthma: United States, 1980–1999. *MMWR, 51,* 1–13.

SUGGESTED READINGS

National Asthma Education and Prevention Program. (1993). *Management of asthma in pregnancy* (Publication No. 93–3279). Bethesda, MD: National Heart, Lung, and Blood Institute, National Institutes of Health.

National Asthma Education and Prevention Program. (1995). *Nurses: Partners in asthma care* (Publication No. 95–3308). Bethesda, MD: National Heart, Lung, and Blood Institute, National Institutes of Health.

National Asthma Education and Prevention Program. (1996). *Considerations for diagnosing and managing asthma in the elderly* (Publication No. 96–3662). Bethesda, MD: National Heart, Lung, and Blood Institute, National Institutes of Health.

National Asthma Education and Prevention Program. (1997). *Expert panel report 2: Guidelines for the diagnosis and management of asthma* (Publication No. 97–4051). Bethesda, MD: National Heart, Lung, and Blood Institute, National Institutes of Health.

National Asthma Education and Prevention Program. (1997). *Practical guide for the diagnosis and management of asthma* (Publication No. 97–4053). Bethesda, MD: National Heart, Lung, and Blood Institute, National Institutes of Health.

National Asthma Education and Prevention Program. (2002). Expert panel report: Guidelines for the diagnosis and management of asthma: Update on selected topics-2002. *Journal of Allergy and Clinical Immunology, 110*, S141–S219.

Upper Respiratory Tract Infections

Marianne Kwiatkowski, Enid Silverman, and Diane Dudas Sheenan

INTRODUCTION

Upper respiratory infections account for the greatest number of annual ambulatory patient visits. A sore throat (pharyngitis) is the fourth most common complaint seen in ambulatory practice and most patients diagnosed with mononucleosis need only education and supportive care. Sinusitis, whether acute or chronic, affects 12% of all adults. In the United States antibiotic usage contributes significantly to pneumococcal antibiotic resistance.

UPPER RESPIRATORY INFECTIONS (URI)

I. Overview
    Upper respiratory infections (URI) are the most common acute illness for which a patient visits their health care provider. It is the most common cause of absenteeism in school and work in the United States.
    A. Definition
        The common cold is a mild, self-limited syndrome caused by viral infection.
    B. Etiology
        Several viruses are responsible for the common cold and each has different seasonal peaks.
        1. Rhinoviruses (89 different serotypes) are identified in 25%–30% of colds, with seasonal peaks in early fall and mid to late spring. Transmission of the rhinovirus is through physical contact of virus-contaminated nasal drainage. The virus can survive on the hand for as long as 4 hours.

2. The coronavirus is identified in 10%–15% of colds, with seasonal peak in midwinter.

3. Other causative agents include influenza and parainfluenza, and the rest are unknown.

4. In young children respiratory syncytial viruses and adenovirus are common but both are rare in adults.

C. Pathophysiology

The virus causes a transient vasoconstriction of the mucous membrane followed by vasodilation and edema with mucous production. The incubation period is 48 to 72 hours. The symptoms last about 1 week but may persist for as long as 2 weeks.

D. Incidence

The common cold occurs in adults 2–4 times per year and 4–8 times a year in children. This is the most frequently managed diagnoses in primary care clinics. The incidence decreases with age.

E. Considerations across the life span

1. Pediatric: The common cold is often mistreated with antibiotics in the pediatric population. Parents should be educated on the viral cause of the common cold and the correct therapies. Anyone under 21 should not be treated with aspirin-containing products.

2. Pregnancy: After the first trimester, pregnant patients can treat their cold symptoms with pseudoephedrine, acetaminophen, and saline nasal sprays.

3. Elderly: The elderly often have other chronic diseases that will affect the therapies used for treatment of the common cold. Caution in the elderly with a history of hypertension and sympathomimetics medication. Also caution with antihistamines in patients with a history of asthma, hypertension, glaucoma, renal disease, cardiac disease, hyperthyroidism, and prostatic obstruction.

F. Complications/sequelae

1. Acute sinusitis
2. Pharyngitis
3. Otitis media
4. Mastoiditis
5. Tonsillitis
6. May lead to lower respiratory infection
7. Bacterial coinfection is rare (Makela et al., 1998)

I. Assessment

A. History: The common cold is characterized by one or more of the following

1. Rhinorrhea
2. Nasal obstruction
3. Sneezing
4. Sore throat
5. Cough
6. Hoarseness

    B. Physical exam
1. Nasal drainage clear and nasal mucosa may be pale and boggy
2. Ears with tympanic membrane translucent with good mobility
3. Sinuses without tenderness to palpation
4. Lymph nodes may be enlarged
5. Lungs clear to auscultation
    C. Diagnostic tests: Diagnosis is based on the history and other testing is usually not required.

II. Common therapeutic modalities
Symptom management is the focus of the treatment.
    A. Antihistamines such as chlorpheniramine reduce rhinorrhea and sneezing but have minimal effects on the other symptoms and may cause sedation.
    B. Anticholinergics such as nasal ipratropium bromide significantly reduce rhinorrhea and sneezing if taken two sprays three to four times per day in each nostril. Insurance may not cover this prescription.
    C. Sympathomimetics such as phenylpropanolamine, pseudoephedrine, and phenylephrine reduce nasal obstruction and rhinorrhea. However, prolonged use can cause a rebound effect. Those with hypertension should avoid these drugs.
    D. Non-steroidal anti-inflammatories are useful for relief of fever and myalgias but may increase viral excretion (Sperber et al., 1992).
    E. Antitussives such as dextromethorphan can be used for treatment of a nonproductive cough. For a productive cough use guaifenesin.
    F. Herbal therapies: Vitamin C may decrease the duration and severity of the common cold but the correct dose has yet to be determined. Zinc lozenges also may be effective in reducing the severity and duration of the common cold. With vitamin C and zinc lozenges, the best effect is seen when it is started at the onset of symptoms.
    G. Home-based therapies using steam or cool mist help to liquefy secretions. Hot soup and increasing fluid intake increase nasal clearance. Normal saline nasal lavage and throat gargle provide symptomatic relief.

III. Patient education: Counseling regarding hand-hand transmission and the importance of handwashing. Infants and children should not share toys with a child who has a URI.

INFLUENZA

I. Overview
    A. Definition: Commonly known as the flu, a self-limiting acute viral illness with seasonal peaks.
    B. Etiology: The influenza virus continually changes over time. People are susceptible to the flu virus throughout their lifetime. If the influenza virus undergoes an abrupt change a new subtype of the virus suddenly emerges. This occurs with influenza type A. Thus a large number of

people are at risk due to lacking antibody protection. This may result in geographical increase in morbidity and mortality. This event is called a *pandemic.*

C. Pathophysiology: The influenza virus is transmitted person to person via talking, coughing, or sneezing. The incubation period is 18 to 72 hours. The flu is characterized by abrupt onset of fever, cough, chills, headache, myalgias, malaise, and arthralgias. The illness usually lasts 1–2 weeks.

D. Incidence: The influenza virus infection is highest in young children and decreases with age. Over a lifetime, individuals develop partial immunity because of prior infections.

E. Considerations across the life span
   1. Pediatric: In a number of children the first sign of influenza is a febrile confusion. Other children present with a nonspecific febrile illness or with a respiratory illness such as croup or bronchitis. Also gastrointestinal complaints are common, such as nausea, vomiting, diarrhea, and abdominal pain as part of influenza.
   2. Pregnancy: There is an increased risk of hospitalization for cardiorespiratory disorders during the second and third trimester (Neuzil, Reed, Mitchell, Simonsen, & Griffin, 1998). Also during pandemics there is an increased risk of mortality for pregnant women and increased risk of miscarriage, still birth, and premature birth.
   3. Elderly: The highest number of mortality/morbidity occurs in the elderly.

F. Complications/sequelae
   1. Airway hyperreactivity, which includes: cough, dyspnea, and wheezing that may last 3–8 weeks after the influenza and occasionally may last 4–6 months.
   2. Pneumonia
      a. Influenza viral pneumonia
      b. Secondary bacterial pneumonia
   3. Reye's syndrome
   4. Myositis
   5. Rhabdomyolysis
   6. Encephalitis
   7. Guillain-Barré syndrome

II. Assessment
   A. History
      1. Fever up to 106°F
      2. Headache
      3. Myalgias
      4. Cough
      5. Nasal drainage
      6. Sore throat
      7. Malaise

    B. Physical exam
      1. Flushed face
      2. Clear nasal drainage
      3. Tender cervical lymph nodes
      4. Occasionally rales in the chest
    C. Diagnostic tests
      1. Viral culture
      2. Rapid diagnostic test detects the influenza virus in 30 minutes

III. Common therapeutic modalities
    A. Antiviral medication used in treating uncomplicated influenza
      1. Amantadine is effective against influenza A with little or no effect on influenza B
        a. Taken within 48 hours of onset of symptoms. Reduces the duration of fever and other symptoms.
        b. Approved for treatment in ages 1 year and older
        c. Also indicated for prophylaxis against influenza A when the flu vaccination is contraindicated
      2. Rimantadine is effective against influenza A with little or no effect on influenza B.
        a. Taken within 24–48 hours of onset of symptoms
        b. Reduces the duration of fever and other symptoms
        c. Approved for treatment in ages 1 year and older
        d. Also indicated for prophylaxis against influenza A when the flu vaccination is contraindicated
      3. Zanamivir is effective against influenza A and B.
        a. Taken within 48 hours of onset of symptoms
        b. Reduces the duration of fever and other symptoms by 1 day
        c. Route of administration is oral inhalation
        d. Approved for treatment in ages 7 years and older
        e. Used with caution in patients with underlying chronic respiratory disease
      4. Oseltamivir is effective against influenza A and B.
        a. Taken within 48 hours of onset of symptoms
        b. Reduces the duration of fever and other symptoms by 1 day
        c. Approved for treatment in ages 1 year and older
        d. Used with caution in patients with underlying chronic respiratory disease
    B. Non-steroidal anti-inflammatories are useful for relief of fever and myalgias.
    C. Prevention with yearly influenza vaccine.
      1. 65 years and older
      2. History of chronic disease in patients of any age
      3. Patients who are immunosuppressed or have diabetes
      4. Residents of long-term care homes
      5. People who are in close contact of any of the above populations

PHARYNGITIS

I. Overview
  A. Definition: Commonly known as a sore throat. Defined as an inflammation of pharynx and surrounding tissues. The fourth most common symptom seen in medical practice.
  B. Etiology
    1. Infectious
      a. Bacterial
        i. Group A beta-hemolytic streptococci
        ii. *Neisseria gonorrhoea*
        iii. *Corynebacterium diphtheriae*
      b. Viral (most common cause)
        i. Rhinovirus, coronavirus, adenovirus, influenza A and B
        ii. Epstein-Barr, herpes simplex, and parainfluenza
      c. Atypical agents
        i. *Mycoplasma pneumoniae*
        ii. *Chlamydia trachomatis*
      d. Fungal
        i. *Candida albicans*
    2. Non-infectious
      a. Tracheal intubation
      b. Mucositis of chemotherapy
      c. Allergic rhinitis and/or postnasal drip
    3. Common pathogens include
      a. Group A and B beta-hemolytic streptococci (10%–15% of cases)
      b. *Mycoplasma pneumoniae* (10%–15%)
      c. *Chlamydia pneumoniae* (10%–15%)
    4. Less common pathogens include
      a. *Corynebacterium haemolyticum*
      b. Rhinovirus, coronavirus, adenovirus, influenza A and B, Epstein-Barr virus, herpes simplex, and parainfluenza
    5. Approximately 1/3 of patients have no pathogen identified despite an extensive workup.
    6. Food-borne outbreaks of pharyngitis have been attributed to group C and G streptococci.
  D. Incidence: Accounts for 40 million clinic visits annually
  E. Considerations across the life span
    1. Adults
      a. Important to identify and treat group A streptococcal infections in adults, especially those with a history of prior rheumatic fever.
      b. *Chlamydia pneumoniae* should be considered.
  F. Complications/sequelae
    1. Peritonsillar abscess
    2. Pharyngeal abscess
    3. Epiglottis

        4. Rheumatic fever

        5. Glomerulonephritis

II. Assessment

  A. History

      1. Sore throat, malaise, fever, headache, and anorexia

      2. Gonococcal pharyngitis should be considered in patients who complain of sore throat in association with urethritis, vaginitis, or proctitis

  B. Physical exam

      1. Classic symptoms of temperature elevation, tender tonsillar lymph nodes, and creamy white exudate on tonsils are noted in only 10% of cases.

      2. Cough and rhinorrhea are usually not present with a strep throat.

      3. Rare scarlatiniform rash (scarlet fever) is only clinical feature specific for group A streptococcal infection.

         a. This rash is characterized by a diffuse red blush first appearing on the trunk and then spreading centrifugally and acquiring a sandpaper texture.

         b. Seven days later the skin desquamates in large sheets especially over the palms and soles.

      4. Small oral vesicles or ulcers on the pharynx, tonsils, or posterior buccal membrane are noted with Coxsackievirus A, herpangina, and aphthous stomatitis.

  C. Diagnostic tests

      1. Diagnosis requires a throat culture.

      2. Rapid strep test kits have adequate specificity, but sensitivity is less than that of a correctly performed throat culture.

      3. Symptomatic family contacts of patients with positive streptococcal pharyngitis should receive throat cultures.

III. Common therapeutic modalities

  A. Viral pharyngitis-symptomatic treatment

  B. Bacterial pharyngitis due to Group A Beta hemolytic streptococcus

      1. Preferred treatment (to ensure compliance) for streptococcal pharyngitis is parenteral benzathine penicillin 1.2 million units × one dose.

      2. Oral therapy regimens include: penicillin V 250 mg TID for 10 days.

      3. For patients allergic to penicillin, erythromycin 250 mg every 6 hours for 10 days.

      4. All patients with tonsillar exudate, tender anterior cervical adenopathy, and a temperature greater than 100° F should be treated while awaiting results of throat culture.

      5. Antibiotic treatment should be routinely started on these three patient groups.

         a. Patients with a history of rheumatic fever not currently on prophylaxis

         b. Young patients with strong family history of rheumatic fever

      c. New cases of pharyngitis in patients living in close proximity such as military bases and dormitories

    6. Treatment for gonococcal pharyngitis

      a. Ceftriaxone 250 mg IM times one dose

      b. Erythromycin 500 mg PO QID × 10 days

      c. Spectinomycin should not be used

      d. Cotreatment for presumed concomitant chlamydial infection should include doxycycline 100 mg BID for 7 days or azithromycin 1 gm PO × 1 dose only

SINUSITIS

I. Overview

  A. Definition

    Bacterial, allergic, or fungal infection of one or more of paranasal sinuses when normal drainage is impaired due to blockage of one or more ostia. Symptoms that last less than 1 month are indicative of acute sinusitis, while symptoms of longer duration may indicate chronic sinusitis.

  B. Etiology

    1. Sinusitis can be a complication of

      a. Viral URI (0.5%)

      b. Dental abscess (10%)

    2. Non-infectious causes include

      a. Nasal polyps, anatomic nasal obstruction (i.e., deviated septum) and foreign bodies

      b. Barotrauma from swimming and diving

      c. Naso-feeding tubes

    3. Patients who are immune compromised are at increased risk.

    4. Patients with cystic fibrosis may have chronic sinusitis and polyps.

    5. Overuse of decongestants can be associated with sinusitis.

  C. Pathophysiology

    1. Occlusion of the sinus ostia usually from mucosal swelling or mechanical obstruction

      a. Mucosal inflammation is most often related to viral infections or allergic rhinitis.

      b. If the obstruction persists, chronic sinusitis develops.

    2. Causative agents. Acute sinusitis is associated with the following

      a. *Streptococcus pneumoniae*

      b. *Hemophilus influenzae*

      c. *Moraxella catarrhalis*

    3. Chronic sinusitis is associated with

      a. *Staphylococcus aureus*

      b. Anaerobes including gram-positive *cocci* and *Bacteroides* species

    4. Nosocomial sinusitis is associated with

      a. *Pseudomonas aeruginosa*

      b. Enteric gram-negative bacilli

      c. *S. aureus*

      d. *S. epidermidis* and *enterococci*

  D. Incidence: accounts for greater than 16 million clinic visits per year. Affects 12% of adults.

  E. Considerations across the life span

    1. In children *Moraxella catarrhalis* is most common pathogen.

    2. Children may have additional symptoms of irritability or vomiting related to gagging on the mucous.

    3. In younger children or children with subacute sinusitis, anaerobes are infrequently found.

    4. Adenoid hypertrophy in children may cause chronic sinusitis.

    5. Transillumination is not useful in the pediatric patient.

  F. Complications/Sequelae

    1. Neurologic meningitis, periorbital infections, subdural empyema, epidural abscess, and brain abscess

    3. Osteomyelitis

    4. Orbital cellulitis

II. Assessment

  A. History

    1. Upper respiratory infection that has lasted more than 5–7 days

    2. Barotrauma

    3. New symptoms

      a. Dental or facial pain

      b. Nasal congestion and drainage

      c. Diminished sense of smell and/or cough

      d. Headache

  B. Physical exam

    1. Examination of pharynx, nose, ears for edema and erythema.

    2. Examination of external nares for mucopus suggestive of sinusitis

    3. Examination of teeth/mouth for teeth grinding, dental disease, and malodorous breath

    4. Percussion over maxillary and frontal sinuses may exacerbate tenderness

  C. Diagnostic tests

    1. Plain film imaging is usually unnecessary and is relatively unsensitive.

    2. Transillumination of sinuses may be useful in adults.

    3. CT scanning is also nonspecific.

    4. MRI is useful when fungal infections/tumors are considered.

    5. Sinus aspiration for complicated sinusitis, immunocompromised patients who have failed to respond to multiple courses of empiric therapy.

III. Common therapeutic modalities

  A. Antibiotic therapy (first line)

    1. Ampicillin or Amoxicillin 250–500 mg qid for 10 days

    2. Trimethoprim-sulfamethoxazole (Bactrim 2 tablets bid for 10 days)

B. PCN-allergy patients
   1. Erythomycin/sulfamethoxazole (Pedizole): children, 50/150 mg/kg/day
C. Broader spectrum agents
   1. Amoxicillin/clavulanate (Augmentin) 875 mg bid
   2. Cefuroxime acetyl (Ceftin) 250 mg bid
   3. Clarithromycin (Biaxin) 500 mg bid
   4. Azithromycin (Zithromax) 500 mg on day 1 and 250 mg days 2–5
D. Intranasal corticosteroids
E. Symptomatic relief
   1. Decongestant sprays should be used short term due to a rebound effect.
   2. Steam and saline inhalation
   3. Use of oral decongestants prior to flying
F. Analgesic therapy

INFECTIOUS MONONUCLEOSIS

I. Overview
   A. Definition: An acute febrile illness characterized by fever, pharyngitis, splenomegaly, and lymphadenopathy.
   B. Etiology: Epstein-Barr virus (EBV1) a herpes virus
   C. Pathophysiology: Infection with the virus is extremely common. The spread is often by oral contact first infecting the throat. The B lymphocytes generate a T-cell response that results in atypical lymphocytosis, which is characteristic of this disease.
   D. Incidence
      1. Primarily affects those between the ages of 15–25.
      2. 50% of college students are found to have antibodies to EBV. Each year, 12% of those who do not have antibodies develop the course of clinical mononucleosis.
      3. Overall incidence is approximately 50:100,000 persons per year.
   E. Considerations across the life span
      Primarily a disease of children, teenagers and young adults. Rarely seen after age 30.
   F. Complications and sequelae
      Severe complications are rare but do exist. They include encephalitis, meningitis, peripheral neuropathy, Guillain-Barré syndrome, and bacterial super infections and splenic rupture. There have been rare deaths linked to splenic rupture, severe pharyngitis, and airway obstruction.
II. Assessment
   A. History: The triad of symptoms is pharyngitis, fever, and lymphadenopathy (especially posterior cervical nodes). Also malaise, mild jaundice. Patients may complain of cough, headache, anorexia.
   B. Physical examination: Lymphadenopathy, splenomegaly, hepatomegaly, moderate to severe erythema of throat, tonsillar enlargement

C. Diagnostic tests
   1. Monospot-positive
   2. CBC hematocrit is usually normal; WBC is usually elevated and characterized by an absolute lymphocytosis with over 10% of total white cell population comprised of atypical lymphocytes. The platelet count is usually normal to slightly decreased.
   3. Liver profile may note increase in hepatitic enzymes.
   4. Heterophil antibodies: highest titers in first week of clinical illness.
III. Common therapeutic modalities
   No specific treatment is needed except for patient education and supportive care. Patients should avoid strenuous activity. If the spleen is tender/enlarged, contact sports should be avoided. Corticosteroids for severe pharyngitis to reduce inflammation and prevent airway obstruction.

OTITIS MEDIA

I. Overview
   A. Definition: Inflammation of the middle ear. Often called acute otitis media (AOM). Can be classified into 5 categories.
      1. Acute infection without effusion
      2. Acute infection with effusion (fluid in the middle ear)
      3. Subacute otitis media: An effusion that persists for 3 weeks to 3 months when acute otitis has not been effectively treated.
      4. Recurrent acute otitis: Documented resolution between 3 episodes within a 6-month period.
      5. Chronic otitis media: An effusion persists after 3 months.
   B. Etiology: Several pathogens are responsible for otitis media. The most common causes are *Streptococcus pneumoniae* (40%–50%), followed by *Haemophilus influenzae* (20%–30%) and *Moraxella catarrhalis* (10%–15%). Viruses (such as RSV and coronavirus). Other bacteria including *Streptococcus pyogenes* and *Staphylococcus aureus* result in some cases.
   C. Pathophysiology: An infection or allergy results in edema and congestion of the mucosa of the nasopharynx, eustachian tube, and middle ear. Eustachian tube dysfunction impedes the flow of middle ear secretions. Negative pressure can increase the pull of fluid into the middle ear. As these secretions increase, microbial pathogens grow and cause infection.
   D. Incidence: Roughly 2/3 of all children will have one episode by the age of two, one third of which will have more than three. OMs occur most frequently in winter months in children <7 years old, with the highest incidence in children between 6 months and 3 years of age. Active or passive smoking can increase the risk. Higher incidences seen in congenital disorders and craniofacial abnormalities, such as cleft palate. Boys and Native American children are also at an increased risk.

E. Considerations across the life span
   1. Pediatric: This population has a higher rate of occurrence. Infants are predisposed if bottle-fed and fed in a supine position. Using a pacifier can increase the risk. Day care attendance and school attendance increase the risk of infection and the likelihood of drug-resistant infections.
   2. Elderly: Conductive hearing loss may be an overlooked symptom of otitis media due to age and preexisting hearing loss.
   3. Pregnancy: Uncommon in adult population; however, amoxicillin is in pregnancy risk category B.
F. Complication/Sequelae: Commonly seen after viral URIs and related to allergic rhinitis.

II. Assessment
   A. History: Otitis media is characterized by one or more of the following symptoms: ear pain, tugging at the ear in the preverbal infant or child, fever, irritability, hearing loss, tinnitus, and dizziness. Associated symptoms are nasal congestion, headache, sore throat, cough, and hearing loss.
   B. Physical exam
      1. Ears: auricle, ear canal, and eardrums. Pressing firmly behind the ear may cause tenderness. Using an otoscope, the bony landmarks of the incus, umbo, or maleus may be obscured or absent. The cone of light reflex may be absent. The tympanic membrane may be full or bulging. The tympanic membrane (TM) may be hyperemic due to infection or crying. Decreased or absent mobility of the TM by pneumatic otoscopy may also be a finding. A fever may be present.
      2. Neck: Lymphadenopathy may be present.
      3. Lungs: clear to auscultation
   C. Diagnostic tests: Diagnosis is based on the appearance of the TM and mobility with pneumatic otoscopy. Other testing is not required. However, in cases of treatment failure tympanocentesis or culture of the middle ear fluid drainage is important to determine appropriate treatment. For clients with otitis media with effusion or recurrent otitis media, consider sinus X-rays. Special work-up for an infant less than 3 months of age with a high fever should include CBC with differential.

III. Common therapeutic modalities: Some cases can spontaneously resolve and symptomatic treatment alone is acceptable in children >2 years of age who present in stable condition.
   A. Analgesics, such as acetaminophen and ibuprofen, are appropriate.
   B. Warm oil eardrops, normal saline nose drops may be helpful.
   C. Antibiotics, of which the FDA has approved 16 agents. Amoxicillin is the initial drug of choice and the best oral antimicrobial agent for acute OM. It has been proven to be safe, clinically effective, and inexpensive. The recommended dose is 40–45 mg/kg/day divided in 3 doses to achieve peak middle ear fluid concentrations to eradicate the microbe. Standard duration of treatment is 10 days; however, recent research demonstrates a 5-day course is acceptable treatment for children over the age of two.

The second line of treatment is higher doses of amoxicillin (80–90 mg/kg/day divided in 3 doses), especially in treatment failure after 3 days of therapy. Other agents include amoxicillin-clavulanate, ceftriaxone (single or 3 dose IM injections), cefuroxime axetil, clindamycin, trimethoprim-sulfamethoxazole (TMP-SMX), and erythromycin. In the United States, antibiotics primarily prescribed for acute otitis media contribute significantly to pneumococcal antibiotic resistance development. Accordingly the following guidelines are recommended.

1. Trimethoprim-sulfamethoxazole, the macrolides, and most cephalosporins should not be prescribed for AOM.
2. Amoxicillin should be dosed from 80 to 90 mg/kg/day for high-risk children.
3. A treatment course of 5–7 days (instead of 10–14 days) for children over 2.
4. If treatment failure occurs, cefuroxime axetil, ceftriaxone, or high-dose amoxicillin-clavulanate.

  D. Chemoprophylaxis is indicated for otitis-prone children, those with recurrent ear infections (children who have 3 or more in 6 months, 4 episodes a year, and those with a positive family history of otitis or infants plagued with ear infections beginning at less than 12 months of age). Amoxicillin (20 mg/kg/d) or sulfisoxazole (50 mg/kg/d) is used at half the therapeutic dose, given once daily for daily prophylaxis. This preventive therapy is safe and effective, often used for 3–6 months or during winter and spring seasons.
  E. Referral for tympanostomy tube placement should occur if a child has chronic bilateral effusions for greater than 3 months with bilateral hearing loss, language developmental delay, hearing loss of 20 decibels, or failure of the antibiotic prophylaxis to prevent recurrent otitis media.
IV. Patient education includes information regarding breast-feeding, which may be a preventative factor in the occurrence of otitis media. In addition, elevating the infant's head during feeding can be protective against OM. Elimination of pacifier by age 1.
 V. Home care considerations
  A. Practice good hand washing techniques especially after coughing and sneezing.
  B. Teach adults and children to cover their mouths with disposable tissues when they cough and blow their nose with disposable tissues.
  C. Use tissue once and then immediately throw away.
  D. Do not allow children to share toys that they put in their mouths.
  E. Smoking cessation for patient and other household members is vital.

WEB SITES

http://www.mayohealth.org
http://www.cdc.gov/ncidod/diseases/flu

http://www.aafp.org
http://www.healthcyclopedia.com
http://www.uihealthcare.com/vh/

REFERENCES

Makela, M., Puhakka, T., Ruuskanen, O., Leinonen, M., Saikku, P., Kimpimaki, M., et al. (1998). Viruses and bacteria in the etiology of the common cold. *Journal of Clinical Microbiology, 36*(2), 539–542.

Neuzil, K. M., Reed, G. W., Mitchell, E. F., Simonsen, L., & Griffin, M. R. (1998). Impact of influenza on acute cardiopulmonary hospitalizations in pregnant women. *American Journal of Epidemiology, 148,* 1094–1102.

Sperber, S. J., Hendley, O., Hayden, F. G., Riker, D. K., Sorrentino, J. V., & Gwaltney, J. M. (1992). Effects of naproxen on experimental rhinovirus colds: A randomized, double-blind, controlled trail. *Annuals of Internal Medicine, 117,* 37–41.

SUGGESTED READINGS

American Academy of Pediatrics. (2006). In G. Peter (Ed.), *Red book: Report of the Committee of Infectious Diseases* (27th ed.). Elk Grove Village, IL: Author.

Barker, L. R., Burton, J. R., & Zieve, P. D. (Eds.). (1995). *Principles of ambulatory medicine.* Baltimore: Williams and Wilkins.

Centers for Disease Control. (2000). *Influenza.* Retrieved from shttp://www.cdc.gov

Cox, N., & Stubbarao, K. (1999). Influenza. *The Lancet, 345,* 1277–1282.

Dykewicz, M. S., & Spector, S. L. (1999). Sinusitis guidelines, part 1: The diagnostic workup. *The Journal of Respiratory Disease, 20*(12), 825–828.

Dykewicz, M., & Spector, S. (2000). Sinusitis guidelines, part 2: The approach to management. *The Journal of Respiratory Diseases, 21*(2), 138–142.

Garland, M., & Hahmeyer, K. (1998). The role of zinc lozenges in the treatment of the common cold. *The Annals of Pharmacotherapy, 32,* 63–69.

Graham, M. V., & Uphold, C. R. (1994). Problems of the ears, nose, sinuses, throat, and mouth. In M. V. Graham & C. R. Uphold (Eds.), *Clinical guidelines in child health* (pp. 220–265). Gainesville, FL: Barmarrae Books.

Grimm, W., & Muller, H. (1999). A randomized controlled trial of the effect of fluid extract of Echinacea purpurea on the incidence and severity of colds and respiratory infection. *The American Journal of Medicine, 106,* 138–143.

Hall, C. B. (1999). Respiratory syncytial virus: A continuing culprit and conundrum. *Journal of Pediatrics, 135*(2), 2–7.

Hayen, F. G., Atmar, R. L., Schilling, M., Johnson, C., Poretz, D., Paar, D., et al. (1999). Use of the selective oral neuraminidase inhibitor oseltamivir to prevent influenza. *The New England Journal of Medicine, 341*(18), 1336–1343.

Hemilä, H. (1997). Vitamin C supplementation and common cold symptoms: Factors affecting the magnitude of the benefit. *Medical Hypotheses, 52*(2), 171–178.

Jader, R. (2002). Respiratory and allergic diseases: From upper respiratory tract infection to asthma. *Primary Care: Clinics in Office Practice, 29,* 231–261.

Kontiokari, T., Koivunen, P., Niemela, M., Pokka, T., & Uhari, M. (1998). Symptoms of acute otitis. *Pediatric Infectious Disease Journal, 17*(8), 676–679.

Mossad, S. (1998). Treatment of the common cold. *British Medical Journal, 317,* 3336.

Niederman, M. S., Sarosi, G. A., & Glassroth, J. (Eds.). (1994). *Respiratory infections: A scientific basis for management.* Philadelphia: W. B. Saunders Co.

Rodriguez, W. J. (1999). Management strategies for respiratory syncytial virus infection in infants. *Journal of Pediatrics, 135*(2), 45–50.

Spector, S. L., & Bernstein, I. L. (1998). Executive summary of sinusitis practice: Parameters. *Journal of Allergy and Clinical Immunology, 102*(6), S107–S144.

Tigges, B. B. (2000). Acute otitis media and pneumococcal resistance: Making judicious management decisions. *The Nurse Practitioner, 25,* 69–87.

Wald, E. R. (1998). Microbiology of acute and chronic sinusitis in children and adults. *American Journal of the Medical Sciences, 316*(1), 13–20.

Cystic Fibrosis

18

Linda Tirabassi and Gwen McDonald

I. Introduction
   A. Definition
      1. CF is the most common life-shortening, autosomal recessive genetic disorder in the Caucasian population. If two individuals that are carriers conceive, there is a 25% chance with each pregnancy of having an infant with CF, a 50% chance of having an infant who is a carrier for CF, and a 25% chance of having an infant who carries no CF genes.
      2. CF is a progressive chronic multi-system condition that has no cure to date. The progressive nature of the individual's lung disease mainly determines quality and duration of life.
      3. Predicted survival age in the United States is now 33.4 years with 39.5% of individuals 18 years or older (Grosse, Boyle, Botkin, & Comeau, 2002).
   B. Etiology
      1. In 1989, the gene responsible for CF was identified as located on the long arm of chromosome 7.
      2. CF is caused by mutations that alter the functioning of a protein called cystic fibrosis transmembrane conductance regulator (CFTR). CFTR is expressed in epithelial cells lining the ducts of exocrine glands of many organ systems, including lungs, pancreas, intestines, vas deferens, and sweat glands. Normally, CFTR helps to control the flow of ions and substrates across the apical surface of the cell membrane thereby controlling the hydration of secretions in the gland's lumen. Abnormal function alters the ion permeability of the cell membrane, creating an imbalance of ions and water whereby the secretions are improperly hydrated (Mickle & Cutting, 1998). Mucociliary transport is decreased in the lungs, predisposing individuals to respiratory infections.

3. To date, the identified mutations of the Cystic Fibrosis Transmembrane Conductance Regulator (CFTR) gene approximate 1,000 (Orenstein, 2002). At the present time, available laboratory genotyping can identify 86 of these mutations. Of these the Δ F508 mutation is the most common and tends to be associated with pancreatic insufficiency. In the United States 23 mutations account for 80.7% of the CF alleles (Mickle & Cutting, 1998).

C. Risk factors
   1. Known family history is a risk factor for CF because it is genetically transmitted. Biological relatives of affected individuals are referred to genetic counseling so they may make informed choices regarding family planning.
   2. Risk factors for more rapid decline in pulmonary function include frequent childhood respiratory infections, pancreatic insufficiency, poor nutritional status, and exposure to respiratory irritants, such as secondhand smoke.
   3. Medicaid coverage as a proxy for lower socioeconomic status has been found to be associated with higher mortality despite no difference in number of outpatient visits or access to specialty care (Schecter, Shelton, Margolis, & Fitzsimmons, 2001).
   4. FEV_1 <30% predicted, a partial pressure of arterial O_2 <55 mm Hg or a partial pressure of arterial CO_2 >55 mm Hg have been associated with 2-year mortality rates >50% (Kerem, Reisman, Corey, Canny, & Levison, 1992). Because an individual must expect up to a 2-year wait for lung transplant, these data are often used to guide timing for lung transplant workup.

D. Pathophysiology
   1. Clinical manifestation of the disease can be found in all organs having epithelial membranes. Abnormal sodium and chloride transport results in the dehydration of secretions with subsequent ductal obstruction.
   2. Sino-Pulmonary disease
      a. Upper respiratory
         i. Paranasal Sinus Disease: Paranasal cavity opacification is considered nearly a universal finding on radiologic reviews of CF sinus disease (Nishioka & Cook, 1996). This is believed to be a result of altered viscoelastic properties of mucus secretion leading to mechanical obstruction of the sinuses. Symptoms include nasal stuffiness, headaches, maxillary pain and pressure, postnasal drip, snoring, mouth breathing, poor sleep habits, and impaired smell acuity.
         ii. Inflammatory nasal polyps are commonly seen in children with CF, less often in adults.
         iii. Sinus cavities become colonized with similar organisms to those found in the lungs, resulting in a chronic low-grade sinusitis with episodic flares of acute sinusitis.

b. Lower respiratory

   i. Initial presentation can be with bronchiolitis, pneumonia, chronic cough, and asthma-like symptoms.

   ii. Inflammatory changes are seen in small airways even prior to bacterial colonization (Cantin, 1995). This has been demonstrated by bronchoalveolar lavage (BAL) in asymptomatic infants.

   iii. As time progresses, mucus accumulation and inflammation affect the larger airways. Bronchial infections develop, which eventually lead to bronchiectasis typically affecting upper lobes earlier than lower lobes.

   iv. Airways are initially colonized by *Staphylococcus aureus* and *Hemophilius influenza*. With disease progression *Pseudomonas aeruginosa* eventually infects the lungs and, once present, usually is not eradicated. There is a predilection of CF airways for colonization of *Pseudomonas aeruginosa* that is incompletely understood. This pathogen is responsible for the majority of pulmonary exacerbations in CF. Other pathogens that may both colonize the lungs and cause disease include *Stenotrophomonas maltophilia, Achromobacter xylosoxidans, Burkholderia cepacia, Aspergillus fumigatus*, and *Mycobacterium avium*.

   v. The characteristic mucus of CF is tenacious and purulent, causing a cycle of chronic inflammation, mucus obstruction of the airways, and infection. Inability to mobilize secretions provides opportunity for increased bacterial growth, resulting in acute pulmonary exacerbations alternating with periods of wellness.

   vi. Increasingly frequent episodes of infection contribute to worsening bronchiectasis, development of blebs and bullae, marked obstructive lung disease, and loss of pulmonary function, ultimately resulting in end-stage lung disease.

3. Gastrointestinal and nutritional abnormalities

   a. Meconium Ileus (MI) may be present at birth due to dehydration and inspissation of stool in the newborn.

   b. Pancreatic dysfunction

   i. Pancreatic insufficiency (PI) occurs in about 85% of individuals, notably those with two copies of the delta F508 mutation. Obstruction of the pancreatic ducts prevents the release of digestive enzymes (lipase, amylase, and protease) into the duodenum, resulting in malabsorption of fats, proteins, complex carbohydrates, and the fat-soluble vitamins (A, D, E, and K).

   ii. Protein/calorie malnutrition of varying degrees results from pancreatic dysfunction. Failure to thrive, manifested by poor linear growth and poor weight gain, is a common presentation in infancy. In severe malnutrition, hypoproteinemia and edema may be present.

    iii. Acute pancreatitis occurs, episodically, in about 10% of pancreatic sufficient individuals, and may be the precipitating problem leading to the diagnosis of CF. It is presumably due to pancreatic ductal obstruction (Drurie & Forstner, 1999).

    iv. Hepatobiliary abnormalities

  c. Focal biliary cirrhosis is pathognomonic with CF. Eosinophilic material is found to occlude the small bile duct (Shalon & Adelson, 1996). These lesions are limited to the bile ducts, rendering most individuals asymptomatic with a firm enlarged liver as the only sign. Biliary sludging and elevations in liver function tests (LFTs) are common and, if persistent, may be treated with Ursodiol. The prevalence of gall stones increases with age, with a prevalence as high as 20% in adults (Colombo et al., 1999). In some patients, focal biliary cirrhosis may progress to multilobar biliary cirrhosis, portal hypertension, esophageal varices, and liver failure.

4. Sweat gland abnormalities

  a. Reduced reabsorption of sodium and chloride from sweat results in excessive loss of Na and Cl.

5. Reproductive abnormalities

  a. Male: Congenital absence of the vas deferens (CAVD) is present in 95% to 98% of men with CF due either to a primary congenital abnormality or to atresia from a buildup of secretions (Boyland, 2001). CAVD can be a presenting symptom of milder variants of CF. Sperm are produced in the testes but their numbers and motility are reduced and they are unable to reach the urethra due to absence of the vas. Sexual function is otherwise normal.

  b. Female: Reproductive organs are anatomically normal. Reported lower fertility rate is thought to be a result of ovulatory cycle disruption, secondary amenorrhea, and thickened cervical mucus that can act as a barrier to spermatic movement into the uterus (Boyland, 2001).

E. Incidence of CF

1. Varies with ethnicity (Mickle & Cutting, 1998).

2. 50% diagnosed by 6 months and 90% by 8 years.

3. 39.5% of the 22,732 individuals with CF documented in the 2001 Cystic Fibrosis Foundation Registry (CFF) were >18 years of age (Grosse et al., 2002). It is predicted that by 2010, the majority of the CF population will be adults (Fiel, Fitzsimmons, & Schidlow, 1994).

F. Considerations across the life span

1. General considerations

  a. The age and developmental level of each individual must be addressed in order to foster progress and mastery of normal psychosocial and developmental tasks. The unique challenges of each developmental level, superimposed with chronic illness, require strategies to balance normalcy with the demands of management of CF.

b. There are a number of CF-related conditions that tend to emerge at certain ages as the disease progresses. Knowledge of these and of how to monitor for these complications is essential.

2. Pediatric issues
   a. CF diagnosis is often devastating for families due to expectations of the child's shortened life span and the genetic nature of the disease; access to accurate information is essential. Referral to a CF center is indicated; parental support groups and family education play key roles.
   b. Sweat testing of biologic siblings is recommended to identify as yet asymptomatic CF in other family members.
   c. Siblings are at risk for increased emotional strain due to diversion of parental time and attention to the CF-affected child, whose care regimen can dominate family activities. Siblings may experience survivor guilt.
   d. The core importance of nutrition to normal growth, weight gain, and respiratory health can set parents up for huge power struggles with the CF-affected child over food intake/enzyme use.
   e. Education and involvement of teachers and other caregivers is critical to assuring optimal self-care during school hours and after school care. Adjustment of school schedules and assignments may be necessary to accommodate treatment of exacerbations.

3. Adolescent issues
   a. Pubertal delay and short stature may result from malnutrition and chronic infection, and can negatively impact adolescent self-esteem, especially in boys.
   b. Adolescent focus on not being different can negatively impact both development of peer relationships and adherence to the needed self-care regimen.
   c. Recurrent exacerbations/illness and the time needed for daily self-care may negatively impact school performance and may require tutoring at home.
   d. Sexual health interventions must include discussion of likely male infertility, prevention of unplanned pregnancies, and STDs. Emphasis on avoiding other high-risk behaviors (e.g., smoking, drugs) is also important, as for any adolescent. Whereas earlier educational efforts focused on parents, education efforts now re-focus on the adolescent and must cover the spectrum of CF disease and self-care.
   e. Decisions regarding who and when to tell about one's CF emerge. Individuals often fear a potential boyfriend/girlfriend will abandon the relationship when he/she learns of their serious illness.
   f. Planning for the transition from pediatric care to adult care is essential, beginning near 12 years of age (Schidlow & Fiel, 1990). This

aspect of care is gaining more attention because people with CF are now living well into adulthood.

i. The provision of age-appropriate care in an age-appropriate setting is now considered the standard of care and is a necessary prerequisite for accreditation of a CF center by the CFF.

ii. Transition facilitates the development and mastery of normal developmental tasks. Transition involves implementation of a planned process that begins at time of diagnosis, accelerates during adolescence and emphasizes age-appropriate incremental increases in self-care behaviors. Necessary components of successful transition include: commitment of both pediatric and adult health teams, excellent communication between health teams, involvement of the family in the transition process, gradual introduction to the adult health team, and when the adult team is new to CF care, education of the adult providers to optimize their current knowledge about CF management.

iii. Adult providers tend to be more experienced in dealing with adult CF complications, reproductive issues, adult developmental issues such as career choices, vocational rehab, disability, and medical insurance coverage, and with end of life issues.

iv. Possible barriers to successful transition include the emotional bonds of the pediatric caregivers with the patient and family, lack of trust of the adult care team, and ambivalence about the transition process. The adult care team may have concerns regarding both the cost and intensity of care for the high resource utilization of this medically complex population. The patient and family may struggle with letting go of a long-term relationship with the caregivers who have followed them for most of their life. Trust issues emerge and control issues may surface when care shifts from the pediatric approach to the adult approach.

4. Adult issues
   a. Education and career planning
      i. Young adults with CF are encouraged to pursue either technical or academic preparation for the careers of their choice regardless of the possibility of a shortened life span. In 2001, 62% of individuals with CF were high school graduates and 28% were college graduates (Grosse et al., 2002).
      ii. Recurrent exacerbations/illness and the time needed for daily self-care may challenge one's ability to manage full-time work.
      iii. Jobs that minimize one's exposure to airway irritants and to persons prone to frequent viral respiratory infections (e.g., young children), that allow flexibility in one's work schedule, that provide potential for more sedentary roles as disease progresses, and that provide health insurance are preferred.

iv. With disease progression, referral to vocational rehab and/or information regarding disability or job retraining is important.

b. Dating, marriage

i. Decisions regarding who and when to tell about one's CF continue to be a key issue. Individuals often fear a potential partner will abandon the relationship when he/she learns of the partner's serious illness.

ii. Marriage or committed partnerships are encouraged and widely embraced by adults with CF; 36% of adults with CF are married or living together (Grosse et al., 2002).

c. Reproductive decision making

i. Biological fatherhood is now possible, though costly, using new reproductive technologies. The technique involves microscopic epididymal spermatic aspiration and intracytoplasmic spermatic injection (MESA/ICSI).

ii. Adoption may be difficult because many agencies will not place a child in a family where one parent is likely to die prematurely.

iii. Issues to be considered when contemplating parenthood include: likelihood of the child having CF; availability of someone to provide child care when the CF-affected parent is ill or hospitalized; ability of the surviving parent to manage child care if the CF-affected parent dies; and ability of a young child to cope with the premature death of a parent.

d. Pregnancy in CF

i. In recent years there has been a dramatic increase in the number of reported pregnancies (3 in 1989; 180 in 2001) (Grosse et al., 2002).

ii. Pre-pregnancy FEV_1 > 50% predicted, pancreatic sufficiency, and absence of *B. cepacia* were found by Tullis and associates to be associated with better survival rates (Gilljam et al., 2000).

iii. Women with CF who become pregnant have survival that is no worse than those who do not become pregnant (Goss, Rubenfeld, Fitzsimmons, & Aitken, 1999).

iv. A pregnant woman with CF is at high risk for developing gestational diabetes (Orenstein, Rosenstein, & Stern, 2000).

v. Choice of antibiotics is limited during pregnancy because of possible teratogenic effects on the fetus, thus rigorous airway clearance becomes even more important to prevent or reduce the frequency of exacerbations. Inhaled antibiotics are often used in lieu of IV.

vi. Nausea and anorexia are common during pregnancy, and if weight gain is suboptimal, total parental nutrition (TPN) should be implemented. The appetite usually returns post partum.

vii. Due to the increased metabolic demands of lactation, a woman choosing to breastfeed must be able to increase her caloric intake by an additional 25%.

5. Across the life span, age and developmentally sensitive information regarding progression of disease process and severity of illness must be addressed.

   a. Discussions about end of life/quality of care issues including life-sustaining treatments, transplant, durable power of attorney for medical decisions, advanced directives, wills, and end of life care are individualized with each person with CF, their family, and significant other.

   b. Counseling around end of life/quality of care issues is imperative and needs to include both the practical aspects of planning outlined above and the emotional supportive aspects needed to facilitate final closure.

   c. Patients, families, and significant others need reassurance that medication for symptom management, control for intrac dyspnea and pain/anxiety will be available at the final stage, as needed.

   d. A peaceful death is often difficult to achieve for those who die while listed for transplant due to the overriding focus on "continuing the fight" in hopes that donor organs become available (refer to chapter 42 "End of Life Issues" and chapter 40 "Patient Advocacy").

6. Elderly considerations are not applicable at present.

G. Cultural issues

  1. Facilitate development of educational materials in native language and/or with modifications consistent with specific cultural beliefs.

  2. Provide support for those in cultural minority because CF is predominately seen in Caucasians. Attempt to link families to culturally matched families for support.

H. Cystic fibrosis related complications

  1. Pulmonary

    a. Hemoptysis: more commonly seen in adolescents and adults

     i. Blood streaking is commonly associated with a CF exacerbation; treatment is with appropriate antibiotics.

     ii. Major hemoptysis is defined as acute bleeding of >240 cc/24 hour period or recurrent bleeding of 100 cc or more over a short period of time (3–7 days). It occurs in approximately 1% of CF patients annually. It is associated with chronic airway inflammation causing markedly enlarged and tortuous bronchial arteries that erode through the airway wall (Yankaskas, Egan, & Mauro, 1999).

     iii. Most major bleeds are acute and self-limiting. Interventions include: minimizing mechanical stress to airway (i.e., hold airway clearance, suppress cough), antibiotics, discontinuation of any medication causing platelet dysfunction. Vitamin K is administered if PT/INR is elevated. In severe cases,

IV Premarin may be administered and if this fails IV Pitressin and blood transfusion may be required (Schidlow et al., 1993). Bronchoscopy may be indicated to identify the site of bleeding and, if conservative measures are unsuccessful in stopping hemoptysis, bronchial artery embolization may be required.

iv. Major hemoptysis may be a life-threatening event. Patients are advised to go immediately to the nearest ER. Individuals who have experienced significant hemoptysis require much reassurance due to the fear of recurrence.

b. Pneumothorax

    i. Experienced by approximately 5%–8% of patients, more commonly in adolescent and adult years, and can be life-threatening (Schidlow et al., 1993). Rupture of cysts or subpleural blebs results in air leaks or a unilateral pneumothorax usually affecting the upper lobes. Presenting symptoms include sudden onset of chest pain and dyspnea.

    ii. Treatment: For small leaks, serial X-rays and oxygen administration may be all that is needed. Nasal oxygen increases the oxygen pressure gradient between the pleura and the lungs and accelerates the reabsorption of air from the pneumothorax. If the air leak occurs in conjunction with an exacerbation, IV antibiotics are initiated. The goal is re-expansion of the lung. More aggressive therapy, such as thoracostomy and suction, blebectomy or chemical pleurodesis, may be indicated. Treatment has become more complex with the advent of lung transplant, since pleural sclerosing complicates removal of the native lung and is therefore a relative contraindication for a later lung transplant.

c. Allergic Bronchopulmonary Aspergillosis (ABPA)

    i. An inflammatory reaction to the pathogen *Aspergillus fumigatus,* is seen in 5% to 15% of adults (Knutson & Slavin, 1992)

    ii. A work up for ABPA may be initiated when a poor response to routine aggressive therapy for a pulmonary exacerbation is evident, or in the presence of persistent pulmonary symptoms of wheezing, increased cough, shortness of breath, rust-colored sputum, and acute deterioration of pulmonary status.

    iii. Diagnosis is made on basis of specific criteria which include markedly elevated serum IgE (>1000 IU/mL), elevation in peripheral blood eosinophils, positive aspergillus serum precipitins, positive skin test to aspergillus, presence of aspergillus in sputum, wheezing, and new pulmonary infiltrates on chest X-ray.

    iv. Treatment is directed at reducing inflammation, usually with oral steroids, while monitoring IgE levels and overall response. Weaning off steroid therapy ensues as the patient improves. Refractory cases may require systemic itraconazole and longer-term steroids, with monitoring for common potential side effects from steroids.

    v. Colonization with aspergillus is a relative contraindication for lung transplant as invasive aspergillosis may occur post-operatively due to immunosupression (Gilligan, 1999).

d. Non-tuberculous mycobacterium (NTM) infection

    i. NTM colonization is seen in up to 20% of older CF patients but does not usually cause disease and rarely requires treatment. Nonresponse to usual antibiotic treatment for a CF exacerbation increases suspicion for mycobacterial disease, for which treatment includes appropriate antimycobacterial agents.

e. Respiratory failure (refer to chapter 26)

    i. CF individuals can present in acute respiratory failure that is reversible; however, most present with progressive, slow deterioration to chronic respiratory failure. Pulmonary hypertension and right-sided heart failure may develop.

    ii. Goals of therapy include improvement of ABGs and of symptoms associated with reduced PaO_2 and elevated $PaCO_2$.

    iii. Treatment includes: long-term oxygen therapy, initially with exercise and at night, eventually continuously. Because CF patients, even when markedly compromised, often maintain a high functional level including work and travel, assessment of oxygen needs during air travel may be indicated and oxygen prescribed based on the nomogram calculating PaO_2 at 8,000 feet as described by Dillard, Moores, Bilello, and Phillipa (1995). Bi-level nasal positive pressure ventilation (NPPV) is implemented when $PaCO_2 > 52$ and symptoms of hypercapnea (morning headaches, restless sleep, nightmares) develop. A sleep study documenting >5 minutes of desaturations below 88% while using the prescribed O_2 flowrate is also required for insurance reimbursement. Because it can extend life by several months, bi-level NPPV is often considered a "bridge to transplant." Mask fitting must be done by a skilled clinician to prevent an initial negative experience.

    iv. Transplant is considered for patients who wish to pursue this option and for whom no clear contraindications exist (see chapter 38).

2. Gastrointestinal

a. Distal Intestinal Obstruction Syndrome (DIOS) (formerly known as meconium ileus equivalent) is seen in about 15% of patients. It can occur at any time, but is more commonly seen in older children and adults (Shalon & Adelson, 1996).

    i. Dehydration, inadequate enzyme supplementation, and change of diet have all been implicated as precipitating factors. A mass of stool forms in the ileocecal region extending distally.

      ii. Complaints of "constipation" must be addressed to distinguish between DIOS and normal constipation and to ensure appropriate treatment. Presenting symptoms include crampy abdominal pain, abdominal distention, right lower quadrant mass, anorexia, vomiting, and presence of air-fluid levels with small bowel dilation on abdominal film.

      iii. Treatment includes Golytely by nasogastric tube (NG) or by mouth (PO). If fully obstructed the patient is made nothing by mouth (NPO), an NG tube is placed and gastrograffin enemas are administered. Miralax twice a day can be used as a preventive therapy for individuals prone to recurrent DIOS.

  b. Intussusception is rare overall but occurs mostly in older patients in association with DIOS.

  c. Rectal prolapse is seen in approximately 20% of infants and young children as a consequence of malnutrition and large, bulky stools (Drurie & Forstner, 1999).

  d. Gastroesophageal reflux (GER/GERD), with or without esophagitis, is reported in about 20%–50% of individuals of all ages (Gaskin, 2000).

      i. Reflux results from chronic cough, chest hyperinflation, and increased trans-diaphragmatic pressure gradient, from tilting during postural drainage, and from inappropriate lower esophageal sphincter relaxation (Cucchiara, Santamaria, & Andreotti, 1991).

      ii. Management includes preventive measures such as avoidance of food at bedtime, avoidance of caffeine, elevation of head of bed on blocks, and use of agents that suppress gastric acid or promote gastric emptying. Fundoplication, as a surgical intervention, may be necessary when medical therapy fails.

  e. Acute pancreatitis: Episodes tend to occur only in pancreatic sufficient individuals and are characterized by abdominal pain and elevation in serum amylase and lipase. Episodes are managed by pain medication and by reducing fat intake. Pancreatic insufficiency may develop eventually due to damage from recurrent attacks.

  f. Although rare, there is a more prevalent occurrence of GI malignancy in adult individuals with CF.

3. Cystic Fibrosis Related Diabetes (CFRD)

  a. Overall prevalence is reported as 5% to 15% with prevalence in adults as high as 30% (Robbins & Ontjes, 1999). Average onset is between 18–21 years of age, with incidence increasing with age. Onset is usually insidious and ketoacidosis is rare (Moran, 2000).

  b. The primary cause of diabetes in CF is diminished insulin secretion. This results because exocrine tissue is replaced by fat and fibrosis, destroying many of the islet cells.

  c. Patients typically present with unexplained weight loss, polyuria, polydipsia, and/or symptoms of glucose intolerance.

    d. Diagnostic criteria for CFRD are
       i. A 2-hour Plasma Glucose > 200 mg/dl during a 75 g OGTT or
      ii. Fasting Plasma Glucose > 126 mg/dl on two or more occasions or
     iii. Fasting Plasma Glucose > 126 mg/dl plus casual glucose level > 200 mg/dl or
     iv. Casual glucose levels (without regard to time of day or last meal) 200 mg/dl on two or more occasions, in association with symptoms (Moran et al., 1999).
    e. Care differs from that of Type 1 and Type 2 diabetes because of its different pathophysiology, and the complex nutritional and medical problems associated with CF.
    f. Treatment includes dietary and insulin therapy. Oral agents are generally not indicated. Overall caloric intake is not limited; rather patients are encouraged to consume a high carbohydrate and fat diet with adjustments in insulin to cover intake. Consistent daily eating patterns are encouraged. Patients are often taught to do carbohydrate counting matching appropriate doses of short-acting insulin to carbohydrate intake.
    g. Referral to an endocrinologist and a diabetes nurse educator with experience in CFRD, when available, is encouraged.
4. Hepatobiliary complications
    a. Multilobular biliary cirrhosis, esophageal varices, liver failure
       i. Progressive liver disease may result in esophageal varices that can bleed. Variceal bleeds can be life threatening, and a transjugular intrahepatic portosystemic shunt (TIPS) may be needed to reduce portal pressures in management of the older child and adult. In younger children stabilization of varices is accomplished with banding or sclerosing procedures. Propanolol may also be used in both children and adults.
      ii. Liver transplantation may be indicated for severe hepatic failure.
    b. Cholecystitis/cholelithiasis are common in CF due to sludging of bile in the biliary tree. Presenting symptom is abdominal pain and, occasionally, jaundice. If URSO is ineffective in altering stone formation, lithotripsy or cholecystectomy may be indicated (Tapson & Kussin, 1997).
5. Salt loss syndrome: Results from reduced reabsorption of sodium and chloride from sweat, with excessive sodium and chloride losses, increased risk of dehydration, electrolyte abnormalities, and heat prostration. Preventive measures include increased fluid and salt intake, especially during hot weather.
6. Osteoporosis is increasingly being identified as a complication in CF, with early bone loss beginning in adolescence. Severity of bone loss tends to correlate with both severity of illness and nutritional state. The causes are multifactorial and likely include malabsorption,

malnutrition, inadequate calcium, inadequate vitamin D, delayed puberty, reduced activity level, steroid use, and reduced sun exposure (Aris et al., 2000; Robbins & Ontjes, 1999). Multiple large cross-sectional studies suggest a prevalence of osteopenia and osteoporosis in adults to be as high as 66% (Hardin, 2002). Symptoms are silent until a fracture occurs.

    a. Kyphosis, sometimes seen in CF, can worsen in association with muscle weakness, increased lung volume, and poor posture.

    b. Treatment of osteoporosis includes adequate calcium and vitamin D intake, with use of supplements as needed, estrogen or testosterone injections if levels are low, and increased weight-bearing exercise. Vitamin D levels should be maintained between 30–60 ng/ml.

    c. Preexisting osteoporosis is a risk factor for patients seeking lung transplant. This is worsened by steroid immunosupressive therapy and increases the risk for spontaneous fractures (Ott & Aitken, 1998). Treatment may include aggressive use of bone resorption inhibitors such as alendronate and/or calicitonin (Aris et al., 2000; Howarth, 2002; Paradowski & Egan, 1999).

  7. Rheumatic disorders

    a. Hypertrophic Pulmonary Osteoarthropathy (HPOA) is the association of digital clubbing with chronic proliferative periostitis of long bones (legs and arms). Onset is during early adulthood, with a prevalence of up to 8% (Noone & Bresnihan, 1999). Symptoms usually worsen in association with exacerbations and include painful swelling of wrists, knees, and ankles.

    b. Episodic acute asymmetric arthropathies are seen in 2% to 8% of young adults with CF, sometimes in association with a cutaneous vasculitis (Noone & Bresnihan, 1999). These usually occur independent of a CF exacerbation.

    c. Vasculitis: Usually presents as purpural lesions on the lower extremities, in older patients, often in association with arthropathy. It is believed to be an immune mediated mechanism related to chronic infection. Usually resolves spontaneously (Noone & Bresnihan, 1999). Some patients may require pretreatment with colchicine or low dose steroids for 2–3 days prior to initiating antibiotic therapy and continuing throughout the IV course to prevent/minimize lesions. Referral to a rheumatologist may be indicated for patients with severe or recurring vasculitis.

II. Assessment

  A. General approach

    1. There exists a vast range of clinical manifestations of CF. Phenotype and genotype are not good correlates for disease severity or prognosis, nor does the value of the sweat test prognosticate the course.

    2. The assessment and treatment of CF is complex and is best managed through a multidisciplinary team approach. The core team is usually

comprised of the following: pulmonologist, RN, registered dietitian, medical social worker, respiratory care practitioner, and physical therapist. In pediatrics, child life specialists are vital adjunctive members of the CF care team.

3. Care is ideally provided in a Cystic Fibrosis Foundation Accreditated Speciality Center with consultations from GI, endocrine, hepatology, genetics, ENT, OB/GYN, mental health professionals, and other specialties as indicated.

4. The Cystic Fibrosis Foundation published clinical practice guidelines in 1997, to provide health care practitioners with Standards of Care to manage CF and its complexities. The guidelines are minimum standards. More frequent assessment and monitoring may be indicated based on the individual's severity of disease and care needs.

B. Respiratory

1. Baseline history needs to include a description of cough, sputum, hemoptysis, dyspnea, wheezing, sinus symptoms, general activity, and exercise tolerance.

2. Query also regarding exposure to environmental irritants, airway clearance technique used, description of a regular exercise program, frequency of exacerbations requiring antibiotics, other respiratory therapies (e.g., oxygen therapy, NPPV), and a review of all medications.

3. Determine if there is a current history consistent with a "pulmonary exacerbation," defined as the presence of 4 or more of the following findings: increased work of breathing, increased cough, change in volume and/or color of sputum (usually more green or gray), increased chest congestion, new or increased hemoptysis, decreased appetite and/or weight loss, fatigue, dyspnea, a decrease in spirometry by 10%, fever >38° C, changes in chest X-ray from baseline, and increased sinus symptoms with increased drainage (Orenstein et al., 2000).

4. Query regarding past history of spontaneous pneumothorax, massive hemoptysis, or respiratory failure requiring intubation.

5. Query regarding sinus symptoms which include nasal stuffiness, post-nasal drip, headache, and sinus tenderness.

C. GI/nutrition

1. A dietary history is obtained, and includes information on feeding/eating patterns, behavioral issues around eating, any recent changes in appetite or weight, and use of oral or feeding tube supplements.

2. Additional history includes stool pattern and characteristics, presence of nausea/vomiting (including post-tussive), complaints of heartburn, bloating, early satiety, adherence to pancreatic enzyme and vitamin supplement regimen, and use of complimentary/alternative supplements.

D. Presence of pain

1. Pain is a frequent manifestation in CF and may include the sinus area manifested as headaches, or pain in chest and lungs, in various areas

of the GI tract, or in joints. Pain assessment must be incorporated into each routine assessment.

E. Physical exam may reveal a range of findings

  1. Pulmonary

    a. Increased anterior/posterior chest diameter

    b. Digital clubbing of the fingers and toes

    c. Increased work of breathing and use of accessory muscles; infants may have chest retractions and nasal flaring

    d. Decreased oxygen saturation at rest and/or with activity

    e. On auscultation, crackles, diminished breath sounds, prominent central airway sounds, and wheezing with a prolonged expiratory phase

    f. On nasal exam, rhinitis, nasal obstruction, polyps, purulent discharge, dry lips and, in children, allergic "shiners" are frequent signs of sinus disease

  2. GI/nutrition

    a. In general, individuals may appear thin, pale, undernourished, and of small stature; however, with enzymes, anti-reflux medications, and aggressive nutritional therapy, improved nutrition and normal growth is achievable.

    b. Growth parameters including weight, length, and head circumference are monitored and plotted on a growth chart at all visits for infants; weight and height are monitored and plotted for children and adolescents. Weight is closely monitored during acute exacerbations. In the adult years, weight is also monitored carefully and plotted against ideal body weight. Anthropometrics, including mid-arm circumference and triceps skin fold thickness, is performed annually to assess changes in fat and muscle stores. BMI is often monitored, especially for patients seeking lung transplant with the goal of BMI > 18.

    c. Abdominal exam, including auscultation of bowel sounds and abdominal palpation for liver and spleen size and texture, masses, tenderness and/or distention, is done at least annually and more often if indicated. A rectal exam is performed if indicated.

  3. Other

    a. Presence of enteric feeding tubes and/or venous access devices are noted (for example a percutaneous endoscopically placed gastrostomy tube [PEG], skin level G-tube, implanted venous access device or peripherally inserted percutaneous central catheter [PICC]).

F. Psychosocial assessment is conducted at least annually, and focuses on general coping including use of denial, adequacy of support systems, individual/family functioning, appropriateness of educational and/or work roles, and adequacy of insurance coverage.

  1. Despite the burden CF brings an individual, most people appear to fare remarkably well psychologically (Davis, Drumm, & Konstans,

1996). Consensus is lacking in the literature, however, regarding psychological adjustment. With disease progression, coping skills may be severely taxed and patterns of denial, nonadherence, anxiety, and depression may emerge.

2. In a review article, Abbott and Gee (1998) provide a summary of the psychosocial literature related to coping, adherence, and quality of life in CF. Key points include

   a. Adherence is not associated with employment, age at diagnosis, number of years doing treatments, number of acute care episodes or clinic visits, but rather with loneliness and isolation.

   b. Worsening severity of illness is associated with reduced adherence.

   c. Individuals who use optimism as a coping strategy were more likely to be adherent.

   d. Those individuals who worry more about their CF tend to be more adherent.

3. Prevalence of depression was reported by the CFF patient registry as 1.6% for individuals less than 18 years old and 8.8% for those greater than 18 years of age (M. Brooks, personal communication, December 4, 2002).

G. Diagnostic tests

1. Diagnosis of CF is based on the following

   a. Presence of one or more characteristics consistent with CF combined with positive laboratory evidence of a CFTR abnormality as documented by

      i. A positive sweat chloride test (greater than 60 mmol/L) on two separate occasions, conducted by a lab with expertise in performing sweat tests. OR

      ii. Identification by DNA mutation analysis of two copies of the CF gene (80%–85% of persons will have two identifiable gene mutations). OR

      iii. Positive nasal potential difference (nasal PD), which is primarily used in research settings.

   b. A positive newborn screening blood test, immunoreactive trypsinogen, is suggestive of CF and confirmed by a sweat test or mutation analysis. Wisconsin and Colorado now screen all newborns for CF using this test.

   c. In 2% of patients, there is an "atypical" phenotype, which consists of sino-pulmonary disease, pancreatic sufficiency, and a sweat chloride between 40 and <60 mmol/L (Rosenstein & Zeitlin, 1998). When this occurs, further work up is indicated to provide evidence of CFTR dysfunction. Nasal PD on two separate days may provide this evidence. Otherwise close clinical follow-up and laboratory re-evaluation is recommended for those who lack conclusive evidence of CFTR dysfunction.

    d. In utero, the diagnosis is based on identification of two mutations from chorionic villous sampling or amniocentesis. Such testing is usually done when there is a known family history of CF or with fetal echogenic bowel findings on routine ultrasound.

2. Carrier testing is encouraged for family members of affected individuals. CF carrier screening is offered to individuals with a family history; reproductive partners of individuals with CF; couples in whom one or both partners are Caucasian and are planning a pregnancy or seek prenatal care; and is available for those in lower risk racial and ethnic groups (American College of Obstetricians and Gynecologists & American College of Medical Genetics, 2001).

3. Recommendations for basic preventive and maintenance care monitoring are outlined by the CFF (1997). These include annual blood tests to assess renal and hepatic function, diagnostic tests to monitor respiratory and nutritional status, screening tests for CFRD and osteoporosis, and a variety of additional tests as clinically indicated.

    a. Respiratory monitoring
        i. Spirometry quarterly; full PFTs as needed
        ii. Respiratory tract cultures and sensitivities annually and with each CF exacerbation; fungal and NTM culture annually. Synergy testing periodically for patients with multi-resistant organisms
        iii. Chest radiograph, A/P and lateral views every 2 to 4 years, and as clinically indicated; chest CT as indicated in more advanced disease
        iv. CBC with differential annually and as indicated to assess for infection related elevation in WBC
        v. Immunologic work-up for ABPA if suspected
        vi. Oximetry at rest, with exercise and at night for patients with advanced disease to assess need for supplemental oxygen and NPPV
        vii. Exercise testing as indicated for patients with more advanced disease
        viii. Arterial blood gases as indicated
        ix. Blood cultures, as indicated, for fevers, to rule out central line infection

    b. GI/hepatic monitoring
        i. LFTs annually to assess for early liver/gallbladder disease
        ii. Abdominal X-ray, CT scan, or ultrasound to assess for GI complications such as DIOS and cholecystitis
        iii. Serum lipase/amylase to rule out acute pancreatitis
        iv. EGD (esophagogastroduodenoscopy), ph study, and, as indicated, gastric emptying study to assess for GERD/esophagitis/hiatal hernia
        v. EGD to assess for esophageal varices secondary to cirrhosis

c. Nutrition monitoring
   i. Weight, height, and head circumference in infants with each visit, plotted on growth chart; weight and height with each visit plotted on growth chart; weight each visit for adults; height annually until growth stops (approximately 20 years)
   ii. Anthropometric measurements annually to assess lean muscle mass, fat stores; vitamin A, D, and E levels, albumin/prealbumin at least annually to assess nutrition and monitor response to nutritional management (vitamin D levels may vary due to sun exposure)
   iii. 72-hour fecal fat analysis as indicated to establish pancreatic function related to malabsorption
   iv. Iron studies to differentiate iron deficiency anemia from anemia of chronic disease for individuals with low Hgb/Hct levels
d. Sinus disease: Sinus CT to assess need for surgery
e. CFRD
   i. Diabetes screening annually for patients over 16 years, every 2 years for patients 10–16 years (screening can include OGTT or serial fasting and 2-hour postprandial blood glucose levels)
   ii. Annual urinalysis to assess for proteinuria/glucosuria
   iii. HgA1C as indicated for known diabetic patients to assess adequacy of glucose control (though value of test is questionable at present)
   iv. OGTT early in pregnancy and repeated at frequent intervals throughout to assess for gestational diabetes
   v. Ophthalmologic exam and further tests of renal function annually
f. Osteoporosis
   i. Baseline DEXA for adolescents and adults, and repeated every 2–4 years; follow-up DEXAs done more often if on oral steroids or with known osteoporosis to assess response to therapy
   ii. Annual calcium, phosphorus, and vitamin D levels to monitor risk for osteoporosis
   iii. Free testosterone level, drawn prior to 9 A.M. for all males with known osteoporosis, and repeated at intervals if on androgen replacement therapy
g. Specific treatment monitoring for
   i. IV aminoglysides require an initial peak and trough level, BUN, and creatinine, drawn at third to fourth dose, with at least weekly surveillance of trough levels, BUN, and creatinine (with peak goals higher than for non-CF individuals due to more rapid metabolism of drug in those with CF); of note, as a general rule peak and trough levels are not drawn from IV lines, including PICCs and indwelling implanted venous access devices. Audiograms to 12,000 htz at baseline and after each 2 to 4 courses of IV aminoglycosides, to assess for high frequency hearing loss.

      ii. High dose ibuprofen: initial pharmacokinetics, BUN, creatinine

      iii. BUN and creatinine repeated every 6 months; pharmacokinetics repeated every 2 years and if weight increases by 25% or more

      iv. Patients who are on low dose coumadin for DVT prophylaxis: protime and INR within 2 to 3 days of starting on TMP-SMZ or quinolones

      v. Patients on prednisone daily or every other day for greater than 3 months: an osteoporosis assessment, BP, and growth parameters in children, and an ophthalmologic exam annually

III. Common therapeutic modalities

General treatment goals are aimed at prevention and to reduce pulmonary infection, slow the progression of lung disease, and promote growth and development. Intensity of interventions is dictated by the severity of illness.

  A. Goals of management include

    1. Slow the progression of lung disease by controlling infection and promoting airway clearance

    2. Promote normal growth and development by optimizing nutrition

    3. Preserve quality of life and normalcy by preventing and managing complications, by promoting daily exercise and activities, and by encouraging developmentally appropriate behavioral milestones

  B. Specific medical therapies

    1. Airway Clearance (indicated for all individuals): In infancy aerosolized medications are delivered by a compressor-powered nebulizer, followed by chest physical therapy session including postural drainage, chest percussion, vibration, and rib shaking. As children get older the airway clearance technique that demonstrates the most benefit is incorporated into the daily regimen. Adolescents and adults utilize approaches that can be done independently (see chapter 40).

    2. Sinus irrigations: Saline sinus irrigations are initiated with the onset of acute sinus flares. If symptoms are unresolved, antibiotic irrigations, and/or nasal steroids are often added. Surgical intervention to clean out sinuses is indicated when patient response to medical therapy is not effective.

    3. Diet and nutrition

      a. Though dietary needs of individuals may vary, a high calorie, high protein, and liberal fat diet is usually recommended. Caloric needs of individuals with CF can be as high as 130%–150% of the RDA (Smith, Ballew, & Ebie, 1999).

      b. Infants usually take a special formula, Pregestimil, which is more easily absorbed because of the medium chain triglyceride (MCT) oil. They are advanced to solids as any other infant.

      c. When poor weight gain is exhibited, oral nutrition supplementation is recommended and if this fails enteral nutritional support through a feeding tube is recommended.

4. Medications
   a. Routine respiratory medications usually include aerosolized bronchodilators and antiinflammatory agents, administered by nebulizer or MDIs/DPIs to decrease airway inflammation and increase mucociliary clearance. Nasal anti-inflammatory sprays are used to decrease inflammation in the upper respiratory system.
   b. For pancreatic insufficient individuals, routine GI medications include daily supplemental fat soluble vitamins (A, D, E, and K in water soluble form). Pancreatic replacement enzymes are taken prior to each meal, with snacks, and with liquid nutrition supplements. The dose should not exceed 2500 U of lipase/kg/meal.
   c. Antibiotics
      i. Though most often used for treatment of acute exacerbations, antibiotics may also be used as preventive or suppressive therapy (Elborn et al., 2000; Szaff, Hoiby, & Flensborg, 1983). CF centers in Denmark routinely implement an aggressive antibiotic regimen at the first emergence of pseudomonas in the hope of eradicating the organism (Frederiksen, Koch, & Hoiby, 1997), and also administer regularly scheduled antibiotic courses as suppressive therapy. Potential problems associated with use of chronic antibiotic therapy include development of antibiotic resistance and the emergence of pseudomonas colonization in individuals previously colonized only with staph.
      ii. Antibiotics from two different classes of drugs active against *P. aeruginosa* (e.g., aminoglycosides, β-lactams, quinolones, cephalosporins with anti-pseudomonal activity) are administered in tandem to achieve a synergistic effect and slow the emergence of resistant organisms.
      iii. Oral antibiotics have a role depending on the organisms cultured, the severity of symptoms and overall condition of the individual. Quinolones (e.g., ciprofloxacin, levaquin) are useful and often given in conjunction with an IV antibiotic.
      iv. Parenteral antibiotics are indicated when the response to oral antibiotics is not adequate, there are unrelenting symptoms or marked worsening of pulmonary symptoms. An IV antibiotic course is usually 14–21 days. Good venous access is essential to complete therapy, therefore a PICC is commonly placed; sometimes an implanted venous access device (e.g., Portacath) is recommended.
      v. Inhaled antibiotics are typically used as prophylaxis but can also be used to treat an acute exacerbation. Because they are delivered directly to the site of infection with only small amounts absorbed systemically, higher doses can be used. This may offer a treatment advantage for those patients reported to be resistant to the drug. Similarly, those who have experienced

high frequency hearing loss from aminoglycosides in the past may tolerate inhaled aminoglycosides without further hearing damage. Inhaled antibiotics may also be used during pregnancy with minimal risk to the fetus. Efficacy of an inhaled antibiotic is contingent on reaching the site of infection. It may not be useful when the locus of infection is more peripherally located.

■ Aerosolized TOBI, a high dose inhaled solution of tobramycin allows for deposition of the drug directly at the site of infection, reducing systemic side effects. It is rotated on a "28 day on and a 28 day off" schedule to discourage emergence of drug resistance. This therapy has decreased hospitalizations by controlling the density of *P. aeruginosa* in sputum (Ramsey et al., 1999).

■ Gentamicin or colistin (Colymycin-M) may also be used as either prophylaxis or to treat exacerbations. The administration of these two drugs by inhalation is considered "off label" (i.e., the formulations are not officially approved for inhaled administration). Colistin must be carefully reconstituted using 3–4 cc of preservative-free saline or water; gentle mixing minimizes foaming. Patients may require premedication with a bronchodilator to prevent wheezing or chest tightness with use.

d. Additional medications

   i. DNase or Pulmozyme is a mucolytic enzyme administered via nebulizer that breaks down the viscoelastic properties in sputum caused by excessive amounts of neutrophil DNA. It should be administered before airway clearance, preferably in the morning.

   ii. Anti-inflammatory agents

   ■ Non-steroidal anti-inflammatories, such as high dose ibuprofen, decrease overall inflammation of the lungs. They are rarely used in adults due to marginal efficacy and increased risk for side effects; efficacy is greatest in young patients with mild disease (Konstan, Byard, Hoppel, & Davis, 1995). Patients must be closely monitored for side effects and to assure adequate blood levels.

   ■ Azithromycin, a macrolide antibiotic, has recently been reported to have a role in the treatment of CF. It is postulated that it modulates the host inflammatory response to infection and/or directly affects virulence factors of bacteria, specifically *P. aeruginosa*. This agent was given 3 times/week with dosing based on body weight to individuals with CF greater than 6 years of age. The study reported a decrease of hospital days of approximately 50%, a 6% improvement in FEV_1, and weight gain. Minimal side effects were reported.

Further studies are underway to determine the long-term benefits and risks (B. Marshall, personal communication, December 4, 2002).

- Oral corticosteroids may be required short term (e.g., during an acute exacerbation) for individuals with a "reactive airway/asthmatic" component, and for treatment of ABPA. Doses are tapered as soon as clinically indicated. Inhaled steroids may be needed for long-term use in those with hyper reactive airways.

iii. H2 receptor antagonists create a less acidic duodenal environment and are used both as treatment for GERD and to enhance enzyme efficacy by facilitating the release of pH sensitive microtablets.

iv. Gastric acid secretion inhibitors and prokinetic agents are used to treat gastroesophageal reflux.

v. Gallstone dissolution agents, such as Ursodiol, are used to improve the hepatic metabolism of essential fatty acids (Taketomo, Hodding, & Kraus, 1999) and reduce biliary sludging.

vi. Adolescents and adults with low dietary calcium intake are routinely advised to add calcium supplements to equal a total daily intake of 1500 mg of elemental calcium.

vii. Oxygen: With disease progression, patients will require oxygen either continuously, nocturnally, or during exercise to maintain oxygen saturation levels. The need for oxygen is often perceived by patients as a negative hallmark in the progression of CF pulmonary disease; increased psychosocial support and education is indicated (King, 1999).

5. Preventive care: Annual influenza vaccines are recommended.

6. Exercise is strongly encouraged, and both strengthening and aerobic exercise programs are incorporated into daily care.

7. Surgical interventions
   a. General surgical interventions are performed as clinically indicated and may include sinus surgery, laparoscopic cholecystectomy, laparoscopic fundoplication, implantation of a venous access device, and so forth.
   b. Lung transplant (refer to chapter 38)
      i. The first successful heart/lung and lung transplant performed for CF was done in 1983 and 1987 respectively. Today lung transplant is available at a number of centers around the world.
      ii. Cadaveric bilateral lung transplant and living related lobar lung transplants are the two accepted approaches. Single lung transplant is not an option because of severity of infection in the remaining native lung.
      iii. One-year, 3-year and 5-year survival rates are currently 81%, 60%, and 45% respectively (United Network for Organ Sharing, n.d.), although statistics vary between transplant centers.

iv. It is emphasized that the transplant recipient is trading one disease entity for another, that is, the pulmonary CF management is traded for posttransplant immunosuppression and ongoing management.

v. Timing of referral for transplant evaluation is critical since the average wait time for cadaveric lungs is 18 months to 2 years.

vi. Usual criteria include: $FEV_1 < 30\%$ predicted, increasing frequency of exacerbations, increasing functional impairment, severe hypoxemia and hypercarbia, and/or rapidly progressing, irreversible lung disease.

vii. Relative contraindications include: severe osteoporosis, prior pleurodesis, severe malnutrition, mechanical ventilation, severe co-existing liver disease with varices, colonization with *B. cepacia* or mycobacterium.

viii. Absolute contraindications include: demonstrated non-adherence to prescribed therapies, an inadequate support system, chemical abuse, smoking, serious psychiatric illness, positive HIV or hepatitis B status as evidenced by positive surface antigen and active mycobacterium tuberculosis (Yankaskas & Mallory, 1998).

f. Liver transplant: A small number of individuals may require liver transplant if they develop progressive hepatic failure with uncontrolled ascites and recurrent esophageal variceal hemorrhaging that is not controlled by medical interventions (Orenstein et al., 2000).

IV. Home care/continuity of care

A. Assess current knowledge base about maintenance care, management plan, and follow-up plan.

1. Review signs of pulmonary exacerbations and appropriate patient response.

2. Review all routine medications and new medications. Request that home medications are brought in for review. If on antibiotics, emphasize importance of completing the prescribed course. Review signs of allergic response. Review preferred sequence for nebulized medications and respiratory treatments: bronchodilator → DNase → airway clearance → inhaled antibiotic → steroids.

3. For home IV antibiotics, assess ability to perform care, verify home schedule, instruct on maintenance of venous access system, flush technique, and problem solving/safety. Instruct on plan for home supply company and home health agency to follow up with home care as indicated.

4. Review airway clearance technique and frequency of home care regimen.

5. Review self care regimen for acute and chronic sinusitis, including irrigation and administration of nasal steroids.

B. Determine if patient has the most efficient compressor and nebulizer to deliver aerosol medications. Some medications (notably TOBI and Pulmozyme) require a specific type of nebulizer and compressor. Some medications may be delivered by MDIs/DPIs in an effort to increase adherence and to decrease total time of treatments. Have caregiver/individual bring compressor to clinic for evaluation periodically. Make sure the filter on the compressor is changed per manufacturer's recommendations.

C. Consider developmental level of patient and provide education to facilitate adherence at each developmental level change.

D. Review self-care strategies to promote mastery of developmental skills appropriate to individual.

E. Special attention is needed for meal preparation to meet the recommended nutrition and caloric needs. Educate/strategize plan to effectively meet nutritional plans and goals. Consider including child life specialist for assisting with behavioral program/rewards for younger children. Consult dietitian for specialized education.

F. Acknowledge that home care is compounded when there is more than one family member in the home with CF. Provide support as needed.

G. Assess support systems and ability of the primary caregiver/significant other to assist with home care as indicated. Provide proactive problem solving as indicated.

H. Review environmental irritants, smoking cessation and effects of second-hand smoke and allergy proofing the home as indicated.

V. Long-term issues

A. Educate regarding the importance of quarterly visits to CF Center (CFF, 1997).

B. Anticipate and provide information to support life transitions, that is, starting "out of home" childcare, starting or changing school (grade advancement), adult care setting, entering college, and/or beginning employment.

C. Refer to disabled students program/office, vocational rehabilitation for adults, and so forth, as needed (Betz, 1999).

WEB SITES

Cystic Fibrosis Foundation: http://www.cff.org
General Web site: http://www.cysticfibrosis.com
Canadian Cystic Fibrosis Foundation: http://www.ccff.ca/
Cystic Fibrosis Resource Center: http://www.cysticfibrosis.co.uk/cystic.htm
Cystic Fibrosis Nursing Web site: http://www.choa.org/cfnurse
Information and support for transplant individuals: http://www.2ndwind.org
A special resource for people living with CF: http://www.mycysticfibrosis.com
A Web site targeted to patients and families discussing interventions for pain for CF: http://www.cfcenter.uab.edu/paincf6/

REFERENCES

Abbott, J., & Gee, L. (1998). Contemporary psychosocial issues in cystic fibrosis: Treatment adherence and quality of life. *Disability and Rehabilitation, 20*(6/7), 262–271.

American College of Obstetricians and Gynecologists & American College of Medical Genetics. (2001). *Preconception and prenatal carrier screening for cystic fibrosis: Clinical and laboratory guidelines.* Washington, DC: Author.

Aris, R. M., Lester, G. E., Renner, J. B., Winders, A., Denene Blackwood, A., Lark, R. K., et al. (2000). Efficacy of pamidronate for osteoporosis in patients with cystic fibrosis following lung transplantation. *American Journal of Respiratory & Critical Care Medicine, 162,* 941–946.

Betz, C. L. (1999). Adolescents with chronic conditions: Linkages to adult service systems. *Pediatric Nursing, 25*(5), 473–476.

Boyland, D. R. (2001). Sexuality and cystic fibrosis. *American Journal of Maternal Child Nursing, 26*(1), 39

Cantin, A. (1995). Cystic Fibrosis lung inflammation: Early, sustained and severe. *American Journal of Respiratory Critical Care Medicine, 151,* 939–941.

Colombo, C., Crosignani, A., Melzi, M. L., Comi, S., Pizzamiglio, G., & Giunta, A. (1999). Hepatobiliary system. In J. R. Yankaskas & M. R. Knowles (Eds.), *Cystic fibrosis in adults* (pp. 320–374). Philadelphia: Lippincott-Raven.

Cucchiara, S., Santamaria, F., & Andreotti, M. R. (1991). Mechanisms of gastroesophageal reflux in cystic fibrosis. *Archives of Disease in Childhood, 66*(5), 617–622.

Cystic Fibrosis Foundation. (1997). *Clinical practice guidelines for cystic fibrosis.* Bethesda, MD: Author.

Davis, P. B., Drumm, M., & Konstans, M. W. (1996). Cystic fibrosis. *American Journal of Respiratory & Critical Care Medicine, 154,* 1229–1256.

Dillard, T. A., Moores, L. K., Bilello, K. L., & Phillipa, Y. Y. (1995). The preflight evaluation: A comparison of the hypoxic inhalation test with hypobaric exposure. *Chest, 107*(2), 352–357.

Drurie, P. R., & Forstner, G. G. (1999). The exocrine pancreas. In J. R. Yankaskas & M. R. Knowles (Eds.), *Cystic fibrosis in adults* (pp. 375–450). Philadelphia: Lippincott-Raven.

Elborn, D. J., Prescott, R. J., Stack, B. H. R., Goodchild, M. C., Bates, J., Pantin, C., et al., on behalf of the British Thoracic Society Research Committee. (2000). Elective versus symptomatic antibiotic treatment in cystic fibrosis patients with chronic Pseudomonas infections of the lungs. *Thorax, 55*(5), 355–358.

Fiel, S. B., Fitzsimmons, S., & Schidlow, D. (1994). Evolving demographics of cystic fibrosis. *Seminars in Respiratory and Critical Care Medicine, 15*(5), 349–355.

Frederiksen, B., Koch, C., & Hoiby, N. (1997). Antibiotic treatment of initial colonization with pseudomonas aeruginosa postpones chronic infection and prevents deterioration of pulmonary function in cystic fibrosis. *Pediatric Pulmonology, 23*(5) 330–335.

Gaskin, K. (2000). Exocrine pancreatic dysfunction: Cystic fibrosis. In W. A. Walker, P. R. Durie, J. R. Hamilton, J. A. Walker-Smith, & J. B. Watkins (Eds.), *Pediatric gastrointestinal disorders* (3rd ed., pp. 1353–1366). Hamilton Ontario: B. C. Decker.

Gilligan, M. (1999). Microbiology of cystic fibrosis lung disease. In J. R. Yankaskas & M. R. Knowless (Eds.), *Cystic fibrosis in adults* (pp. 160–220). Philadelphia: Lippincott-Raven.

Gilljam, M., Antoniou, M., Shin, J., Dupuis, A., Corey, M., & Tullis, D. E. (2000). Pregnancy and cystic fibrosis: Fetal and maternal outcomes. *Chest, 118*(1), 85–91.

Goss, C. H., Rubenfeld, G. D., Fitzsimmons, S. C., & Aitken, M. L. (1999). Women with cystic fibrosis who get pregnant do not have decreased survival (abstract). *Pediatric Pulmonology, 19*(Suppl), 334.

Grosse, S. D., Boyle, C. A., Botkin, J. R., & Comeau, M. M. (2002). *Cystic Fibrosis Foundation Patient Registry 2001 Annual Report.* Bethesda, MD: Cystic Fibrosis Foundation.

Hardin, D. S. (2002). The prevalence and clinical manifestation of bone disease in CF. *Pediatric Pulmonary, 24*(Suppl), 20–24.

Howarth, C. S. (2002). Treatment of cystic fibrosis bone disease. *Pediatric Pulmonary, 24*(Suppl), 180–181.

Kerem, E., Reisman, J., Corey, M., Canny, G. J., & Levison, H. (1992). Prediction of mortality in patients with cystic fibrosis. *The New England Journal of Medicine, 326*(18), 1187–1191.

King, K. L. (1999, December). Cystic fibrosis and its treatment today. *AARC Times,* 58–63.

Knutson, A. P., & Slavin, R. G. (1992). Allergic bronchopulmonary mycosis complicating cystic fibrosis. *Seminars in Respiratory Infections, 7*(3), 179–192.

Konstan, W. M., Byard, P. J., Hoppel, C. L., & Davis, P. B. (1995). Effect of highdose ibuprofen in patients with cystic fibrosis. *The New England Journal of Medicine, 332*(13), 848–854.

Mickle, J. E., & Cutting, G. R. (1998). Clinical implications of cystic fibrosis transmembrane conductance regulator mutations. In S. B. Fiel. (Ed.), *Cystic fibrosis: Clinics in Chest Medicine,* 443–458.

Moran, A. (2000). Cystic fibrosis-related diabetes: An approach to diagnosis and management. *Pediatric Diabetes, 1,* 41–48.

Moran, A., Hardin, D., Rodman, D., Allen, H. F., Beall, R. J., & Borowitz, D. (1999). Diagnosis, screening and management of cystic fibrosis related diabetes mellitus: A consensus report. *Diabetes Research and Clinical Practice, 45,* 61–73.

Nishioka, G. J., & Cook, P. R. (1996). Paranasal sinus disease in patients with cystic fibrosis. *Otolaryngologic Clinics of North America, 29*(1), 193–205.

Noone P. G., & Bresnihan, B. (1999). Rheumatic disease in cystic fibrosis. In J. R. Yankaskas & M. R. Knowles (Eds.), *Cystic fibrosis in adults.* Philadelphia: Lippincott-Raven.

Orenstein, D. (2002). Cystic fibrosis: A 2002 update. *Journal of Pediatrics, 140*(2), 156–164.

Orenstein, D., Rosenstein, B. J., & Stern, R. C. (2000). *Cystic fibrosis medical care.* Baltimore: Lippincott Williams & Wilkins.

Ott, S. M., & Aitken, M. L. (1998). Osteoporosis in patients with cystic fibrosis. *Clinics in Chest Medicine, 9*(3), 555–567.

Paradowski, L. J., & Egan, T. M. (1999). Lung transplantation for CF. In J. R. Yankaskas & M. R. Knowles (Eds.), *Cystic fibrosis in adults.* Philadelphia: Lippincott-Raven.

Ramsey, B. W., Pepe, M. S., Quan, J. M., Otto, K. L., Montgomery, A. B., & Williams-Warren, J. (1999). Intermittent administration of inhaled tobramycin in patients with cystic fibrosis. *The New England Journal of Medicine, 340*(1), 23–30.

Robbins, M. K., & Ontjes, D. A. (1999). Endocrine and renal disorders in cystic fibrosis. In J. R. Yankaskas & M. R. Knowles (Eds.), *Cystic fibrosis in adults.* Philadelphia: Lippincott-Raven.

Rosenstein, B., & Zeitlin, P. (1998). Cystic fibrosis. *Lancet, 351*, 277–282

Schecter, M. S., Shelton, B. J., Margolis, P. A., & Fitzsimmons, S. C. (2001). The association of socioeconomic status with outcomes in cystic fibrosis patients in the United States. *American Journal of Respiratory & Critical Care Medicine, 163*(6), 1331–1337.

Schidlow, D. V., & Fiel, S. B. (1990). Life beyond pediatrics: Transitions of chronically ill adolescents from pediatric to adult health care systems. *Medical Clinics of North America, 74*(5), 1113–1120.

Shalon, L. B., & Adelson, J. W. (1996). Cystic fibrosis: Gastrointestinal complications and gene therapy. *Pediatric Clinics of North America, 43*(1), 157–191.

Smith, J., Ballew, M., & Ebie, R. (1999). Nutrition management of CF. *Support Line, 21*(1), 6–10.

Szaff, M., Hoiby, N., & Flensborg, E. W. (1983). Frequent antibiotics therapy improves survival of cystic fibrosis patients with chronic pseudomonas aeruginosa infection. *Acta Paediatrica Scandinavica, 72*, 651–657.

Taketomo, C. K., Hodding, J. H., & Kraus, D. M. (1999). *Pediatric dosage handbook* (6th ed.). Hudson (Cleveland/Akron), OH: Lexi-Comp.

Tapson, V. F., & Kussin, P. S. (1997). Cystic fibrosis. In R. H. Goldstein, J. J. O'Connell, & J. B. Karlinsky (Eds.), *A practical approach to pulmonary medicine.* New York: Lippincott-Raven.

United Network for Organ Sharing. (n.d.). Retrieved from http://www.unos.org

Yankasas, J. R., Egan, T. M., & Mauro, M. A. (1999). Major complications. In J. R. Yankaskas & M. R. Knowles (Eds.), *Cystic fibrosis in adults.* Philadelphia: Lippincott-Raven.

Yankaskas, J. R., & Mallory, G. B. (1998). Lung transplantation in cystic fibrosis: Consensus conference statement. *Chest, 113*(1), 217–226.

Bronchiectasis

Marilyn Borkgren and Cynthia Gronkiewicz

INTRODUCTION

1. Clinical features of bronchiectasis include cough, daily mucus hypersecretion, and recurrent respiratory tract infections with or without hemoptysis.
2. The most common complication of bronchiectasis is bronchopulmonary infection predominantly due to *Haemophilus influenza, Streptococcus pneumoniae, Staphylococcus aureus,* and *Pseudomonas* species.
3. High-resolution computed tomography of the chest, with 90% sensitivity and specificity, is the principal diagnostic tool for bronchiectasis.
4. The goals of medical therapy are prevention and control of infection and maintenance of airway patency to minimize or avoid disease progression.
5. Treatment of bronchiectasis includes bronchodilator medications, bronchial hygiene measures, antibiotics tailored to infectious organisms, and, for some patients, inhaled corticosteroids.

I. Overview
   A. Definition
      1. Bronchiectasis is a chronic pulmonary disease characterized by permanent abnormal dilatation and destruction of the elastic and muscular components of the walls of major bronchi and bronchioles.
      2. Chief clinical features of the disease are cough, daily mucus hypersecretion, dyspnea, and recurrent respiratory tract infections, which may be accompanied by hemoptysis.
   B. Etiology
      1. The primary etiology in the development of ordinary acquired bronchiectasis is inflammatory destruction of the elastic tissue, smooth muscle, and cartilage of bronchial walls usually due to severe preceding

infection(s). Fewer cases are caused by genetic or immune deficiencies or result from inhalation injury.

2. The development of bronchiectasis also requires impaired mucus clearance, airway obstruction, and/or impaired host defense mechanisms.

3. The following conditions are predisposing factors for bronchiectasis (Swartz, 1998; Mysliwiec & Pina, 1999)

   a. Bronchopulmonary infection—*Mycobacterium species,* bacterial (e.g., *Staphylococcus aureus, Bordetella pertussis, Klebsiella pneumoniae, H. influenza*), viral (e.g., measles, HIV, adenovirus, influenza), fungal (histoplasmosis, coccidiomycosis), recurrent aspiration pneumonia

   b. Bronchial obstruction—foreign body aspiration, lung or bronchogenic neoplasm, airway nodules, hilar adenopathy (e.g., sarcoidosis), mucus impaction (e.g., allergic bronchopulmonary aspergllosis), broncholith, external compression by vascular aneurysm

   c. Immunodeficiency states—hypogammaglobulinemia, IgG subclass deficiency, selective IgA deficiency

   d. Other congenital syndromes—cystic fibrosis, alpha1-antitrypsin deficiency, primary ciliary dyskinesia (e.g., Kartagener's syndrome), Young's syndrome (azoospermia and chronic sinopulmonary infections)

   e. Inhalation injury—smoke, ammonia, sulfur or nitrogen dioxide

   f. Rheumatologic disease—rheumatoid arthritis, Sjogren's syndrome

   g. Anatomic defects—bronchomalacia, Swyer-James syndrome, bronchial cartilage deficiency (Williams-Campbell syndrome), tracheobronchomegaly (Mounier-Kuhn syndrome)

C. Pathophysiology—An original classification scheme of bronchiectasis describes three anatomic subtypes of the disease (Mysliwiec & Pina, 1999; Reid, 1950). Each of these may cause focal (affecting 1–2 lobes) or diffuse, bilateral disease. The terms are descriptive, but there are no significant clinical, treatment, or prognostic differences among types.

1. In cylindrical (or fusiform) bronchiectasis, affected bronchi are mildly dilated and fail to taper distally.

2. Varicose bronchiectasis refers to bronchi that are generally dilated but have alternating areas of relative constriction and irregular shape, terminating in bulbous distal ends.

3. Saccular (or cystic) bronchiectasis is characterized by severe ballooning or pouching of bronchi peripherally.

4. In all forms of bronchiectasis, there is abnormal dilatation in the subdivisions of bronchi that contain cartilaginous walls.

   a. Chronic or recurrent bronchial inflammation destroys airway elastic and muscular components. This injury is mediated by numerous host factors and cells including immune effector cells, polymorphonuclear neutrophils (PMNs), and PMN-derived proteases, nitric oxide, and inflammatory cytokines (Barker, 2002; Sepper, Konttinen, Kemppinen, Sorsa, & Eklund, 1998).

   b. Neutrophil infiltration causes increased protease activity leading to mucus hypersecretion and airway damage. The blood neutrophil count may correlate with disease severity (Wilson et al., 1998).

   c. Increased concentrations of neutrophil elastase, interleukin, tumor necrosis factor, and prostanoids are found in expectorated sputum (Barker, 2002).

   d. Airway distortion impairs mucous clearance allowing pooling of secretions, bacterial colonization, and intermittent infection.

   e. Surrounding lung parenchyma may also become damaged and fibrotic.

  5. Bronchial arteries become enlarged and tortuous in severe bronchiectasis due to development of anastomoses between the bronchial and pulmonary arterial circulatory beds.

  6. The lag time between inciting injury or infection and the development of chronic bronchiectasis symptoms may exceed 10 years (Nicotra, Rivera, Dale, Shepherd, & Carter, 1995).

  7. Hypoxemia, airflow obstruction, or mixed obstruction and restriction develop as a result of airway disruption and destruction.

D. Incidence/prevalence—Bronchiectasis has become rare in the United States since the development of effective childhood vaccines (particularly against measles and pertussis) and antibiotics, but remains prevalent in less developed parts of the world (Barker, 2002).

  1. The prevalence of bronchiectasis is approximately 60 per 100,000 in the United States (Swartz, 1998).

  2. The annual incidence rate is higher in specific subpopulations including native Alaskan Indians.

  3. Bronchiectasis due to infection is diagnosed predominantly in middle-aged to elderly persons.

  4. Congenital defects causing bronchiectasis generally present in younger patients (Nicotra et al., 1995).

  5. Bronchiectasis occurs more often in females than in males.

  6. The disease affects both smokers and lifelong nonsmokers.

  7. Immunocompromised patient populations developing bronchiectasis include persons with HIV illness and recipients of bone marrow or organ transplants (Fiel, 2000).

E. Considerations across the life span

  1. Pediatric bronchiectasis can occur as a result of foreign body airway obstruction, infection, or hereditary abnormalities.

   a. In children, aspiration of a foreign body (such as food, toy or grass) can produce postobstructive localized bronchiectasis weeks to years after the event (Swartz, 1998).

   b. Cystic fibrosis is the most common cause of childhood bronchiectasis (see chapter 18).

    c. Postinfectious bronchiectasis from pneumonia, measles, or pertussis is no longer common in this country but occurs in poorly developed nations.

  2. The highest frequency of bronchiectasis occurs in patients 60–80 years of age (Nicotra et al., 1995).

F. Complications/sequelae

  1. Recurrent episodes of pneumonia or bronchopulmonary infection comprise the most common complication, and can lead to progression of the underlying disease.

    a. *Haemophilus influenza, Streptococcus pneumoniae,* and *Pseudomonas* species are the predominant aerobic bacteria causing acute infections in bronchiectasis (Fiel, 2000; Nicotra et al., 1995). *Staphylococcus aureus* and resistant strains of *Pseudomonaus* species are common in cystic fibrosis.

    b. Anaerobic infections may also cause significant morbidity.

    c. Both *Mycobacterium tuberculosis* and atypical *Mycobacterial* infections (*Mycobacterium avium-intracellulare*) can initiate, or complicate, bronchiectasis.

  2. Hemoptysis occurs in nearly 50% of patients with bronchiectasis (Mysliwiec & Pina, 1999); major pulmonary hemorrhage and death from exsanguination are rare (Swartz, 1998).

  3. Empyema, lung abscess, and pneumothorax are serious but rare complications of acute infections in bronchiectasis (Luce, 1994).

  4. Progressive respiratory insufficiency and cor pulmonale complicate severe bronchiectasis associated with deteriorating pulmonary function and hypoxemia.

II. Assessment

A. A history of recurrent bronchopulmonary infections and symptoms of chronic productive cough are hallmark features of bronchiectasis. Pain and dyspnea are also common.

  1. The history of acute, even if delayed, onset of bronchiectasis can sometimes be traced to a definite illness, pneumonia, or aspiration event in patients with postobstructive or infectious bronchiectasis. Those patients with underlying congenital or immune disorders usually demonstrate a more insidious disease onset (Luce, 1994).

  2. Cough is present in 90% of patients (Nicotra et al., 1995).

  3. Daily (often purulent) sputum production occurs in 75% of patients and varies in volume from 10–500 ml (Nicotra et al., 1995).

  4. Pleuritic chest pain represents distended peripheral airways or distal pneumonitis adjacent to a visceral pleural surface. This symptom occurs in 50% of bronchiectasis patients (Barker, 2002).

  5. Repeated episodes of fever, pleurisy, and/or sinusitis are also common.

  6. Weakness, dyspnea, and weight loss are seen in patients during infectious exacerbations or those with extensive disease.

  7. The St. George's Respiratory Questionnaire (SGRQ) has been validated as a useful tool for assessment of health-related quality of life

in patients with bronchiectasis (Wilson, Jones, O'Leary, Cole, & Wilson, 1997). Test items are divided into three major areas: symptomatology; activity tolerance; and impact of the condition on daily life including employment, need for medications, and sense of control or panic over one's health.

B. Physical examination findings are neither sensitive nor specific for bronchiectasis.

1. Crackles are the most common adventitious auscultatory finding, followed in frequency by wheezing, rhonchi, and a pleural friction rub (Barker, 2002; Mysliwiec & Pina, 1999; Nicotra et al., 1995).
2. Digital clubbing is rare (Barker, 2002; Mysliwiec & Pina, 1999).
3. Nasal polyps and sinusitis may also be evident (Luce, 1994).
4. Patients may have fetid breath chronically or solely during episodes of purulent sputum production.
5. Generalized weight loss and use of accessory muscles accompany severe disease.

C. Diagnostic tests are used in bronchiectasis to identify potentially treatable causes, to provide functional evaluation at baseline and following treatment, and to differentiate between diseases with similar symptoms and radiographic findings.

1. Radiographic imaging studies are the principal diagnostic tools for bronchiectasis.

   a. The plain chest roentgenogram with frontal and lateral views is abnormal in 50%–90% of patients (Hansell, 1998). Key features are dilated, thickened bronchial walls that appear as parallel markings (tram lines); patchy peribronchial consolidation in generalized bronchiectasis; and thin-walled ring shadows associated with cystic bronchiectasis.

   b. High resolution, non-contrast computed tomography (HRCT) and spiral volumetric scans of the chest have demonstrated 90% sensitivity and specificity for bronchiectasis (van der Bruggen-Bogaarts, van der Bruggen, van Waes, & Lammers, 1996; Grenier, Maurice, Musset, Menu, & Nahum, 1986).

   c. The pattern of CT abnormalities can point to specific bronchiectasis entities (Hansell, 1998).

      i. Upper lobe, central or perihilar distribution suggests allergic bronchopulmonary aspergillosis.

      ii. Predominant upper lobe, bilateral involvement is seen in cystic fibrosis and its variants.

      iii. Middle lobe and lingular involvement or the presence of multiple small lung nodules are often found in the presence of *Mycobacterium avium* infection or colonization (Barker, 2002; Swensen, Hartman, & Williams, 1994).

      iv. Lower lobe predominance is seen in patients developing bronchiectasis following earlier childhood viral infection (Cartier, Kavanaugh, Johkoh, Mason, & Muller, 1999).

v. Lack of bronchial tapering combined with dilatation is more specific for the diagnosis of bronchiectasis than simply the presence of widened airways.

   d. Plain sinus radiograph or CT scan of the sinuses can detect the presence of sinusitis, which frequently coexists with bronchiectasis (Fiel, 2000).

   e. The extent of airway abnormalities on HRCT correlates with pulmonary function impairment (Barker, 2002; Ooi et al., 2002).

2. Bronchoscopy is used to examine airways for obstructing tumors or foreign bodies, to evaluate the degree and site of hemoptysis, and to detect or remove inspissated secretions (Barker & Bardana, 1988; George, Matthay, Light, & Matthay, 1995).

3. Laboratory studies are important in the diagnosis and follow-up of patients.

   a. The complete blood count with cell differential may reveal leukocytosis or increased neutrophil levels during acute exacerbations; anemia may be present in chronic infections (Swartz, 1998).

   b. Quantitative serum immunoglobulin levels of IgA, IgM, IgE, IgG, and IgG subclasses are assessed in patients with recurrent sinopulmonary infections and bronchiectasis (Fiel, 2000); the most common finding is panhypoglobulinemia (Barker & Bardana, 1988). IgG subclass deficiency occurs in only 1%–5% of bronchiectasis patients (Hill, Mitchell, Burnett, & Stockley, 1998).

   c. Sputum smear reveals large numbers of white blood cells and both gram-positive and gram-negative organisms, including *Staphylococcus aureus, Haemophilus influenza, Streptococcus pneumoniae, Moraxella catarrhalis,* and *Pseudomonas aeruginosa. Mycobacterium avium* complex may represent infection or colonization (Farzan, 1997).

   d. Sweat chloride testing is used to screen for cystic fibrosis in young adults with no identifiable predisposing cause for bronchiectasis.

   e. Aspergillus titers are indicated when an *Aspergillus* organism is cultured or if radiographic exam (chest X-ray or HRCT) demonstrates central bronchiectasis (Barker & Bardana, 1988).

   f. A serum alpha-1-antitrypsin level is used to screen for hereditary emphysema in patients with respiratory symptoms or abnormal pulmonary function or radiographic findings.

   g. Ciliary motility studies via electron microscopy analysis of nasal or bronchial cilia can establish or rule out dyskinetic cilia syndromes.

4. Functional assessment of the bronchiectasis patient includes pulmonary function testing with spirometry and lung volumes, and arterial blood gas analysis. Patients with mild to moderate disease may have no abnormalities when tested between exacerbations.

   a. The pattern of airways obstruction (reduced FEV_1 and FEV_1/FVC ratio, and increased residual volume) is common in patients with moderate, diffuse involvement (Swartz, 1998).

    b. Airway hyperresponsiveness can be demonstrated in more than 30% of patients by spirometric improvement following bronchodilator administration or by inhalation challenge testing with methacholine or histamine (Barker, 2002).

    c. Mixed obstruction and restriction including decreased vital capacity and functional residual capacity is seen in advanced disease (Fiel, 2000). Pulmonary function tests are helpful in establishing the degree of airflow impairment but do not distinguish bronchiectasis from other airway abnormalities such as chronic bronchitis or emphysema.

    c. Pulse oximetry at rest and with exercise, and arterial blood gas analysis are used to detect hypoxemia, the most common gas exchange abnormality seen in bronchiectasis. Hypercapnea reflects advanced disease.

  5. Electrocardiogram shows evidence of cor pulmonale only in advanced bronchiectasis (Swartz, 1998).

III. Common therapeutic modalities

The goals of treatment are prevention and control of infection and maintenance of airway patency to minimize ongoing symptoms and long-term disease progression.

  A. Medical interventions

    1. Inhaled bronchodilators may be helpful in diffuse small airway disease; beta adrenergic agents dilate airways and improve ciliary activity (Swartz, 1998).

    2. Antimicrobial therapy for treatment of acute infectious exacerbations is based on results of sputum gram stain and culture.

      a. The selection of oral vs. intravenous route is based on the identified organism(s), antimicrobial sensitivity, severity of clinical presentation, and desired length of therapy. The use of prophylactic cyclical antibiotic courses is not routinely recommended. A recent limited meta-analysis suggests a small benefit for the use of prolonged antibiotics (range 4 weeks to 1 year) in the treatment of bronchiectasis (Evans, Bara, & Greenstone, 2003).

      b. For patients with infections unresponsive to oral or intravenous antibiotics, or as an adjunct to treatment, nebulized (aerosolized) antibiotics may be considered. Aerosolized antibiotics provide a high concentration of medication at the site of infection with low systemic absorption (Lin et al., 1997). While they reduce the colonizing microbial load in the lungs, improve symptoms, and may prevent disease progression, potential adverse effects are bronchospasm and chest tightness (Currie, 1997).

       i. Short-term aerosolized Gentamycin decreases gram-negative colonization and reduces the airway inflammatory response (Lin et al., 1997).

       ii. Limited evidence suggests long-term efficacy and safety of inhaled antibiotics (Ceftazidime or Tobramycin) in those with

Pseudomonas aeruginosa infection reflected by decreased hospital days and admissions (Orriols et al., 1999).

   iii. Aerosolized Tobramycin 300 mg twice daily reduced sputum *Pseudomonas* density. However, no significant change was seen in pulmonary function; and adverse events including increased dyspnea, non-cardiac chest pain, and wheezing were noted (Barker et al., 2000). This approach is currently FDA approved only for patients with cystic fibrosis but is prescribed for broader groups of bronchiectasis patients.

3. Corticosteroids reduce the airway inflammatory response in bronchiectasis.

   a. Inhaled beclomethasone diproprionate decreases both cough and sputum production in this population (Elborn et al., 1992).

   b. High dose inhaled fluticasone reduces sputum inflammatory indices in severe non-cystic fibrosis bronchiectasis (Tsang et al., 1998).

4. Oxygen therapy is prescribed as indicated for patients with hypoxemia at rest, during sleep, and/or with activity.

5. Gamma globulin replacement for immunoglobulin deficiency may be effective in reducing the frequency and severity of sinopulmonary infections (George et al., 1995).

6. Effective reduction and removal of bronchial secretions by a variety of available methods is critical in patients with bronchiectasis. The approach selected should be based upon an individual's self-care abilities, motivation, breath control, neuromuscular status, preferences, needs, and financial resources (Langenderfer, 1998).

   a. Effective cough

   b. Percussion and postural drainage

   c. Autogenic drainage

   d. Positive expiratory pressure (PEP) therapy

   e. Flutter valve

   f. Vest therapy

   g. Humidification (by cold water, jet nebulizers) as an adjunct to chest physiotherapy enhanced sputum production (Conway, Fleming, Perring, & Holgate, 1992).

7. Aerosolized recombinant human DNase may lyse the DNA that causes the sputum to be highly viscous. Initial studies for cystic fibrosis are promising, but this therapy is not FDA approved in non-CF bronchiectasis (O'Donnell, Barker, Ilowite, & Fick, 1998; Wills et al., 1996).

8. Non-invasive intermittent positive pressure ventilation (NIPPV) is an alternative to tracheostomy for respiratory failure due to advanced bronchiectasis. Although no significant reduction in hospital days or gas exchange occurred, short-term benefits such as improved sleep quality and improved daytime activity levels have been shown (Gacouin et al., 1996; Leger et al., 1994).

B. Surgical intervention
   1. Surgical resection
      a. Candidates for surgical resection include patients with massive hemoptysis, recurrent and refractory symptoms, anatomically limited disease distribution, and adequate cardiopulmonary reserve (Agasthian, Deschamps, Trastek, Allen, & Pairelero, 1996; Annest, Kratz, & Crawford, 1982). Surgical options include lobectomy, segmentectomy, and pneumonectomy (Ashour et al., 1999). Life-threatening hemoptysis may also be managed by bronchial artery embolization if interventional radiology service is immediately available (Barker, 2002).
      b. Preoperative evaluation includes, but is not limited to, bronchoscopy, pulmonary function testing, high-resolution computed tomography, and studies evaluating lung perfusion and pulmonary artery flow (Ashour, 1999).
   2. Lung or heart-lung transplantation
      a. Patients with bronchiectasis comprise <5% of the lung or heart-lung transplantation population, based on published series from numerous centers (McFadden et al., 1995; Medalion et al., 1996; Montoya, 1994; Sarris et al., 1994).
      b. Morbidity and survival data in this group are comparable to outcomes in other recipient diagnostic groups.

IV. Home care considerations
   A. Provide continuity of care post-hospitalization to reduce recurrence and frequency of acute exacerbations.
      1. Evaluate patient's knowledge regarding bronchiectasis, treatment plan, and self-care abilities.
         a. Instruct on early signs of pulmonary or sinus infection: change in amount or color of sputum or nasal drainage, hemoptysis, increased dyspnea, fever, chills, fatigue, headache, chest pain.
         b. Emphasize importance of completing full course of antimicrobial therapy to prevent relapse or development of resistant strains of organisms; include education on proper delivery of intravenous and/or aerosolized antibiotics (Conway, 1996).
         c. Teach patient and significant other effective airway clearance techniques to remove secretions and optimize ventilation. In addition to postural drainage and chest percussion, the patient may be instructed on proper use of the Flutter or PEP devices. The Vest is an alternative to chest percussion.
      2. Identify socioeconomic barriers to long-term therapy.
         a. Establish presence of significant others or support persons to aid in home bronchial hygiene routine.
         b. Investigate insurance coverage for nebulized or intravenous home antibiotics and durable medical equipment.
         c. Evaluate the individual's ability to use the nebulizer, oxygen, or airway clearance devices outside the home.

    d. Pursue availability of compassionate use medication trials and eligibility requirements.

  B. Advocate health maintenance and promotion to prevent acute exacerbations and to prevent long-term pulmonary deterioration.

    1. Educate on avoidance of potential lung irritants: secondhand smoke, dust, noxious fumes, occupational exposures, and respiratory infections.

    2. Identify community resources such as support groups, lung associations, research centers, and home health agencies.

    3. Provide annual influenza vaccination and pneumococcal vaccination as indicated.

    4. Inform patient of variety of pharmacologic and non-pharmacologic smoking cessation strategies and aids.

    5. Refer to dietitian for optimal plan for nutrition and fluid intake.

REFERENCES

Agasthian, T., Deschamps, C., Trastek, V. F., Allen, M. S., & Pairelero, P. C. (1996). Surgical management of bronchiectasis. *Annals of Thoracic Surgery, 62,* 967–980.

Annest, L. S., Kratz, J. M., & Crawford, F. (1982). Current results of treatment of bronchiectasis. *Journal of Thoracic and Cardiovascular Surgery, 83,* 546–550.

Ashour, M., Al-Kaftan, K., Rafay, M. A., Saja, K. F., Hajjar, W., Al-Fraye, A. R., et al. (1999). Current surgical therapy of bronchiectasis. *World Journal of Surgery, 23,* 1096–1104.

Barker, A. F. (2002). Bronchiectasis. *New England Journal of Medicine, 346,* 1383–1393.

Barker, A. F., & Bardana, E. J. (1988). Bronchiectasis: Update of an orphan disease. *American Review of Respiratory Disease, 137,* 969–978.

Barker, A. F., Couch, L., Fiel, S. B., Gotfried, M. K., Ilowite, J., Meyer, K. C., et al. (2000). Tobramycin solution for inhalation reduces sputum *Pseudomonaus aeruginosa* density in bronchiectasis. *American Journal of Respiratory and Critical Care Medicine, 162,* 481–485.

Cartier, Y., Kavanaugh, P. V., Johkoh, T., Mason, A. C., & Muller, N. L. (1999). Bronchiectasis: Accuracy of high-resolution CT in the differentiation of specific diseases. *American Journal of Roentgenology, 173,* 47–52.

Conway, A. (1996). Home intravenous therapy for bronchiectasis patients. *Nursing Times, 92,* 34–35.

Conway, J. H., Fleming, J. S., Perring, & Holgate, S. T. (1992). Humidification as an adjunct to chest physiotherapy in aiding tracheobronchial clearance in patients with bronchiectasis. *Respiratory Medicine, 86,* 109–114.

Currie, D. C. (1997). Nebulisers for bronchiectasis. *Thorax, 52*(Suppl 2), S72–S74.

Elborn, I. S., Johnston, B., Allen, F., Clarke, J., McGarry, J., & Varghese, G. (1992). Inhaled steroids in patients with bronchiectasis. *Respiratory Medicine, 86,* 121–124.

Evans, D., Bara, A., & Greenstone, M. (2003). Prolonged antibiotics for purulent bronchiectasis. *Cochrane Database Systematic Reviews, 4*(CD001392).

Farzan, S. (1997). Bronchiectasis. In *A Concise Handbook of Respiratory Diseases* (4th ed.). Stamford, CT: Apple and Lange.

Fiel, S. (2000). Bronchiectasis: The changing clinical scenario. *Journal of Respiratory Diseases, 21,* 666–681.

Gacouin, A. R., Desrues, B., Lena, H., Quinquenel, M. L., Dassonville, J., & Delaval, P. (1996). Long-term nasal intermittent positive pressure ventilation in sixteen consecutive patients with bronchiectasis: A retrospective study. *European Respiratory Journal, 9,* 1246–1250.

George, R. B., Matthay, M. A., Light, R. W., & Matthay, R. A. (1995). *Chest medicine: Essentials of pulmonary and critical care medicine* (3rd ed.). Baltimore: Williams and Wilkins.

Grenier, P., Maurice, F., Musset, D., Menu, Y., & Nahum, H. (1986). Bronchiectasis: assessment by thin-section CT. *Radiology, 161,* 95–99.

Hansell, D. M. (1998). Bronchiectasis. *Radiology Clinics of North America, 36,* 107–128.

Hill, S. L., Mitchell, J. L., Burnett, D., & Stockley, R. A. (1998). IgG subclassess in the serum and sputum from patients with bronchiectasis. *Thorax, 53,* 463–468.

Langenderfer, B. (1998). Alternatives to percussion and postural drainage. *Journal of Cardiopulmonary Rehabilitation, 18,* 283–289.

Leger, P., Bedicam, J. M., Cornette, A., Reybet-Degat, O., Langevin, B., Polu, J. M., et al. (1994). Nasal intermittent positive pressure ventilation: Long-term follow-up in patients with severe chronic respiratory insufficiency. *Chest, 105,* 100–105.

Lin, H., Cheng, H., Wang, C., Liu, C., Yu, C., & Kuo, H. (1997). Inhaled gentamycin reduces airway neutrophil activity and mucus secretion in bronchiectasis. *American Journal of Respiratory and Critical Care Medicine, 155,* 2024–2029.

Luce, J. M. (1994). Bronchiectasis. In J. F. Murray & J. A. Nadel (Eds.), *Textbook of respiratory medicine* (pp. 1398–1417). Philadelphia: W. B. Saunders.

McFadden, P. M., Ochsner, J. L., Emory, J. B., VanMeter, C. H., Pridjian, A. K., Young, G. S., et al. (1995). Lung transplantation in Louisiana: Report of the first twenty lung transplants performed in the state. *Journal of the Louisiana State Medical Society, 147,* 37–42.

Medalion, B., et al. (1996). Early experience in lung transplantation. *Israel Journal of Medical Science, 32,* 292–296.

Montoya, A. (1994). Survival and outcome after single and bilateral lung transplantation. Loyola Lung Transplant Team. *Surgery, 116,* 712–718.

Mysliwiec, V., & Pina, J. S.(1999). Bronchiectasis: The other obstructive lung disease. *Postgraduate Medicine, 106,* 123–131.

Nicotra, M. B., Rivera, M., Dale, A. M., Shepherd, R., & Carter, R. (1995). Clinical, pathophysiologic, and microbiologic characterization of bronchiectasis in an aging cohort. *Chest, 108,* 955–961.

O'Donnell, A. E., Barker, A. F., Ilowite, J. S., & Fick, R. B. (1998). Treatment of idiopathic bronchiectasis with aerosolized recombinant human DNase I. *Chest, 113,* 1329–1334.

Ooi, G. C., Khong, P. L., Chan-Yeung, M., Ho, J. C. M., Chan, P. K. S., & Lee, J. C. K. (2002). High-resolution CT quantification of bronchiectasis: clinical and functional correlation. *Radiology, 225,* 663–672.

Orriols, R., Roig, J., Ferrer, J., Sampol, G., Rosell, R., Ferrer, A., et al. (1999). Inhaled antibiotic therapy in non-cystic fibrosis with bronchiectasis and chronic bronchial infection by *Pseudomonaus aeruginosa. Respiratory Medicine, 93,* 476–480.

Reid, L. M. (1950). Reduction in bronchial subdivision in bronchiectasis. *Thorax, 5,* 233–247.

Sarris, G. E., Smith, J. A., Shumway, N. E., Stinson, E. B., Dyer, P. E., Robbins, R. C., et al. (1994). Long-term results of combined heart-lung transplantation: The Stanford experience. *Journal of Heart Lung Transplantation, 13,* 940–949.

Sepper, R., Konttinen, Y. T., Kemppinen, P., Sorsa, T., & Eklund, K. K. (1998). Mast cells in bronchiectasis. *Annals of Medicine, 30,* 307–315.

Swartz, M. N. (1998). Bronchiectasis. In A. P. Fishman (Ed.), *Pulmonary diseases and disorders* (3rd ed., pp. 2045–2070). New York: McGraw Hill Health Professions Division.

Swensen, S. J., Hartman, T. E., & Williams, D. E. (1994). Computed tomographic diagnosis of *Mycobacterium avium-intracellulare* complex in patients with bronchiectasis. *Chest, 105,* 49–52.

Tsang, K. W. T., Ho, P., Lam, W., Ip, M. S. M., Chan, K., Ho, C., et al. (1998). Inhaled fluticasone reduces inflammatory indices in severe bronchiectasis. *American Journal of Respiratory and Critical Care Medicine, 158,* 723–727.

Van der Bruggen-Bogaarts, B. A., van der Bruggen, H. M., van Waes, P. F., & Lammers, J. W. (1996). Assessment of bronchiectasis: Comparison of HRCT and spiral volumetric CT. *Journal of Computer Assisted Tomography, 20,* 15–19.

Wills, P. J., Wodehouse, T., Corkeny, K., Mallon, K., Wilson, R., & Cole, P. J. (1996). Short-term recombinant human DNase in bronchiectasis. *American Journal of Respiratory and Critical Care Medicine, 154,* 413–417.

Wilson, C. B., Jones, P. W., O'Leary, C. J., Cole, P. J., & Wilson, R. (1997). Validation of the St. George's Respiratory Questionnaire in bronchiectasis. *American Journal of Respiratory and Critical Care Medicine, 156,* 536–541.

Wilson, C. B., Jones, P. W., O'Leary, C. J., Hansell, D. M., Dowling, R. B., Cole, P. J., et al. (1998). Systemic markers of inflammation in stable bronchiectasis. *European Respiratory Journal, 12,* 820–824.

Interstitial Lung Disease — 20

Kathleen O. Lindell

INTRODUCTION

Interstitial lung disease is actually a broad category of lung diseases that affect the interstitium of the lung. There are 130–180 defined interstitial lung diseases, which are frequently classified according to etiology. They are most commonly restrictive lung diseases with widespread structural damage and alterations in pulmonary function. Primary symptoms include cough and progressively increasing dyspnea, especially related to activity. Goals of treatment include the elimination of causes, if known, and prevention of disease progression by suppressing the chronic inflammatory response. Nursing interventions are focused on assisting the patient to achieve and maintain the highest functional level possible and assisting them to meet their psychosocial needs.

I. Interstitial lung disease
   A. Definition—a category of lung diseases that affect the interstitium of the lung
      1. Pulmonary interstitium
         a. Provides the connective-tissue structure that supports the lung
         b. Is responsible for the lung's normal elasticity
      2. They are most commonly restrictive lung diseases with widespread structural involvement and alterations in pulmonary function.
      3. Primarily affects the lung parenchyma, with little affect on the airways.
   B. Etiology
      1. Etiology is identified in only about 35% of cases (Kersten, 1989).
      2. Determining etiology represents one of the challenges of differential diagnosis of ILD. Among the most common identifiable causes of ILD are occupational and environmental exposures. Systemic diseases

such as those of autoimmune origin and complications of previous medical therapy must also be considered. Other possible etiologies are listed on Table 20.1.

C. Pathophysiology

   1. Injury to the lung, no matter the source, causes characteristic pathologic changes that represent a common response, due to the lungs limited capacity to react to injury (Fauci, 1998).

Table 20.1	Possible Etiologies of Interstitial Lung Disease

Known Origin

Occupational and Environmental
   Inorganic dusts: silica, asbestos, chalk, kaolin or china clay, coal dust, cobalt
   Organic dusts (Hypersensitivity pneumonitis or extrinsic allergic alveolitis)
   Microbial—examples:
      Bacterial—farmer's lung
      Fungal—farmer's lung, hot-tub lung
      Animal/Insect proteins—examples:
         birdbreeder's disease, animal handler's lung, bird droppings, feathers, serum
         pelts, urine, serum
      Chemical fumes—examples:
         silo-filler's disease, nitrogen dioxide,
         ammonia, chlorine, sulfur dioxide, hydrochloric acid

Drugs, Poisons, Radiations
   Chemotherapeutic agents (busulfan, bleomycin, methotrexate)
   Antibiotics (nitrofurantoin, sulfasalazine)
   Cardiovascular drugs (Amidarone, Tocainide)
   Anti-inflammatories (Gold salts, Penicillamine)
   Neurotropics/Psychotropics
   Miscellaneous
      Paraquat, cocaine
      Radiation, oxygen

Rheumatologic and Autoimmune Diseases
   Systemic lupus erythematosus
   Rheumatoid arthritis
   Wegener's granulomatosis
   Churg-Strauss syndrome
   Goodpasture's syndrome

Others
   Chronic left ventricular failure, mitral stenosis, neoplastic diseases of the lung,
      pulmonary veno-occlusive disease, blood or fat emboli

| **Table 20.1** | Possible Etiologies of Interstitial Lung Disease (*continued*) |

Unknown Origin

Sarcoidosis
Pulmonary alveolar proteinosis
Desquamative interstitial pneumonia (DIP)
Acute interstitial pneumonia (AIP, Hamman-Rich Syndrome)
Lymphaangioliomyomaatosis (LAM)
Histocytosis (eosinophilic granuloma)
Chronic eosinophilic pneumonia
Idiopathic bronchiolitis obliterans with organizing pneumonia (BOOP)
Diffuse idiopathic pulmonary fibrosis or
   Usual interstititial pneumonia (UIP) &
   Crytogenic fibrosing alveolitis

Source: Adapted from Nicholson, A. G., Colby, T. V., Dubois, R. M. Hansell, D. M., & Wells, A. U. (2000). The prognostic significance of the histologic pattern of interstitial pneumonia in patients presenting with the clinical entity of cryptogenic fibrosing alveolitis. *American Journal of Respiratory and Critical Care Medicine, 162,* 2213–2217.

2. Most interstitial diseases pass through a series of pathological changes that represent different stages of a disease (Kersten, 1989).
   a. Alveolitis—an injury to the alveolar and/or endothelial cells occurs, and local and circulating inflammatory cells move to the site in response (Nicholson, Colby, Dubois, Hansell, & Wells, 2000).
   b. Fibrosis—the chronic inflammation progresses to scarring and the development of fibrotic tissue—what is called *stiff lung*.
   c. Loss of alveolar-capillary units—fibrotic changes result in distortion and disruption of gas-exchange units, with resultant physiologic symptoms. Ultimately this may result in large cystic spaces separated by thick bands of fibrous tissue called *honeycomb lung* (Nicholson et al., 2000)
3. This course is highly variable. The process may evolve over 1 to 10 or more years. There may be a steady progression of the disease, or it may be characterized by exacerbations and remissions
4. Dyspnea is due to the increased work of breathing—primarily due to the stiffness of the lungs and by excessive minute ventilation and may be amplified by hypoxemia (Baum, 1989).
D. Incidence
   1. More than 10 million people in the United States are affected by one of the interstitial diseases.
   2. 100,000 are admitted to the hospital each year with chronic interstitial fibrosis (Baum, 1989).
   3. Estimated 15% of diseases in patients seen by pulmonologists.

4. ILD may affect people of any age or race.
   a. Institial pulmonary fibrosis (IPF) develops most frequently in patients over age 60.
   b. Connective diseases and sarcoidosis usually occur under age 50.
   c. Environmental etiologies are not age specific.

E. Considerations across the life span
   1. Pediatric
      a. Actual incidence in children unknown, less information than adults.
      b. Aspiration syndromes represent a common etiology, other etiologies include bronchopulmonary dysplasia, congenital disorders, HIV.
      c. Concern about open lung biopsy in children but it is generally well tolerated and accurate diagnosis frequently leads to change in treatment (Coren, Nicholson, Goldstraw, Rosenthal, & Bush, 1999).
      d. Weight loss and failure to thrive noted with advanced disease.
      e. Hydroxychloroquine often used for treatment because of low toxicity. Cylclyphoshamide used less than in adults due to sterility issues.
   2. Pregnancy—incidence unknown, rare case reports only
   3. Elderly
      a. Progressively increasing breathlessness
      b. Often incorrectly attributed to the general aging process or lack of physical conditioning

F. Complications/Sequelae
   1. Clinical deterioration is common and may be life-threatening.
   2. Although complications may be resultant from the disease process, frequently there are also significant adverse reactions to the medical treatment of the disease.
   3. Hypoxemia is a major contributor to mortality in ILD (Nicholson et al., 2000).
   4. See Table 20.2 for progression and complications of ILD.

II. Assessment—early diagnosis is crucial.
   A. History—Presentation
      1. Cough—usually dry but occasionally productive of scant mucous
      2. Progressively increasing breathlessness
         a. Non-variable, related to exercise
         b. Quantify dyspnea—stairs, on a scale
         c. Usually persistent (not variable as asthma or CHF)
      3. Fatigue, even in the absence of dyspnea
      4. Chest discomfort
      5. Social history with emphasis on tobacco and drug use
      6. Medical history with emphasis on drugs
      7. Occupational exposures
      8. Environmental exposures (Nicholson et al., 2000). Disease onset may be immediate to 20 or more years after exposure
         a. Vent system

Table 20.2	Progression and Complications of Interstitial Lung Disease

Progression if disease process not controlled
  Symptoms
    Increasing dyspnea or cough, reduced exercise capacity
  Physical exam
    Progression of crackles from basilar to diffuse
    Worsening right-sided heart failure
  Diagnostics
    Worsening hypoxemia with increasing supplemental oxygen requirements
    Progressive volume lung loss, honeycombing
    Progressive right-sided cardiomegaly
Complications of ILD
  Infection
  Pneumothorax
  Lung cancer
  Pulmonary Hypertension
  Cor Pulmonale
  Pulmonary embolism
  Hypertension
Complication of treatment
  Infection
  Respiratory and peripheral muscle weakness
  Osteoporosis
  Cataracts
  Fluid & electrolyte imbalances
  Hyperglycemia
  Bone marrow suppression

Source: Adapted from Nicholson, A. G., Colby, T. V., Dubois, R. M. Hansell, D. M., & Wells, A. U. (2000). The prognostic significance of the histologic pattern of interstitial pneumonia in patients presenting with the clinical entity of cryptogenic fibrosing alveolitis. *American Journal of Respiratory and Critical Care Medicine, 162,* 2213–2217.

      b. Hot tubs, pools
      c. Pets—birds most common
      d. Water damage
      e. Cooling systems
      f. Fumes—gas
   B. Physical exam
      1. Altered respirations with activity
         a. Rapid, shallow respirations
         b. Ranges from mild to severe respiratory distress
      2. Clubbing
      3. Possible systemic symptoms, such as fever, weight loss
      4. Skin and joint alterations secondary to connective tissue disease

5. Fine mid-to-end inspiratory crackles
6. Rubs
7. Cyanosis (late)
8. Wheezes (not commonly)
9. Hemoptysis (not commonly)

C. Diagnostic tests—differential diagnosis is a diagnostic challenge

1. Pulmonary function tests (PFT): usually a restrictive impairment, low diffusing capacity
   a. Diffusing capacity and lung volumes, in particularly total lung capacity, are good indicators of severity/progression.
   b. Monitor effectiveness of treatment
2. Arterial desaturation/hypoxemia
   a. Not at rest until late stages but rapid decline with exercise
   b. Also a very good indicator of severity
3. Chest radiography
   a. May present as abnormal chest X-ray with the absence of symptoms
   b. 30% have changes on their initial visit
   c. May be normal even with symptomatic ILD (10%)
   d. Appears as diffuse involvement (found to be "patchy" at autopsy)
   e. Honeycombing, reticular, nodular, or ground glass pattern in the low to mid regions
   f. Poor indicator of disease progression
4. Systemic disease differential—serum studies
   a. Erythrocyte sedimentation rate (ESR)
   b. Antinuclear antibody test (ANA), rheumatoid factor (RF)
   c. Immunologic testing
   d. Fungal panel
   e. Hypersensitivity panel
5. Exercise physiology testing to evaluate physiologic severity
6. CT Scan—insufficient for diagnosis, but assists with differential by use of high resolution, thin section
7. Broncho alveolar lavage (BAL)—useful with some types of ILD but limited
8. Open lung biopsy
   a. Surgical lung biopsy (open thoracotomy or video-assisted thoracoscopy) is recommended in most patients unless contraindication to surgery exists (American Thoracic Society, 2000).
   b. Even experts demonstrate a low sensitivity for diagnosis using clinical or radiological parameters when compared with open lung biopsy (Raghu et al., 1999).
9. Video-assisted thoroscopic surgery (VATS)—may be procedure of choice to obtain tissue for biopsy: fewer complications, less recovery time.

III. Common therapeutic modalities

Goal of therapy: elimination of cause if known, and prevention of disease progression by suppressing the chronic inflammatory response and reversing the deposition of fibrotic tissue (Nicholson et al., 2000)

A. Treatment of underlying cause and cessation of known exposures
   1. Earliest possible diagnosis is essential.
   2. Accurate and exhaustive history to determine etiology and eliminate adverse occupational or environmental exposures.
   3. Smoking cessation.
B. Control of inflammation
   Immunosuppression is the cornerstone of drug therapy although there are few controlled trials demonstrating long-term efficacy.
   1. Corticosteroids
      a. Response varies—near complete response to limited or no response
      b. Benefits must be balanced against risks
         Side effects, such as osteoporosis with possible compression fractures, hyperglycemia, cataracts
   2. Cytotoxic medications, such as cyclophosphamide, azathioprine, cyclosporin
      a. Used to decrease the dose of steroids
      b. May be added to take advantage of different types of anti-inflammatory action
      c. Frequently limited by bone marrow toxicity
      d. Benefits must be balanced against risks
         Side effects, such as bone marrow toxicity, secondary cancers, ILD
   3. Dose and length of therapy will depend on response, side effects and the specific ILD. A discernible objective response to therapy may or may not be evident until the patient has received 3 months of therapy and if possible should be continued at least 6 months (American Thoracic Society, 2000).
   4. Usually suppression—not cure. Takes days to weeks to months.
C. Supportive care, treatment of complications and sequelae
   1. Oxygen therapy
      a. May significantly improve a patient's sense of well-being and help to prevent hypoxia-related complications (i.e., cor pulmonale)
      b. Initially with exercise only
      c. Potential for extremely high flow rates
   2. Pulmonary rehabilitation/exercise
      a. Maintain functional level, weight control, bone mass
      b. Tertiary health promotion
      c. Overall improvement in sense of well-being
   3. Early management of bacterial infections to reduce further damage
   4. Lung transplantation (current waiting list is 18–24 months)
IV. Nursing diagnoses, outcomes, and interventions
   A. Nursing diagnoses
      1. Altered breathing pattern related to decreased lung and chest wall compliance. Respiratory system tries to compensate through rapid, shallow breathing to reduce tidal volume and work of breathing.
      2. Alteration in comfort related to dyspnea.

Dyspnea is due to the increased work of breathing—primarily due to the stiffness of the lungs and by excessive minute ventilation and may be amplified by hypoxemia (Baum, 1989).

3. Impaired gas exchange related to changes in the interstitial structure of the lung.
4. Activity intolerance related to dyspnea on exertion.
5. Anxiety related to inability to breathe and unknown aspects of disease.
6. Knowledge deficit related to disease process and diagnostic tests.

B. Outcomes for patients with interstitial lung disease
   1. Compliance with follow-up so that changes in treatment are made as progression through stages occurs
   2. Maintenance of normal oxygenation
   3. To achieve and maintain the highest functional level possible for as long as possible
   4. An acceptable level of comfort for the patient achieved both physically and psychosocially through all stages of progression

C. Interventions—Different than obstructive diseases which involve the airways
   1. Education (Dettenmeier, 1992)
      a. Coordination of diagnostic studies and medical therapies
      b. Education of disease pathophysiology, progression, and treatment
      c. Need for early reporting to physician of changes in condition
      d. Assist in learning to live with a chronic lung disease
   2. Assist with smoking cessation.
   3. Management of dyspnea
      a. Monitor ABGs and ambulatory oximetry. Give oxygen as ordered.
      b. Breathing techniques
         i. Interstitial—emphasize deep breathing exercises, do *not* try to decrease ventilatory rate during activity
         ii. Obstructive—pursed lip and diaphragmatic breathing
      c. Morphine should be considered for terminal patients for severe breathlessness. Nebulized or p.o. morphine may be considered (Farncombe & Chater, 1993).
   4. Assist patient in achieving and maintaining highest functional level possible
      a. Monitor functional status—evaluate for self-care deficits.
      b. Monitor nutritional status.
      c. Refer to pulmonary rehabilitation.
      d. Assist with ADLs as needed.
   5. Monitoring progression
      a. Frequently evaluate respiratory status. Monitor compliance and effect of therapies (PFTs, oximetry).
      b. Quality of life status may be helpful. Current quality of life tools used for other respiratory diseases such as the SF-36, QWB, CRQ,

SGRQ may be applied to patients with ILD (Chang, Curtis, Patrick, & Raghu, 1999).

    c. Hospice may be considered for terminal stages.

V. Home care considerations

    1. Varied due to the different stages of ILD (minimal effect on ADL to devastating effect)

    2. Oxygen therapy

        a. Initially with exercise only

        b. Becomes a challenge as extremely high flow rates of oxygen are needed as disease progresses to end stages

        c. High flow needs especially great in a portable system so that patient can leave the home for as long as possible

        d. Consider transtracheal oxygen delivery

    3. Living with a chronic lung disease, including terminal stages

WEB SITES

http://www.healthlinkusa.com
http://www.lung.ca
http://www.lungusa.org
http://www.mayohealth.org
http://www.medhelp.org
http://www.mtsinai.org
http://www.nationaljewish.org
http://www.nhlbi.nih.gov

REFERENCES

American Thoracic Society. (2000). Idiopathic pulmonary fibrosis: Diagnosis and Treatment: International consensus statement. *American Journal of Respiratory and Critical Care Medicine, 161*(2 Pt 1), 646–664.

Baum, G. L. (Ed.). (1989). *Textbook of pulmonary diseases* (4th ed.). Boston: Little, Brown.

Chang, J. A., Curtis, J. R., Patrick, D. L., & Raghu, G. (1999). Assessment of health-related quality of life in patients with interstitial lung disease. *Chest, 116*(5), 1175–1182.

Coren, M. E., Nicholson, A. G., Goldstraw, P., Rosenthal, M., & Bush, A. (1999). Open lung biopsy for diffuse interstitial lung disease in children. *European Respiratory Journal, 14*(4), 817–821.

Dettenmeier, P. A. (1992). *Pulmonary nursing care.* St. Louis: Mosby.

Farncombe, M., & Chater, S. (1993). Case studies outlining use of nebulized morphine for patients with end-stage chronic lung disease and cardiac disease. *Journal of Pain and Symptom Management, 8*(4), 221–225.

Fauci, A. (Ed.). (1998). *Harrison's principles of internal medicine* (14th ed.). New York: McGraw-Hill.

Kersten, L. D. (Ed.). (1989). *Comprehensive pulmonary nursing.* Philadelphia: Saunders.

Nicholson, A. G., Colby, T. V., Dubois, R. M. Hansell, D. M., & Wells, A. U. (2000). The prognostic significance of the histologic pattern of interstitial pneumonia in patients presenting with the clinical entity of cryptogenic fibrosing alveolitis. *American Journal of Respiratory and Critical Care Medicine, 162,* 2213–2217.

Raghu, G., Mageto, Y. N., Lickhart, D., Schmidt, R. A., Wood, D. E., & Godwin, J. D. (1999). The accuracy of the clinical diagnosis of new-onset idiopathic pulmonary fibrosis and other interstitial lung disease: A prospective study. *Chest, 116*(5), 1168–1174.

Pneumonias

Janet Harris

INTRODUCTION

Mortality from pneumonia ranges from <1% in healthy patients with Community Acquired Pneumonia (CAP) to 50% in severe CAP admitted to the ICU (American Thoracic Society [ATS], 2001); attributable mortality is 11%–33% in ICU patients with Hospital Acquired Pneumonia (HAP). Colonization of the respiratory tract represents a dynamic balance between host defenses and microbes. Understanding colonization is key to understanding pneumonia. Aspiration is the primary route of bacterial entry into the lungs (Centers for Disease Control [CDC], 1994; CDC, 1997; Niederman, 1990; Niederman, Craven, Fein, & Schultz, 1990). Patients most vulnerable to acquiring pneumonia include extremes in age (neonates and elderly), individuals with chronic illnesses, and critically ill patients.

I. Overview

Pneumonia is the sixth leading cause of death in the United States, the second most common nosocomial infection, and the leading cause of death from nosocomial infections (CDC, 1999). Annually, 4.8 million cases on pneumonia are reported (1.8 cases per 100 persons; CDC, 2001). The annual direct cost of diagnosing and treating pneumonia exceeds $2 billion (Wenzel, 1989).

A. Definition: Inflammatory response of the host to the uncontrolled multiplication of microorganisms invading the lower respiratory tract (Griffin & Meduri, 1994; Lerner, 1980; Skerrett, 1994). Accumulation of neutrophils and other effector cells in the peripheral bronchi and alveolar spaces (Skerrett, 1994). The Centers for Disease Control and Prevention (CDC) definitions for pneumonia are outlined in Table 21.1 (CDC, 1989a).

The views of the author are her own and do not reflect the official policy or position of the Department of the Army, the Department of Defense, or the United States Government.

Table 21.1	Centers for Disease Control and Prevention (CDC)

Pneumonia must meet one of the following criteria

1. Rales or dullness to percussion on physical examination of chest *and* any of the following
   a. New onset of purulent sputum or change in character of sputum
   b. Organism isolated from blood culture
   c. Isolation of pathogen from specimen obtained by transtracheal aspirate, bronchial brushing, or biopsy
2. Chest radiographic examination shows new or progressive infiltrate, consolidation, cavitation, or pleural effusion *and* any of the following:
   a. New onset of purulent sputum or change in character of sputum
   b. Organisms isolated from blood culture
   c. Isolation of pathogen from specimen obtained by transtracheal aspirate, bronchial brushing, or biopsy
   d. Isolation of virus or detection of viral antigen in respiratory secretions
   e. Diagnostic single antibody titer (IgM) or fourfold increase in paired serum samples (IgG) of pathogen
3. Patient ≤12 months of age has two of the following: apnea, tachypnea, bradycardia, wheezing, rhonchi, or cough, *and* any of the following:
   a. Increased production of respiratory secretions
   b. New onset of purulent sputum or change in character of sputum
   c. Organism isolated from blood culture
   d. Isolation of pathogen for specimen obtained by transtracheal aspirate, bronchial brushing, or biopsy
   e. Isolation of virus or detection of viral antigen in respiratory secretions
   f. Diagnostic single antibody titer (IgM) or fourfold increase in paired serum samples (IgG) of pathogen
   g. Histopathologic evidence of pneumonia
4. Patient ≤12 months of age has chest radiologic examination that shows new or progressive infiltrate, cavitation, consolidation, or pleural effusion, *and* any of the following:
   a. Increased production of respiratory secretions
   b. New onset of purulent sputum or change in character of sputum
   c. Organism isolated from blood culture
   d. Isolation of pathogen for specimen obtained by transtracheal aspirate, bronchial brushing, or biopsy
   e. Isolation of virus or detection of viral antigen in respiratory secretions

Source: Definitions of Pneumonia (CDC, 1989b).

1. Hospital-acquired pneumonia (HAP) (nosocomial pneumonia)—"There is no evidence that the infection (pneumonia) was present or incubating at the time of hospital admission" (CDC, 1989a, p. 1058)
2. Community-acquired pneumonia (CAP)—Pneumonia that develops outside of the hospital or health care institution.

B. Etiology
  1. Hospital-acquired pneumonia
     a. Bacterial
        i. Frequently polymicrobial, with more than one organism identified in over 30% of patients (CDC, 1989a, 1997; Chastre et al., 1988; Harris, Joshi, Morton, & Soeken, 2000; Jimenez et al., 1989; Rello, Ausina, Castella, Net, & Prats, 1992; Torres et al., 1989). The causative organism(s) varies by patient type.
        ii. Gram-negative bacilli the predominant organisms (isolated in over 50% of HAP; CDC, 1997, 1999)
            ■ *Pseudomonas aeruginosa* (12%–22%)
            ■ *Enterobacter* sp. (8%–13%)
            ■ *Klebsiella pnsumoniae* (5%–8%)
            ■ *Escherichia coli* (3%–5%)
        iii. Gram-positive organisms (CDC, 1997, 1999)
            ■ *Staphylococcus aureus* (11%–25%)
            ■ Methicillin-resistant *Staphylococcus aureus (MRSA)*
            ■ *Enterococcus* sp. (1%–2%)
            ■ *Streptococcus pneumoniae*
        iv. Other bacterial pathogens
            ■ *Legionella* species (1%–14%), risk of developing depends on the type and duration of exposure and the individuals health status, with patients with immunosuppression and chronic health problems at an increased risk (CDC, 1997).
            ■ *Haemophilus influenzae*
     b. Viral—20% of HAP (CDC, 1997)
        i. Respiratory syncytial virus (RSV), most common in infancy and early childhood
        ii. Influenza—typically occurs in the winter, December through April
        iii. Other viruses—Adenoviruses, measles virus, parainfluenza virus, rhinoviruses, and varicella-zoster virus
     c. Fungus
        i. Aspergillus species: greatest risk in highly immunocompromised patients and patients with preexisting lung disease (CDC, 1997)
        ii. *Candida albicans* (1.5%–6.3%) (CDC, 1997)
  2. Community-acquired pneumonia
     a. Bacterial
        i. Causative organism is not known in approximately 50% of cases (ATS, 2001; Campbell, 1999).
        ii. *Streptococcus pneumoniae* is the most common cause (ATS, 2001; Bartlett et al., 2000; Campbell, 1999; Marrie, 1998b; Ruiz et al., 1999). *Streptococcus pneumoniae* is the most common pathogen associated with mortality (ATS, 2001; Bartlett et al., 2000). Increased incidence of drug-resistant *Streptococcus*

255

pneumoniae (DRSP) in recent years, particularly in individuals age 65 or older (ATS, 2001; Campbell, 1999).

   iii. Other frequently found bacteria include: *H. influenzae, Klebsiella pneumoniae,* and *Staphylococcus aureus* (MRSA is a rare cause of CAP).

   iv. *Legionella* species

  b. Viral—reported in approximately 10% of CAP (Ruiz et al., 1999)

   i. Influenza—greatest risk in the very young, the elderly, immunocompromised patients, and patients with chronic conditions such as heart and lung disease (ATS, 2001)

   ii. Other viruses—include adenoviruses, RSV, measles virus, parainfluenza viruses, rhinoviruses, and varicella-zoster virus (ATS, 2001)

  c. Atypical pathogens

   i. *Pneumosystis carinii*—common in HIV-infected patients

   ii. *Chlamydia pneumoniae*—Intracellular parasite responsible for 6%–10% of CAP (Cassell, 1999; Peeling & Brunham, 1996)

   iii. *Mycoplasma pneumoniae*—Most common cause of CAP in young adults, particularly military recruits (Farzan, 1997; Ruiz et al., 1999)

C. Pathophysiology

  1. Bacterial pneumonia (Figure 21.1)

   A theoretical model depicting the pathogenesis of bacterial pneumonia (nosocomial) was postulated by the CDC's Hospital Infection Control Practices Advisory Committee and modified by the author based

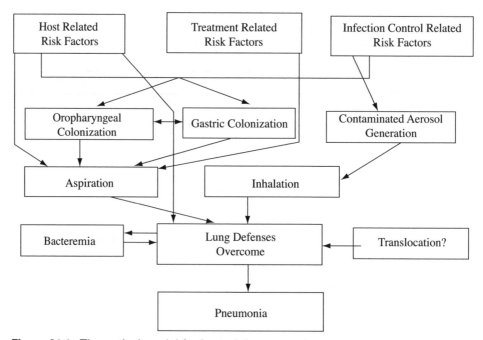

Figure 21.1. Theoretical model for bacterial pneumonia.

on empirical data (CDC, 1997; Harris et al., 2000; Harris & Miller, 2000). Although the model was originally developed for hospital acquired bacterial pneumonia, the principles also apply to bacterial CAP.

a. Pulmonary defenses overwhelmed—Pneumonia develops when pulmonary defense mechanisms are either overwhelmed to impaired allowing rapid multiplication of microorganisms (CDC, 1997; Huxley, Viroslav, Gray, & Pierce, 1978)

b. Routes of microbial entry

    i. Aspiration is the primary route of bacterial entry into the lungs (CDC, 1994, 1997; Niederman, 1990; Niederman, Craven, Fein, & Schultz, 1990). Approximately 45% of healthy individuals aspirate during their sleep (Huxley et al., 1978); however, infection rarely develops because the bacteria are cleared by the pulmonary defense mechanisms. Aspiration of large quantities of material increases the likelihood that the pulmonary defense mechanisms will be exceeded. Characteristics (pH, bacterial content, etc.) of the aspirate may increase the risk of pneumonia.

    ii. Inhalation is the second route of entry of microorganisms into the lower respiratory tract. Normally, the upper respiratory host defenses prevent particles from reaching the lower respiratory tract. If respiratory equipment is contaminated with microorganisms, the organisms become aerosolized, bypass the protective mechanisms of the upper airways, and are inhaled directly into the lower respiratory tract.

    iii. Hematogenous spread from a distant site—The pulmonary circulation, with its dense network in the walls of the alveoli, provides a potential portal of entry for microbes. Bacteria from a distant infection site can migrate through the pulmonary circulation, creating an opportunity for pneumonia (CDC, 1994, 1997). However, bacteremia is considered a rare cause of pneumonia (CDC, 1994; 1997).

    iv. Translocation of bacterial toxins and bacteria from the gut lumen—Ischemic mucosal injury in the gut allows passage of bacteria from the lumen of the gastrointestinal tract to the mesenteric lymph nodes and the lung (CDC, 1994, 1997; Fiddian-Green & Baker, 1991).

c. Colonization—the persistence of microorganisms, other than flora normal for the site, in the absence of clinical evidence of infection (Bonten et al., 1994; Johanson & Dever, 1998)

    i. Oropharyngeal colonization—the persistence of microorganisms, other than normal flora, in the oropharynx, with no clinical evidence of infection (Bonten et al., 1994; Johanson & Dever, 1998). When antibiotics or other mechanisms destroy normal oropharyngeal flora, the binding sites usually occupied by normal flora are susceptible to colonization by pathogenic organisms. Once the oropharynx is colonized with pathogenic

257

Table 21.2 | Risk Factors Associated With Oropharyngeal Colonization

Risk Factor	References
Prior Antibiotic Therapy	(Johanson, Pierce, Sanford, & Thomas, 1972)
Increased Age	(Lowry, Carlisle, Adams, & Feiner, 1987; Valenti, Trudell, & Bentley, 1978)
Depressed Level of Consciousness	(Valenti et al., 1978)
Endotracheal Intubation	(Johanson et al., 1972)
COPD	(Johanson et al., 1972)
Nasogastric Tube	(Valenti et al., 1978)
Acidosis	(Johanson et al., 1972)
Alcoholism	(Johanson et al., 1972; Mackowiak, Martin, Jones, & Smith, 1978)
Diabetes mellitus	(Johanson et al., 1972; Mackowiak et al., 1978)
Malnutrition	(Higuchi & Johanson, 1980; Niederman et al., 1984)
Severity of Illness	(Johanson et al., 1972; Kerver et al., 1987)
Smoking	(Niederman et al., 1983)
Dental Plaque	(Fourrier, Duvivier, Boutigny, & Roussel-Delvallez, 1998)

Source: Reprinted with permission: Harris, J. R., & Miller, T. H. (2000). Preventing Nosocomial Pneumonia: Evidenced-Based Practice. *Critical Care Nurse, 20*(1), 54.

organisms, these organisms are available for aspiration into the lower respiratory tract. Risk factors for oropharyngeal colonization are outlined in Table 21.2.

ii. Gastric colonization—the presence of microorganisms in the stomach in the absence of infection (Bonten et al., 1994). A linear relationship exists between stomach pH and gastric colonization (DuMoulin, Paterson, Hedley-Whyte, & Lisbon, 1982). Patients with a gastric pH < 4 do not have gastric colonization, while gastric colonization occurred in patients with a gastric pH > 4 (DuMoulin et al., 1982). Gastric colonization potentates retrograde colonization of the oropharynx. Risk factors for gastric colonization are outlined in Table 21.3.

iii. Colonization of equipment (respiratory)—the presence of microorganisms on respiratory equipment. If respiratory equipment becomes colonized with microorganisms, these organisms become aerosolized and are inhaled directly into the lower respiratory tract (CDC, 1997; Craven, Steger, Barat, & Duncan, 1992; Niederman, 1990).

d. Risk factors (see Tables 21.4 and 21.5)

i. Host–related: individual characteristics, which alter an individual's risk of developing pneumonia

| Table 21.3 | Risk Factors Associated With Gastric Colonization |

Risk Factor	References
Gastric Acid Neutralization Histamine Type 2 Blockers	(Dirks et al., 1987; Donowitz, Wenzel, & Hoyt, 1982; DuMoulin et al., 1982; Pingleton, Hinthorn, & Liu, 1986)
Antacids	(Dirks et al., 1987; Donowitz et al., 1982; DuMoulin et al., 1982; Pingleton et al., 1986)
Enteral Feedings	(Dirks et al., 1987; Donowitz et al., 1982; DuMoulin et al., 1982; Pingleton et al., 1986)
Achlorhydria	(Drasar, Shiner, & McLead, 1969)
Ileus or upper gastrointestinal Disease	(Dirks et al., 1987; Donowitz et al., 1982; DuMoulin et al., 1982; Pingleton et al., 1986)

Source: Reprinted with permission: Harris, J. R., & Miller, T. H. (2000). Preventing Nosocomial Pneumonia: Evidenced-Based Practice. *Critical Care Nurse, 20*(1), 54.

    ii. Treatment-related: procedures or therapies that increase the patient's risk of developing pneumonia.

    iii. Infection control–related: the spread of microorganisms on the hands of providers or caregivers, from the environment, or on equipment.

2. Viral pneumonias—Usually follow community outbreaks of the virus; spread from person to person by direct deposit of droplets infected with the virus on mucosal membranes (CDC, 1997).

3. Legionnaires' disease—a multisystem illness with pneumonia resulting from exposure to contaminated water (CDC, 1997). *Legionella* species are commonly present in natural and man-made water environments. Factors that increase the likelihood of colonization of *Legionella* species in man-made water environments (cooling towers, evaporative condensers, potable-water distribution systems) include temperatures of 25–42° C, stagnation, and sediment (CDC, 1997).

4. Chlamydiae pneumonia—Spread by person to person on respiratory droplets (Peeling & Brunham, 1996). Infections are generally mild or asymptomatic but can be severe, particularly in the elderly. Outbreaks can occur in schools, military barracks, and nursing homes (Cassell, 1999; Peeling & Brunham, 1996).

5. Aspergillosis—"Fungi commonly found in soil, water, and decaying vegetation . . . has been cultured from unfiltered air, ventilation systems, contaminated dust dislodged during hospital renovation and construction, horizontal surfaces, food, and ornamental plants" (CDC, 1997, p. 12). Inhalation of fungal spores is the primary route of entry (CDC, 1997).

259

| Table 21.4 | Risk Factors Associated With Hospital-Acquired Pneumonia |

Host Related Risk Factors	References
Increased Age	(Antonelli et al., 1994; Celis et al., 1988; Harris et al., 2000; Hoyt et al., 1993; Joshi, Localio, & Hamory, 1992; Kollef, 1993; Windsor & Hill, 1988)
Altered Level of Consciousness	(Andrews, Coalson, Smith, & Johanson, 1981; Celis et al., 1988; Chevret, Hemmer, Carlet, Langer, & the European Cooperative Group on Nosocomial Pneumonia, 1993; Craven et al., 1986; Cunnion et al., 1996; Helling, Evans, Fowler, Hays, & Kennedy, 1988; Hoyt et al., 1993; Joshi et al., 1992; Langer et al., 1987; Rello et al., 1992; Rodriguez et al., 1991; Salemi, Morgan, Kelleghan, & Hiebert-Crape, 1993; Torres et al., 1990; Walker, Kapelanski, Weiland, Stewart, & Duke, 1985)
COPD	(Celis et al., 1988; Craven et al., 1992; Ephgrave et al., 1993; Garibaldi, Britt, Coleman, Reading, & Page, 1981; Gaynes, Bizek, & Mowry-Hanley, 1991; Jimenez et al., 1989; Salemi et al., 1993; Torres et al., 1990)
Severity of Illness	(Chevret et al., 1993; Cunnion et al., 1996; Harris et al., 2000; Hoyt et al., 1993; Joshi et al., 1992; Kollef, 1993; Rodriguez et al., 1991; Salemi et al., 1993; Sariego, Brown, Matsumoto, & Kerstein, 1993; Torres et al., 1990)
Malnutrition	(Cunnion et al., 1996; Garibaldi et al., 1981; Gorse, Messner, & Stephens, 1989; Niederman et al., 1984; Windsor & Hill, 1988)
Shock	(Hoyt et al., 1993; Rodriguez et al., 1991; Walker et al., 1985)
Blunt Trauma	(Hoyt et al., 1993; Walker et al., 1985)
Severe Head Trauma	(Baraibar et al., 1997; Harris et al., 2000; Hoyt et al., 1993; Rodriguez et al., 1991)
Chest Trauma	(Harris et al., 2000; Helling et al., 1988; Hoyt et al., 1993; Rodriguez et al., 1991)
Smoking	(Celis et al., 1988; Garibaldi et al., 1981; Salemi et al., 1993; Windsor & Hill, 1988)
Dental Plaque	(Fourrier et al., 1998)

Treatment Related Risk Factors	References
Mechanical Ventilation	(Antonelli et al., 1994; Celis et al., 1988; Chevret et al., 1993; Cunnion et al., 1996; Gaynes et al., 1991; Haley et al., 1981; Harris et al., 2000; Joshi et al., 1992; Kollef et al., 1997; Langer et al., 1987; Langer, Mosconi, Cigada, Mandelli, & The Intensive Care Unit Group of Infection Control, 1989; Salemi et al., 1993; Torres et al., 1990; Walker et al., 1985)

Table 21.4	Risk Factors Associated With Hospital-Acquired Pneumonia (*continued*)

Treatment Related Risk Factors	References
Reintubation or Self-extubation	(Harris et al., 2000; Torres et al., 1990)
Bronchoscopy	(Joshi et al., 1992; Torres et al., 1990)
Nasogastric Tube	(Celis et al., 1988; Cunnion et al., 1996; Harris et al., 2000; Joshi et al., 1992; Salemi et al., 1993)
Presence of Intra-cranial Pressure (ICP) monitor	(Craven et al., 1986; Harris et al., 2000)
Prior Antibiotic Therapy	(Craven et al., 1986; Kollef et al., 1997; Kollef, 1993; Rello et al., 1994; Walker et al., 1985)
Elevated gastric pH Histamine Type2 Blockers Antacid Therapy Enteral Feedings	(Craven et al., 1986; Gaynes et al., 1991; Joshi et al., 1992; Salemi et al., 1993)
Head Surgery	(Harris et al., 2000; Salemi et al., 1993)
Upper Abdominal or Thoracic	(Baraibar et al., 1997; Craven, Connolly, Lichtenberg, Primeau, & McCabe, 1982; Harris et al., 2000; Hoyt et al., 1993)
Surgery	(Celis et al., 1988; Haley et al., 1981; Harris et al., 2000; Hooten, Haley, White, Morgan, & Carroll, 1981; Hoyt et al., 1993; Joshi et al., 1992; Windsor & Hill, 1988)
Supine Position	(Kollef, 1993; Torres et al., 1992)

Infection Control Related Risk Factors	References
Poor Hand Washing	(CDC, 1994; CDC, 1997; Maki, 1978)
Changing Ventilator Tubing < 48 Hours	(Craven et al., 1986)

Source: Reprinted with permission: Harris, J. R., & Miller, T. H. (2000). Preventing Nosocomial Pneumonia: Evidenced-Based Practice. *Critical Care Nurse, 20*(1), 55.

D. Incidence—Sixth leading cause of death in the United States
   1. Hospital-acquired pneumonia
      a. Second most common hospital-acquired (nosocomial) infection (CDC, 1999)
      b. Leading cause of death from hospital-acquired infections (CDC, 1999). Rate: 4 episodes/1000 admissions in nonteaching hospitals versus 7 episodes per 1000 admissions in teaching hospitals (Craven & Steger, 1997)
      c. Incidence varies by type of patient
         i. ICU patients at greatest risk, 9%–45% of ICU patients develop HAP (CDC, 1999; Craven & Steger, 1997; Harris et al., 2000).

| Table 21.5 | Risk Factors for Community-Acquired Pneumonia (CAP) |

Risk Factor

Age
  Very young (<2 years old)
  >65 years of age

Smoking

Alcohol abuse

Comorbidities
  Pulmonary Diseases
  Cardiovascular Diseases
  Hepatic Diseases
  Renal Diseases
  Central Nervous System Diseases
  Immunosuppression

ii. Pediatric ICU 5.7 episodes/1000 ventilator days (lowest ICU rate) (CDC, 1999)
iii. Burn ICU 16.9 episodes/1000 ventilator days (highest ICU rate) (CDC, 1999)

2. Community-acquired pneumonia
   a. 4 million people per year, resulting in 1.4 million hospital admissions (ATS, 2001)
   b. Rate: 12 episodes per 1000 persons in the United States (Marrie, 1998a)

E. Considerations across the life span
   1. Pediatric
      a. Prevention
         i. Yearly influenza vaccination (CDC, 1984)
            Children with chronic illnesses (cardiovascular, pulmonary, metabolic diseases, renal dysfunction, anemia, immunosuppression) that required follow-up during the preceding year
         ii. Pneumococcal vaccination
            Children >2 years of age with chronic illnesses associated with increased risk of pneumococcal disease (asplenia; nephrotic syndrome; cerebrospinal fluid leaks; immunosuppression; asymptomatic or symptomatic HIV infection) (CDC, 1989b)
      b. Diagnosis
         i. Clinical symptoms include fever, headache, abdominal pain, cough, and crepitating; tachypnea (respiratory rate > 50 breaths/minute) (Sinaniotis, 1999)

        ii. Wheezing in viral and myocoplasma pneumonias (Sinaniotis, 1999)

  2. Pregnancy

    Prevention—Influenza vaccine is considered safe for pregnant women, however recommend waiting until the second or third trimester to minimize the possibility of teratogenicity (CDC, 1984)

  3. Elderly

    a. Prevention

        i. Yearly influenza vaccination (CDC, 1984)

          All individuals >65 years of age

          Individuals <65 years old with chronic illnesses (cardiovascular, pulmonary, metabolic diseases, renal dysfunction, anemia, immunosuppression)

        ii. Pneumoccoal vaccination (5–6 yr.) (CDC, 1989b)

          All individuals >65 years of age

          Individuals <65 with chronic illnesses (cardiovascular disease; pulmonary disease, diabetes milieus, alcoholism, cirrhosis, asymptomatic and symptomatic HIV infection, splenic dysfunction, nephrotic syndrome, chronic renal failure, immunosuppression)

    b. Diagnosis

        i. May not exhibit the classic symptoms of increased temperature, increased WBC, cough, crackles, or consolidation on chest X-ray (Feldman, 1999; Harris et al., 2000)

        ii. Frequently see confusion, lethargy, weakness, anorexia, and failure to thrive (Feldman, 1999)

        iii. Respiratory rate > 26 breaths/minute—good indicator of pneumonia (Feldman, 1999)

F. Complications/sequelae

  1. Failure to respond to therapy

    a. Incorrect diagnosis—investigate other causes

    b. Incorrect antibiotic coverage

  2. Mortality—ranges from <1% in healthy patients with CAP to 50% in severe CAP admitted to the ICU (ATS, 2001); attributable mortality of 11%–33% in ICU patients with HAP

    a. Pneumonia with gram-negative bacilli, particularly *Pseudomonas aureginosa* has the highest mortality rate (CDC, 1997; Ruiz et al., 1999)

    b. Legionnaires' disease—up to a 40% mortality rate (CDC, 1997)

    c. *Streptococcus pneumoniae* in CAP (Ruiz et al., 1999)

  3. Secondary infections and other complications

    a. Bacteremia (10% of patients with pneumonia have positive blood cultures) (Marrie, 1998a)

    b. Sepsis

    c. Lung abscess

    d. Empyema

    e. Acute respiratory distress syndrome (ARDS)

II. Assessment
  A. History
    1. Duration and extent of fever (if any)
    2. Chills
    3. Pleuritic chest pain
    4. Cough
    5. Sputum production (characteristics—color, odor, usually purulent)
    6. Dyspnea
    7. Weight loss
    8. Identification of risk factors, including comorbidities
    9. Identification of potential environmental risks
    10. Change in mental status (particularly in elderly)
    11. Onset of symptoms, abrupt versus gradual
  B. Physical exam
    1. Fever usually present, some may be hypothermic; some patients particularly the elderly may not have an elevated temperature
    2. Crackles heard on auscultation over the affected area of the lung
    3. Bronchial breathe sounds—sign of consolidation
    4. Dullness to percussion present in approximately 20% of patients
    5. Presence of nasal flaring and expiratory grunt
    6. Use of accessory muscles to breathe
    7. Tachypnea
    8. Tachycardia
  C. Diagnostic tests
    1. CAP: Patients to be treated as outpatients (80% of all CAP; Bernstein, 1999)
      a. Chest radiograph
      b. Complete white blood count
      c. Oxygen saturation by pulse oximetry
      d. In COPD patients, sputum specimen for culture (ATS, 2001)
      e. Value of sputum Gram stain is controversial in patients with mild to moderate CAP to be treated as outpatient. American Thoracic Society (ATS, 2001) recommends only in COPD patients. IDSA (Infectious Disease Society of America; 1999) recommends in all patients.
    2. HAP and CAP requiring hospitalization
      a. Chest radiograph
      b. Complete white blood count
      c. Electrolytes and creatinine
      d. Oxygen saturation by pulse oximetry,
      e. Sputum for gram stain and culture (specimen should be cultured only if it has more than 25 polymorphonuclear neutrophils and less than 10 squamous epithelial cells per low-power field)
      f. Two sets of blood cultures
      g. Culture of pleural fluid if indicated
      h. Diagnostic antibody titers may be indicated

    i. Bronchoscopy with bronchial lavage or bronchial brush specimen may be indicated to assist with diagnosis and identification of causative organism.

III. Common therapeutic modalities

  A. Antibiotic therapy initiated as soon as possible

    1. Initially empiric based on suspected organism as determined by patient history and applicable risk factors

    2. Antibiotic therapy adjusted as necessary based on identification of causative organism and response of patient

    3. Guidelines are available for treatment of HAP and CAP from the American Thoracic Society and the Infectious Diseases Society of America (ATS, 1996, 2001; Bartlett et al., 2000; Bernstein, 1999; Campbell Jr., 1999)

  B. Supportive care

    1. Oxygen therapy

    2. Hydration

    3. Nutritional support

    4. Mechanical ventilation may be required in severe cases

    5. Rest

    6. Airway clearance techniques

    7. Nonsteroidal anti-inflammatory drugs (NSAIDs) for fever/aches

IV. Nursing diagnoses, outcomes, and interventions (see Table 21.6)

Table 21.6 | Nursing Diagnoses, Patient Outcomes, and Interventions

Diagnoses	Patient Outcomes	Interventions
1. Impaired gas exchange related to ventilation/ perfusion inequality resulting from pneumonia	Maintain adequate oxygenation/ventilation ■ O_2 Saturation >90%, (>88% if underlying lung disease) ■ Skin, mucous membrane, and nail bed color normal ■ Respiratory rate normal for age ■ Heart rate normal for age	■ Monitor vital signs and temperature; assess use of accessory muscles ■ Monitor for signs of hypoxia and hypoxemia ■ Monitor mental status ■ Administer oxygen ■ May require mechanical ventilation to maintain adequate oxygenation ■ Monitor SaO_2 or ABGs as indicated ■ Assess/monitor closely for orthostatic hypotension ■ Position to maximize oxygenation (Good lung down

(continued)

Table 21.6 | Nursing Diagnoses, Patient Outcomes, and Interventions (*continued*)

Diagnoses	Patient Outcomes	Interventions
		position, semifowlers, etc.) Monitor respiratory status and oxygenation closely during position changes
2. Infection of pulmonary parenchyma related to inability of the pulmonary defense mechanisms to clear invading organisms	No evidence of infection ■ WBC within NL ■ Afebrile ■ Lungs clear to auscultation ■ No chills ■ Mental status normal ■ Respiratory rate within NL	■ Administer antibiotics as ordered (initiate antibiotics as soon as possible after suspected diagnosis) ■ Monitor for nonresponse to antibiotic therapy (continued fever or hypothermia, chills, WBC >11,000 or <4,000, worsening respiratory status) ■ Assist in the identification of the causative organism as indicated (primarily in HAP and CAP requiring hospitalization; blood cultures, sputum gram stain & culture, titers)
3. Ineffective airway clearance related to copious secretions	■ Airway maintained	■ Pulmonary toilet; cough and deep breathe, chest percussion with postural drainage (if tolerates) ■ Auscultate lungs ■ Suctioning of secretions as indicated ■ Monitor for hypoxia and hypoxemia ■ Monitor chest X-ray results and ABGs as indicated
4. Ineffective breathing pattern related to infection of the lung parenchyma	■ Patient verbalizes breathing is comfortable ■ Skin, mucous membrane and nail bed color normal ■ Afebrile ■ Respiratory rate normal for age ■ Able to breathe without the use of accessory muscles	■ Assess respiratory status: rate, rhythm, depth, auscultate lung fields, use of accessory muscles ■ Pulmonary toilet; cough and deep breathe, chest percussion with postural drainage (if tolerates) ■ Instruct in relaxation techniques
5. Alteration in nutrition, less than body	■ Maintains weight or adequate weight gain for age (pediatrics)	■ Weigh daily ■ Assess mucous membranes, skin turgor, and electrolytes

Table 21.6 Nursing Diagnoses, Patient Outcomes, and Interventions (*continued*)

Diagnoses	Patient Outcomes	Interventions
requirements related to pneumonia, stress, and intubation (if required)	■ Oral intake adequate ■ Moist mucous membranes ■ Good skin turgor	■ Monitor intake and output ■ Administer diet or intravenous therapy as ordered ■ Dietary consult to calculate caloric requirements
6. Activity intolerance related to impaired oxygenation	■ Patient able to resume normal activities	■ Pace activities ■ Allow adequate rest between activities ■ Monitor for signs of orthostatic hypotension
7. Alteration in comfort related to pleuritic pain	■ Patient verbalizes relief from pain	■ Administer analgesics as ordered to provide pain relief

V. Home care considerations
  A. Equipment considerations
     1. Patients receiving at home nebulizer treatments should be taught about infection control issues and proper care of the nebulizer to prevent colonization and subsequent inhalation of microorganisms
     2. Antibiotic therapy—may receive intravenous antibiotics at home
  B. Caregiver considerations—monitor for signs of failure to respond to therapy and worsening respiratory status indicating the need for hospitalization (Feldman, 1999)
     1. Respiratory rate > 30 breaths/minute
     2. Fever continues after 72 hours
     3. Cyanosis
     4. Tachycardia > 140 beats/minute
     5. Confusion
     6. Systolic hypotension <90 mm Hg
     7. Diastolic hypotension <60 mm Hg

WEB SITES

Agency for Healthcare Research and Quality: http://www.ahrq.gov/
American Association of Respiratory Care (AARC): http://www.aarc.org/
American College of Chest Physicians: http://www.chestnet.org/
American Lung Association: http://www.lungusa.org/
American Thoracic Society: http://www.thoracic.org/
British Thoracic Society: http://www.brit-thoracic.org.uk/

Canadian Thoracic Society: http://www.lung.ca/cts/
Centers for Disease Control and Prevention: http://cdc.gov/
National Guideline Clearinghouse: http://guideline.gov/
National Institute of Allergy and Infectious Diseases: http://www.niaid.nih.gov/
  default.htm/
National Institutes of Health: http://nih.gov/
Society of Critical Care Medicine: http://www.sccm.org/

REFERENCES

American Thoracic Society. (1996). Hospital-acquired pneumonia in adults: Diagnosis, assessment of severity, initial antimicrobial therapy, and preventive strategies. *American Journal of Respiratory and Critical Care Medicine, 153*, 1711–1725.

American Thoracic Society. (2001). Guidelines for the management of adults with community-acquired pneumonia. *American Review of Respiratory Diseases, 163*, 1730–1754.

Andrews, C. P., Coalson, J. J., Smith, J. D., & Johanson, W. G., Jr. (1981). Diagnosis of nosocomial bacterial pneumonia in acute, diffuse lung injury. *Chest, 80*(3), 254–258.

Antonelli, M., Moro, M. L., Capelli, O., De Blasi, R. A., D'Errico, R. R., Conti, G., et al. (1994). Risk factors for early onset pneumonia in trauma patients. *Chest, 105*, 224–228.

Baraibar, J., Correa, H., Mariscal, D., Gallego, M., Valles, J., & Rello, J. (1997). Risk factors for infection by Acinetobacter baumannii in intubated patients with nosocomial pneumonia. *Chest, 112*, 1050–1054.

Bartlett, J. G., Dowell, S. F., Mandell, L. A., File, T. M., Jr., Musher, D. M., & Fine, M. J. (2000). Practice guidelines for management of community-acquired pneumonia in adults. *Clinical Infectious Diseases, 31*, 347–382.

Bernstein, J. M. (1999). Treatment of community-acquired pneumonia—ISDA Guidelines. *Chest, 115*(3), 9S–13S.

Bonten, M. J. M., Gaillard, C. A., van Tiel, F. H., Smeets, H. G. W., van der Geest, S., & Stobberingh, E. E. (1994). The stomach is not a source for colonization of the upper respiratory tract and pneumonia in ICU patients. *Chest, 105*, 878–884.

Campbell, G. D., Jr., (1999). Commentary on the 1993 American Thoracic Society guidelines for the treatment of community-acquired pneumonia. *Chest, 115*, 14S–18S.

Cassell, G. H. (1999). Infectious causes of chronic inflammatory diseases and cancer. *Emerging Infectious Diseases, 4*(3), 42–56.

Celis, R., Torres, A., Gatell, J. M., Almela, M., Rodriguez-Roisin, R., & Agusti-Vidal, A. (1988). Nosocomial pneumonia: A multivariate analysis of risk and prognosis. *Chest, 93*(2), 318–324.

Centers for Disease Control. (1984). Recommendation of the Immunization Practices Advisory Committee (ACIP) Prevention and Control of Influenza. *Morbidity and Mortality Weekly Report, 33*(19), 253–260, 265–266.

Centers for Disease Control. (1989a). CDC definitions for nosocomial infections, 1988. *American Review of Respiratory Diseases, 139,* 1058–1059.

Centers for Disease Control. (1989b). Recommendations of the Immunization Practices Advisory Committee Pneumococcal Polysaccharide Vaccine. *Morbidity and Mortality Weekly Report, 38*(5), 64–68, 73–78.

Centers for Disease Control. (1994). Guideline for prevention of nosocomial pneumonia. *Infection Control and Hospital Epidemiology, 15*(9), 587–627.

Centers for Disease Control. (1997). Guidelines for prevention of nosocomial pneumonia. *Morbidity and Mortality Weekly Report, 46*(RR-1), 1–80.

Centers for Disease Control. (1999). *National nosocomial infections surveillance (NNIS) system report, data summary form January 1990–May 1999, Issued June 1999.* Atlanta, GA: National Center for Infectious Diseases, Centers for Disease Control and Prevention.

Centers for Disease Control. (2001). Fast stats. *National Vital Statistics Report, 48*(11), 1–106.

Chastre, J., Fagon, J. Y., Soler, P., Domart, Y., Pierre, J., & Dombret, M. C. (1988). Diagnosis of nosocomial bacterial pneumonia in intubated patients undergoing ventilation: Comparison of the usefulness of broncheoalveolar lavage and the protected specimen brush. *American Journal of Medicine, 85,* 499–506.

Chevret, S., Hemmer, M., Carlet, J., Langer, M., & the European Cooperative Group on Nosocomial Pneumonia. (1993). Incidence and risk factors of pneumonia acquired in intensive care units. *Intensive Care Medicine, 19,* 256–264.

Craven, D. E., Connolly, M. G., Jr., Lichtenberg, D., Primeau, P. J., & McCabe, W. R. (1982). Contamination of mechanical ventilators with tubing changes every 24 or 48 hours. *New England Journal of Medicine, 306*(25), 1504–1509.

Craven, D. E., Kunches, L. M., Kilinsky, V., Lichtenberg, D. A., Make, B. J., & McCabe, W. R. (1986). Risk factors for pneumonia and fatality in patients receiving continuous mechanical ventilation. *American Review of Respiratory Diseases, 133,* 792–796.

Craven, D. E., & Steger, K. A. (1997). Hospital-acquired pneumonia: Perspectives for the healthcare epidemiologist. *Infectious Control Hospital Epidemiology, 18*(11), 783–795.

Craven, D. E., Steger, K. A., Barat, L. M., & Duncan, R. A. (1992). Nosocomial pneumonia: Epidemiology and infection control. *Intensive Care Medicine, 18,* S3–S9.

Cunnion, K. M., Weber, D. J., Broadhead, W. E., Hanson, L. C., Pieper, C. F., & Rutala, W. A. (1996). Risk factors for nosocomial pneumonia: Comparing adult critical-care populations. *American Journal of Respiratory and Critical Care Medicine, 153,* 158–162.

Dirks, M. R., Craven, D. E., Celli, B. R., Manning, M., Burke, R. A., Garvin, G. M., et al. (1987). Nosocomial pneumonia in intubated patients given sucralfate as compared with antacids or Histamine type 2 blockers. *New England Journal of Medicine, 317*(22), 1376–1382.

Donowitz, L. G., Wenzel, R. P., & Hoyt, J. W. (1982). High risk of hospital-acquired infection in the ICU patient. *Critical Care Medicine, 10*(6), 355–357.

Drasar, B. S., Shiner, M., & McLead, G. M. (1969). The bacterial flora of the gastrointestinal tract in healthy and achlorhydric persons. *Gastroenterology, 56,* 71–79.

DuMoulin, G. C., Paterson, D. G., Hedley-Whyte, J., & Lisbon, A. (1982). Aspiration of gastric bacteria in antacid-treated patients: A frequent cause of postoperative colonisation of the airway. *Lancet, 30,* 242–246.

Ephgrave, K. S., Kleiman-Wexler, R., Pfaller, M., Booth, B., Werkmeister, L., & Young, S. (1993). Postoperative pneumonia: A prospective study of risk factors and morbidity. *Surgery, 114,* 815–821.

Farzan, S. (1997). *A concise handbook of respiratory diseases.* Stamford, CT: Apple & Lange.

Feldman, C. (1999). Pneumonia in the elderly. *Clinics in Chest Medicine, 20*(3), 563–573.

Fiddian-Green, R. G., & Baker, S. (1991). Nosocomial pneumonia in the critically ill: Product of aspiration or translocation? *Critical Care Medicine, 19*(6), 763–769.

Fourrier, F., Duvivier, B., Boutigny, H., & Roussel-Delvallez, M. (1998). Colonization of dental plaque: A source of nosocomial infections in intensive care unit patients. *Critical Care Medicine, 26*(2), 301–308.

Garibaldi, R. A., Britt, M. R., Coleman, M. L., Reading, J. C., & Page, N. L. (1981). Risk factors for postoperative pneumonia. *American Journal of Medicine, 70,* 677–680.

Gaynes, R., Bizek, B., & Mowry-Hanley, J. (1991). Risk factors for nosocomial pneumonia after coronary artery bypass graft operations. *Annals of Thoracic Surgery, 51,* 215–218.

Gorse, G., Messner, R. L., & Stephens, N. D. (1989). Association of malnutrition with nosocomial infection. *Infection Control and Hospital Epidemiology, 10*(5), 194–203.

Griffin, J. J., & Meduri, G. U. (1994). New approaches in the diagnosis of nosocomial pneumonia. *Medical Clinics of North America, 78*(5), 1091–1121.

Haley, R. W., Hooten, T. M., Culver, D. H., Emori, T. G., Hardison, C. D., Quade, D., et al. (1981). Nosocomial infections in U.S. Hospitals, 1975–1976: Estimated frequency by selected characteristics of patients. *American Journal of Medicine, 70,* 947–959.

Harris, J. R., Joshi, M., Morton, P. G., Soeken, K. L. (2000). Predictors of nosocomial pneumonia in critically ill trauma patients. *AACN Clinical Issues, 11*(2), 198–231.

Harris, J. R., & Miller, T. H. (2000). Preventing nosocomial pneumonia: Evidenced-based practice. *Critical Care Nurse, 20*(1), 51–66.

Helling, T. S., Evans, L. L., Fowler, D. L., Hays, L. V., & Kennedy, F. R. (1988). Infectious complications in patients with severe head injury. *Journal of Trauma, 28*(11), 1575–1577.

Higuchi, J. H., & Johanson, W. G., Jr. (1980). The relationship between adherence of *Pseudomonas aeroginosa* to upper respiratory cells in vitro and susceptibility to colonization in vivo. *Journal of Laboratory and Clinical Medicine, 95*(5), 698–705.

Hooten, T. M., Haley, R. W., White, J. W., Morgan, W. M., & Carroll, R. J. (1981). The joint associations of multiple risk factors with the occurrence of nosocomial infection. *American Journal of Medicine, 70,* 960–970.

Hoyt, D. B., Simons, R. K., Winchell, R. J., Cushman, J., Hollingsworth-Fridlund, P., Holbrook, T., et al. (1993). A risk analysis of pulmonary complications following major trauma. *Journal of Trauma, 35*(4), 524–531.

Huxley, E. J., Viroslav, J., Gray, W. R., & Pierce, A. K. (1978). Pharyngeal aspiration in normal adults and patients with depressed consciousness. *American Journal of Medicine, 64,* 564–568.

Jimenez, P., Torres, A., Rodriguez-Roisin, R., De La Bellacasa, J. P., Aznar, R., Gatell, J. M., et al. (1989). Incidence and etiology of pneumonia acquired during mechanical ventilation. *Critical Care Medicine, 17*(9), 882–885.

Johanson, W. G., Jr., & Dever, L. L. (1998). Microbial flora and colonization of the respiratory tract. In A. P. Fishman (Ed.), *Fishman's pulmonary diseases and disorders* (Vol. 2, pp. 1883–1890). New York: McGraw-Hill.

Johanson, W. G., Jr., Pierce, A. K., Sanford, J. P., & Thomas, G. D. (1972). Nosocomial respiratory infections with Gram-negative bacilli: The significance of colonization of the respiratory tract. *Annals of Internal Medicine, 77,* 701–706.

Joshi, N., Localio, A. R., & Hamory, B. H. (1992). A predictive risk index for nosocomial pneumonia in the intensive care unit. *American Journal of Medicine, 93,* 135–142.

Kerver, A. J. H., Rommes, J. H., Mevissen-Verhage, E. A. E., Hulstaert, P. F., Vos, A., Verhoef, J., et al. (1987). Colonization and infection in surgical intensive care patients: A prospective study. *Intensive Care Medicine, 13,* 347–351.

Kollef, M., Sharpless, L., Vlasnik, J., Pasque, C., Murphy, D., & Fraser, V. (1997). The impact of nosocomial infections on patient outcomes following cardiac surgery. *Chest, 112*(3), 666–675.

Kollef, M. H. (1993). Ventilator-associated pneumonia: A multivariate analysis. *JAMA, 270*(16), 1965–1970.

Langer, M., Cigada, M., Mandelli, M., Mosconi, P., Tognoni, G., & ICU Collaborative Group for Infection Control. (1987). Early onset pneumonia: A multicenter study in intensive care units. *Intensive Care Medicine, 13,* 342–346.

Langer, M., Mosconi, P., Cigada, M., Mandelli, M., & The Intensive Care Unit Group of Infection Control. (1989). Long-term respiratory support and risk of pneumonia in critically ill patients. *American Review of Respiratory Diseases, 140,* 302–305.

Lowry, F. D., Carlisle, P. S., Adams, A., & Feiner, C. (1987). The incidence of nosocomial pneumonia following urgent endotracheal intubation. *Infection Control, 8*(6), 245–248.

Mackowiak, P. A., Martin, R. M., Jones, S. J., & Smith, J. W. (1978). Pharyngeal colonization by Gram-negative bacilli in aspiration-prone persons. *Archives of Internal Medicine, 138,* 1224–1227.

Maki, D. G. (1978). Control of colonization and transmission of pathogenic bacteria in the hospital. *Annals of Internal Medicine, 89,* 777–780.

Marrie, T. (1998a). Acute bronchitis and community-acquired pneumonia. In A. P. Fishman (Ed.), *Fishman's pulmonary diseases and disorders* (Vol. 2, pp. 1985–1995). New York: McGraw-Hill.

Marrie, T. J. (1998b). Community-acquired pneumonia: epidemiology, etiology, treatment. *Infectious Disease Clinics of North America, 12*(3), 723–740.

McEachern, R., & Campbell, G. D., Jr. (1998) Hospital-acquired pneumonia: Epidemiology, etiology, and treatment. *Infectious Disease Clinics of North America, 12*(3), 761–779.

Niederman, M. S. (1990). Gram-negative colonization of the respiratory tract: Pathogenesis and clinical consequences. *Seminars in Respiratory Infections, 5*(3), 173–184.

Niederman, M. S., Craven, D. E., Fein, A. M., & Schultz, D. E. (1990). Pneumonia in the critically ill hospitalized patient. *Chest, 97*(1), 170–181.

Niederman, M. S., Merril, W. W., Ferranti, R. D., Pagano, K. M., Palmer, L. B., & Reynolds, H. Y. (1984). Nutritional status and bacterial binding in the lower respiratory tract in patients with chronic tracheostomy. *Annals of Internal Medicine, 100,* 795–800.

Niederman, M. S., Rafferty, T. D., Sasaki, C. T., Merrill, W. W., Matthay, R. A., & Reynolds, H. Y. (1983). Comparison of bacterial adherence to ciliated and squamous epithelial cells obtained from the human respiratory tract. *American Review of Respiratory Diseases, 127,* 85–90.

Parodi, S., & Goetz, M. B. (2002). Aerobic gram-negative bacillary pneumonias. *Current Infectious Disease Reports, 4*(3), 249–256.

Peeling, R. W., & Brunham, R. C. (1996). Chlamydiae as pathogens: New species and new issues. *Emerging Infectious Diseases, 2*(4), 306–319.

Pingleton, S. K., Hinthorn, D. R., & Liu, C. (1986). Enteral nutrition inpatients receiving mechanical ventilation. *American Journal of Medicine, 80,* 827–832.

Rello, J., Ausina, V., Castella, J., Net, A., & Prats, G. (1992). Nosocomial respiratory tract infections in multiple trauma patients. *Chest, 102*(2), 525–529.

Rello, J., Torres, M., Ricart, J., Valles, J., Gonzalez, J., Artigas, A., et al. (1994). Ventilator-associated pneumonia by *Staphylococcus aureus. American Journal of Respiratory and Critical Care Medicine, 150,* 1545–1549.

Rodriguez, J. L., Gibbons, K. J., Bitzer, L. G., Dechert, R. E., Steinberg, S. M., & Flint, L. M. (1991). Pneumonia: Incidence, risk factors, and outcome in injured patients. *Journal of Trauma, 31*(7), 907–914.

Ruiz, M., Ewig, S., Marcos, M. A., Martinez, J. A., Arancibia, F. A., Mensa, J., et al. (1999). Etiology of community-acquired pneumonia: impact of age, comorbidity, and severity. *American Journal of Respiratory and Critical Care Medicine, 160,* 397–405.

Salemi, C., Morgan, J. W., Kelleghan, S. I., & Hiebert-Crape, B. (1993). Severity of illness classification for infection control departments: A study in nosocomial pneumonia. *American Journal of Infection Control, 21*(3), 117–126.

Sariego, J., Brown, J. L., Matsumoto, T., & Kerstein, M. D. (1993). Predictors of pulmonary complications in blunt chest trauma. *International Surgery, 78,* 320–323.

Sinaniotis, C. A. (1999). Community-acquired pneumonia: Diagnosis and treatment. *Pediatric Pulmonology. Supplement, 18,* 144–145.

Skerrett, S. J. (1994). Host defenses against respiratory infection. *Medical Clinics of North America, 78*(5), 941–966.

Torres, A., Aznar, R., Gatell, J. M., Jimenez, P., Gonzalez, J., Ferrer, A., et al. (1990). Incidence, risk, and prognosis factors of nosocomial pneumonia in mechanically ventilated patients. *American Review of Respiratory Diseases, 142,* 523–528.

Torres, A., Puig De La Bellacasa, J., Xaubet, A., Gonzalez, J., Rodriguez-Roisin, R., Jimenez de Anta, M. T., et al. (1989). Diagnostic value of quantitative cultures of bronchoaveolar lavage and telescoping plugged catheters in mechanically ventilated patients with bacterial pneumonia. *American Review of Respiratory Disease, 140,* 306–310.

Torres, A., Serra-Batlles, J., Ros, E., Piera, C., Puig de la Bellacasa, J., Cobos, A., et al. (1992). Pulmonary aspiration of gastric contents in patients receiving mechanical ventilation: The effect of body position. *Annals of Internal Medicine, 116,* 540–543.

Valenti, W. M., Trudell, R. G., & Bentley, D. W. (1978). Factors predisposing to oropharyngeal colonization with gram-negative bacilli in the aged. *New England Journal of Medicine, 298,* 1108–1111.

Walker, W. E., Kapelanski, D. P., Weiland, A. P., Stewart, J. D., & Duke, J. H., Jr. (1985). Patterns of infection and mortality in thoracic trauma. *Annals of Surgery, 201*(6), 752–757.

Wenzel, R. P. (1989). Hospital-acquired pneumonia: Overview of the current state of the art for prevention and control. *European Journal of Clinical Microbiology and Infectious Disease, 8,* 56–60.

Windsor, J. A., & Hill, G. L. (1988). Risk factors for postoperative pneumonia. *Annals of Surgery, 208*(2), 209–214.

Lung Cancers

Karen Leaton and Donna J. Wilson

INTRODUCTION

I. Definition: Lung cancer is the uncontrolled growth of abnormal cells, which may occur in the lining of the trachea, bronchi, bronchioles, or alveoli. Ninety-five percent of lung cancers are bronchogenic (arise from the epithelial lining of the bronchial tree).

II. Cause
    A. Carcinogenesis
        1. *Initiation* by a carcinogen (cancer-causing agent), for example, cigarette smoke, asbestos, or coal dust
        2. *Promotion* by a secondary factor, for example, number of years smoking or number of cigarettes smoked
        3. *Progression,* that is, the growth of pre-malignant cells and their ability to metastasize
    B. Lifestyle risk factors: Smoking
        1. Most common risk factor: 85% of people are or were former smokers
        2. Environmental tobacco smoke (secondhand smoke)
            a. About 3,400 lung cancer deaths in nonsmoking adults.
            b. Nonsmokers chronically exposed to secondhand smoke may have as much as a 24% increased risk for developing lung cancer.
    C. Occupational risks
        1. Radon
        2. Asbestos fibers (insulation and shipbuilding)
            a. 7 times increased risk of death in asbestos workers
            b. Asbestos exposure combined with cigarette smoking act synergistically to produce an increased risk of lung cancer
        3. Arsenic (copper refining and pesticides)

4. Beryllium (airline industry and electronics)
5. Metals (nickel or copper)
6. Chromium
7. Cadmium
8. Coal tar (mining)
9. Mustard gas
10. Air pollution: diesel exhaust
11. Radiation
12. Tuberculosis
D. Biological risks
1. Sex/age
   a. Males have a greater risk of lung cancer than do females, although incidence rate is declining significantly in men, from high of 102 per 100,000 in 1984 to 77.8 per 100,000 in 2002.
   b. Lung cancer incidence doubled in females from 1975 to 2000 and now has stabilized.
   c. Increased risk is associated with increasing age.
   d. 70% of all lung cancers diagnosed in individuals over the age of 65 and the number of cases diagnosed at 50 or earlier are increasing.
2. Family history: Lung cancer in one parent increases their children's risk of the diagnosis of lung cancer before age 50.
3. Genetic predisposition: Genetic susceptibility is a contributing factor in those that develop lung cancer at a younger age.
   a. A single gene for lung cancer has not been identified.
   b. Abnormalities of p53 gene, a tumor-suppressor gene, has been suggested to be mutated in many people with lung cancer.
   c. EGFL6 gene identified as potential tumor marker (Yeung et al., 1999).
   d. Her-2 expression in non-small cell lung cancer
4. Race
   a. African Americans, native Hawaiians, and non-Hispanic whites have greater risk of lung cancer.
   b. Black men between the age of 35 and 64 years of age have twice the risk compared to non-Hispanic Whites.
5. Chronic inflammation, chronic obstructive pulmonary disease (COPD), pulmonary fibrosis
   a. Tuberculosis: Scarring of healthy lung tissue may lead to lung cancer development.
   b. Pulmonary fibrosis: Silica is the probable lung carcinogen.
   c. COPD: Airflow limitation results in a 6.44 times greater risk for lung cancer compared with the risk associated with absence of ventilatory impairment.
III. Incidence of lung cancer
   A. 213,380 new cases in 2007
      1. 30% of all cancer types
      2. Incidence rate is decreasing in men and stable in females.

    B. 160,390 deaths in 2007
      1. 57% of all cancer deaths
      2. Most common cause of cancer death in both men and women.
    C. Decreasing incidence and mortality rates in men are most likely related to decreased adult smoking rates over the previous three decades.
IV. Pathophysiology: Non-Small Cell Lung Cancer (87% of all cases of lung cancer)
    A. Squamous cell (epidermoid forms in the lining of the bronchial tubes)
      1. Most common type of lung cancer in men
      2. Decreasing incidence in last two decades
      3. Typically develops in segmental bronchi, causing bronchial obstruction and regional lymph node involvement
      4. Symptoms are related to obstruction
        a. Nonproductive cough
        b. Pneumonia
        c. Atelectasis, that is, a collapsed lung
        d. Chest pain is a late symptom associated with bulky tumor
        e. Pancoast Tumor, or pulmonary sulcus tumor, begins in the upper portion of the lung and commonly spreads to the ribs and spine causing classic shoulder pain that radiates down the ulnar nerve distribution
      5. Treatment
        a. Surgical resection is preferred before the development of metastatic disease.
        b. Chemotherapy and radiation therapy to decrease the incidence of recurrence.
    B. Adenocarcinoma
      1. Most common form in Unites States
      2. Increasing incidence in females
      3. Occurs in non-smokers
      4. Develops in the periphery of the lungs and frequently metastasizes to brain, bone, and liver
      5. Symptoms
        a. No symptoms with small peripheral lesions
        b. Identified by routine chest radiograph/CT scan
      6. Treatment
        a. Surgical resection
        b. Chemotherapy and radiation therapy to decrease the incidence of recurrence
    C. Bronchioalveolar (BAC)
      1. Form near the lung's air sacs
      2. BAC may have abnormal gene in their tumor cells
      3. Targeted chemotherapy treatment appears to be effective
    D. Large cell
      1. 10% of all lung cancer cases
      2. Bulky peripheral tumor

3. Metastasizing to brain, bone, adrenal glands, or liver
4. Symptoms related to obstruction or metastatic spread
   a. Pneumonitis
   b. Pleural effusions
5. Treatment
   a. Surgical resection: Limited because of the often aggressive course of this tumor type
   b. Chemotherapy and radiation therapy: Palliative role to minimize symptoms of advanced disease

V. Pathophysiology: Small-Cell Lung Cancer
   A. Oat cell carcinoma
      1. 13% of all lung cancers
      2. Most aggressive type
      3. Greater tendency to metastasize than Non-Small Cell Lung Cancer
      4. Strongly related to cigarette smoking
      5. Often occurs within the mainstem bronchi and segmental bronchi; 80% of cases have hilar and mediastinal node involvement.
      6. Symptoms
         a. Paraneoplastic syndrome: Syndrome of inappropriate antidiuretic hormone (SIADH)
         b. Hyponatremia, fluid retention, weakness, and fatigue
         c. Ectopic adrenocorticotropic hormone (ACTH) production
         d. Hypokalemia, hyponatremia, hyperglycemia, lethargy, and confusion
      7. Treatment
         a. Surgery rarely indicated even in those with limited stage disease because of the need for immediate systemic therapy.
         b. Chemotherapy and radiation therapy offers the best hope for prolonged survival and quality of life. Majority of the patients respond to chemotherapy and radiation therapy but recurrence rate is very high.
         c. Two-thirds of patients demonstrate evidence of extensive disease at the time of diagnosis.
   B. Non-bronchogenic carcinomas—Undifferientated non-small cell lung cancer (NSCLC)
      1. <5% of all lung cancers combined
         a. Mesothelioma—a rare tumor of the parietal pleura directly associated with exposure to asbestos
         b. Bronchial adenoma (Carcinoid)
         c. Fibrosarcoma

VI. Complications/sequelae
   A. Early stage and localized disease—may be asymptomatic
      1. Symptoms are often medically treated and attributed to conditions such as bronchitis, pneumonia, and chronic obstructive pulmonary disease.
         a. Cough
         b. Wheezing

      c. Increased sputum production

      d. Hemoptysis

      e. Dyspnea

      f. Pneumonia

      g. Pleural effusions

B. Advanced disease predominant at time of diagnosis related to tumor growth and compression of adjacent structures

  1. Symptoms

      a. Chronic cough

      b. Dyspnea

          i. Loss of alveolar space from tumor

         ii. Bronchial obstruction

        iii. Pleural effusion

        iv. Pneumonia

         v. Lymphangitic spread

        vi. Hemoptysis

       vii. Bronchospasm

      viii. COPD

      c. Weight loss

      d. Increased sputum production

      e. Hemoptysis

      f. Hoarseness (involvement of the laryngeal nerve)

      g. Pleural effusions and atelectasis

      h. Chronic pain

      i. Pain over the shoulder and medial scapula

      j. Arm pain with or without muscle wasting along ulnar distribution

      k. Horner's syndrome with ptosis, miosis, hemifacial anhydrosis

      l. Clubbing, hypertrophic osteoarthropathy

      m. Bone pain

      n. Fatigue

      o. Dysphagia from esophageal compression

      p. Wheezing or stridor

      q. Phrenic nerve paralysis with elevated hemidiaphragm

      r. Arrhythmias and heart failure (from pericardial involvement)

      s. Hypoxia related to lymphangitic spread

      t. Superior Vena Cava syndrome

          i. Swelling of the face, neck and upper extremities

         ii. Related to compression of blood vessels in the neck and upper thorax

  2. Extrathoracic spread of disease

      a. Adrenal glands (50%)

      b. Liver (30%)

      c. Brain (20%)

      d. Bone (20%)

      e. Kidneys (15%)

      f. Scalene lymph nodes

3. Prognosis remains poor and has improved very slightly despite medical advances: <14% combined 5-year survival rate.

VII. Assessment

A. History

1. Smoking history
2. Other risk factors (family history, occupational risks)
3. Associated diseases (COPD, tuberculosis, emphysema)
4. Symptom description and onset

B. Physical examination

1. Lung auscultation
2. Respiratory rate and depth
3. Palpitation of supraclavicular area for tumor or lymphatic involvement, or both
4. Clubbing
5. Nicotine stains to skin, hair, teeth

C. Diagnostic tests

1. Chest radiographs—plain anterior-posterior and lateral views not reliable to find lung tumors in their earliest stage.
2. Chest Computed Tomography (CT)—three-dimensional image of the lungs and lymph nodes (can detect tumors as small as 5 millimeters). CT is only about 80% accurate in predicting mediastinal node involvement.
3. Spiral computed tomography of the chest.
4. Magnetic Resonance Imaging (MRI) 92% accuracy in the diagnosis of mediastinal invasion.
5. Positron Emission Tomography (PET) scan is based upon increased glucose metabolism in cancer cells. The PET scan uses a glucose analogue radiopharmaceutical to identify increased glycolysis in tumor tissues. The PET scan is a highly sensitive test in the diagnosis and staging of lung cancer.
6. Bronchoscopic detection of tumor autofluorescence could improve cure rates in selected groups at high-risk (see Photodynamic Therapy).
7. Sputum cytology
8. Percutaneous transthoracic needle biopsy
9. Fine-needle aspiration or biopsy
10. Bronchoscopy (needle or brush for cytology)
11. Mediastinoscopy (evaluate lymph node involvement)
12. Scalene node biopsy (evaluate lymph node involvement)
13. Photodynamic therapy (experimental)
   An injection of a light-sensitive agent with uptake by cancer cells, followed by exposure to a laser light within 24 to 48 hours, will result in fluorescence of cancer cells or cell death. Especially helpful in identifying developing cancer cells or "carcinoma in-situ." Also used to determine the extent of disease and the response to treatment.

D. Assessment of distant metastasis
   1. Abdominal CT (identify adrenal or liver metastasis)
   2. Head CT
   3. MRI (brain)
   4. Bone scan
   5. Thoracentesis (detect malignant cells in the pleural fluid)

VIII. Staging
   A. TNM (tumor, nodes, metastases) system of staging (see Table 22.1)
   B. Stage grouping (see Table 22.2)
      1. Stage IA, IB
         a. Most common form of early lung cancer located only in the lungs
         b. Detected on routine chest X-ray in patients who present for unrelated medical condition or routine examination.
         c. Treatment-surgical resection
      2. Stage IIA, IIB
         a. Tumors in the lung and lymph nodes (hilar and bronchopulmonary nodes).
         b. Treatment-surgical resection and adjuvant radiation or chemotherapy, or both.
         c. Induction chemotherapy before surgery is being investigated.
         d. Patients with significant co-morbid disease surgery may not be an option.
      3. Stage IIIA
         a. Cancer in the lung and lymph nodes on the same side of the chest
         b. T3 tumors involving the mainstem bronchi produce hemoptysis, dyspnea, wheezing, atelectasis, and postobstructive pneumonia
         c. T3 tumors involving the pericardium or diaphragm may be symptomatic but those involving the chest wall usually cause pain.
         d. Nodal disease is often asymptomatic, if extensive nodal disease may cause compression of the proximal airways and superior vena cava syndrome.
         e. Treatment—selected cases surgical resection (T3NO-1), commonly multi-modality therapy with chemotherapy being primary form of treatment; multiple trials of combined chemotherapy, radiation with or without surgery are under investigation.
      4. Stage IIIB
         a. Cancer has spread to the lymph nodes on the opposite side of the chest.
         b. T4 tumors invade the mediastinum structures, and/or malignant pleural effusions. N3—metastases.
         c. Treatment—chemotherapy and radiation therapy; in rare exceptions, surgery may be considered.

Table 22.1 | TNM Descriptors

Primary tumor (T)

TX Primary tumor cannot be assessed, or tumor proven by the presence of malignant cells in sputum or bronchial washings but not visualized by imaging or bronchoscopy

T0 No evidence of primary tumor

Tis Carcinoma in situ

T1 Tumor 3 cm in greatest dimension, surrounded by lung or visceral pleura, without bronchoscopic evidence of invasion more proximal than the lobar bronchus[a] (i.e., not in the main bronchus)

T2 Tumor with any of the following features of size or extent:
    3 cm in greatest dimension
    Involves main bronchus, 2 cm distal to the carina
    Invades the visceral pleura
    Associated with atelectasis or obstructive pneumonitis that extends to the hilar region but does not involve the entire lung.

T3 Tumor of any size that directly invades any of the following: chest wall (including superior sulcus tumors), diaphragm, mediastinal pleura, parietal pericardium; or tumor in the main bronchus, 2 cm distal to the carina, but without involvement of the carina; or associated atelectasis or obstructive pneumonitis of the entire lung

T4 Tumor of any size that invades any of the following: mediastinum, heart, great vessels, trachea, esophagus, vertebral body, carina; or tumor with a malignant pleural or pericardial effusion,[b] or with satellite tumor nodule(s) within the ipsilateral primary-tumor lobe of the lung

Regional lymph nodes (N)

NX Regional lymph nodes cannot be assessed

N0 No regional lymph node metastasis

N1 Metastasis to ipsilateral peribronchial and/or ipsilateral hilar lymph nodes, and intrapulmonary nodes involved by direct extension of the primary tumor

N2 Metastasis to ipsilateral mediastinal and/or subcarinal lymph node(s)

N3 Metastasis to contralateral mediastinal, contralateral hilar, ipsilateral, or contralateral scalene, or supraclavicular lymph node(s)

Distant metastasis (M)

MX Presence of distant metastasis cannot be assessed

M0 No distant metastasis

M1 Distant metastasis present[c]

[a] The uncommon superficial tumor of any size with its invasive component limited to the bronchial wall, which may extend proximal to the main bronchus, is also classified T1.

[b] Most pleural effusions associated with lung cancer are due to tumor. However, there are a few patients in whom multiple cytopathologic examinations of pleural fluid show no tumor. In these cases, the fluid is non-bloody and is not an exudate. When these elements and clinical judgment dictate that the effusion is not related to the tumor, the effusion should be excluded as a staging element and the patient's disease should be staged T1, T2, or T3. Pericardial effusion is classified according to the same rules.

[c] Separate metastatic tumor nodule(s) in the ipsilateral nonprimary-tumor lobe(s) of the lung also are classified M1.

Source: Mountain, C. (1997). Revision in the international system for staging lung cancer. *Chest, 111:* 1710–1717.

Table 22.2	Stage Grouping: TNM Subsets

Stage	TNM Subset
0	Carcinoma in situ
IA	T1N0M0
IB	T2N0M0
IIA	T1N1M0
IIB	T2N1M0
	T3N0M0
IIIA	T3N1M0
	T1N2M0
	T2N2M0
	T3N2M0
IIIB	T4N0M0
	T4N1M0
	T4N2M0
	T1N3M0
	T2N3M0
	T3N3M0
	T4N3M0
IV	Any T Any N M1

Staging is not relevant for occult carcinoma, designated TXN0M0.

Source: Mountain, C. (1997). Revision in the international system for staging lung cancer. *Chest, 111:* 1710–1717.

5. Stage IV
    a. Evidence of metastatic disease. Treatment often palliative (to relieve symptoms).
    b. Clinical trials may offer some survival benefit.

IX. Common methods of treatment
  A. Surgery—the treatment of choice for non-small cell lung cancer, Stage IA, IB, IIA, IIB, and selected cases of Stage IIIA
    1. Lobectomy—removal of a lobe of the lung
    2. Pneumonectomy—removal of one lung
    3. Wedge resection or segmentectomy—for patients with inadequate pulmonary reserve who cannot tolerate lobectomy
    4. Video assisted thoroscopic surgery (VATS)
    5. Palliative surgery
      a. Laser or tracheobronchial stent placement
      b. De-bulking of tumor
    6. Before surgery
      a. Patient understands surgical procedure, incision, placement of chest tube(s)

b. Smoking cessation before surgery to reduce pulmonary complications

c. Pain control

d. Bronchodilators

e. Coughing and deep-breathing exercises

f. Early ambulation after surgery

7. After surgery

a. Assess respiratory function (respiratory rate, level of dyspnea, use of accessory muscles, and arterial blood gases)

b. Monitor chest tube drainage and air leaks

c. Monitor oxygen saturation at rest and ambulation

d. Assess pain control

e. Chest physical therapy (bronchial drainage positions, deep breathing, coughing)

f. Early ambulation

g. Monitor for atrial arrhythmias

h. Discharge planning and home care arrangements

B. Chemotherapy—Researchers are continually looking at different ways of combining new and old drugs for advanced non-small cell lung cancer.

1. Non-Small Cell Lung Cancer

a. Customize treatment

i. Erlotinib (Tarceva) for people whose tumors have epidermal growth factor receptors, a genetic mutation

ii. Gefitinib (Iressa) effective in people whose lung tumors have similar genetic mutations

b. Targeted treatments for advanced non-small cell lung cancer

i. Sunitinib (Sutent) works by cutting off blood supply and blocking the cancer cells their ability to grow

ii. Sorafenib (Nexavar) suppresses receptors for vascular endothelial growth factor platelet derived growth factor—plays a critical role in the growth of blood vessels that feed the cancer (angiogensis)

c. Combined methods are the treatment of choice for selected cases of stage IIIA and IIIB

i. Cispatin

ii. Paclitaxel and Gemcitabine

iii. Gemcitabine and Vinorelbine

iv. Carboplatin and Paclitaxel and radiation

v. Cisplatin and Vinblastine and radiation

d. Stage IV

i. Carboplatin and Paclitaxel

ii. Carboplatin and Gemcitabine

iii. Cisplatin and Vinorelbine

iv. Docetaxel and Gemcitabine

v. Pemetrexed

      vi. Chemotherapy combined with Cetuximab (Erbitux): Cetux-
imab binds to epidermal growth factor receptors (EGFR), preventing a series of reactions in the cell that lead to lung cancer

   e. Progression of disease: Single-agent Docetaxel, Gemcitabine, Paclitaxel

   f. Investigational—New treatment approaches are being investigated all the time.

      i. Mage-A3 vaccine and non-small cell lung cancer

      ii. Bortezomib (Velcade)—proteasome inhibitors—destroys cancer
cells

  2. Small-Cell Lung Cancer

   a. Limited-stage disease

      i. Pulmonary resection stage I or stage II

      ii. Etoposide and Cisplatin and Radiation

      iii. Etoposide and Carboplatin

   b. Extensive stage disease: Etoposide and Carboplatin +/− Paclitaxel,
Adriamycin, Cyclophosphamide

   c. Investigational: Vaccine-autologous dendritic cell-adenovirus p53

  3. Complications of chemotherapy treatment

   a. Myelosuppression (infection, anemia, bleeding)

   b. Nephrotoxicity

   c. Nausea and vomiting

   d. Mucositis (inflammation of the mucous membranes)

   e. Fatigue

   f. SIADH and hyponatremia

   g. Hypotension

   h. Anaphylaxis

   i. Alopecia (hair loss)

   j. Neurotoxicity (peripheral neuropathies, central nervous system
[CNS] toxicity)

   k. Cardiomyopathy, arrhythmias, congestive heart failure, myocardial infarction

   l. Pneumonitis or pulmonary fibrosis

   m. Taste changes

  4. Patient education: chemotherapy

   a. Chemotherapeutic agents

   b. Treatment schedule

   c. Adverse effects of drugs

C. Radiation therapy

  1. External beam radiotherapy—Used as an adjunct to surgery to decrease tumor size, to cure patients considered inoperable for medical
or pathologic reasons, or to decrease symptoms.

   a. Radiation after surgery

      i. To improve resectability of tumor

      ii. To sterilize microscopic disease

b. Radiation after surgery
   i. To treat disease confined to one hemithorax with hilar or mediastinal nodal metastasis
   ii. To reduce local recurrence (if positive surgical margins exist)
c. Prophylactic Cranial Irradiation: Limited disease Small-Cell Lung Cancer to reduce reoccurrence in CNS
2. Brachytherapy—Placement of radioactive sources (seeds or catheter) directly into or adjacent to a tumor
   a. Intraoperative: reduce local recurrence
   b. Symptom palliation
      i. Relief of pain from bone metastases
      ii. Hemoptysis
      iii. Superior Vena Cave Syndrome
      iv. Airway obstruction
3. Complications of radiation therapy
   a. Dyspnea
   b. Cough, initial increase in mucus production, and then dry cough
   c. Fatigue
   d. Skin erythema
   e. Esophagitis and dysphagia
   f. Pneumonitis
   g. Lung fibrosis
4. Patient education: radiation therapy
   a. Indelible markings
   b. Treatment schedule
   c. Site-specific adverse effects (within treatment field)
D. Treatment alternatives
1. Neoadjuvant is therapy given before the primary therapy to improve effectiveness (e.g., chemotherapy or radiation before surgery)
2. Adjuvant treatments are equally beneficial and often given concurrently or immediately following one another to maximize effectiveness (e.g., surgery and adjuvant chemotherapy after surgery)
3. Multimodality is therapy that combines more than one method of treatment (e.g., concurrent chemotherapy and radiation, such as, Adjuvant and Neoadjuvent)
X. Home care considerations
A. After lung surgery
1. Smoking cessation
2. Control of incisional pain
3. Wound care
4. Breathing exercises and coughing
5. Pursed lip breathing exercises
6. Maintain fluid intake
7. Maintaining your nutrition
8. Resume activity
9. Regaining arm and shoulder function

B. During and after radiation therapy
   1. Monitor side effects of radiation therapy and report any change in symptoms
   2. Dyspnea
   3. Fatigue is common lasting 4–6 weeks after therapy
   4. Good nutrition
   5. Liquid diet supplement during periods of esophagitis
   6. Avoid wearing tight clothes
   7. Skin care
C. During and after chemotherapy, advise patients
   1. To identify all treatment related side effects and report changes
   2. Fatigue may last weeks to months
   3. To plan their day, and allow for periods of rest
   4. Try activities such as yoga, exercise, meditation, and guided imagery
   5. Keep a diary and document symptoms, activity level, nutrition, treatments, and emotions
   6. To monitor effectiveness of pain medications
   7. To monitor for any signs of infection, such as an increased temperature, redness or swelling, and that the latter symptoms may not be present during weeks of impaired immunity following chemotherapy administration
   8. Monitor weight change and appetite
   9. Nutritional supplements
D. Pulmonary rehabilitation programs
   1. Exercise strengthening
   2. Breathing exercises
   3. Walking program
   4. Nebulizers/Aerosol medication delivery
   5. Disease specific instruction and support
E. Support groups
   1. Lung Cancer specific
   2. Better Breathers Club—a support group sponsored by the American Lung Association for patients with chronic lung disease
F. Hospice
   1. Dignified dying
   2. Pain management
   3. End of life issues
   4. Patient/family support

WEB SITES

ALCASE (Alliance for Lung Cancer Advocacy, Support and Education): http://www.alcase.org
American Cancer Society: http://www.cancer.org
American Lung Association: http://www.lungusa.org

Cancer Care: http://www.cancercare.org
Cancer Information Network: http://www.cancernetwork.com
National Cancer Institute: http://www.cancernet.nci.nih.gov/cancertopics

REFERENCES

Mountain, C. (1997). Revision in the international system for staging lung cancer. *Chest, 111,* 1710–1717.

Yeung, G., Mulero, J., Berntsen, R., Loeb, D., Drmanac, R., & Ford, J. (1999). Cloning of a novel epidermal growth factor repeat containing gene EGFL6: Expressed in tumor and fetal tissues. *Genomics, 62,* 304–307.

SUGGESTED READINGS

Bach, P. B., Kelley, M. J., Tate, R. C., & McCrory, D. C. (2003). Screening for lung cancer: A review of the current literature. *Chest, 123,* 5, 725–825.

Balduych, B., Hendriks, J., Lauwers, P., & Van Schil, P. (2007). Quality of life evolution after lung cancer surgery: A prospective study in 100 patients. *Lung Cancer, 56,* 423–431.

Bepler, G. (1999). Lung cancer epidemiology and genetics. *Journal of Thoracic Imaging, 14,* 228–234.

Bezjak, A., Tu, D., Seymour, L., Clark, G., Trajkovic, A., Zukin, M., et al. (2006). Symptom improvement in lung cancer patients treated with erlotinib: Quality of life analysis of the National Cancer Institute of Canada Clinical Trials Group Study BR.21. *Journal of Clinical Oncology, 20*(24), 3831–3837.

Brown, J. K., & Radke, K. J. (1998). Nutritional assessment, intervention, and evaluation of weight loss in patients with non-small cell lung cancer. *Oncology Nursing Forum, 25,* 547–553.

Chandra, V., Allen, M. S., Nichols, F. C., Deschamps, C., Cassivi, S. D., & Pairolero, P. C. (2006). The role of pulmonary resection in small cell lung cancer. *Mayo Foundation for Medical Education and Research, 81*(5), 619–624.

Dales, R., Stark R., & Raymond, S. (1990). Computed tomography to stage lung cancer: Approaching a controversy using meta-analysis. *American Review of Respiratory Disease, 141,* 1096–1101.

Davey, S., McCance, K., & Budd, M. (1994). The Pulmonary System. In K. L. McCance, & S. E. Huether (Eds.), *Pathophysiology: The biologic basic for disease in adults and children* (pp. 1180–1187). St. Louis: Mosby.

Downey, R. J. (1999). Surgical management of lung cancer. *Journal of Thoracic Imaging, 14,* 266–269.

Early Lung Cancer Cooperative Study. (1984). Early lung cancer detection: Summary and conclusions. *American Review of Respiratory Disease, 130,* 565–570.

Friedberg, J. S., & Kaiser, L. R. (1997). Epidemiology of lung cancer. *Seminars in Thoracic and Cardiovascular Surgery, 9,* 56–59.

Henschke, C. I., Yankelevitz, D. F., Libby, D. M., Pasmantier, M. W., Smith, J. P., & Miettinen, O. S. (2006). Survival of patients with stage I lung cancer detected on CT screening. *New England Journal of Medicine, 355,* 1763–1771.

Hilderly, L. J. (1996). Radiation therapy for lung cancer. *Seminars in Oncology Nursing, 12,* 304–311.

Gridelli, C., Maione, P., Del Gaizo, F., Colantuoni, G., Guerriero, C., Ferrara, C., et al. (2007). Sorafenib and Sunitinib in the treatment of advanced non-small cell lung cancer. *Oncologist, 12,* 191–200.

Jemal, A., Siegel, R., Ward, E., Murray, T., Xu, J., Smigal, C., et al. (2006). Cancer statistics. *Cancer Journal for Clinicians, 56,* 106–130.

Jemel, A., Siegel, R., Ward, E., Murray, T., Xu, J., & Thun, M. J. (2007). Cancer statistics 2007. *Cancer Journal for Clinicians, 57,* 43–46.

Johnson, J. R., Cohen, M., Sridhara, R., Chen, Y. F., Williams, G. M., Duan, J., et al. (2005). Approval summary for erlotinib for treatment of patients with locally advanced or metastatic non-small cell lung cancer after failure of at least one prior chemotherapy regimen. *Clinical Cancer Research, 11*(18), 6414–6421.

Kelly, K., & Mikhaeel-Kamel, N. (1999). Medical treatment of lung cancer. *Journal of Thoracic Imaging, 14,* 257–265.

Kraev, A., Rassias, D., Vetto, J., Torosoff, M., Ravichandran, P., Clement, B. S., et al. (2007). Wedge resection vs. lobectomy. *Chest, 131,* 136–140.

Lind, J. (1992). Lung cancer. In J. C. Clark & R. F. McGee (Eds.), *Core curriculum for oncology nursing* (Vol. 3, 2nd ed., pp. 403–412). Philadelphia: W. B. Saunders.

Losito, J. M., Murphy, S. O., Thomas, L. (2006). The effects of group exercise on fatigue and quality of life during cancer treatment. *Oncology Nursing Forum, 33*(4), 821–825.

Meier, E. (1999). Despite state tobacco settlements, unresolved issues remain. *ONS News, 14,* 10.

Pass, H. I., Carbone, D. P., Johnson, D. H., Minna, J. D., Turrisi, A. T. (Eds.). (2004). *Lung cancer: Principles and practice* (3rd ed.). Philadelphia: Lippincott Williams & Wilkins.

Reuters Medical News. (2000, May 21). Diesel fuel might cause 125,000 cancer cases. Retrieved from www.oncology.medscape.com/reuters/prof/2000/03/03.16/pb03160d

Ryan, L. S. (1996). Psychosocial issues and lung cancer: A behavioral approach. *Seminars in Oncology Nursing, 12,* 318–323.

Sazon, D., Santiago, S., & Soo Hoo, G. (1996). Fluorodeoxyglucose-Positron Emission Tomography in the detection and staging of lung cancer. *American Journal of Respiratory and Critical Care Medicine, 153,* 417–421.

Spruit, M. A., Janssen, P. P., Willemsen, S. C. P., Hochstenbag, M. H., & Wouters, E. F. M. (2006). Exercise capacity before and after an 8-week multidisciplinary inpatient rehabilitation program in lung cancer patients: A pilot program. *Lung Cancer, 52,* 257–260.

Tockman, M. S., Anthonisen, N. R., & Wright, E. C. (1987). Airway obstruction and the risk for lung cancer. *Annals of Internal Medicine, 106,* 512–518.

Tootla, J., & Easterling, A. (1989). PDT: Destroying malignant cells with laser beams . . . photodynamic therapy. *Nursing, 19,* 48.

Webster, J. S. (1992). Sociodemographic and attitudinal changes affecting cancer care. In J. C. Clark & R. F. McGee (Eds.), *Core curriculum for oncology nursing* (Vol. 2, 2nd ed., pp. 195–203). Philadelphia: W. B. Saunders.

Wilson, L. (1992). Pulmonary malignant neoplasms. In S. A. Price, & L. M. Wilson (Eds.), *Pathophysiology: Clinical concepts of disease process* (pp. 593–598). St. Louis: Mosby.

Pulmonary Thromboembolism

23

Christine Archer-Chicko

INTRODUCTION

This chapter will focus primarily on pulmonary thromboembolism including predisposing factors, sources of emboli, clinical presentation, diagnostic evaluation, and treatment. We will present information on thrombotic emboli and only briefly mention the other types of pulmonary emboli as they have very different clinical presentations. Deep vein thrombosis (DVT) will be discussed only as it applies to the pulmonary vasculature. The pathogenesis, diagnostic evaluation, and treatment of DVT is extensive and beyond the scope of this chapter.

I.   Overview
   A. Definition: Pulmonary embolism (PE)
      1. The movement of a clot(s) or insoluble substance from the systemic venous circulation through the right side of the heart to then lodge in one or more of the branches of the pulmonary arterial tree.
      2. Because the lung functions to filter the blood, it is not uncommon for small clots to occur periodically (and asymptomatically), even in healthy individuals.
      3. Pulmonary thromboembolism becomes a serious and potentially life threatening condition when a clot(s) travels into the pulmonary vessels and causes the individual to become symptomatic with hemodynamic or respiratory compromise. The danger to the patient is not only from clots that have already traveled but also from those that may still be released from the deep veins.
   B. Etiology: Palevsky, Kelley, and Fishman (1998) originally described a triad of predisposing factors responsible for the development of thromboemboli.

1. Venous stasis (alternation in normal blood flow) involves local accumulation of activated coagulation factors and low blood flow.
   a. Immobility, long distance travel
   b. Prolonged bedrest
   c. Sluggish circulatory states (congestive heart failure, chronic venous insufficiency, polycythemia)
   d. Extensive and long surgical procedures, particularly those involving the abdomen or pelvis
   e. Anesthesia—promotes venous dilation and stasis
   f. Central venous catheters (also damages vessel wall)
   g. Prior venous thrombosis
2. Alternation in the constitution of blood: Hypercoagulability
   a. Predisposing venous thrombosis
      i. Hormonal changes of pregnancy
      ii. Estrogen use
      iii. Certain malignancies
   b. Conditions that decrease fibrinolytic activity
      i. Antithrombin III deficiency
      ii. Protein C and Protein S deficiency
      iii. Factor V Leiden disease
      iv. Plasminogen deficiency
      v. Hyperhomocystinemia
      vi. Increased levels of antiphospholipid antibodies
   c. Other
      i. Anticardiolipin antibody syndrome
      ii. Nephrotic syndrome
      iii. Essential thrombocytosis
      iv. Heparin-induced thrombocytopenia
      v. Inflammatory bowel disease
      vi. Paroxysmal nocturnal hemoglobulinuria
      vii. Disseminated intravascular coagulation
3. Injuries to the vascular endothelium: Vessel wall injury
   a. Exposure of the underlying collagen starts the mechanisms of hemostasis, coagulation, and fibrinolysis, which contribute to the formation of a thrombus.
   b. Surgery
   c. Trauma/fractures

C. Etiology: Sources of emboli
   1. Blood clots: Deep veins of the leg
      a. Accounts for at least 90% of clinically significant pulmonary emboli
      b. Usually begins behind a valve in the calf veins and then propagates upward toward the right heart
   2. Blood clots: Pelvic veins
      a. May be a source of thromboemboli in women especially if any of the following conditions: recent pelvic inflammatory disease,

recent childbirth, recent gynecologic surgery, or clinical signs of pelvic pathology

    b. Men may develop thrombi with prostate cancer or after prostate surgery

  3. Other non-thrombotic types of pulmonary emboli

    a. Particulate matter

      i. Tissue

      ii. Fibers

      ii. Parasites

      iv. Catheter fragments

    b. Liquid droplets

      i. Amniotic fluid embolism

      ii. Fat embolism

    c. Air embolism

D. Pathophysiology: Factors

The effects of pulmonary emboli range from clinically insignificant to life threatening. Three factors determine the extent of the physiologic effects.

  1. The nature of the emboli, the amount of the vascular bed affected, and the size of the affected pulmonary vessels

  2. The patient's pre-existing cardiopulmonary status

  3. The degree of secondary effects that follow after the emboli lodge in the pulmonary bed (local release of chemical mediators)

E. Pathophysiology: Effects

When a thrombus migrates and lodges in a pulmonary vessel, several pathologic effects occur as a result of the mechanical obstruction and also because specific chemical mediators such as histamine, serotonin and prostaglandins are released from the thrombus.

  1. With the mechanical obstruction

    a. Forward blood flow through the vessel stops.

    b. Perfusion of the downstream pulmonary capillaries ceases.

    c. If ventilation to the corresponding alveolar unit continues, the region of lung physiologically functions as dead space.

    d. The pulmonary vascular resistance increases, which increases the pulmonary artery pressure, and can result in right heart failure (cor pulmonale) with hypotension, lightheadedness/syncope, or hypotensive shock.

  2. When chemical mediators are released.

    a. Bronchoconstriction of small airways occurs and contributes to hypoxemia.

    b. Vasoconstriction of the pulmonary arteries and arterioles adds to the compromise of the pulmonary vascular bed.

  3. Additional pathologic effects that make the lung susceptible to atelectasis and volume loss

    a. Synthesis of surfactant in the affected lung region diminishes leaving it more susceptible to alveolar collapse and atelectasis.

    b. Hypocapnia causes secondary bronchoconstriction.

F. Incidence
   1. Annually more than 600,000 cases of pulmonary thromboembolism occur in the United States.
   2. 70% of those cases are undiagnosed and result in 30% mortality.
   3. When PE is accurately diagnosed and treated, mortality falls to under 10%.
   4. Some patients die suddenly and the disease is detected at autopsy.
G. Types/classification of pulmonary thromboembolism
   1. Specific features of acute, nonmassive pulmonary emboli
      a. Most common clinical presentation of PE
      b. Difficult to diagnose because signs and symptoms are frequently vague and nonspecific
      c. The severity and persistence of the patient's dyspnea usually correlates with the extensive nature of the embolization
      d. Symptoms persist even when the patient is sleeping
      e. Syncope may be present and signify large, central clot
      f. Recurrent episodes of dyspnea in patients predisposed to venous thrombosis should alert the clinician to suspect thromboembolic disease
      g. Chest X-ray (CXR) is often normal, however, it may display any one of the following subtle abnormalities:
         i. an elevated hemidiaphragm related to the reduced lung volume on the ipsilateral side
         ii. an area of consolidation—usually wedge-shaped and pleural based
         iii. a small pleural effusion
         iv. Fleischner's lines—plate-like areas of atelectasis at the lung bases which appear as streaks parallel to the diaphragm
         v. Hampton's hump—a peripheral wedge-shaped infarct
         vi. Westermark's signs—large areas of the lung appear without vascular markings
   2. Specific features of acute, massive pulmonary emboli
      a. Occurs in a small percentage of patients
      b. Truly life-threatening as it causes hemodynamic instability
      c. Causes shock and severe pulmonary hypertension as a result of the extensive clot burden occluding the pulmonary vascular bed
   3. Specific features of multiple pulmonary emboli
      Two clinical scenarios
      a. Patient has repeated episodes of venous thromboemboli and/or pulmonary emboli followed by gradual onset of pulmonary hypertension. Patient eventually dies suddenly or slowly from cor pulmonale and heart failure.
      b. Patient is diagnosed with syndrome of multiple pulmonary emboli yet no prior history of thrombosis or embolism. Patient becomes incapacitated over months to years as a result of shortness of breath (SOB), chest pain and anxiety. A lung biopsy (or at autopsy)

reveals widespread occlusive disease from thromboemboli in the arteries and arterioles of the lungs.

    i. It is important to note that this type of pulmonary emboli is not caused from showering of multiple emboli. It is the result of widespread distribution of uniform thrombotic lesions in the pulmonary microcirculation. The pathology is believed to arise from a local malfunction of the pulmonary vascular endothelium.

    ii. This disease process leads to chronic pulmonary hypertension.

4. Specific features of unresolved pulmonary emboli

    a. Patients whom have survived large pulmonary emboli may have unresolved clot occluding a segment of the pulmonary vascular bed.

    b. CXR reveals enlarged central pulmonary arteries and occasionally areas of pruning over the affected lung.

    c. Ventilation-Perfusion scans show a high probability pattern.

    d. Angiography confirms the organized, unresolved clot.

H. Considerations across the life span

1. Pediatric

    a. PE is uncommon in the pediatric population.

2. Pregnancy

    a. PE is uncommon but can cause maternal death. The incidence is 1 per 1,000 pregnancies and 1 per 3,000 deliveries.

    b. PE remains the leading cause of pregnancy-related maternal death in developed countries.

    c. There is an increased risk of DVT in pregnancy due to several mechanisms.

        i. Hormones decrease vascular tone, especially in the third trimester.

        ii. The enlarging uterus compresses the iliac veins and/or the inferior vena cava (IVC).

        iii. Coagulation factors increase by the third trimester, and there is a reduction in coagulation inhibitory factors causing a hypercoagulable state.

    d. All diagnostic studies, including CT scan and pulmonary angiography, may be performed without significant risk to the fetus.

    e. Making the diagnosis of PE in a pregnant woman is no different from diagnosing a nonpregnant woman.

    f. An accurate diagnosis of PE is essential, as a long-term course of heparin will be required.

    g. The treatment for PE in pregnancy is heparin (unfractionated heparin or low molecular weight heparin) because it does not cross the placenta and it is not found in breast milk in any significant amounts.

    h. Coumadin is contraindicated in the first and third trimester of pregnancy because of deleterious effects.

      i. At the time of labor and delivery, subcutaneous injections should be held at the onset of regular contractions and intravenous heparin should be stopped 4–6 hours before delivery.

  3. Elderly

    a. The incidence of thromboembolic events increases with age. One study calculated the cumulative probability for a venous thromboembolic event to be 0.5% at the age of 50 years and 10.7% at the age of 80 years.

    b. Older patients are more likely to have less cardiopulmonary reserve as a result of natural aging and perhaps from intrinsic disease. Therefore, a PE in this population can have very serious effects.

I. Complications/sequelae

  1. Acute complications: Hemodynamic

    a. Pulmonary hypertension (increased PVR)

    b. Cor pulmonale (right heart failure)

    c. Arrhythmias

    d. Decreased cardiac output, hypotension, syncope, or shock

    e. Cardiac arrest/myocardial infarction

  2. Acute complications: Respiratory

    a. Decreased pulmonary perfusion (possible pulmonary infarction), increased dead space, altered ventilation/perfusion, worsened physiologic shunt, atelectasis, alveolar collapse, or hypoxemia

    b. Respiratory failure

  3. Acute complications: Complications of therapy

    a. Bleeding

    b. Allergic reaction to thrombolytic agent

    c. Heparin induced thrombocytopenia (HIT)

  4. Long-term complications

    a. Pulmonary hypertension (from unresolved or recurrent emboli) Progressive dyspnea and functional limitation

    b. Venous insufficiency Venous stasis, peripheral edema, possible ulcerations

    c. Complications of therapy

      i. Bleeding

      ii. Nontherapeutic anticoagulation, or recurrent PE/DVT

      iii. Poor compliance to therapeutic regimen

      iv. Heparin induced osteoporosis

II. Assessment

  A. History

    1. Common signs and symptoms

      a. Patient symptoms vary depending on the amount and size of the embolism. A few, small emboli in a patient with normal pulmonary vascular bed may cause no hemodynamic compromise. On the other hand, large emboli that lodge in the major pulmonary vessels may produce profound hemodynamic effects such as hypotension, bradycardia, pulmonary hypertension, and a decrease in cardiac output.

b. The patient's underlying cardiopulmonary status will also determine the extent of the hemodynamic effect. In a patient with a normal cardiovascular status, more than one-half of the pulmonary vasculature needs to be affected by emboli before hemodynamic compromise will occur. Conversely, patients with pre-existing cardiovascular disease will become symptomatic with a much smaller amount of emboli affecting their pulmonary vascular bed.

c. The signs and symptoms of PE are notoriously vague and difficult to rely upon; therefore, diagnostic testing should be initiated if a pulmonary thromboembolism is suspected.

d. Pulmonary thromboembolism should be considered whenever a patient presents with unexplained dyspnea or unexplained hypoxemia.

e. Signs and symptoms vary widely. The classic syndrome of dyspnea, pleuritic chest pain, and tachypnea is not typically seen. In fact, most emboli occur without sufficient clinical findings to suggest the diagnosis.

f. Acute, nonmassive PE (symptoms present suddenly)
   i. Tachycardia
   ii. Pleuritic chest pain or diffuse chest discomfort
   iii. Dyspnea
   iv. Cough
   v. Hemoptysis
   vi. Anxiety, apprehension, restlessness
   vii. Light headedness, syncope

g. Acute, massive PE (symptoms present suddenly)
   i. Severe pulmonary hypertension and hemodynamic instability: hypotension, tachycardia, pale, weak, diaphoretic, dull chest pain, nauseated, oliguric, dyspnea
   ii. Cardiac arrest may occur
   iii. Impaired thought processes, impending feeling of doom, or loss of consciousness
   iv. Anxiety, apprehension, restlessness

h. Multiple pulmonary emboli
   i. Progressive dyspnea
   ii. Progressive right heart failure

i. Unresolved pulmonary emboli
   i. Progressive dyspnea
   ii. Progressive right heart failure

2. Past medical history
   Any precipitating factors present

3. Medications
   Using oral contraceptives with estrogen or hormone replacement therapy

4. Substance abuse
   i. Any injection drug use currently or in the past
   ii. Any smoking currently or in the past

5. Family history
   i. Anyone in the family diagnosed with blood clots in the legs or lungs
   ii. Anyone in the family diagnosed with heart or lung disease
B. Physical exam: The physical exam may be relatively unimpressive.
   1. Vitals: tachycardia, tachypnea, BP may be unstable, low pulse oximetry recording
   2. General: pale, anxious, apprehension
   3. Head eyes ear nose throat (HEENT): increased jugular venous pressure (JVP)
   4. Respiratory: dyspnea, cough, hemoptysis depends upon presence of lung disease—rales are possible, may have decreased sounds or some wheezing
   5. Pleural friction rub
   6. Cardiovascular (CV): increased pulmonic component of the second heart sound
      a. Visible/palpable pulmonary artery in the second left intercostal space
      b. Right ventricular S3 gallop and tricuspid insufficiency murmur at left lower sternal border
   7. Lightheadedness, syncope
   8. Abdomen (ABD): enlarged liver (hepatic congestion) is possible
   9. Extremities: phlebitis (palpable cord, tenderness, warmth, redness, local swelling), Homan's sign may be present in affected lower extremity (pain with dorsiflexion), ankle edema is possible
C. Diagnostic tests
   The most important factor in diagnosing a PE is considering PE as a possible diagnosis. If you do not think of PE as a possibility, you will never order the diagnostic tests which would confirm the diagnosis.
   1. EKG
      a. Nonspecific ST-T wave changes and sinus tachycardia are most common.
      b. Atrial arrhythmias may be seen.
      c. A pattern of RV strain S1Q3T3 may be seen in cases of massive PE.
   2. ABG
      a. Nondiagnostic for thromboembolic disease—A patient without underlying lung disease may have a normal PaO_2 despite having a PE. Therefore, normal ABGs do not rule out a PE.
      b. Conversely, abnormal ABGs with no apparent cause should alert the clinician to consider a PE and to obtain a V/Q scan.
   3. CXR
      a. Typically is unremarkable or only reveals a nonspecific abnormality—an infiltrate, effusion, atelectasis or elevated hemidiaphragm.
      b. Classic finding of a peripheral wedge-shaped infarct (Hampton's hump) or decreased vascularity (Westermark's sign) is uncommon.

4. Ventilation-perfusion lung scan (V/Q scan)
   a. Has been regarded as a pivotal diagnostic test for PE.
   b. The Prospective Investigation of Pulmonary Embolism Diagnosis (PIOPED) was a NIH-sponsored, multicenter study evaluating the sensitivity and specificity of the V/Q scan. In addition, the study also considered the importance of clinical suspicion for PE in combination with V/Q scans in correctly diagnosing pulmonary thromboembolism. The study found that a high number of patients with PE had nondiagnostic V/Q scans in association with a high level of suspicion (PIOPED Investigators, 1990).
   c. The PIOPED study generated a wealth of information on pulmonary embolism and provides the background for many of today's standards of care.
   d. Several other important points from the PIOPED and related studies include
      i. As the severity of cardiopulmonary disease increases, the V/Q scan diagnostic capability decreases.
      ii. If the ventilation part of a V/Q scan cannot be performed, obtaining only the perfusion part is helpful if the perfusion scan is high probability, low probability, or normal.
      iii. When a lung scan is nondiagnostic (and the patient is hemodynamically stable), it is beneficial to evaluate the lower extremities to determine the need for anticoagulation.
   e. Interpretation of ventilation-perfusion scans is performed by noting the presence and size of defects and comparing the ventilation and perfusion defects.
   f. PE make perfusion defects that are unmatched by the ventilation defects. Therefore, a negative V/Q scan rules out the diagnosis of clinically significant PE.
   g. Scans are classified into 4 categories.
      i. Normal—No perfusion defects. Perfusion corresponds to lung fields viewed on chest X-ray.
      ii. High probability—Has multiple perfusion defects of at least 25%–75% of a segment unmatched by ventilation defects. High probability scans are fairly insensitive. In the PIOPED study, high probability scans were found in only 41% of patients with embolism documented by angiogram.
      iii. Intermediate or Indeterminate probability—Difficult to categorize as high or low probability; non-diagnostic.
      iv. Low probability—Perfusion defect of less than 25% of a segment in a patient with a normal chest X-ray.
5. Chest CT scan
   a. Chest CT scans: helical (spiral) and electron beam can visualize the pulmonary vascular bed to the level of the segmental arteries.
   b. Both types of scan can be done rapidly such that following injection of contrast, the opacification of the vasculature can be seen.

299

    c. Low sensitivity for detecting emboli at the segmental and more distal levels.

    d. At present, a positive scan can be used as the basis to treat a patient, however a negative scan does not exclude PE and should not be used as the reason for withholding anticoagulation or stopping the patient's evaluation.

6. Chest MRI

    a. May become a new method for visualizing emboli, however, at present, less available than CT scanners.

    b. Does not require the use of intravenous contrast.

    c. Similar to the chest CT scan, MRI is better at detecting emboli in the central and segmental levels and less accurate with smaller more distal emboli.

    d. Disadvantages include: expensive, not widely available, and time consuming.

7. Transthoracic or transesophageal echocardiography with color flow Doppler mapping

    a. May provide information about the presence of large emboli in the main pulmonary arteries.

    b. The transthoracic echocardiogram can show acute tricuspid regurgitation or abnormal right ventricular volume or contractility that occurs in patients with clinically significant PE.

    c. The transesophageal echocardiogram may reveal abnormal flow patterns in the main pulmonary arteries.

8. Pulmonary angiogram

    a. Most accurate diagnostic study (considered the gold standard) for evaluation of pulmonary embolism.

    b. Commonly used when the V/Q scan is nondiagnostic and the level of clinical suspicion is high.

    c. Pulmonary angiogram should not be performed in hemodynamically unstable patients.

    d. There are two characteristic findings signifying embolism.

       i. Intralumenal filling defect (visualized in two views)

      ii. Cutoff of the radiopaque stream (confirming occlusion)

    e. Study involves a right heart catheterization and intravenous injection of contrast material which does carry some small risk of complications. (If an experienced angiographer performs the study, the risk is minimal.) The contrast opacifies the pulmonary arteries and vascular bed. Optimally, biplane angiography is used to provide views in two planes with each contrast injection, which is helpful in accurately visualizing emboli.

    f. Angiogram can detect emboli as small as 0.5 mm.

    g. Normal angiogram can exclude the diagnosis of embolism in all but the minute vessels of the lung or in vessels where there is incomplete occlusion.

    h. Relative contraindications include: renal insufficiency and significant bleeding risk.
        i. For patients with renal insufficiency, a pulmonary angiogram may be safely performed if the patient is adequately hydrated before, during, and after the procedure.
        ii. To reduce the risk of bleeding, coagulation studies should be normal or near normal and the platelet count should be at least 75,000/mm^3.
    i. A pulmonary angiogram should be performed by an experienced angiographer
    j. Complications include cardiopulmonary compromise, renal failure, bleeding, groin hematomas requiring transfusion, and contrast reaction. Death as a direct result of the procedure is rare (0.2% mortality).
    k. Major flaws of procedure: invasive, technically complex, expense, limited availability.

III. Common therapeutic modalities
    A. Anticoagulation
    For the most updated review of the literature regarding management of thromboembolic disorders and dosing recommendations, refer to the Sixth American College of Chest Physicians (ACCP) Consensus Conference on Antithrombotic Therapy (Hirsh et al., 2001).
    B. Prophylactic or chronic therapy
      1. Should be used in medical conditions and surgical procedures that predispose a patient to developing a deep vein thrombosis.
      2. Mechanical methods are not really effective to prevent venous stasis.
        a. Elevation of foot of bed
        b. Performing leg exercises
        c. Frequent position changes
      3. Use of intermittent pneumatic compression stockings is somewhat effective against venous stasis.
        a. Heparin
          i. Action: Binds to the heparin-antithrombin complex and inactivates a number of coagulation enzymes
          ii. Dosing: The usual dose is 5000 units subcutaneously every 8–12 hrs. It may be started 2 hours before surgery and continued until the patient is ambulatory.
          iii. Has been associated with bleeding complications and thrombocytopenia
        b. Low molecular weight heparin (LMWH)
          i. Action: Similar to heparin, yet LMWHs are smaller molecules and therefore have trouble binding to the antithrombin complex
          ii. Not associated with side effects as heparin
          iii. Dosing: Low dose subcutaneously daily. (Note: There are several LMWHs available, and they are not interchangeable. Dosing is individualized.)

      c. Coumadin

         i. Action: Interferes with the activation of vitamin K dependent clotting factors

         ii. Dosing: Maintain INR 2.0–3.0

         iii. Effectiveness of therapy may be altered by drug interactions, inaccuracies in lab testing, patient noncompliance, miscommunication between patient and physician, levels of dietary vitamin K, and hepatic dysfunction. (Note: The list of drug interactions with Coumadin is extensive.)

C. Acute therapy: Heparin

  1. Should be started when there is suspicion of a PE and the diagnostic evaluation is underway

  2. Should not be discontinued until the evaluation is completed and negative or alternative therapies have been started

  3. Dosing

    a. Administered as a bolus (5,000 units) given to achieve a therapeutic drug level quickly then, a continuous infusion is started at 1,200–1500 units/hour.

    b. It is important to check a PTT within 4–6 hours after initiating Heparin therapy to verify that a therapeutic level has been achieved.

    c. The dose of Heparin is very individualized based on the patient's rate of metabolism and coagulant activity. (Some patients appear to be Heparin resistant at the beginning of therapy and require large doses to obtain a therapeutic level.)

    d. There are weight-based dosing nomograms and computer dosing programs to assist in guiding therapy.

    e. The target PTT is 1.5–2.0 times normal.

    f. Dosing changes should be followed by a PTT in 4–6 hours.

    g. The half-life of Heparin is approximately 90 minutes in patients with active thrombosis.

    h. After two consecutive therapeutic PTTs have been documented, it is reasonable to monitor the level once daily.

    i. Monitoring platelet counts every 1–3 days to detect thrombocytopenia (Heparin-induced thrombocytopenia or HIT).

    j. Patients should be treated for a minimum of 5 days and receive overlapping therapy with Coumadin.

D. Acute therapy: Warfarin (Coumadin)

Should be initiated while heparin therapy is ongoing. Overlap both therapies because it takes 36 hours for Coumadin to effect the INR and it may take 5–7 days to achieve full anticoagulation.

  1. Dosing: INR 2.0–3.0 is as effective as a more intense regimen (INR 3.0–4.5) and associated with less bleeding complications.

  2. The duration of Coumadin therapy depends on the individual patient's clinical situation. Six months of therapy is recommended; however, for patient's with continuing, unresolvable risk factors (cancer,

　　　hypercoagulable states, recurrent PE, congestive heart failure, venous
　　　stasis), lifetime anticoagulation may be necessary.
　　　　a. The major risk factor is bleeding.
　　E. Thrombolytic therapy
　　　1. Used for treatment of major pulmonary thromboembolism. (Patients
　　　　with hemodynamic instability and respiratory compromise caused by
　　　　PE should be treated with thrombolytic therapy.)
　　　2. It is less clear if thrombolytic therapy is appropriate for nonmassive
　　　　PE and large DVT.
　　　3. These agents are administered without the simultaneous use of other
　　　　antithrombotic medications such as aspirin and heparin.
　　　4. The optimal dosing regimen has not yet been established; thrombo-
　　　　lytic agents are administered on an individual basis.
　　　5. Before thrombolytic therapy is initiated, patients must be thoroughly
　　　　evaluated for risk factors of major hemorrhage. The decision to pro-
　　　　ceed with therapy should be individualized and based on careful eval-
　　　　uation of both the risks and benefits.
　　　6. Two approaches to determining the duration of therapy
　　　　a. Repeated imaging with therapy continuing as long as there is evi-
　　　　　dence of clot dissolution
　　　　b. Monitoring for circulating clot lysis indicators
　　　7. May be administered as a peripheral continuous intravenous infu-
　　　　sion, intermittent bolus injection, or as catheter directed at the pul-
　　　　monary thromboembolism.
　　　8. When the course of thrombolytic therapy is completed, standard an-
　　　　ticoagulation is initiated.
　　　9. Complications of thrombolytic therapy
　　　　a. Bleeding
　　　　　i. A greater risk of bleeding than heparin therapy
　　　　　ii. Common sites of bleeding: vascular puncture sites, GI, retro-
　　　　　　peritoneal, and intracranial
　　　　b. Fever
　　　　c. Allergic reactions—flushing, urticaria, hypotension
　　　　d. Other—nausea, vomiting, myalgias, headaches
　　　　e. If bleeding occurs during therapy, the severity, duration, and cause
　　　　　will determine its management.
　　　　　i. Intracranial hemorrhage is an emergency and warrants an im-
　　　　　　mediate neurosurgical consult at the first sign of altered men-
　　　　　　tal status or focal neurologic finding.
　　　　　ii. Clinically significant bleeding warrants discontinuation of
　　　　　　treatment with the thrombolytic and administration of cryo-
　　　　　　precipitate and/or fresh frozen plasma.
　　　　　iii. Bleeding from vascular puncture sites can usually be controlled
　　　　　　with compression dressings or manual pressure.
　　F. Thrombolytic therapy: Streptokinase
　　　1. Derived from beta-hemolytic *streptococci*

303

2. Converts circulating plasminogen to plasmin
3. Possesses antigenic properties and therefore, requires a loading dose to overcome neutralizing antibodies from prior streptococcal infections. In addition, it cannot be readministered for at least 6 months because circulating antibodies may inactivate the drug and develop severe allergic reactions.
4. Recommended dosing (according to the Food and Drug Administration)
   a. Loading dose: 250,000 IU over 30 minutes followed by
   b. Hourly infusion: 100,000 IU/hr for 24 hrs
   c. Has the ability to dissolve thrombi, but also causes systemic thrombolytic state, which places the patient at risk for hemorrhage

G. Thrombolytic therapy: Tissue-type plasminogen activator (t-PA)
1. Produced by recombinant DNA technology
2. Binds to a fibrin clot and converts plasminogen to plasmin, which then dissolves the clot
3. Despite a high affinity for fibrin, t-PA still has systemic lytic effects.
4. Proper dosage is crucial to avoid complications. A dose of 0.50–0.75 mg/kg IV is sufficient to cause degradation of fibrinogen and only slight systemic fibrinolysis.
5. Recommended dosing (according to the Food and Drug Administration)
   a. No loading dose
   b. Hourly infusion: 50 mg/hr for 2 hrs
   c. Results in more rapid clot lysis as compared to the 24-hour Streptokinase regimen.

H. Surgical management: Inferior vena cava (IVC) interruption
Small filters may be placed percutaneously or surgically to prevent recurrent pulmonary emboli.
1. Indications for use
   a. When anticoagulation is strongly contraindicated
   b. When the patient develops a recurrent PE despite anticoagulation
2. Because of relative safety with placement of the IVC filter, it has been used for PE prevention in other situations including suspicion of floating proximal end of a thrombus and some high risk cases.
3. High risk cases include
   a. Elderly patients with hip surgery and prior DVT
   b. Patients with minimal cardiopulmonary reserve and/or pulmonary hypertension
   c. Patients with prior DVT requiring thrombolysis
   d. Trauma patients
4. There are six designs, but the two most frequently placed are: Greenfield filter, Bird's nest filter
5. Following placement of an IVC filter the incidence of PE is 1.9%–2.4%
6. Use of the Greenfield filter for a 12-month period revealed the following complications (Greenfield, Proctor, Cho, & Cutler, 1994).

     a. 4% had recurrent PE

     b. 3% had occlusion of the filter (2 patients had resolution over time)

     c. 10% had filter arm asymmetry at the time of placement

     d. 5% had suboptimal placement

     e. 1% had hematoma at the insertion site

     f. 1% had filter migration

     g. No procedural-related deaths

I. Surgical removal: Transvenous catheter embolectomy

  1. Involves the use of a specially designed percutaneous catheter to mechanically extract or disrupt the embolus and reduce the size into smaller pieces, which can travel into the distal vascular bed.

  2. May be used in conjunction with catheter directed thrombolytic therapy to achieve faster clot resolution.

  3. Indications

     a. Patients who are not candidates for open surgery

     b. Patients who are not candidates for systemic thrombolytic therapy

  4. Greenfield and colleagues had a 76% success rate with catheter embolectomy in 46 patients with massive PE (Greenfield et al., 1994). Complications included:

     a. 15% wound hematoma

     b. 11% pulmonary infarct

     c. 6% recurrent DVT

     d. 4% pleural effusion

     e. 4% myocardial infarction

  5. Catheter technology continues to improve with the development of catheter tips with rotating heads, saline jets, suction to remove debris, and the ability to place a self expanding stent.

J. Surgical removal: Surgical embolectomy

  1. Involves emergent removal of fresh thrombotic material from the large pulmonary vessels.

  2. Performed by a surgical procedure utilizing cardiopulmonary bypass.

  3. Indications

     a. For patients in whom thrombolytic therapy is contraindicated

     b. For patients in whom thrombolytic therapy is ineffective

     c. For patients with acute, massive PE

  4. The optimal surgical candidate has subtotal obstruction of the main pulmonary artery or one of its major branches with reversible pulmonary hypertension.

  5. The goal of this surgical procedure is to prevent death from major pulmonary artery obstruction, which ceases blood flow to the lungs and causes acute right heart failure.

  6. Placement of an IVC filter before closing the chest is recommended by Greenfield.

  7. Postoperative care is similar to care for patients who have had open cardiac surgery.

a. Vasoactive medications may be used to support cardiac output.

b. Renal failure and ischemic brain damage may become apparent as a result of inadequate circulation in the preoperative period.

8. Survival mortality rates vary greatly between 40% and 92%.

9. The outcome ultimately depends upon the patient's preoperative circulation. If cardiac arrest occurs as a result of the embolism, the mortality rate is higher.

10. Brain damage, cardiac arrest, and sepsis are the leading causes of death.

11. With increasingly effective thrombolytic therapy, the justification of this procedure has been questioned. The decision to proceed with surgery should be made on an individual basis.

K. Surgical removal: Thromboendarterectomy

1. An innovative surgical procedure performed to remove chronic thromboembolic material from the pulmonary arteries and its branches. It involves the use of cardiopulmonary bypass, deep hypothermia, and circulatory arrest. The beneficial effects of this procedure include: improved blood flow distribution, reduced pulmonary arterial pressures, and relief from right heart failure.

2. Indications

a. Patients with unresolved thromboemboli (documented by unchanged V/Q scans over 8 to 12 weeks despite anticoagulation) and functional limitation (NYHA Class III or IV).

b. All cases must have evidence that the proximal extent of the organized thrombotic material is at least the level of the lobar pulmonary arteries so that a plane of dissection can be established.

3. Postoperative care is similar to other open heart surgery cases with a few important differences.

a. Patients are mechanically ventilated to maintain arterial oxygen saturations over 95 torr and carbon dioxide tensions below 35 torr. Frequently, high levels of inspired oxygen (FiO_2 80–100) and 5–10 cm of positive end expiratory pressure (PEEP) is needed to ensure even distribution of airflow and to reduce reperfusion pulmonary edema.

b. Prostaglandin E1 is administered as a continuous infusion at 0.5–1.0 mcg/min to prevent pulmonary arterial constriction.

c. Diuretics are used to reduce interstitial edema, which contributes to shunting and decreased lung compliance.

4. Complications specific to this procedure

a. Reperfusion pulmonary edema

i. A process similar to acute respiratory distress syndrome (ARDS) that results in the pulmonary secretions becoming proteinaceous and blood tinged, increased interstitial markings on chest X-ray, and decreased lung compliance.

ii. Physiologic consequences include worsened physiologic shunt, decreased alveolar surfactant, increased atelectasis, and increased work of breathing.

           iii. Treatment consists of ventilatory support with increased FiO_2 and PEEP, aggressive diuresis, positioning and chest physiotherapy, and protection from infection.

      b. Malignant pulmonary hypertension

        A severe complication in which the pulmonary arterial pressures progressively rise postoperatively for unknown reasons despite pharmacologic therapies. Eventually, the patients develop worsened right heart failure and low cardiac output and die.

      c. Hemorrhagic lung

      d. Neurologic disorders related to circulatory arrest and deep hypothermia.

      e. Operative mortality is –5.4%–20%, which is an improvement in the last several years as a result of surgeon experience and better patient selection.

      f. Risk factors for operative death include: preoperative pulmonary vascular resistance >1100 dynes/sec, prolonged ventilator dependence (>5 days), presence of ascites, and need for more than four blood transfusions.

      g. Following surgery, patients receive lifelong anticoagulation with both Coumadin and low-dose aspirin. (The goal prothrombin time is an INR of 2.8–3.5.)

  L. Outcomes

    1. PE may occur as a single event or as recurrent episodes.

      a. An acute, first event may cause death, severe or mild symptoms, or no symptoms at all.

      b. Generally, the size of the emboli corresponds to the severity of the physiologic consequences with larger emboli creating more symptoms.

      c. There is more risk of recurrent emboli within the first 4–6 weeks.

    2. Short-term successful outcome following an initial PE episode is related to whether anticoagulation therapy is started. (Initiation of therapy may be dependent upon whether the diagnosis was made in a timely manner or not.)

    3. The mortality of untreated PE is 25%–30%. With appropriate therapy, the incidence of recurrent PE is less than 8%.

    4. A massive PE may have been preceded in the last few weeks by several episodes of small PEs that were undiagnosed.

    5. Following an acute episode of PE, the prognosis is dependent upon revascularization of the pulmonary vascular bed. Several factors can influence a patient's prognosis: adequacy of anticoagulation, advanced age, cancer, stroke, and cardiopulmonary disease.

IV. Home care considerations

  A. Signs/symptoms to report to physician

    1. Any shortness of breath or chest discomfort

    2. Any change in functional level

B. Adopt healthy lifestyle
  1. Avoid long periods of sitting or immobility, especially on long car trips or airline flights. Walk and exercise legs every few hours when traveling.
  2. Eliminate oral contraceptive use if at risk for developing a thromboembolism.
  3. Avoid smoking.
C. Coumadin therapy
  1. Importance of compliance with therapy
    a. Take Coumadin as prescribed by your physician.
    b. Do not switch back and forth from generic to brand name; take one form consistently.
    c. Obtain routine labwork to monitor therapy as directed by your physician.
  2. Monitor self for bleeding
    a. Observe for bleeding gums, frequent nosebleeds, blood in stool or urine, excessive vaginal bleeding.
    b. Report any bleeding to physician immediately.
  3. Wear Medic Alert bracelet
  4. Avoid aspirin and aspirin containing products
D. Low molecular weight heparin therapy

REFERENCES

Greenfield, L. J., Proctor, M. C., Cho, K. J., & Cutler, B. S. (1994). Extended evaluation of the titanium Greenfield vena caval filter. *Journal of Vascular Surgery, 20,* 458–464.

Hirsh, J., Dalen, J. E., & Guyatt, G. (2001). The sixth (2000) ACCP guidelines for antithrombotic therapy for prevention and treatment of thrombosis. *Chest, 119*(1), 15–25.

PIOPED Investigators. (1990). Value of the ventilation/perfusion scan in acute pulmonary embolism. Results of the Prospective investigation of Pulmonary Embolism Diagnosis. *Journal of the American Medical Association, 263,* 2753–2759.

SUGGESTED READINGS

American Thoracic Society. (1999). The diagnostic approach to acute venous thromboembolism: Clinical practice guideline. *American Journal of Respiratory and Critical Care Medicine, 160,* 1043–1066.

Arcasoy, S. M., & Kreit, J. W. (1999). Thrombolytic therapy of pulmonary embolism: A comprehensive review of current evidence. *Chest, 115,* 1695–1710.

European Society of Cardiology. (2000). Task Force Report: Guidelines on diagnosis and management of acute pulmonary embolism. *European Heart Journal, 21,* 1301–1334.

Greenfield, L. J., Proctor, M. D., Williams, D. M., & Wakefield, T. M. (1994). Pulmonary angiography and the diagnosis of pulmonary embolism. *Journal of Vascular Surgery, 18,* 450–453.

Hansson, P. O., Welin, L., Tibblin, G., & Eriksson, H. (1997). Deep vein thrombosis and pulmonary embolism in the general population: The study of men born in 1913. *Archives of Internal Medicine, 157*(15), 1665–1670.

Hirsch, J., Warkentin, T. E., Shaughnessy, S. G., Anand, S. S., et al. (2001). Heparin and low-molecular-weight-heparins: Mechanisms of action, pharmacokinetics, dosing, monitoring, efficacy, and safety. *Chest, 119, 1*(suppl), 64S–94S.

Hirsch, J., Dalen, J. E., Anderson, D. R., Poller, L., Bussey, H., Ansell, J. et al. (2001). Oral anticoagulants: Mechanism of action, clinical effectiveness, and optimal therapeutic range. *Chest, 119*(1 Suppl), 8S–21S.

Marini, J. J., & Wheeler, A. P. (Eds.). (1997). Venous thrombosis and pulmonary embolism. *Critical care medicine: The essentials* (pp. 364–376). Baltimore: Williams & Wilkins.

Palevsky, H. I. & Edmunds, L. H. (1997). Pulmonary thromboembolism. In L. H. Edmunds (Ed.), *Cardiac surgery in the adult* (pp. 1319–1343). New York: McGraw-Hill.

Palevsky, H. I., Kelley, M. A., & Fishman. A. P. (1998). Pulmonary thromboembolic disease. In A. P. Fishman, J. A. Elias, J. A. Fishman, M. A. Grippi, L. R. Kaiser, & R. M. Senior (Eds.), *Fishman's pulmonary diseases and disorders* (pp. 1297–1329). New York: McGraw-Hill.

Palmer, S. M. & Tapson, V. F. (1999). New approaches to the diagnosis of pulmonary embolism. *Hospital Physician, 35*(6), 23–32.

Tai, N. R. M., Atwal, A. S., & Hamilton, G. (1999). Modern management of pulmonary embolism. *British Journal of Surgery, 86*(7), 853–868.

Weinberger, S. E. (Ed.). (1998). *Pulmonary embolism: Principles of pulmonary medicine.* Philadelphia: W. B. Saunders.

Adult Obstructive Sleep Apnea 24

Terri E. Weaver

I. Introduction
   A. Definition: Presence of >5 obstructed breathing events/h sleep documented by overnight monitoring and either
      1. excessive daytime sleepiness unexplained by other factors
      2. presentation of two or more symptoms unrelated to other factors
         a. choking or gasping during sleep
         b. recurrent awakenings
         c. unrefreshing sleep
         d. daytime fatigue
         e. impaired concentration (American Academy of Sleep Medicine [AASM], 1999).
      3. Obstructed breathing events include any combination of obstructive apneas/hypopneas or respiratory-related arousals (AASM, 1999).
   B. Etiology
      1. Physical factors: There is emerging evidence that the etiology of OSA has a genetic basis (Ferini-Strambi et al., 1995; Palmer et al., 2003; Pillar & Lavie, 1995; Redline et al., 1995; Strohl, 2003)
   C. Risk factors
      1. Obesity, especially body mass index (BMI) >27
      2. Small upper airway
      3. Ethanol intake as it exacerbates OSA
      4. Young African-Americans may be at increased risk (Redline et al., 1997)
      5. Presence of retrognathia, prognathia, macroglossia
      6. Male gender
      7. Postmenopausal women
   D. Pathophysiology: Repetitive nocturnal upper airway collapse resulting in episodic hypoxemia and sleep fragmentation. Thought to be caused by

anatomic narrowing, upper airway muscle fatigue, and/or lack of central nervous system stimulation to the upper airway. Degree of severity indicated by the respiratory disturbance index (RDI)—the number of respiratory events/hour of sleep or apnea-hyponea index (AHI)—the number of apneas and hypopneas/hour of sleep.

E. Incidence: 4% of male population and 2% female population (Young et al., 1993)

F. Considerations across the life span
   Nocturnal respiratory disturbances increase with age.

G. Potential complications/sequelae
   1. Increased cardiovascular morbidity (Faccenda, Mackay, Boon, & Douglas, 2001; Nieto et al., 2000; Peppard, Young, Palta, & Skatrud, 2000)
   2. Excessive daytime sleepiness (EDS; Gottlieb et al., 1999) associated with
      a. Increased errors and accidents (Bedard, Montplaisir, Malo, Richer, & Rouleau, 1993; Findley, Smith, Hooper, Dineen, & Suratt, 2000; George & Smiley, 1999)
      b. Decrements in neurobehavioral functioning (Bedard et al., 1993; Engleman, Kingshott, Martin, & Douglas, 2000; Kribbs et al., 1993)
      c. Depressed mood (Derderian, Bridenbaugh, & Rajagopal, 1988; Millman, Fogel, McNamara, & Carlisle, 1989)
      d. Reduced functional status and quality of life (Flemons, 2000; Gall, Isaac, & Kryger, 1993; Weaver, Laizner, et al., 1997)

II. Assessment
   A. History
      1. Presence of excessive daytime sleepiness, including history of sleep-related accident
      2. Presence and frequency of snoring, gasping, witnessed apneas
      3. Intellectual deterioration—memory loss, poor judgment, difficulty maintaining attention, disorientation, hallucinations
      4. Personality changes, irritability
      5. Morning headaches
      6. Nocturnal enuresis
      7. Impotence
      8. History of hypertension or cardiovascular disease
      9. Complaint of insomnia
      10. Nocturia
      11. Nocturnal esophageal reflux and heartburn
   B. Physical exam
      1. Obesity, especially body mass index (BMI) >28
      2. Small upper airway and craniofacial abnormalities including high arched high palate, long soft palate placed low, and redundant tissues, tonsillar hypertrophy ("kissing tonsils"), large uvula, retrognathia, micrognathia, underbite, and macroglossia
      3. Nasal septal deviation
      4. Hypertension

C. Diagnostic tests
   1. Polysomnography for detection of sleep disorder including EEG, EMG, EOG, respiratory effort (inductive plethysmography), measurement of oronasal airflow, and pulse oximetry
   2. Multiple Sleep Latency Test (MSLT) to measure objective daytime sleepiness; specifically the latency to sleep (up to 20 minutes) during a series of daytime naps in a darkened room.
   3. Cephalometric radiographs to evaluate relevant cranial and facial structures
   4. Fiberoptic endoscopy and/or video fluoroscopy
III. Common therapeutic modalities
   A. Behavioral modification for sleep hygiene and weight control
   B. Continuous positive airway pressure (CPAP) or Bilevel positive airway pressure (BiPAP)—primary medical treatment modality
   C. Surgery including septoplasty, polypectomy or turbinate reduction, tonsillectomy, adenoidectomy, soft palate resection (uvulopalatopharyngoplasty [UPPP]), mandibular advancement procedures, tongue reduction, and pharyngeal suspension (Woodson et al., 2000)
   D. Oral appliance including tongue retaining as well as mandibular adjustment devices
IV. Interventions
   A. Evaluate and promote sleep hygiene (see "Impaired Sleep")
   B. Provide behavioral interventions to promote weight loss and if necessary decrease in alcohol ingestion and smoking cessation
   C. Evaluate patient adherence to treatment (see "Equipment Considerations")
V. Home care considerations
   A. Equipment considerations
   1. Approximately half of those who use CPAP are non-adherent to treatment (Kribbs et al., 1993; Weaver, Kribbs, et al., 1997). Efforts should be made to assure that the patient understands that the negative consequences of obstructive sleep apnea can be prevented with the nightly use of CPAP treatment. Patients should also be fitted with the mask that is most acceptable to them. The addition of a chinstrap may help alleviate dry mouth in the morning. Warm humidification should be added to CPAP equipment as there is evidence that the use of warm humidification promotes adherence (Massie, Hart, Peralez, & Richards, 1999). Nasal steroids should be prescribed if necessary.
      a. Assessment of patient adherence and treatment outcome should occur during the first week of treatment when non-adherent patterns of use are most likely to be established (Rosenthal et al., 2000; Weaver, Kribbs, et al., 1997).
      b. Patients with less severe disease who are unable to tolerate CPAP treatment should be referred for treatment with either oral appliance or surgery.

313

       c. Those with a history of claustrophobia may have more difficulty using CPAP (Kribbs et al., 1993).
   B. Social supports
       a. AWAKE support group provides support of patients with obstructive sleep apnea

REFERENCES

American Academy of Sleep Medicine. (1999). Sleep-related breathing disorders in adults: Recommendations for syndrome definition and measurement techniques in clinical research. The Report of an American Academy of Sleep Medicine Task Force. *Sleep, 22*(5), 667–689.

Bedard, M. A., Montplaisir, J., Malo, J., Richer, F., & Rouleau, I. (1993). Persistent neuropsychological deficits and vigilance impairment in sleep apnea syndrome after treatment with continuous positive airways pressure (CPAP). *Journal of Clinical and Experimental Neuropsychology, 15*(2), 330–341.

Derderian, S. S., Bridenbaugh, R. H., & Rajagopal, K. R. (1988). Neuropsychologic symptoms in obstructive sleep apnea improve after treatment with nasal continuous positive airway pressure. *Chest, 94,* 1023–1027.

Engleman, H. M., Kingshott, R. N., Martin, S. E., & Douglas, N. J. (2000). Cognitive function in the sleep apnea/hypopnea syndrome (SAHS). *Sleep, 23*(Suppl 4), S102–S108.

Faccenda, J. F., Mackay, T. W., Boon, N. A., & Douglas, N. J. (2001). Randomized placebo-controlled trial of continuous positive airway pressure on blood pressure in the sleep apnea-hypopnea syndrome. *Am J Respir Crit Care Med, 163*(2), 344–348.

Ferini-Strambi, L., Calori, G., Oldani, A., Della Marca, G., Zucconi, M., Castronovo, V., et al. (1995). Snoring in twins. *Respir Med, 89*(5), 337–340.

Findley, L., Smith, C., Hooper, J., Dineen, M., & Suratt, P. M. (2000). Treatment with nasal CPAP decreases automobile accidents in patients with sleep apnea. *American Journal of Respiratory and Critical Care Medicine, 161*(3 Pt 1), 857–859.

Flemons, W. W. (2000). Measuring health related quality of life in sleep apnea. *Sleep, 23*(Suppl 4), S109–S114.

Gall, R., Isaac, L., & Kryger, M. (1993). Quality of life in mild obstructive sleep apnea. *Sleep, 16,* S59–S61.

George, C. F., & Smiley, A. (1999). Sleep apnea & automobile crashes. *Sleep, 22*(6), 790–795.

Gottlieb, D. J., Whitney, C. W., Bonekat, W. H., Iber, C., James, G. D., Lebowitz, M., et al. (1999). Relation of sleepiness to respiratory disturbance index: The Sleep Heart Health Study. *Am J Respir Crit Care Med, 159*(2), 502–507.

Kribbs, N. B., Pack, A. I., Kline, L. R., Smith, P. L., Schwartz, A. R., Schubert, N. M., et al. (1993). Objective measurement of patterns of nasal CPAP use by patients with obstructive sleep apnea. *Am Rev Respir Dis, 147*(4), 887–895.

Massie, C. A., Hart, R. W., Peralez, K., & Richards, G. N. (1999). Effects of humidification on nasal symptoms and compliance in sleep apnea patients using continuous positive airway pressure. *Chest, 116*(2), 403–408.

Millman, R. P., Fogel, B. S., McNamara, M. E., & Carlisle, C. C. (1989). Depression as a manifestation of obstructive sleep apnea: reversal with nasal continuous positive airway pressure. *Journal of Clinical Psychiatry, 50,* 348–351.

Nieto, F. J., Young, T. B., Lind, B. K., Shahar, E., Samet, J. M., Redline, S., et al. (2000). Association of sleep-disordered breathing, sleep apnea, and hypertension in a large community-based study. Sleep Heart Health Study. *Journal of the American Medical Association, 283*(14), 1829–1836.

Palmer, L. J., Buxbaum, S. G., Larkin, E., Patel, S. R., Elston, R. C., Tishler, P. V., et al. (2003). A whole-genome scan for obstructive sleep apnea and obesity. *Am J Hum Genet, 72*(2), 340–350.

Peppard, P. E., Young, T., Palta, M., & Skatrud, J. (2000). Prospective study of the association between sleep-disordered breathing and hypertension. *New England Journal of Medicine, 342*(19), 1378–1384.

Pillar, G., & Lavie, P. (1995). Assessment of the role of inheritance in sleep apnea syndrome. *Am J Respir Crit Care Med, 151*(3 Pt 1), 688–691.

Redline, S., Tishler, P. V., Hans, M. G., Tosteson, T. D., Strohl, K. P., & Spry, K. (1997). Racial differences in sleep-disordered breathing in African-Americans and Caucasians. *Am J Respir Crit Care Med, 155*(1), 186–192.

Redline, S., Tishler, P. V., Tosteson, T. D., Williamson, J., Kump, K., Browner, I., et al. (1995). The familial aggregation of obstructive sleep apnea. *Am J Respir Crit Care Med, 151*(3 Pt 1), 682–687.

Strohl, K. P. (2003). Periodic breathing and genetics. *Respir Physiol Neurobiol, 135*(2–3), 179–185.

Weaver, T. E., Kribbs, N. B., Pack, A. I., Kline, L. R., Chugh, D. K., Maislin, G., et al. (1997). Night-to-night variability in CPAP use over the first three months of treatment. *Sleep, 20*(4), 278–283.

Weaver, T. E., Laizner, A. M., Evans, L. K., Maislin, G., Chugh, D. K., Lyon, K., et al. (1997). An instrument to measure functional status outcomes for disorders of excessive sleepiness. *Sleep, 20*(10), 835–843.

Woodson, B. T., Derowe, A., Hawke, M., Wenig, B., Ross, E. B., Jr., Katsantonis, G. P., et al. (2000). Pharyngeal suspension suture with repose bone screw for obstructive sleep apnea. *Otolaryngol Head Neck Surg, 122*(3), 395–401.

Young, T., Palta, M., Dempsey, J., Skatrud, J., Weber, S., & Badr, S. (1993). The occurrence of sleep-disordered breathing among middle-aged adults. *New England Journal of Medicine, 328*(17), 1230–1235.

Respiratory Muscle Weakness

25

Janet Crimlisk

INTRODUCTION

This chapter summarizes the common respiratory muscle weakness disorders of Multiple Sclerosis (MS), Amyotropic Lateral Sclerosis (ALS), Guillain-Barré Syndrome (GBS), Muscular Dystrophy (MD), Myasthenia Gravis (MG), and Spinal Cord Injury (SCI). The normal response for voluntary and involuntary muscle movement is presented to help understand the pathology of these respiratory muscle weakness disorders. Disease or dysfunction in the muscle, the spinal cord or the central nervous system can cause respiratory muscle weakness. "The cardinal symptom of muscle disease is weakness. A careful clinical analysis usually distinguishes the weakness of primary muscle disease from that caused by problems in the motor unit or the central nervous system" (Brown, 1994, p. 1108).

THE ACT OF BREATHING

I.   Respiratory muscles
- Three muscle groups are essential for normal ventilation.
- The act of breathing is accomplished by these skeletal muscle groups.
- These muscles are innervated by both motor and sensory neurons.
   A.   Group 1—Muscles of inspiration
      1. Inspiratory muscles: diaphragm, external intercostals, accessory muscles of inspiration (sternocleidomastoid, scalenus, and trapezius muscles)
      2. Inspiration: an active process with diaphragm the primary muscle of inspiration
      3. Standing or seated position, diaphragm responsible for one-third of tidal volume (Vt); in supine position, diaphragm responsible for two-third of Vt (Levitsky, 1995)

317

4. Diaphragm innervated by 2 phrenic nerves that exit the spinal cord at 3rd through 5th cervical segments
5. If a nonfunctional diaphragm, due to fatigue or paralysis
   a. Inspiration performed solely by external intercostals and accessory muscles
   b. Paradoxical breathing occurs due to upward displacement of nonfunctioning diaphragm with inward displacement of abdominal wall during inspiration
   c. Paradoxical breathing seen clinically as asynchronous rocking motion of the chest and abdomen; mechanically inefficient.
   d. Hemidiaphragmatic paralysis, one diaphragm leaflet paralyzed; also presents with paradoxical breathing (Levitsky, 1995)
6. Inspiratory muscle weakness leads to loss of sigh volumes and microatelectasis; respiratory muscle failure leads to ventilatory failure, CO_2 retention, and hypoxemia.

B. Group 2—Muscles of expiration
   1. Expiratory muscles: abdominal muscles, internal intercostal muscles
      a. Expiration: passive process; primary abdominal muscles: rectus abdominis, external and internal oblique muscles, transverse abdominis
      b. Active expiration occurs during exercise, speech, singing, coughing, sneezing.
   2. Sign of expiratory muscle weakness: short speech phrases with shallow inspirations

C. Group 3—Upper airway muscles
   1. The human larynx facilitates deglutition, phonation, and respiration.
      a. Larynx functions as a respiratory organ with glottis (vocal cords) opened slightly on inspiration and closed slightly on expiration to regulate the passage of air.
      b. Laryngeal muscles open the glottis prior to diaphragmatic descent, a direct effect from the medullary respiratory center.
   2. Muscles of the oropharynx contract during normal inspiration, which dilates and stabilizes the upper airway during inhalation.

D. Inspiration summary: events occurring in the inspiratory act of tidal breathing (normal quiet breathing)
   1. Brain initiates inspiration
   2. Nerves carry message to inspiratory muscles
   3. Diaphragm and laryngeal muscles contract and simultaneously
      a. Diaphragm descends
      b. Thoracic volume increases
      c. Intrapleural pressure becomes more negative
      d. Air flows into alveoli due to the pressure gradient created

E. Expiration summary: events occurring in the expiratory act of tidal breathing (normal quiet breathing)
   1. Brain ceases inspiratory effort
   2. Inspiratory muscles relax and simultaneously

a. Diaphragm ascends

b. Thoracic volume decreases

c. Intrapleural pressure becomes less negative

d. Air flows out due to the pressure gradient

II. Central nervous system, neural pathways

Control of breathing is initiated in the brain. The muscles of breathing do not contract spontaneously (Figure 25.1).

A. Control of breathing extends from the cerebral hemisphere where basic voluntary function located, to the central homeostatic centers in pons and medulla.

1. Spontaneous automatic breathing generated by groups of neurons located in the reticular formation of the medulla.

2. Apneustic center located in the pons; postulated to be the site of termination of inspiration; apneustic breathing is prolonged inspiratory hold interrupted by occasional expirations.

3. Pneumotaxic center, group of neurons in the midbrain, modulate activity of the apneustic center, balance inspiration with expiration; may modulate responses to stimuli such as hypercapnea and hypoxia (Levitsky, 1995).

B. Spinal pathways from the brain descend in the white matter of the spinal cord to influence the diaphragm, intercostals, and abdominal muscles of inspiration.

1. Motor unit: composed of motor neuron, axon (myelinated nerve fiber), and group of muscle fibers innervated by the axon

2. Neuromuscular junction: area of contact between a nerve and muscle fiber, the axon releases acetylcholine, which contracts the muscle fibers

III. Motor control and disruption of functional levels of spinal cord

▪ Spinal cord disease has a profound effect on pulmonary function.

▪ Breathing difficulty will depend on level of spinal cord injury.

▪ Decreased lung volumes, impaired cough and sigh, atelectasis, pneumonia, and respiratory compromise, including complete loss of respiratory function, can occur.

A. Motor control

1. Sensory tracts of spinal cord transmit information to brain to guide movements.

a. ascending tracts are major sensory (afferent) tracts involved in proprioception and discrimination (i.e., lateral spinothalamic tract transmits pain impulses).

2. Motor tracts of spinal cord transmit signals from brain to spinal cord to direct and coordinate movements.

a. Descending tracts are major motor (efferent) tracts involved in voluntary (pyramidal or corticospinal tracts) and involuntary (extrapyramidal tracts) movement

3. Spinal reflexes are reflexes to a stimulus that occur at each level of the spinal cord.

a. Usually involuntary conduction over a reflex arc (i.e., deep tendon reflexes)

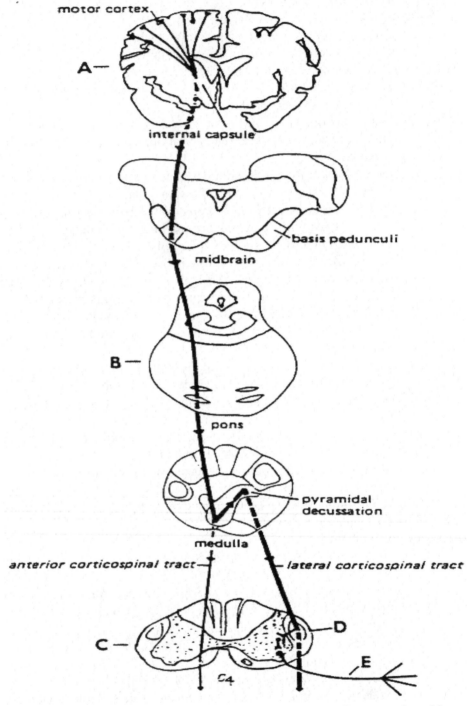

Figure 25.1. Levels of motor symptom and sites of sensory influence on breathing. A. Cerebral hemisphere—voluntary, emotional. B. Pons and medulla—central homeostatic reflexes. C. Spinal cord—basic motor and sensory reflexes. D. Anterior horn—motor neuron. E. motor axion.

B. Lower motor neurons and upper motor neurons (Figure 25.2)
  1. Lower motor neurons (LMN)
     a. LMNs in anterior gray horns of the spinal cord; final common pathway for all skeletal muscles.
     b. LMNs originate in the anterior horn cells at each segment of the spinal cord, exit the spinal cord to form spinal nerves and branches of peripheral nervous system; axons of anterior horn cells are the only motor fibers terminating in skeletal muscles.
  2. Examples of LMN injuries
     a. Reflex arc: Sensory and motor loop of LMN; damage to anterior horn cells will cause paralysis of associated muscles and arc with reflex muscle contractions lost.
     b. Examples of LMN lesions: Anterior horn cell destruction (polio), peripheral nerve damage, spinal cord injury.
     c. LMN injury evident in lesions below T12/L1 (conus medullaris/cauda equina); spinal cord ends at lower border of L1 vertebrae; spinal nerve roots extend to the coccyx.
     d. LMN lesions: Loss of reflex arc and voluntary and involuntary muscle innervation present with
        i. Flaccid paralysis
        ii. Absent or decreased reflexes below the level of injury
        iii. Severe muscle atrophy
  3. Upper motor neurons (UMN)
     a. Long tracts from brain to spinal cord with cell bodies located in motor strip of the cerebral cortex; axons lie in either pyramidal (corticospinal, corticobulbar) or extrapyramidal (reticulospinal) tracts
     b. UMN synapse with LMN in anterior horn cell of spinal cord at each segmental level.
     c. UMN lesions present with exaggerated responses
        i. Hyperactive reflexes
        ii. Spastic paralysis
        iii. Positive plantar reflex (Babinski)
        iv. Minimal muscle atrophy.
     d. Damage to the UMN system from brain down to and including T 12/L1 segments of spinal cord create UMN lesion (i.e.. MS, SCI)
  4. Segmental innervation of respiratory muscles
     a. Effects on pulmonary function based on level of spinal cord lesion; specific respiratory muscles innervated at segmental level shown in Table 25.1.
     b. C5 Lesions affect diaphragm function; C3 lesions and above produce bilateral diaphragmatic paralysis requiring mechanical ventilation; accessory muscles affected in high cervical cord lesions.
     c. Lesions of lumbar area have little or no effect on ventilation or cough.

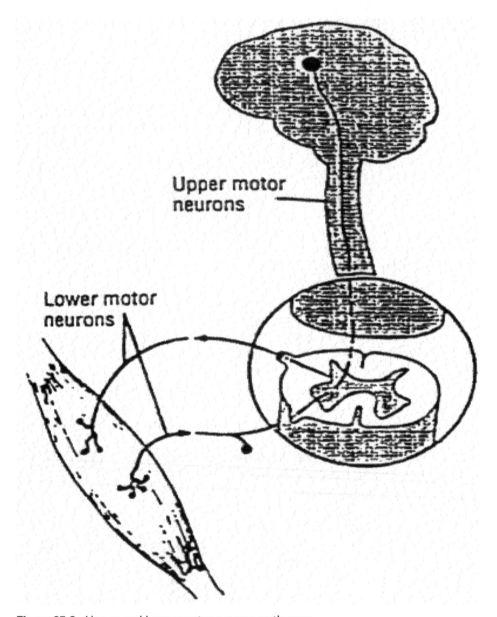

Figure 25.2. Upper and lower motor neuron pathways.

Reproduced with permission from Emick-Herring, B. (Ed.). (1993). Normal motor control and neurophysiological approaches. In A. E. McCourt (Ed.), *The specialty practice of rehabilitation nursing: A core curriculum* (3rd ed., p. 31). Skokie, IL: Rehabilitation Nursing Foundation.

Table 25.1	Respiratory Muscles Presented by Descending Segmental Innervation Sites and Muscle Function	
Respiratory Muscles	**Segmental Innervation Sites**	**Muscle Function**
Laryngeal Muscles	Brainstem C2–C5 Cranial Nerve X (vagus) Cranial Nerve XI (spinal accessory)	Contraction of upper airway muscles opens pharynx & larynx for air flow on inspiration
Sternocleidomastoid	C1–C3, Cranial Nerve IX (glossopharyngeal)	Attaches to manubrium of sternum to help elevate upper rib cage
Trapezius	C3–C4, Cranial Nerve XI (spinal accessory)	Attaches to scapula to help elevate shoulder girdle for inspiration
Diaphragm	C3–C5	Each hemidiaphragm is supplied by corresponding phrenic nerves arising from C3–C5 of spinal cord
Scalenus	C3–C8	Elevates 1st and 2nd ribs during forced inspiration
Intercostals	T1–T11	Facilitate ability to cough and deep breathe; intercostal muscles are continuous with the oblique muscle of the abdominal wall
Rectus Abdominis	T6–T12	Major muscles of expiration; produces effective cough

Adapted from: Schmitt, J., Midha, M., & McKenzie, N. (1991). Medical Complications of Spinal Cord Disease. In R. M. Woolsey, & R. R. Young (Eds.), Neurologic Clinics (p. 780). Philadelphia: W. B. Saunders.

NEUROMUSCULAR DISEASES

Multiple Sclerosis

I.   Overview Multiple Sclerosis (MS)
- Neurologic degenerative disease; disorder of the central nervous system (CNS) myelin (Table 25.2)
- Most common demyelinating disease; a disease of young adults (Olek, 2004)
- Chronic recurrent inflammatory disorder of the CNS (Multiple Sclerosis Council Clinical Practice Guidelines [MSCCPG], 2001)

Table 25.2 Respiratory Muscle Weakness Disorders. An overview by disease, site of injury, respiratory muscle involvement, management, and natural course of the disease.

Disease	Site of Injury	Prominent Signs & Symptoms	Respiratory Muscle Involvement	Management	Course of the Disease
Multiple Sclerosis	CNS myelin sheaths destroyed	Fatigue, muscle weakness, ataxia, paresthesias	Thoracic site: inspiratory muscles	Symptomatic	Chronic, may be progressive; remissions, exacerbations
ALS	Motor neuron damaged: UMN, LMN	Muscle atrophy, bulbar palsy	Diaphragm, bulbar involvement	Symptomatic	Chronic, progressive; ventilator support
Guillain-Barré Syndrome	Peripheral nerve myelin destroyed	Ascending paralysis, starting in lower limbs	Diaphragm, bulbar Involvement	Symptomatic	Acute disease; ventilator support; recovery expected
Muscular Dystrophy	Skeletal muscle deteriorates	Muscle weakness, proximal muscles first	Diaphragm, Restrictive pulmonary disease possible	Symptomatic	Chronic, progressive; genetic counseling recommended
Myasthenia Gravis	Neuromuscular junction: destruction of acetylcholine at postsynaptic sites	Muscle weakness, fatigue, dysarthria, dysphagia; muscle weakness T with activity, with rest	Respiratory muscles, bulbar paralysis	Mestinon therapy-prolongs acetylcholine at motor end plate	Chronic, progressive; remissions, exacerbations
Spinal Cord Injury	Spinal cord destruction, level of injury varies; UMN, LMN Lesions	Motor, sensory involvement; paralysis, paresis, spasticity	Diaphragm, intercostals, abdominals, depending on injury	Symptomatic	Chronic; permanent

A. Definition

Multiple sclerosis is a chronic demyelinating disease of the CNS with destruction of the myelin sheath covering nerve fibers; when the lesions heal *multiple sclerotic plaques* are seen, which gives the disease its name (Ross, 1999).

1. There are four classifications of MS (Olek, 2004; Ross, 1999).
    a. Relapsing remitting MS: most common (90%); episodes of remission and exacerbation with no progression between episodes
    b. Primary progressive MS: uncommon (10%); continual progression of the disease
    c. Secondary progressive MS: 40%–50% start with relapsing remitting and develop secondary progression in which the disease continues with or without relapses
    d. Progressive relapsing MS: rare; progression of the disease with relapses and worsening of disease occurring between relapses
2. The relapsing form of disease is generally associated with a better prognosis than the progressive disease (Olek, 2004).

B. Etiology

1. Cause unknown; considered an autoimmune disorder.
2. MS may be autoimmune response to viral infection in genetically susceptible person.
3. Epidemiologic evidence suggests MS is an acquired disease with a long period between exposure and development of signs and symptoms.

C. Pathophysiology

1. MS involves the white matter of brain and spinal cord; myelin sheaths destroyed by lymphocytes with inflammation, edema, and demyelination.
2. Early in disease the areas of demyelination heal without nerve damage; as disease progresses scarring and sclerotic plaques develop with permanent damage

D. Incidence and clinical manifestations

1. 8,000 new cases annually; young adults, 20–40 years of age; insidious, gradual onset; course of the disease highly variable depending on lesions and type of MS
2. Prevalent in temperate zones, highly developed countries; Caucasians higher incidence than blacks; women more affected than men (1:2 ratio; Ross, 1999); life expectancy more than 25 years (Rosebrough, 1998)
3. Frequent signs and symptoms: fatigue, weakness, visual disturbances, tremor, ataxia, and paresthesias (Chusid, 1985); depression, anger, euphoria.
4. Fatigue is now recognized as the most common symptom of MS, 75%–95% of patients experience fatigue (MSCCPG, 1998; Lisak, 2001).
5. Cervical spinal cord involvement: gait weakness, numbness in hands, Lhermitte's sign (flexing neck produces tingling down to the legs; Taylor, 1999).
6. Thoracic involvement: numbness in the rib cage/waist.

7. Neurogenic bowel and bladder symptoms occur with lumbar/sacral involvement.

E. Considerations across the life span
1. Pediatrics: MS rare in this age group
2. Pregnancy: remissions during pregnancy; risk for exacerbations during postpartum (Ozuna, 2004)
3. Elderly: MS can present as a chronic progressive spinal cord disease with asymmetric spastic paraperesis and sensory deficits (Adams & Salam-Adams, 1991); cervical spondylosis needs to be excluded.

F. Complications and sequelae
1. Day-to-day variability; may progress rapidly to total disability and dependence
2. Cognitive impairment, pain with paresthesias, bowel and bladder dysfunction, altered sexual functioning, heat sensitivity, fatigue (Rosebrough, 1998)
3. Death from pneumonia and complications of immobility (Ozuna, 2004)

II. Assessment
A. History: Include history of viral infections, recent stress, extremes of heat and cold, pregnancy; medications; functional health pattern.
B. Physical exam: general condition, cognitive ability, focused review of skin (pressure ulcers), neurologic (ataxia, nystagmus, tremors, spasticity, hyperreflexia, poor coordination), and musculoskeletal (muscle weakness, paresis, paralysis, dysarthrias, spasms) systems (Ozuna, 2004).
C. Diagnostic tests: no definitive tests; diagnosis by exclusion; CSF fluid analysis may help if active disease; CT and MRI may identify sclerotic plaques.

III. Common therapeutic modalities
A. Threefold Treatment: Management of symptoms; acute relapses; and reduction in frequency of relapses. Newer disease-modifying agents are available for acute relapses and reduction in relapses (MSCCPG, 2001).
1. Symptomatic management: Pharmacological treatment for tremors, spasticity and paresthesias with anticonvulsants, antispasmodics and antidepressants; physical therapy (PT) and occupational therapy (OT) for passive stretching and range of motion (ROM) exercises (Ozuna, 2004; Lisak, 2001); bowel and bladder programs.
2. Acute relapses: High dose methylprednisone (500–1000 mg) standard therapy for acute exacerbation given over 3–7 days with or without a prednisone taper (Olek, 2004).
3. Reducing relapses: Disease modifying agents, the immunomodulators, Interferon beta 1-b (Betaseron) and Interferon beta 1-a (Avonex, Rebif), for relapsing remitting MS decreased the number and severity of relapses; Glatiramer acetate (Copolymer 1, Copaxone) believed to prevent damage to myelin; IV immunoglobulin reported to reduced exacerbations (Olek, 2004; MSCCPG, 2001; Ross, 1999).

B. Rehabilitation program: Rehabilitation aimed at maintaining optimum level of independence; involves interdisciplinary team of rehabilitation specialists.

IV. Home care considerations

A. Home care to help patient adjust to illness, avoid triggers that precipitate the disease and maintain self care activities.

B. PT to relieve spasms and increase coordination

C. Bowel and bladder programs

D. National MS Society local chapter can offer a variety of services.

Amyotrophic Lateral Sclerosis

I. Overview Amyotrophic Lateral Sclerosis (ALS)

■ Primary motor neuron disease (Table 25.2)

■ Most common form of motor neuron disease in adults (Thompson & Swash, 2001)

■ Characterized by loss of motor neurons in brain stem and spinal cord (Francis, Bach, & Delisa, 1999)

A. Definition

ALS, Lou Gehrig's Disease; neurodegenerative disease of upper and lower motor neurons; 5%–10% of cases familial, four major subtypes of ALS (Francis et al., 1999)

1. Classical ALS: 90% of all ALS; UMN and LMN involvement
2. Progressive muscular atrophy: LMN only; affects limb and trunk muscles only
3. Progressive bulbar palsy: rare; affect bulbar musculature only
4. Primary lateral sclerosis: UMN only, affects limb, trunk or bulbar musculature

B. Etiology

Cause unknown; believed to be multifactorial; genetic, environmental, and autoimmune causes being researched (Francis et al., 1999); 5%–10% inherited (Brown, 2004)

C. Pathophysiology

Motor neurons gradually degenerate in motor cortex and lateral cortico-spinal tract, giving it its name *lateral sclerosis*.

1. Progression to LMN involvement with destruction of anterior horn cells.
2. Bulbar function deteriorates more slowly than limb strength or respiration.
3. Sensory system largely unaffected in ALS and cognition remains intact.

D. Incidence and clinical manifestations

1. 1–3 per 100,000 annually; ages of onset 40–70 years old; men more than women (ratio 2:1; Francis et al., 1999).
2. Clinical presentation varies considerably depending on motor neurons affected.

   a. Initial presentation: asymmetric focal weakness in one limb

       b. LMN involvement: weakness of hands and forearms, atrophy, cramps, fasciculations

       c. UMN involvement: hyperreflexia, loss of dexterity, muscle stiffness, spasticity

       d. Bulbar symptoms: dysarthria, dysphagia, fasciculations of the tongue

       e. Respiratory symptoms with upper extremity weakness and diaphragm involvement

       f. Depression common throughout the illness

   E. Considerations across the life span

      1. Pediatric: may occur teenage years; younger patients survive longer (Francis et al., 1999)

      2. Pregnancy: no literature on the effects of ALS and pregnancy

      3. Elderly: Incidence after age 70 equal in men and women; bulbar involvement 43% in persons over 70 (Francis et al., 1999); late onset associated with more rapid progression

   F. Complications and sequelae

      1. Progresses to tetraplegia; 50% mortality in first 3 years of onset

      2. Mean duration from onset of disease to death or ventilator dependency is 2–4 years; survival 10 years or more without ventilator support has been reported in 8%–22% of patients (Francis et al., 1999)

II. Assessment

   A. History: Include history related to weakness; decreased cough and speech ability; dyspnea on exertion (DOE); muscle cramping, stiffness, spasticity; swallowing difficulty; medications; functional health pattern

   B. Physical: General condition, cognitive ability; focused review of neurological (dexterity, fasciculations, hyperreflexia), bulbar (dysphagia, dysarthria), respiratory (dyspnea, tachypnea, decreased diaphragmatic movement), and musculoskeletal (muscle weakness/wasting, paralysis) systems.

   C. Diagnostic tests

      1. The El Escorial criteria for diagnosis of ALS, developed by the World Federation of Neurology, indicates a definitive diagnosis if progressive UMN and LMN signs in 3 of 4 regions (bulbar, cervical, thoracic, lumbosacral) in the absence of electrophysiological or neuroimaging evidence of other disease processes (Francis et al., 1999)

      2. Disorders that mimic ALS must be ruled out; testing may include EMG, nerve conduction studies, MRI of brain and spinal cord, pulmonary function tests, ABGs, muscle biopsy

III. Common therapeutic modalities

There is no known cure; management is aimed at symptomatic treatment, rehabilitation needs, and clinical trials of pharmacologic agents.

   A. Symptomatic management

      1. Communication: Speech deficits the first bulbar effects; speech training includes rate, articulation, respiration efficiency, tongue strengthening, and diaphragmatic exercises; communication devices and environmental control units (ECU) may be used.

2. Swallowing and nutrition: Poor caloric intake and dehydration occur with bulbar involvement; pureed diet, chin-touch position for swallowing, aspiration precautions may be insufficient; a permanent gastrostomy may be necessary.
3. Mobility and ADL-PT: mobility adjuncts, wheelchair use and training; OT: upper extremity bracing, adaptive equipment, safety skills, energy conservation, environmental control units.
4. Pain, fatigue, abnormal sleep pattern
   a. Baclofen, including intrathecal baclofen, is the drug of choice for muscle cramps and stiffness due to spasticity; analgesics and narcotics for severe pain
   b. Fatigue: generalized tiredness; sleep deprivation common from abnormal nocturnal movements, myoclonus, respiratory muscle weakness, pharyngeal hypotonia, orthopnea (Ferguson, Strong, Ahmad, & George, 1996)

B. Respiratory management
   1. Evaluate respiratory status: vital capacity, SpO_2, and peak cough flows
   2. Inspiratory muscle aids
      a. Inspiratory muscle training (IMT) devices: inhale against resistance, improves muscle strength and endurance
      b. Glossopharyngeal breathing (GPB): 6 gulps (50–150 cc/gulp) in one breath to achieve a tidal volume of approximately 600 cc; useful in non-bulbar ALS and as backup in event of sudden ventilator failure. (American College of Chest Physicians [ACCP], 1998)
      c. Mechanical pneumobelt: abdominal bladder inflates for inspiration and deflates for expiration; noninvasive support to assist diaphragmatic activity and decrease work of breathing (Bach, 1994; Branson, Hess, & Chatburn, 1999)
      d. Mouthpiece IPPV (intermittent positive pressure breathing) used for intermittent deep breaths (Bach, 1994)
   3. Expiratory muscle aids
      a. Manual assisted cough "quad cough," huff cough, PEP (positive expiratory pressure therapy), and flutter valve used in management of airway secretions (American Association of Respiratory Care, 1993; Bach, 1994; Branson et al., 1999)
      b. Mechanical oscillation devices: high frequency chest wall compressions (ThAIRapy vest); oscillating motion helps mobilize secretions (ACCP, 1998)
      c. Mechanical insufflation-exsufflation (in-exsufflator): device to deliver deep positive insufflation followed by passive negative exsufflation; administered by mouthpiece or tracheal tube; clears large amounts of secretions (ACCP, 1998; Bach, 1994)
      d. Intrapulmonary percussive ventilator (IPV) manually triggers high frequency percussive breaths; offers aerosol medication administration; increases secretion mobilization (Bach, 1994; Branson et al., 1999)

4. Mechanical ventilation: Decision requires careful consideration; ethical, financial and quality of life issues; noninvasive nocturnal ventilation an option (Goldberg, 1999).

5. Noninvasive positive pressure ventilation used for intermittent nocturnal support; shown to reduce morning headache, improve vital capacity, and decrease respiratory fatigue (Sherman & Paz, 1994).
   a. External negative pressure ventilation devices: chest cuirass, pulmowrap; both uncomfortable; skin breakdown possible due to need for tight chest seal
   b. Positive pressure devices: delivered through nose or face mask; most common device used is BiPAP (bimodal positive airway pressure); provides inspiratory pressure assist triggered by the patient's inspiratory effort

6. Continuous mechanical ventilation and tracheostomy
   a. Portable battery powered ventilators with pressure, volume cycling and intermittent mechanical ventilation; custom fit to wheelchair
   b. Speech alternatives
      i. In-line expiratory valve, the Passy-Muir Valve
      ii. Tracheostomy tube cuff leak
      iii. "Talking trach" tube
      iv. Computerized communication devices

C. Pharmacologic interventions
   1. Symptomatic
      a. Theophylline: strengthen respiratory muscles (Sherman & Paz, 1994)
      b. Anticholinergic agents: decrease oral secretion if bulbar involvement; protect lung from aspiration of these secretions
      c. Expectorants, mucus controlling agents, aerosolized bronchodilators, and antibiotics, as indicated
      d. Annual flu vaccine and pneumococcal vaccines
   2. Future directions and research
      a. In 1998, FDA approved the first drug to slow the degenerative process; Riluzole (Rilutek) inhibits glutamine release, resulted in small positive effect of survival (Thompson & Swash, 2001).
      b. Neutrophic factors: involved in growth, survival of motor neurons (Francis et al., 1999).
         i. Myotrophin, a neutrophic, pending FDA approval.
         ii. Intrathecal neutrophic agents and delivery routes are in clinical trials.
         iii. Antiepileptic, gabapentin, showed slowing of functional deterioration.
         iv. Antioxidants and gene therapy in research
         v. Combination therapy to attack multiple pathways promising

IV. Home care considerations
   A. Support

Devastating illness; support patient's cognitive and emotional function; help patient and family with grieving related to loss of function and to eventual demise.

B. Respiratory support
Respiratory home care equipment; respiratory therapy services; patient, family and patient care attendant training to care for patient on mechanical ventilator, including chest physical therapy and airway management

C. Rehabilitation needs
Enormous rehabilitation needs; multidisciplinary team approach includes a physiatrist, neurologist, rehabilitation nurse, respiratory specialists, speech therapists, PT, OT, psychologists, and social service providers; inpatient acute rehabilitation care and follow-up outpatient rehabilitation therapy important to ensure optimal health and quality of life. (See spinal cord injury [SCI] for environmental, home care modifications, patient care attendant.)

Guillain-Barré Syndrome

I. Overview Guillain-Barré Syndrome (GBS)
   - Acute inflammatory demyelinating disease of the peripheral nervous system (Table 25.2)
   - Polyneuropathy, a syndrome of diffuse lesions of the peripheral nerves
   - Characterized by progressive muscle weakness and areflexia
   - Most common cause of acute flaccid paralysis in healthy people (DeLisser, 2003)

   A. Definition
   Also called acute inflammatory demyelinating polyradicular neuropathy (AIDP); an acute postinfectious polyneuropathy with ascending paralysis; rapidly progressing and potentially fatal (Logigian, 1994)

   B. Etiology
   Etiology unknown; believed to be cell-mediated immune reaction directed at peripheral nerves

   C. Pathophysiology (Figure 25.3)
   1. Generally preceded by a viral infection, trauma, gastroenteritis, surgery, or viral immunization (DeLisser, 2003; Warms, 2004).
   2. These stimuli thought to affect immune system causing destruction of peripheral nerve myelin sheaths and damage to nerve impulse transmission.
   3. Typically the weakness is ascending and progressive with loss or diminished deep tendon reflexes (DeLisser, 2003; Scheinberg, 1986).
   4. Bulbar muscles may become involved; progression involves lower brainstem with facial, abducens, oculomotor, hypoglossal, trigeminal and vagus nerves affected (cranial nerves VII, VI, III, XII, V, X).
   5. In recovery phase, remyelination occurs slowly and returns in a descending proximal to distal pattern (Warms, 2004).

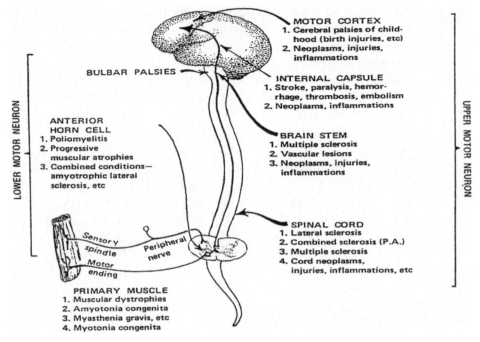

Figure 25.3. Motor pathways.

Reproduced with permission from Chusid, J. G. (1985). *Correlative neuroanatomy and functional neurology* (19th ed., p. 190). Los Altos, CA: Lange Medical.

D. Incidence and clinical manifestations
1. Affects both genders equally; 20–50 years of age; course of the disease variable
2. Onset develops 1–3 weeks after an infection, other stimuli; weakness of lower extremities occurring over hours to days, peaking about the 14th day (Warms, 2004)
3. Mildest form: flaccid weakness of lower limbs with little upper extremity involvement; improvement begins in 2–3 weeks with 85% recovering completely (Scheinberg, 1986)
4. More severe form: involves all four limbs, respiratory muscles, and bulbar muscles; regression of paralysis may take up to a year
5. Sympathetic, parasympathetic systems affected; respiratory muscle paralysis, abnormal vagal responses (bradycardia, heart block), hypertension due to autonomic dysfunction
6. Facial weakness, eye movement difficulties, dysphagia, and paresthesias of the face occur with bulbar involvement
7. 25% require ventilatory support; 10% mortality from respiratory failure or dysrhythmias
8. Pain common with paresthesias, muscle cramps, hyperesthesias; pain worse at night
E. Considerations across the life span
1. Pediatric: GBS is rare

2. Pregnancy: no literature on GBS in pregnancy
    3. Elderly: although rare it may occur in the elderly
  F. Complications and sequelae
    1. Respiratory failure due to respiratory muscle paralysis
    2. Immobility due to paralysis may cause paralytic ileus, DVT, pulmonary emboli, nutritional deficiencies, skin breakdown
II. Assessment
  A. History
    Include history of recent respiratory or gastrointestinal infections, trauma or immunizations; medications, functional health pattern.
  B. Physical
    General condition, cognitive ability; focused review of neurological (distal extremity weakness, paresthesias, hypesthesias), bulbar (dysphagia), respiratory (dyspnea, tachypnea), and musculoskeletal (muscle aches, cramps, weakness, paralysis) systems
  C. Diagnostic tests
    1. Diagnosis based on history and clinical signs; after 7–10 days, the CSF will show elevated protein (7 g/L, normal is 0.15–0.45 g/L); EMG and nerve conduction studies are markedly abnormal in the affected extremities indicating reduced nerve conduction velocity from demyelination (DeLisser, 2003; Warms, 2004).
III. Common therapeutic modalities therapy is supportive
  A. Supportive care
    1. Respiratory: monitor respiratory rate, tidal volume, vital capacity and negative inspiratory force to anticipate ventilatory support; continuous mechanical ventilation may be necessary; GBS tend to have normal lung function; ventilator settings aimed at preventing atelectasis, pneumonia; low risk of barotrauma, recommendations are for large tidal volumes (12–15 ml/kg IBW) and high inspiratory flows (ACCP, 1993).
    2. Swallowing and Nutrition: Poor nutritional status, especially if bulbar involvement, may necessitate evaluation of body weight, serum albumin levels, calorie counts, and total parenteral nutrition.
    3. Autonomic Dysfunction: Bradycardia from vagal stimulation, orthostatic hypotension due to muscle atony; monitor for dysrhythmias, hypotension.
    4. Pain: severity of pain from paresthesias may require analgesics.
    5. Mobility and ADL: PT initiated early to prevent hazards of immobility, maintain muscle tone. Adaptive devices, acute rehabilitation program to build up muscle strength and endurance.
  B. Pharmacologic interventions
    1. Plasmapheresis shortens course of disease; more effective when administered early within first 7 days of disease (DeLisser, 2003).
    2. Intravenous immunoglobulin (IVIG) reportedly effective (DeLisser, 2003; Warms, 2004).
    3. Corticosteroids have not shown to be beneficial and no longer have a role (DeLisser, 2003).

IV. Home care considerations
  A. Residual problems, relapses uncommon; complete recovery seen; plan for rehabilitation, home care services, insurance and disability coverage if slow recovery process.
  B. Rehabilitation, home care services focus on patient's specific functional limitations

Muscular Dystrophy

I. Overview Muscular Dystrophy (MD)
  ▪ Childhood neuromuscular disorder; a group of congenital disorders characterized by progressive muscle weakness. (Table 25.2)
  ▪ Duchenne Muscular Dystrophy (DMD) is the most common.
  A. Definition
    MD is a genetically determined disease of muscles associated with progressive weakness. Muscular Dystrophy subtypes
    1. Duchenne Muscular Dystrophy (DMD) affects proximal muscles first, associated with the most severe clinical symptoms (Darras, 2003).
    2. Limb Girdle Dystrophy (LGD) presents with slow progression of shoulder and pelvic girdle weakness.
    3. Myotonic Muscular Dystrophy (MMD) characterized by myotonia, cataracts, mental deficiency, testicular atrophy; facial muscles involved with absence of facial expression due to muscle weakness.
  B. Etiology
    Etiology unclear; thought to be genetic, possibly neurogenic or an enzyme abnormality (Scheinberg, 1986)
  C. Pathophysiology (Figure 25.3)
    Current theory: muscle membrane unable to maintain proper biochemical environment for cells; loss, destroyed muscle fibers and haphazard arrangement of fibers seen on muscle biopsy; skeletal muscle function deteriorates; DMD and MMD restrictive pulmonary syndrome occurs.
  D. Incidence and clinical manifestations
    1. MD individuals have relatively normal muscle function early in life.
    2. DMD: sex linked, genetic disorder; 1 in 3000 boys; Infants normal at birth; symptoms of gait; mobility problems seen at age 3; weakness of upper extremities appear late; mental retardation in half of children; DMD can be mild to severe with cardiomyopathy, restrictive lung disease (Melvin, Lacy, & Eyck, 1998).
    3. LGD: autosomal recessive disorder; progressive weakness of proximal arms and legs; age of onset varies; in later stages, diaphragmatic weakness common.
    4. MMD: autosomal dominant disorder; may be diagnosed in adulthood; myotonia; progressive wasting of facial, neck, and distal limb muscles; cardiac disease; mental retardation; cataracts; pharyngeal,

laryngeal, and respiratory muscle weakness (Brown, 1994; Scheinberg, 1986).

E. Considerations across the life span
   1. Pediatric: DMD presents in first 3–6 years of life, LGD late adolescence, MMD may not be diagnosed until adulthood (Scheinberg, 1986).
   2. Pregnancy: Babies of mothers with MMD may have hypotonia and floppiness with weak respiratory and sucking. In DMD, females are carriers in the X-linked disorder; genetic counseling is available (Brown, 1994).
   3. Elderly: Mortality in adolescence and young adulthood; older adult survivors are seen.

F. Complications and sequelae
   1. DMD
      a. Rapid course; loss of ability to ambulate around 9 years of age
      b. Respiratory insufficiency occurs in the second or third decade; respiratory failure a major cause of death (Hahn et al., 1997; Lyager, Steffenson, & Juhl, 1995).
      c. First sign of respiratory dysfunction is reduction in expiratory muscle strength, that is, decrease in vital capacity and maximum expiratory pressure (Hahn et al., 1997).
   2. LGD
      a. Recurrent respiratory infection, severe diaphragmatic weakness with chronic hypercapnea
      b. Expiratory muscles weak with a decrease in vital capacity (Gigliotti et al., 1995).
      c. Slow course
   3. MMD: ventilatory failure and cardiac dysfunction
   4. Considerable variability in severity of the dystrophies; death seen in adolescence and mid-20s, long-term survival seen in LGD (Brown, 1994)

II. Assessment
   A. History
      Include history of familial disorders of muscle weakness disorders, mental retardation, mobility ambulation, frequent pneumonias; medications, functional health pattern.
   B. Physical
      Focus on respiratory (pharyngeal, laryngeal muscle weakness; tachypnea, dyspnea), musculoskeletal (waddle gait, lumbar lordosis, Gower's sign [pushing up on thighs to stand]), and cardiac (tachycardia, conduction defects, EKG abnormalities) systems (Scheinberg, 1986).
   C. Diagnostic tests
      1. Lab tests: elevated CPK from dying muscle cells (Melvin et al., 1998).
      2. EMG and muscle biopsies: not type specific; do show distinct differences between myopathic versus neurogenic disease.

III. Common therapeutic modalities
   These disorders remain untreatable; management supportive.

A. Supportive care
  1. Respiratory
      a. Monitor respiratory status, VC, and anticipate respiratory supports.
      b. Inspiratory muscle training useful in early stages of DMD (Bach, 1996).
      c. Nocturnal respiratory failure occurs; nocturnal noninvasive ventilation options include: mouthpiece or nasal mask: CPAP, BiPAP, IPPV; rarely tracheostomy and oxygen (Barthlen, 1997).
      d. Pneumobelt and glossopharyngeal breathing also considered.
      e. Negative pressure ventilators (chest shells, pneumowrap) provide effective ventilation in older children without having to resort to tracheostomy (ACCP, 1998).
      f. Respiratory failure may progress to requiring continuous ventilatory support in some cases. (See ALS for description of ventilator information.)
  2. Mobility and ADL (see ALS); Lightweight ankle orthoses for plantar flexion; long leg braces for standing or walking (Darras, 2003)
B. Pharmacologic interventions
  1. Prednisone appears to improve strength and function with DMD; Oxandrolene, an anabolic steroid, has similar effects to prednisone but fewer side effects (Darras, 2003).
  2. Methylphenidate structurally related to amphetamine and a CNS stimulant; successfully used to combat excessive daytime sleepiness in MMD (Barthlen, 1997).
  3. Experimental gene therapies currently under evaluation (Darras, 2003).
IV. Home care considerations
  A. Rehabilitation focus: maintain muscle strength; increase functional ability, independence
  B. Schooling: combined placement; special education (Melvin et al., 1998)
  C. Support groups offer patient and family opportunity to grieve and learn coping mechanisms; family counseling, genetic counseling important

Myasthenia Gravis

I. Overview Myasthenia Gravis (MG)
  ▪ Chronic progressive disease of neuromuscular junction; distinguished by muscle weakness, fatigue (Table 25.2)
  ▪ Affects motor end plate at myoneural junction; term derived from Greek and Latin words for "grave weakness."
  ▪ The cardinal feature of the illness is fatigue as the muscle weakness increases (Allan, 2003).
  A. Definition
      Autoimmune neuromuscular disorder; weakness of voluntary muscles, proximal muscles more affected than distal; affinity for muscles innervated

by bulbar system: face, lips, eyes, tongue, throat, neck (Chusid, 1985; Rosebrough, 1998).

B. Etiology

Believed autoimmune system attacks acetylcholine receptors on the postsynaptic muscle membrane blocking the transmission of nerve impulses (Ross, 1999).

C. Pathophysiology (Figure 25.3)

At the neuromuscular junction receptor sites antibody-mediated autoimmune response occurs with destruction of postsynaptic sites; insufficient depolarization of the muscle results in weakness (Seybold, 1994).

D. Incidence and clinical manifestations

1. 5 cases per 100,000; any age, race, geographic site; familial cases rare (Seybold, 1994)

2. Young female adults and older males, 6:4 ratio (Rosebrough, 1998); age of onset: women 20–30 years old, men over age of 60-years-old (Allan, 2003)

3. Onset of symptoms gradual or sudden; progressive the first 5–7 years after onset of initial symptoms; characterized by remissions and exacerbations; severity of the muscle weakness varies; muscle weakness increases with activity and decreases with rest.

4. Thymus gland abnormalities seen in MG patients; 10% present with thymomas; increased incidence of autoimmune diseases such as lupus, rheumatoid arthritis, polymyositis, and thyroid disease (Seybold, 1994)

5. Factors precipitating myasthenic muscle weakness: infection, fever, temperature extremes, trauma, pregnancy, stress, and strenuous exercise (Ross, 1999; Rosebrough, 1998)

6. Classic manifestations: muscle weakness, fatigability, dysarthria, dysphagia, eye muscle weakness, ptosis, drooling, difficulty swallowing, choking, and blurred vision

7. Life-threatening "myasthenic crisis" when respiratory function impaired (Allan, 2003); muscles in neck and extremities affected; sensation, reflexes, and coordination remain intact.

E. Considerations across the life span

1. Pediatric: All ages from infant to elder; women more affected in the 0–30 age group (Ross, 1999; Scheinberg, 1986).

2. Pregnancy: Pregnancy ameliorates MG; effects of pregnancy unpredictable (Chusid, 1985). MG mothers may transmit a transient form of MG to their infant at birth, these symptoms subside within a few days (Seybold, 1994).

3. Elderly: The elderly male has higher incidence of MG.

F. Complications and sequelae

1. Respiratory failure and bulbar paralysis due to muscle weakness are complications.

2. Cholinergic crisis caused by excessive medication: increased muscle weakness, fasciculations around mouth, lips; diarrhea, cramping, sweating, drooling.

3. Myasthenic crisis caused by insufficient or ineffective medications: increased muscle weakness, anxiety, apprehension, respiratory difficulties; a neurologic emergency and must be differentiated from cholinergic crisis; myasthenic crisis with sudden death from respiratory failure may occur; survival of a crisis is followed by a remission (Ross, 1999).

4. Factors precipitating crisis: stress change in MG medication schedule, skipping medications, alcohol intake, inadequate sleep.

5. Pharmacologic sensitivities: quinine, succinlylcholine, and morphine increase weakness; aminoglycosides have a neuromuscular blocking influence; sedatives and narcotics administer with caution.

II. Assessment

A. History

Include history of muscle weakness that increases with activity and decreases with rest; dysphagia, visual difficulties, fatigue; medications, functional health pattern.

B. Physical

Focus on neurologic (ptosis, ocular muscle weakness, dysphagia, dysarthria), musculoskeletal (muscle weakness, fatigue, lack of endurance) and respiratory (tachypnea, dyspnea) systems (Seybold, 1994).

C. Diagnostic tests

1. Acetylcholine receptor antibody (AchR-ab) titers elevated in 90%. EMG: reduction of muscle potential and delay of neuromuscular transmission can identify specific muscle groups affected (Allan, 2003; Ross, 1999).

2. Anticholinesterase testing, using tensilon or neostigmine, indicative of neuromuscular junction dysfunction if, after administration of the medication, there is improvement in muscle strength (Allan, 2003; Ross, 1999; Seybold, 1994).

III. Common therapeutic modalities

No known cure. Treatment to prolong remissions.

A. Short-term treatment

1. Pharmacologic strategies: drugs to prolong life of acetylcholine at the motor-end plate provide temporary relief of symptom; cholinesterase inhibitors (neostigmine or pyridostigmine) used to prevent breakdown of acetylcholine; dosage varies with the patient's symptomatic response, sensitivity to the drug and side effects.

2. Mestinon (pyridostigmine): common anticholinesterase medication (onset of action 30 minutes, peaks in 2 hours, lasts 4 hours), given in divided doses 30–45 minutes before meals to assure ability to chew and swallow (Augustus, 2000); a long-acting form given at night used for bulbar or respiratory weakness at night or on awakening; identify optimum dosing to prevent weakness; side effects include abdominal cramping, diarrhea, bradycardia, blurred vision, muscle weakness, fatigue.

3. Taking doses close together inadvisable: it may initiate a cholinergic crisis from overdose; excessive anticholinesterase dosing can induce

muscle weakness by desensitizing receptor sites; treatment is withdrawal of medications for 24–48 hours, ventilatory support if needed.

4. Plasmapheresis treatment aimed at reducing the number of circulating antibodies found in the blood; useful in decreasing symptoms preoperatively, for short-term relief of symptoms and during acute respiratory crisis

5. Intravenous human immune globulin (IVIG) effective for acute disease; lasts for several weeks; has also been used to prevent myasthenic crisis (Rosebrough, 1998).

B. Long-term therapy

1. Immunosuppresive therapy: prednisone, azathioprine (Imuran), or cyclophasphamide (Cytoxan). Steroid therapy and Imuran frequently used; cytoxan reserved for cases refractory to other types of treatment because of its side effects (Augustus, 2000; Rosebrough, 1998).

2. Thymectomy performed in patients with thymoma; believed thymus gland influences immune modulation; thymectomy may or may not improve the MG; this surgery may be recommended in the absence of thymoma; younger patients with a recent onset (1–3 years) tend to have the best long-term results.

3. Long-term supportive care; prevention of infection, respiratory care, mobility adjuncts.

IV. Home care considerations

A. Spontaneous remissions occur frequently; relapse is the rule; spontaneous remissions lasting 1 year or longer in 20% of patients (Rosebrough, 1998); plan rehabilitation services, home care services, disability coverage, and health insurance.

B. The Myasthenia Gravis Foundation is a resource for patients and family.

SPINAL CORD INJURY

I. Overview Spinal Cord Injury (SCI)
- Injury to the spinal cord, generally result of direct trauma (Table 25.2).
- Injury mid-thoracic level or higher will have respiratory muscle weakness or paralysis.

A. Definition

SCI commonly a traumatic insult to the spinal cord (SC) that results in varying levels of motor, sensory, and autonomic dysfunction (National Spinal Cord Injury Statistical Center [NSCISC], 2003; Figure 25.4).

1. Tetraplegia (from the Greek *tettares,* meaning "four," and *plegia,* meaning "to strike"; formerly called *quadriplegia*)

a. Loss of motor and sensory function in cervical segments of SC causing impairment in all four extremities, the arm, trunk, legs, and pelvic organs.

b. "High tetraplegia" C2–C4 injury; profound injury, ventilator dependent, requires 24-hour caregiver

c. "Low tetraplegia" C5–C8 injury; ventilatory function impaired

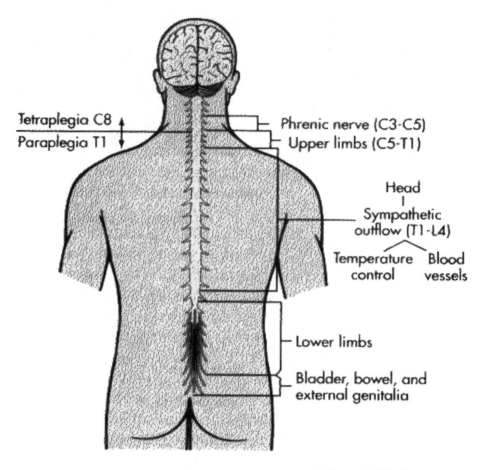

Figure 25.4. Symptoms, degree of paralysis, and potential for rehabilitation depend on the level of the lesion.

Reproduced with permission from Lewis, S. M., Heitkemper, M. M., & Dirksen, S. R. (2004). *Medical-surgical nursing* (6th ed., p. 1612). Boston: Mosby.

     2. Paraplegia (from the Greek, indicating lower limbs)
        a. Loss of motor, sensory function in thoracic, lumbar or sacral segments with impairment in trunk, legs, pelvic organs
        b. T12 to sacral vertebrae affected
  B. Etiology
    Traumatic SCI primarily caused by motor vehicle accidents (41%); acts of violence, especially gunshot wounds second largest cause, followed by falls, and recreational sports.
  C. Pathophysiology (Figure 25.3)
     1. Injury from spinal cord trauma results from lack of blood supply with resultant hypoxia; spinal cord rarely torn or transected since it is wrapped in tough dura layers.
     2. Spinal cord damage due to autodestruction of the cord; progressive tissue destruction occurs within hours with decreased perfusion, petechial hemorrhages in the gray matter, hematoma, edema, and

within 4 hours, infarction of the gray matter; release of biochemicals with ischemia, necrosis, and edema cause permanent damage within 24 hours (Warms, 2004).

3. Edema: primary cause of cord compression; end result is same as mechanically severing the cord; necrosis complete in 48 hours.

4. The injury to the spinal cord can be complete or incomplete.
   a. Complete injury results in loss of both motor and sensory function below the level of injury
   b. Incomplete injury has some spinal tracts intact; finding of any sensations is consistent with incomplete injury; types of incomplete injury include anterior cord syndrome (loss of anterior two-thirds of cord), central cord syndrome (damage to central cord fibers), Brown-Sequard Syndrome (hemi-cord damage), and posterior cord syndrome (posterior damage).

5. Spinal cord injury is identified as either upper motor neuron (UMN) or lower motor neuron (LMN) damage.
   a. UMN injury is seen in lesions above T12 segments with an intact motor reflex arc and spastic paralysis below the level of injury.
   b. LMN injury is seen in lesions below T12 with flaccidity and paralysis and loss of motor reflex arc at the level of injury.

D. Incidence and clinical manifestations

1. Incidence: 11,000 new cases annually; young adults (16–30 years old) more affected; 80% male; Black and Hispanic men at higher risk (NSCISC, 2003). Risk taking behaviors may affect the incidence of SCI.

2. Factors affecting survival rate include level of lesions, extent of paralysis, age, medical complications; psychological factors predictive of survival include alcohol abuse and poor self-care (DeVito, Krause, & Lammertse, 1999).

3. Life expectancy increased due to medical advances and prevention of complications. Prognosis for survival somewhat less than for persons of the same age without SCI (NSCISC, 2003).

4. Assessing impairment: American Spinal Injury Association (ASIA) Impairment Scale was developed to reflect severity of impairment after SCI.
   a. Level A: Complete—no sensory or motor function preserved
   b. Level B: Incomplete—sensory function preserved
   c. Level C: Incomplete—motor function preserved
   d. Level D: Incomplete—motor function preserved with muscle strength ≥ 3
   e. Level E: Normal—normal sensory and motor function

5. Functional outcomes, respiratory muscle strength by level of complete injury (Table 25.1)
   a. C2–C4 tetraplegia: High cervical cord injury with no strength in any limb, ventilator dependent with all respiratory muscles paralyzed.
   b. C5–C6 tetraplegia have some bicep function, can feed self with adaptive devices; C6 injury have intact wrist extension; diaphragm

and accessory muscles spared, intercostals, and abdominals impaired.

c. C7–C8 tetraplegics have some tricep muscle function; inspiratory intercostal muscles and expiratory abdominal muscles affected

d. T1–T12 thoracic paraplegics have modified independence with upper extremity function intact; intercostal or abdominal muscle impairment based on level of injury; low thoracic paraplegic have intact abdominals and intercostals, which improve cough and secretion clearance.

e. Lumbar paraplegics have upper extremity function and some strength in lower extremities with no respiratory muscle impairment.

6. Spinal shock occurs at time of trauma.

a. Reflex inhibition with the entire cord below the level of injury failing to function.

b. Resultant shock presents with hypotonia, hypotension, bradycardia, warm dry extremities, and immediate loss of motor and sensory activity and flaccid paralysis below the level of injury.

c. Spinal shock lasts generally 7–10 days but can last longer.

d. Spasticity, hyperreflexia, and reflex bladder emptying are indications the spinal shock has ended.

E. Considerations across the life span

1. Pediatric: All age groups; children unrestrained in motor vehicle accidents at great risk.

2. Pregnancy: Women with SCI at risk for autonomic dysreflexia during labor.

3. Elderly: Central cord syndrome is more common in older adults. This syndrome is frequently a result of hyperextension of an osteoarthritic spine.

F. Complications and sequelae

1. Autonomic dysreflexia

a. Life threatening complication of SCI at or above T6 level; uninhibited sympathetic response occurs from a noxious stimulus (Figure 25.5).

b. Neurological emergency; sympathetic hyper-response with vasoconstriction below the level of injury with inability of stimuli to travel past the injury.

c. Parasympathetic stimulation in compensatory manner above level of injury with vasodilation.

d. Unchecked, sudden paroxysmal hypertension, as high as 300/160, symptoms of severe pounding headache, bradycardia, sweating, flushing and distress occur. Death results from a stroke or cerebral hemorrhage.

e. Immediate intervention with removal of noxious stimuli, usually bladder distension, will resolve the problem, and the BP will return to normal limits.

When a spinal cord injury is at T8 or higher, an irritant below the level of injury can stimulate the autonomic nervous system to an exaggerated, dangerously unopposed response. Here, a full bladder triggers a sympathetic response (red line). The sympathetic response causes vasoconstriction, so the BP rises. The patient may also notice gooseflesh or pallor below the level of injury. The sympathetic response also constricts the bladder neck. However, the sympathetic response cannot cross the injured area of the cord to communicate with the parasympathetic system, so the BP continues to rise dangerously. Meanwhile, the baroreceptors in the carotids detect the rising BP and try to compensate by stimulating a parasympathetic response (blue line). The vagus nerve responds to the parasympathetic signals and slows the heart rate. Above the level of injury, the patient feels other parasympathetic effects: vasodilation, headache, flushing, sweating, and nasal congestion.

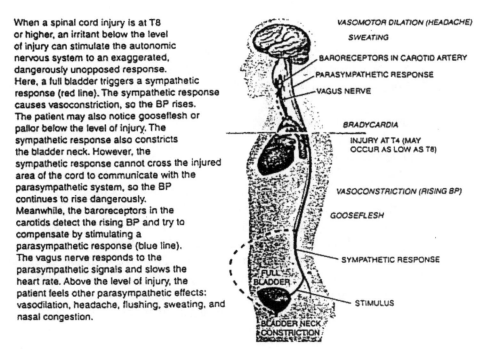

VASOMOTOR DILATION (HEADACHE)
SWEATING
BARORECEPTORS IN CAROTID ARTERY
PARASYMPATHETIC RESPONSE
VAGUS NERVE
BRADYCARDIA
INJURY AT T4 (MAY OCCUR AS LOW AS T8)
VASOCONSTRICTION (RISING BP)
GOOSEFLESH
SYMPATHETIC RESPONSE
FULL BLADDER
STIMULUS
BLADDER NECK CONSTRICTION

Figure 25.5. Autonomic dysreflexia.

Reproduced with permission from Rosebrough, A. (1998). Chronic neurological disorders. In P. A. Chin, D. N. Finocchiaro, & A. Rosebrough (Eds.), *Rehabilitation nursing practice* (pp. 278–307). New York: McGraw-Hill.

    f. If the stimulus can not be identified with immediate intervention, pharmacologic treatment of the hypertension is initiated (Consortium for Spinal Cord Medicine [CSCM], 2001).

2. Cause of death: pneumonia, pulmonary emboli, septicemia (NSCISC, 2003).
3. Orthostatic hypotension from poor vasomotor control, pooling of blood in the extremities.
4. Impaired temperature regulation with poikilothermia (inability to sweat or shiver above the injury).
5. Incidence of DVT 40%; DVT occurs due to venostasis from failure of the venous muscle pump with paralysis and a transient hypercoagulable state (CSCM, 1997).

II. Assessment
  A. History
    Include history of recent trauma, risk taking behavior, use of alcohol, drugs; medications, functional health pattern
  B. Physical
    General condition, cognitive ability and mental health; focused review of neurologic (weakness, paresthesias, paralysis, loss of sensation), respiratory (paradoxical movement, crackles, rhonchi, dyspnea, tachypnea), musculoskeletal (spasticity, muscle strength, cramping); bowel and bladder function.

C. Diagnostic tests
   1. A complete neurological assessment with motor and sensory function to identify neurological level of injury.
   2. X-rays: lateral, supine, and oblique spine; odontoid view if odontoid injury suspected; CT and MRI studies to identify vertebral level of injury.

III. Common therapeutic modalities
   Therapy is mainly supportive.
   A. Initial management
      1. The National Acute Spinal Cord Injury Study 3 (NASCIS III, 1997) found use of high dose methyprednisolone beneficial in acute SCI, if started within 3 hours of injury and continued over 24 hours (Bracken et al., 1998). Recent guidelines from Association of Neurological Surgeons (AANS) indicate the available medical evidence does not support a significant benefit from the administration of methylprednisolone in the treatment of patients after acute spinal cord injury for either 24- or 48-hours duration (American Association of Neurological Surgeons [AANS], 2002). These guidelines are controversial and medical institutions have to identify the specific protocol for their spine injured patients .
      2. Respiratory failure: Patients with SCI typically have normal ventilatory drive and normal lung function; paralyzed inspiratory muscles predisposed to atelectasis from inadequate lung inflation and pneumonia from impaired cough and airway clearance; the American College of Chest Physicians (ACCP) consensus statement recommend large tidal volumes (12–15 ml/kg) with or without PEEP in SCI patients to relieve dyspnea; high inspiratory flow rates (≥60 L/min) may also be required (American College of Chest Physicians [ACCP], 1993); type of ventilatory support, respiratory aids needed will depend on level of injury (see ALS for more information on ventilatory support and respiratory aids).
      3. Immobilization of the cord and surgical procedures to alleviate cord compression are used as immediate therapies (Buckley & Guanci, 1999).
   B. Supportive management
      1. Immobilization
         a. Spinal alignment is the most effective method of spinal cord decompression.
         b. Spinal traction with tong or halo apparatus are used in cervical injuries.
         c. Surgical management indicated for definitive stabilization of cervical injury.
         d. Orthotic devices from halo, sterno-occipito-mandibular-immobilizer orthosis (SOMI), cervical thoracic orthosis (CTO), and thoracolumbar-sacral orthosis (TLSO) may be utilized; these rigid stabilizers may displace the upper airway into slight extension with potential swallowing difficulties.

e. Chest vests sized correctly allow for thoracic expansion without difficulty.

2. Respiratory care
   a. Long-term ventilatory support
      i. Tracheostomy and continuous or nocturnal positive pressure mechanical ventilation necessary in high tetraplegia.
      ii. Phrenic nerve pacing may be an option if there is some intact LMN supply to the diaphragm, expense is significant with initial costs $300,000; maintenance of radio antenna, pacemaker battery changes, and backup ventilation required.
      iii. Non-invasive methods of ventilation for patients with high cord lesions have been used (ACCP, 1998).
      iv. Communication modalities: Passy-Muir valve, computer generated voicing using sip and puff devices, tracheostomy tube cuff leaks for speech.
      v. Weaning from ventilator a goal for patients if some respiratory muscles intact.
   b. Respiratory adjuncts include
      i. Glossopharyngeal breathing, as a backup in case of ventilator malfunction and to improve VC, cough (Bach, 1996)
      ii. Manually assisted cough for secretion clearance (Lucke, 1998; Bach, 1996)
      iii. Chest PT; inspiratory muscle training to improve strength, endurance
      iv. Abdominal binders in sitting position to elevate diaphragm, improve function (Lucke, 1998)
      v. Mechanical adjuncts for secretion clearance: Mechanical Insufflation-Exsufflator; Intrapulmonary Percussive Ventilation (Bach, 1996).

3. DVT prophylaxis
   a. Management includes intermittent pneumatic compression devices, thigh-high graded compression stockings, heparin, or low molecular weight heparin
   b. Vena cava filter placed in selected patients; quad coughing contraindicated in patients with filters since the quad technique can displace the filter.

4. Autonomic dysfunction
   a. In spinal shock, orthostatic hypotension occurs: manage by slowly elevating the patient's head, allowing the patient to "dangle" the legs before getting up, use thigh high compression stockings and abdominal binders to help diminish the BP drop; ephedrine may be indicated (Buckley & Guanci, 1999).
   b. Impaired temperature regulation can present with quad fevers; high temperatures (>104° F) with no consistent source; poikilothermia, body temperature affected by ambient temperature, is

managed by adjusting thermostats to appropriate temperature and using climate control systems.

    c. Autonomic dysreflexia (AD) with severe paroxysmal hypertension can occur in patients with lesions at T6 or above; immediate intervention; sit patient upright, check BP, loosen clothing, check for noxious stimuli causing the dysreflexia (usually bladder distension); topical nitrates, calcium channel blockers used to treat the hypertension; patient and family need to watch for this and be educated in the action plan to manage AD (CSCM, 2001).

5. Pressure ulcers and contractures from paralysis
    a. Skin care program, alternative bed surfaces, and wheelchair cushions
    b. PT to prevent muscle contractures with passive ROM
    c. Orthotic devices to maintain positioning of hands, elbows, knees, ankles
    d. Proper bed positioning; wheelchair use of armrests, leg straps, and footrests

6. Bowel and bladder management
    a. Bowel and bladder programs based on UMN/LMN lesion and patient's ability to do self-care
    b. Bowel regimes: include using the gastrocolic reflex, placing the patient on a commode after breakfast, rectal digital stimulation, rectal suppositories, pharmacologic agents, and enemas
    c. Bladder regimes: include foley/condom catheter, crede maneuver, intermittent catheterization program, timed voiding, bladder ultrasound program, and pharmacologic agents

7. Acute rehabilitation program
    a. SCI programs for acute rehabilitation focus on training the patient and family in self-care.
    b. The *Yes, You Can! A Guide to Self-Care for Persons with Spinal Cord Injury* (3rd ed.), published by the Paralyzed Veterans of America (PVA) is a training manual for patient/family education and is available for purchase at www.pva.org Web site.
    c. Interdisciplinary rehabilitation team composed of psychiatrist, rehabilitation nurses, PT, OT, ST, RRT, recreational therapist, psychologist, social worker and dietician; daily, weekly, long-term goals identified with length of stay.
    d. Community reentry, environmental modifications, wheelchair mobility, sexuality, and psychological issues are all part of the rehabilitation plan.

C. New research

Tremendous research in spinal cord injury aimed, in acute SCI, at interrupting the biochemical cascade of injury, while in chronic SCI, aimed at stimulating repair or regrowth of damaged neural elements (Lammertse, 1997); restorative and regenerative therapies show promise; therapies undergoing research/clinical trials.

1. Acute injury

   GM-1, a ganglioside, to influence motor recovery; 4-AP (aminopyridine), a potassium channel blocker, to improve conduction through the spinal cord (Buckley & Guanci, 1999). There is insufficient evidence to support its benefits clinically (AANS, 2002).

2. Chronic injury

   Schwann cell implantation into the injured spinal cord to promote axonal regeneration; fetal neuronal cell implants to promote axon growth; nerve growth factor (NGF) to produce regeneration of corticospinal neurons (Lammertse, 1997).

IV. Home care considerations

A. Environmental modifications

1. Home modifications for tetraplegics and paraplegics
   a. Wheelchair access, accessible heights of working surfaces, light switch accessibility, wide doorways.
   b. High tetraplegics with no upper extremity function require the most modifications; entrances and hallways wide enough to accommodate a large power wheelchair and possibly a portable ventilator.

2. Environmental Control Units (ECU) are technology-driven systems that access multiple electrical devices to allow for direction of many tasks such as opening doors, turning on lights and TVs; portable ECU mounts on power wheelchairs; integration of ECU into home computers is possible (Caves & Galvin, 2000).

3. Kitchen, bathroom and bedroom modifications undertaken after consultations with the patient/family, PT, OT, MD and vendors and contractors.

4. Ramps, door modifications and elevators or porch lifts considered during home evaluations done by PT, OT; recommendations made to offer optimum functioning with as much independence as possible.

B. Personal care services

1. Personal care needs and light household tasks: family or PCA (personal care attendant) trained by the family; PCA services reimbursed by Medicaid.

2. Address medical coverage, benefits, transportation and income supports early in discharge plan

3. Discuss family support, ability to care for the SCI person; often spouse or family member a permanent caregiver; respite care, PCA can help caregiver that is prone to emotional and physical distress.

SUMMARY

I. Neuromuscular disease and government support

A. U.S. Department of Health and Human Services (USDHHS)

1. Identified Healthy People paradigm as the prevention agenda for the nation.

2. Healthy People 2000 focused on national health promotion and disease prevention
3. The Healthy People 2010 (USDHHS, 2004) is "Healthy People in Healthy Communities"
4. Healthy People 2010 identifies preventable threats to health; public and private sectors address these threats; federal, state, community grants, private sector funding
5. Impacts neuromuscular diseases, respiratory disease, disability and secondary conditions

II. The future

The next 10 years will bring significant research into gene therapy and its impact on neuromuscular diseases as well as more supports for disabled individuals with these devastating diseases that have such significant disability and burden of care.

WEB SITES

Amyotrophic Lateral Sclerosis Newsletter: www.mdausa.org
Department of Health and Human Services gateway: www.healthfinder.gov
Healthy People 2010: www.healthypeople.gov
Multiple Sclerosis National Society: www.nmss.org
Muscular Dystrophy Association: www.mdausa.org
Myasthenia Gravis Information: www.mdausa.org/disease/mg
National Institute of Neurological Disorders and Stroke: www.ninds.nih.gov
National Spinal Cord Injury Association: www.spinalcord.org
New England MS Society Chapter: www.msnewengland.org
Paralyzed Veterans Association: www.pva.org
Spinal Cord Cure Information: www.cureparalysis.org
Spinal Cord Injury Information: www.spinalcord.uab.edu

REFERENCES

Adams, R. D., & Salam-Adams, M. (1991). Chronic nontraumatic diseases of the spinal cord. *Neurologic Clinics, 9,* 748–778.

Allan, W. (2003). Clinical manifestation and diagnosis of myasthenia gravis. *UpToDate, 12*(1). Retrieved March 1, 2004, from www.uptodate.com

American Association of Neurological Surgeons. (2002). Guidelines for the management of acute cervical spine and spinal cord injuries. *Neurosurgery, 50*(3 Suppl), S1–S180.

American Association of Respiratory Care. (1993). AARC Clinical practice Guideline: Directed cough. *Respiratory Care, 38,* 495–499.

American College of Chest Physicians. (1993). Mechanical Ventilation. *Chest, 104,* 1833–1859.

American College of Chest Physicians. (1998, May). Mechanical ventilation beyond the intensive care unit. *Chest, 113* (Suppl).

Augustus, L. (2000). Crisis: Myasthenia Gravis. *American Journal of Nursing, 100,* 24AA–24HH.

Bach, J. R. (1994). Update and perspective on noninvasive respiratory muscle aids. Part 2: The expiratory aids. *Chest, 105,* 1538–1544.

Bach, J. R. (1996). Prevention of morbidity and mortality with the use of physical medicine aids. In Bach J. R. (Ed.), *Pulmonary rehabilitation* (pp. 303–329). Philadelphia: Hanley & Belfus.

Barthlen, M. (1997). Nocturnal respiratory failure as an indication of noninvasive ventilation in the patient with neuromuscular disease. *Respiration, 164*(Suppl 1), 35–38.

Bracken, M. B., Shepard, M. J., Holford, T. R., Leo-Summers, L., Aldrich, E. F., Fazl, L., et al. (1998). Methylprednisolone or tirilazad mesylate administration after acute spinal cord injury: 1-year follow up. Results of the third National Acute Spinal Cord Injury randomized controlled trial. *Journal of Neurosurgery, 89,* 699–706.

Branson, R. D., Hess, D. R., & Chatburn, R. L. (1999). *Respiratory care equipment* (2nd ed.). New York: Lippicott Williams & Wilkins.

Brown, R. H. (1994). Muscle disease. In J. H. Stein (Ed.), *Internal medicine* (4th ed., pp. 1108–1115). Boston: Mosby-Year Book.

Brown, R. H. (2004). Chapter 365: Amyotrophic lateral sclerosis and other motor neuron diseases. Retrieved March 1, 2004, from www.harrisonsonline.com

Buckley, D., & Guanci, M. M. (1999). Spinal cord trauma. *Nursing Clinics of North America, 34,* 661–687.

Caves, K., & Galvin, J. C. (2000). Computer assistive devices and environmental controls. In R. L. Braddom (Ed.), *Physical medicine and rehabilitation* (2nd ed., pp. 488–497). New York: W. B. Saunders.

Chusid, J. G. (1985). *Correlative neuroanatomy and functional neurology* (19th ed.). Los Altos, CA: Lange Medical.

Consortium for Spinal Cord Medicine. (1997). *Clinical practice guidelines: Acute management of autonomic dysreflexia.* Washington: Paralyzed Veterans of America.

Consortium for Spinal Cord Medicine. (2001). *Clinical practice guidelines: Prevention of thromboembolism in spinal cord injury.* Washington, DC: Paralyzed Veterans of America.

Darras, B. T. (2003). Duchenne and Becker muscular dystrophies. *UpToDate, V12.1.* Retrieved March 1, 2004, from www.uptodate.com

DeLisser, H. M. (2003). Guillain-Barre syndrome. *UpToDate, V12.1.* Retrieved March 1, 2004, from www.uptodate.com

DeVito, M. J., Krause, J. S., & Lammertse, D. P. (1999). Recent trends in mortality and causes of death among persons with spinal cord injury. *Archives of Physical Medicine and Rehabilitation, 80,* 1411–1418.

Emick-Herring, B. (Ed.). (1993). Normal motor control and neurophysiological approaches. In A. E. McCourt (Ed.), *The specialty practice of rehabilitation nursing: A core curriculum* (3rd ed., p. 31). Skokie, IL: Rehabilitation Nursing Foundation.

Ferguson, K. A., Strong, M. J., Ahmad, D., & George, C. F. P. (1996). Sleep-disordered breathing in amyotrophic lateral sclerosis. *Chest, 110,* 664–669.

Francis, K., Bach, J. R., & DeLisa, J. A. (1999). Evaluation and rehabilitation of patients with adult motor neuron disease. *Archives of Physical Medicine and Rehabilitation, 80,* 951–963.

Gigliotti, F., Pizzi, A., Durante, R., Gorini, M., Fandelli, I., & Scano, G. (1995). Control of breathing in patients with limb girdle dystrophy: A controlled study. *Thorax, 50,* 962–968.

Goldberg, A. (1999). Clinical indications for noninvasive positive pressure ventilation in chronic respiratory failure due to restrictive lung disease, COPD, and nocturnal hypoventilation: A consensus conference report. *Chest, 116,* 521–534.

Hahn, A., Bach, J. R., Delaubier, A., Renardel-Irani, A., Guillou, C., & Rideau, Y. (1997). Clinical implications of maximal respiratory pressure determinations for individuals with Duchenne muscular dystrophy. *Archives of Physical Medicine and Rehabilitation, 78,* 1–5.

Lammertse, D. P. (1997). Recovery of neurologic function in spinal cord injury: A review of new and experimental therapies. *Topics in Spinal Cord Injury Rehabilitation, 2,* 95–100.

Levitzky, M. G. (1995). *Pulmonary physiology* (4th ed.). New York: McGraw-Hill.

Logigian, E. L. (1994). Demyelinating diseases. In J. H. Stein (Ed.), *Internal medicine* (4th ed., pp. 1095–1104). Boston: Mosby-Year Book.

Lewis, S. M., Heitkemper, M. M., & Dirksen, S. R. (2004). *Medical-surgical nursing* (6th ed., p. 1612). Boston: Mosby.

Lisak, D. (2001). Overview of symptomatic management of multiple sclerosis. *Journal of Neuroscience Nursing, 33,* 224–230.

Lucke, K. T. (1998). Pulmonary management following acute SCI. *Journal of Neuroscience Nursing, 30,* 91–104.

Lyager, S. Steffenson, B., & Juhl, B. (1995). Indication of need for mechanical ventilation in Duchenne muscular dystrophy and spinal muscular atrophy. *Chest, 108,* 779–85.

MacDonnell, K. F., & Segal, M. S. (Eds.). (1977). *Current respiratory care.* Boston: Little Brown.

Melvin, C. L., Lacy, M. L., & Eyck, L. E. S. (1998). Pediatric rehabilitation. In P. A. Chin, D. N. Finocchiaro, & A. Rosebrough (Eds.). *Rehabilitation nursing practice* (pp. 443–473). New York: McGraw Hill.

Multiple Sclerosis Council for Clinical Practice Guidelines. (1998). *Fatigue and multiple sclerosis.* Washington, DC: Paralyzed Veterans of America.

Multiple Sclerosis Council for Clinical Practice Guidelines. (2001). *Disease modifying therapies in multiple sclerosis.* Washington, DC: Paralyzed Veterans of America.

National Spinal Cord Injury Statistical Center. (2003). *Spinal cord injury falls and figures at a glance.* Washington, DC: National Institution on Disability and Rehabilitation Research. Retrieved March 12, 2004, from www.spinalcord.uab.edu

Olek, M. J. (2004). Treatment of multiple sclerosis. *UpToDate, V12.1.* Retrieved March 1, 2004, from www.uptodate.com

Ozuna, J. M. (2004). Chronic neurologic problems. In S. M. Lewis, M. M. Heitkemper, & S. R. Dirksen (Eds.), *Medical-surgical nursing* (6th ed., pp. 1549–1580). Boston: Mosby.

Rosebrough, A. (1998). Chronic neurological disorders. In P. A. Chin, D. N. Finocchiaro, & A. Rosebrough (Eds.), *Rehabilitation nursing practice* (pp. 443–473). New York: McGraw Hill.

Ross, A. P. (1999). Neurologic degenerative disorders. *Nursing Clinics of North America, 34,* 725–742.

Scheinberg, P. (1986). *An introduction to diagnosis and management of common neurologic disorders.* New York: Raven Press.

Schmitt, J., Midha, M., & McKenzie, N. (1991). Medical complications of spinal cord disease. *Neurologic Clinics, 9,* 779–795.

Seybold, M. E. (1994). Diseases of the neuromuscular junction. In J. H. Stein (Ed.), *Internal medicine* (4th ed., pp. 1104–1108). Boston: Mosby-Year Book.

Sherman, M. S., & Paz, H. L. (1994). Review of respiratory care of the patient with amyotrophic lateral sclerosis. *Respiration, 61,* 61–67.

Taylor, P. A. (1999). Diagnosis multiple sclerosis. *Clinician Reviews, 9,* 72.

Thompson, C., & Swash, M. (2001). Amyotrophic lateral sclerosis: Current understanding. *Journal of Neuroscience Nursing, 33,* 245–253.

U.S. Department of Health and Human Services (USDHHS). (2004). Healthy people 2010: Publications: Healthy people in healthy communities. Washington, DC. Retrieved March 12, 2004, from www.healthypeople.gov

Warms, C. (2004). Peripheral nerve and spinal cord problems. In S. M. Lewis, M. M. Heitkemper, & S. R. Dirksen. *Medical-surgical nursing* (6th ed., pp. 1610–1631). Boston: Mosby.

SUGGESTED READINGS

Dawson, D. M. (1994). Demyelinating diseases. In J. H. Stein (Ed.), *Internal medicine* (4th ed., pp. 1087–1091). Boston: Mosby-Year Book.

Finocchiaro, D., & Herzfeld, S. (1998). Neurological deficits associated with spinal cord injury. In P. A. Chin, D. N. Finocchiaro, & A. Rosebrough (Eds.), *Rehabilitation nursing practice* (pp. 278–307). New York: McGraw Hill.

Gilman, S., & Newman, S. W. (1992). *Manter and Gatz's essentials of clinical neuroanatomy and neurophysiology* (8th ed.). Philadelphia: F. A. Davis.

Respiratory Failure

Irene Grossbach

INTRODUCTION

1. Hypoxemia may be due to the following mechanisms: inadequate alveolar ventilation, ventilation-perfusion (V/Q) mismatch, intrapulmonary shunt (right to left shunt), low inspired oxygen concentration, impaired alveolar diffusion, and increased tissue oxygen consumption.
2. Hypercapnia is due to ventilatory or "pump" failure and can be categorized into disorders of the central nervous system, peripheral nervous system, respiratory muscles, chest wall, pleura, upper airways, lower airways, and lung parenchyma.
3. Arterial blood gases may initially be normal or acceptable at the expense of significant increased work of breathing and stress on the cardiopulmonary system. Blood gases will deteriorate with potential cardiopulmonary arrest if there is inadequate or inappropriate management.
4. Individuals with chronic hypercapnic respiratory failure present with increased $PaCO_2$, increased HCO_3, and normalized pH. Examples include COPD, obesity-hypoventilation syndrome. They may be alert and oriented despite severe carbon dioxide retention ($PaCO_2$ greater than 100 mm Hg).
5. Assessments for respiratory failure include observations for signs and symptoms of hypoxemia, hypercapnia, and increased work of breathing. Various drugs and clinical conditions may blunt the normal responses to hypoxemia and hypercapnia.

I. Overview
Acute respiratory failure (ARF) is a common clinical problem that may be caused by multiple disease processes and affects all age groups. Successful management includes recognition/anticipation and prevention of problems

contributing to ARF, making accurate clinical assessments and interpretations, and performing appropriate interventions.

A. Definitions

1. Respiratory failure is an inability to maintain adequate gas exchange.

2. Acute respiratory insufficiency occurs when gas exchange is maintained at an acceptable level only at the expense of significantly increased work on the cardiopulmonary system.

3. Dysfunction in the processes necessary to sustain cell energy production including

   a. ventilation: air movement between lungs and environment

   b. intrapulmonary gas exchange: process where mixed venous blood releases carbon dioxide and becomes oxygenated

   c. gas transport: delivery of adequate quantities of oxygenated blood to metabolizing tissues and carbon dioxide back to lungs

   d. tissue gas exchange: use of oxygen and release of CO_2 by peripheral tissues (Marini & Wright, 1998, p. 919)

4. May be classified into hypoxemic and hypercapnic respiratory failure

5. Hypoxemic respiratory failure

   a. Commonly present with abnormally low PaO_2 and low $PaCO_2$ unless there is also cause for hypercapnic failure.

   b. Primary defect is failure to oxygenate due to lung pathology causing inadequate alveolar gas exchange or inadequate exchange between alveolar gas and pulmonary blood.

   c. Low $PaCO_2$ due to hyperventilation is an attempt to increase the PaO_2.

6. Hypercapnic respiratory failure

   a. Also referred to as *pump failure* or *ventilatory failure*

   b. Impaired alveolar ventilation causing elevation in $PaCO_2$ with relative preservation of PaO_2

7. Acute respiratory failure includes presence of two of the following four factors

   a. acute dyspnea

   b. PaO_2 less than 50 mm Hg while breathing room air

   c. $PaCO_2$ greater than 50 mm Hg.

   d. pH compatible with significant acidosis

   e. Presence of altered mental status plus one or more of above criteria (Hoozen & Albertson, 1998)

8. Respiratory failure may be either acute or chronic process. Chronic ventilatory failure occurs in patients with baseline acid-base derangements (COPD, restrictive lung disease) with hypercapnia (chronic elevation of PCO_2), SpO_2 90% and clinically stable.

9. Many chronically hypercapnic individuals exhibit few or no clinical symptoms to suggest acute respiratory failure because of gradual adaptations to hypercapnia and hypoxemia. Supplemental oxygen to correct hypoxemia ($SaO_2 > 90\%$) and various aggressive interventions to improve ventilation (bronchodilators, steroids, airway clearance

techniques, noninvasive ventilation support, etc.) frequently prevents need for intubation and mechanical ventilation support (American Thoracic Society, 1995; Pauwels, Buist, Calverley, Jenkins, & Hurd, 2001).

II. Pathophysiology/etiology of hypoxemic respiratory failure
  A. Mechanisms contributing to arterial oxygen desaturation are
    1. ventilation-perfusion mismatch
    2. alveolar hypoventilation
    3. intrapulmonary shunting
    4. low inspired oxygen concentration
    5. impaired alveolar diffusion
    6. increased tissue oxygen consumption.
  B. Ventilation-perfusion (V/Q) mismatch: abnormal matching of ventilated areas to perfused areas in the lung. Lung units are poorly ventilated in relation to perfusion; high V/Q units contribute to physiologic dead space but not to hypoxemia.
    1. V/Q mismatch is the most common cause of oxygen desaturation and reversed with supplemental oxygen
    2. Examples include secretions, bronchospasm
  C. Alveolar hypoventilation: lung parencyhma normal; hypoxemia due to elevated carbon dioxide, causing displacement of oxygen.
    1. PaO_2 varies inversely with $PaCO_2$. Increased $PaCO_2$ results in a proportional fall in PaO_2 unless patient is given oxygen therapy. For example, acute rise in $PaCO_2$ from 40 to 70 mm Hg results in proportional fall in PaO_2 from 90 to 52 mm Hg assuming normal A-a (alveolar-arterial) partial pressure gradient for oxygen of 10 mm Hg.
    2. In primary hypoventilation, the $PaCO_2$ and PaO_2 add up to 110–130 Hg on room air. Hypoxemia is due to V/Q mismatch, shunt or diffusion impairments if the sum is less than 110 on room air (Hoozen & Albertson, 1998).
    3. Examples include drug overdose, neuromuscular disease
    4. Treatment focuses on improving ventilation
  D. Intrapulmonary shunting (Qs/Qt) or right to left shunt refers to pulmonary blood flow that does not come in contact with functioning alveoli or is shunted (Qs) in comparison with total blood flow (Qt).
    1. Involved alveolar units are perfused but not ventilated.
    2. Systemic venous blood (deoxygenated blood) passes from right to left side of heart without going through pulmonary capillaries to pick up oxygen. Shunted or deoxygenated blood enters arterial circulation and mixes with oxygenated blood.
    3. Hallmark of shunting-oxygen therapy does not improve hypoxemia; PaO_2 progressively worsens with fewer functioning air sacs.
    4. Most common cause of shunting is atelectasis due to collapsed or fluid-filled alveoli. Other conditions include
      a. pneumonia
      b. acute respiratory distress syndrome (ARDS)

   c. pulmonary embolism
   d. pulmonary edema from left ventricular failure
   e. mitral stenosis
   f. arteriovenous malformations (AVMs) intracardiac right-to-left shunts
5. Hypoxemia associated with V-Q disturbance, hypoventilation and diffusion problems can usually be corrected with supplemental oxygen. 100% oxygen does not correct hypoxemia associated with right-to-left shunt problems >30% (Hoozen & Albertson, 1998).
6. Bedside assessment of oxygen exchange efficiency
   a. Many methods have been devised; no methods completely reliable.
   b. One simple method: PaO_2/FIO_2 ratio: normal = 350 mm Hg; levels as low as 286 clinically acceptable. The lower the PaO_2/FIO_2 number, the more severe the shunt disturbance (Ahrens & Rutherford, 1993).
   c. Value in estimating shunt: helps identify changes and analyze trends in lung function, reveals extent of pulmonary dysfunction induced by clinical condition
   d. $PaO_2/FIO_2 < 200$ = shunt >20% (Marino, 2000)
   e. Affected by changes in SvO_2, not equally sensitive across entire FIO_2 range (Marini & Wheeler, 1997)
E. Low inspired oxygen fraction (FiO_2) due to reduced oxygen concentration provided to patient or higher altitudes (>10,000 feet) reduces barometric pressure; examples: toxic fume inhalation, fires that consume oxygen in combustion
F. Impaired alveolar diffusion: any process that thickens lining separating the alveolus and capillary lumen (interstitial edema, pulmonary fibrosis) or shortened time of red blood cell transit through capillaries (high cardiac output)
G. Increased tissue oxygen consumption: conditions resulting in abnormally high metabolic demands for oxygen relative to oxygen delivery
   1. cardiogenic shock: increase in energy demand (stiff lungs, hyperventilation) and a decrease in supply of blood to respiratory muscles causing muscles to fail with resulting alveolar hypoventilation and respiratory arrest
   2. septic shock
   3. pancreatitis
   4. severe burns
   5. salicylate overdose
   6. cyanide poisoning.
III. Pathophysiology/etiology of hypercapnic respiratory failure
   A. Three major disorders responsible for ventilatory muscle failure
      1. Inadequate ventilatory drive
         a. drug overdose
         b. morbid obesity causing obesity-hypoventilation
         c. sleep apnea
         d. brainstem lesions

      e. sleep deprivation

      f. hypothyroidism

      g. metabolic alkalosis

  2. Ventilatory muscle dysfunction causing neuromuscular weakness, fatigue, failure

      a. neuromuscular diseases: Guillain-Barré Syndrome, Amytrophic Lateral Sclerosis, Myasthenia Gravis, Muscular Dystrophy

      b. critical illness polyneuropathy

      c. phrenic nerve palsy due to thoracic surgery or tumors

      d. infections (botulism, tetanus, poliomyelitis)

      e. diaphragm paralysis drug toxicity (paralytic agents, aminogylcosides)

      f. malnutrition

      g. electrolyte imbalances and mineral deficiencies (hypophosphatemia, hypokalemia, hypomagnesemia, hypocalcemia)

  3. Increased work of breathing due to excessive ventilatory loads

      a. increased airway resistance due to secretions, bronchospasm, tumor, vocal cord paralysis, or other airway obstruction problems

      b. decreased lung compliance due to pneumothorax, pulmonary edema, pleural effusions, obesity, thoracic abnormalities, such as rib fractures and kyphoscoliosis

      c. decreased efficiency of inspiratory muscles due to lung hyperinflation (auto-PEEP or intrinsic PEEP)

      d. hypermetabolic states, which increase carbon dioxide production and minute ventilation requirements

B. Combined hypoxemia and hypercapnic respiratory failure are present in many clinical situations.

  1. Patient with COPD and concurrent respiratory infection may exhibit hypercapnia and hypoxemia due to secretions, bronchospasm, air-trapping or auto-PEEP, rapid shallow breathing.

  2. Patient with neuromuscular disease may have pneumonia or atelectasis due to impaired cough, which results in hypoxemia superimposed on primary hypercapnia.

C. Chronic hypercapnic respiratory failure

  1. Clinical presentation: increased $PaCO_2$, increased HCO_3, normalized pH.

  2. Examples: COPD, obesity-hypoventilation syndrome, neuromuscular diseases.

  3. Chronic and acute hypercapnic respiratory failure can be differentiated by severity of change in pH.

      a. Acute failure: pH drops 0.08 for every 10 mm Hg rise in $PaCO_2$

      b. Chronic failure: pH drops 0.03 for every 10 mm Hg rise in $PaCO_2$ (Christie & Goldstein, 1999)

  4. Carbon dioxide retention develops over weeks to months allowing body to develop compensatory mechanisms including renal response by which kidneys retain bicarbonate to normalize pH. Compensatory metabolic alkalosis is not expected to restore pH to normal.

5. Chronic hypoxemia causes increase in red blood cell mass (polycythemia) to improve tissue oxygen delivery.

6. Patient normally alert, oriented despite high $PaCO_2$ levels. Carbon dioxide narcosis is not present due to gradual increase in carbon dioxide retention.

IV. Clinical assessment

    A. Signs and symptoms of hypoxemia, hypercapnia

        1. Respiratory: dyspnea, increased respiratory rate.

        2. Central nervous system: change in mental status or behavior (e.g., anxiety, restlessness, confusion, irritability, inability to concentrate, loss of judgment, paranoia); picky, combative (e.g., pulls at tubes); signs of CO_2 retention include: lethargy, drowsiness, confusion, coma, muscle tremor/twitching.

        3. Cardiovascular: tachycardia, hypertension, hypotension, redness of skin, sclera and conjunctiva, sweating, arrhythmias, cardiac arrest. Hypoxemia causes pulmonary hypertension, polycythemia, right heart failure.

    B. Signs and symptoms of increased work of breathing

        1. increased respiratory rate, dyspnea, forced abdominal muscle contraction, neck accessory muscle use, discoordination of chest and abdominal muscles

        2. "usual" signs will not present if there are conditions or problems of neuromuscular weakness, paralysis, decreased muscle strength

    C. Clinical criteria for stability/acute care

        1. Stability: normal blood gases, vital signs, work of breathing signs/symptoms normalized, patients normal mental status, behavior

        2. Acute care criteria: pH < 7.35, $PaCO_2$ > patient's normal level, PaO_2 <55–60 mm Hg, increased work of breathing signs, symptoms (increased respiratory rate, dyspnea, forced abdominal muscle contractions on expiration, neck accessory muscle use), unusual anxiety, restlessness, confusion, lethargy, other mental status and behavior changes; diaphoresis, unusual changes in vital signs

        3. Example of ICU admission criteria for COPD exacerbation

           a. Severe dyspnea that responds inadequately to initial emergency therapy

           b. Confusion, lethargy, coma

           c. Persistent or worsening hypoxemia (PaO_2 50 mm Hg), or severe/worsening hypercapnia ($PaCO_2$ 70 mm Hg), or severe/worsening respiratory acidosis (pH < 7.30) despite oxygen therapy

           d. Requires assisted mechanical ventilation (noninvasive techniques or intubation; Pauwels et al., 2001)

    D. Effects of drugs; clinical status on signs symptoms of hypoxemia, hypercapnia

        1. May blunt the normal response to hypoxemia, hypercapnia, therefore, patient does not exhibit usual signs, symptoms.

        2. Examples include narcotics, anesthetics, various cardiac medications that lower heart rate, blood pressure, starvation.

E. Pulse oximeter monitoring
   1. Measures oxygen saturation of hemoglobin (SpO_2).
   2. General goals: maintain SpO_2 90% or greater.
   3. SpO_2 has no direct relationship to adequate ventilation. Patients on oxygen concentrations can maintain normal SpO_2 readings despite severe hypercapnia, acute respiratory acidosis.
   4. SpO_2 readings may be normal in presence of hypotension, inadequate cardiac output or anemia.
F. Respiratory muscle fatigue, respiratory pump failure
   1. Definitions
      a. Work of breathing: energy expenditure or work required to accomplish muscle contraction and quantified in terms of oxygen utilization. Oxygen utilization of respiratory muscles at rest is approximately 2.5% of total body oxygen consumption. Increased work of breathing can significantly increase oxygen consumption.
      b. Respiratory muscle fatigue: inability of muscles to continue generating required force to sustain adequate ventilation; energy demand greater than supply; eventually $PaCO_2$ increases, exhaustive exercise can cause muscle fiber damage.
      c. Clinical example: COPD patient exhibits increased work of breathing due to various factors: increased airway resistance (secretions, bronchospasm), decreased mechanical efficiency (chest hyperinflation, air-trapping, obesity), decreased lung compliance due to infiltrate, pneumonia, muscle weakness due to hyperinflation and/or atrophy and undernutrition. Respiratory muscles are pushed to limits causing hypoventilation, respiratory muscle fatigue.
   2. Clinical signs of respiratory muscle fatigue (in sequence)
      a. Tachypnea, dyspnea
      b. Abdominal paradox
      c. Respiratory alternans
      d. Hypercapnia
      e. Bradypnea
      f. Central apnea
      g. There is a late reduction of respiratory rate, minute ventilation with progressive academia and respiratory rate may be "normal" despite severe acute respiratory acidosis (Cohen, Zagelbaum, Gross, & Macklem, 1982). (Figure 26.1)
      h. Respiratory rate may remain within normal limits during deterioration of respiratory status.
G. Dyspnea (Refer to chapter 10 "Dyspnea")
V. Common therapeutic modalities
   A. Provide emergency airway management as needed to maintain adequate oxygenation and ventilation status.
   B. Manage underlying clinical condition(s) that increase work of breathing, cause hypoxemia and acute carbon dioxide retention.

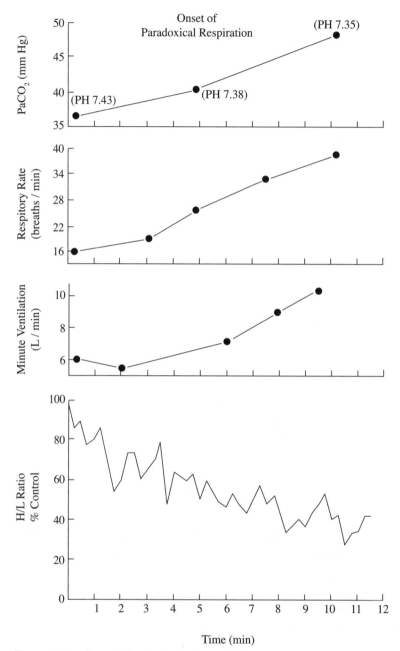

Figure 26.1. Onset of paradoxical respiration.

C. Provide noninvasive positive pressure ventilation support: successfully used in the management of acute respiratory failure.

D. Intubation and mechanical ventilation may be required for patients with impending ARF, those with life-threatening acid-base problems, altered mental status despite aggressive therapies

VI. Home care considerations
   A. Identify various factors or problems contributing to acute respiratory insufficiency/failure
      1. Quality post acute care requires effective discharge planning of multi-disciplinary team.
      2. Patients at risk: deconditioned, elderly, chronic respiratory diseases, immobile, immunocompromised, early postoperative.
      3. Self care abilities and need for assistance with consideration of abilities of caregivers at home or alternative health care settings.
      4. Deficiencies in education including preventive measures, early recognition, management.
   B. Implement appropriate patient/family education. Refer patient/family to home care or alternative care setting.
   C. Refer to chapter 36 "Mechanical Ventilation."

WEB SITES

Pubmed Medline: http://www4.ncbi.nlm.nih.gov/PubMed/clinical.html
www.uptodate.com
www.thoracic.org

REFERENCES

Ahrens, T., & Rutherford, K. (1993). *Essentials of oxygenation-implications for clinical practice.* Boston: Jones and Bartlett Publishers.

American Thoracic Society. (1995). Standards for the diagnosis and care of patients with chronic obstructive pulmonary disease. *American Journal of Respiratory and Critical Care Medicine, 152*(Suppl), 77–120.

Christie, H. A., & Goldstein, L. S. (1999). Respiratory failure and the need for ventilatory support. In R. S. Irwin, F. B. Cerra & J. M. Rippe (Eds.), *Intensive care medicine* (4th ed., pp. 819–831). Philadelphia: Lippincott-Raven.

Cohen, C., Zagelbaum, G., Gross, D., & Macklem, P. T. (1982). Clinical manifestations of inspiratory muscle fatigue. *American Journal of Medicine, 73,* 308–316.

Hoozen, B. V., & Albertson, T. E. (1998). Acute respiratory failure. In J. E. Hodgkin & J. J. Ward (Eds.), *Respiratory care-a guide to clinical practice* (4th ed., pp. 1107–1132). Philadelphia: Lippincott-Raven.

Marini, J. J., & Wheeler, A. P. (1997). *Critical care medicine: The essentials* (2nd ed). Baltimore: Williams & Wilkins.

Marini, J. J., & Wright, L. A. (1998). Acute respiratory failure. In G. L. Baum, J. D. Crapo, B. R. Celli, & J. B. Karlinsky (Eds.), *Textbook of pulmonary diseases* (6th ed., pp. 919–939). Philadelphia: Lippincott-Raven Publishers.

Marino, P. L. (2000). *The ICU book* (2nd ed.). Baltimore: Williams & Wilkins.

Pauwels, R. A., Buist, A. S., Calverley, P. M. A., Jenkins, C. R., & Hurd, S. S. (2001). Global strategy for the diagnosis, management, and prevention of chronic obstructive pulmonary disease. *American Journal of Respiratory and Critical Care Medicine, 163*, 1256–1276.

SUGGESTED READINGS

Matthay, M. A., & Atabai, K. (2000). Acute hypercapnic respiratory failure: neuromuscular and obstructive diseases. In R. B. Goerge, R. W. Light, M. A. Matthay, & R. A. Matthay (Eds.), *Chest medicine: essentials of pulmonary and critical care medicine* (4th ed., pp. 561–575). Philadelphia: Lippincott Williams & Wilkins.

Roussos, C. R. (1990). Respiratory muscle fatigue and ventilatory failure. *Chest, 97*(Suppl), 89–96.

Roussos, C., & Zakynthinos, S. (1996). Fatigue of the respiratory muscles. *Intensive Care Medicine, 22*, 134–155.

Sharpiro, B. A., Harrison, R. A., Kacmarek, R. M., & Cane, R. D. (1990). *Clinical application of respiratory care* (4th ed.). Chicago: Mosby Medical Publishers, Inc.

Cor Pulmonale

27

Elizabeth Burlew

INTRODUCTION

1. Chronic cor pulmonale is a common complication of chronic obstructive pulmonary disease and results from pulmonary hypertension with thromboembolic pulmonary disease being the predominant cause of acute cor pulmonale.
2. Vasodilatory therapy coupled with a low fat, low sodium diet, supplemental oxygen therapy (when indicated), anticoagulation, and judicious use of diuretics are the main treatment strategies for cor pulmonale and pulmonary hypertension.
3. Home therapy with prostacyclin and prostacyclin analogs for pulmonary hypertension and cor pulmonale requires extensive patient education and support to be successful.
4. The definitive treatment for cor pulmonale and pulmonary hypertension is heart-lung (or lung) transplantation.

The prevalence of pulmonary hypertension and cor pulmonale as complications associated with use of the anorectic agents fenfluramine (Pondimin, Fen-phen) and dexfenfluramine (Redux) has heightened public awareness of this disease process. The predominate age group impacted by COPD-associated pulmonary hypertension and cor pulmonale is older males; primary pulmonary hypertension is most common in young to middle-aged females. While the exact incidence remains unknown, autopsy studies suggest that it may be as high as 1 in 1,000. Approximately 400 new cases are diagnosed each year in the United States (Ricciardi & Rubenfire, 1999).

Definitions

1. Acute cor pulmonale—right heart strain or overload due to acute pulmonary hypertension, very frequently due to massive pulmonary embolism

2. Chronic cor pulmonale—hypertrophy, dilatation, and dysfunction of right ventricle secondary to pulmonary hypertension

Etiology

Table 27.1 (Adapted from Wiedemann & Matthay, 1997)

Pathophysiology

I. Right ventricular function
   A. Normal adult right ventricular (RV) is crescent shaped.
   B. Pumping activity is more like bellows compared to concentric contraction of left ventricle (LV).
   C. Thin walls enable RV to handle increases in volume better than increases in pressure.
   D. With chronic pressure loads the mass, structure and function of the RV changes dramatically.
   E. Animal studies demonstrate that the RV can rapidly change structure and function in response to outflow tract obstruction.
      1. RV decompensation occurs along a continuum.
      2. Unlike LV, small increases in outflow tract pressures (pulmonary artery) result in significant decreases in RV stroke volume.
      3. RV systolic pressures of 60–80 mm Hg lead to dilatation and failure resulting in hypotension and systemic hypoperfusion.
   F. Right ventricular ischemia is a limiting factor in response to acute right ventricular overload.
      1. Right coronary artery supplies right ventricular free wall and portion of interventricular septum.
      2. Right coronary artery originates in aorta with left ventricular function and systemic arterial pressure as determinates of right ventricular perfusion in setting of pulmonary hypertension.
II. Structure and function of pulmonary circulation
   A. Thin-walled vessels containing smaller amounts of smooth muscle fibers than systemic vessels
   B. Sparse innervation
      1. Vasomotor responses not sufficiently intense to overload right ventricle to point of producing acute cor pulmonale.
   C. Mechanical obstruction is suggested as the mechanism producing acute cor pulmonale (e.g., pulmonary embolism).
   D. Structural changes in pulmonary vasculature are implied mechanism of chronic cor pulmonale.
      1. Pulmonary vessels stiffer than systemic counterparts
         a. Large vessels can only accept small increases in blood flow.
         b. Pulmonary vascular resistance varies in a U-shaped curve manner with lung volumes.
         c. Pulmonary vascular resistance is highest at extremes of inflation (i.e., full inflation or deflation).

Table 27.1 Etiology of Cor Pulmonale Change

Pulmonary Vascular and Other Diseases	Disorders of Respiratory Drive, Chest Wall, and Neuromuscular Systems	Lung and Alveolar Disorders	Other Causes
Primary arterial wall diseases	Idiopathic hypoventilation	ARDS	High-altitude disease
■ Chronic liver disease		COPD	
■ Granulomatous pulmonary arteritis	Kyphoscoliosis	Cystic fibrosis	Pressure on pulmonary arteries by aneurysms, fibrosis, granulomas, or mediastinal tumors
■ Peripheral pulmonic stenosis	Neuromuscular weakness	Congenital defects	
■ Primary pulmonary hypertension	Sleep apnea syndromes	Infiltrative or granulomatous diseases	
■ Toxin-induced (IV drug abuse)		1. Eosinophilic granuloma	
		2. Idiopathic pulmonary fibrosis	
Blood disorders		3. Malignant infiltration	Surgeries involving lung resection
■ Pulmonary microthrombi		4. Pneumoconiosis	Upper airway obstruction
■ Sickle cell		5. Polymyositis	Use of fenfluramine (Pondimin, Fen-phen) and dexfenfluramine (Redux) associated with increased risk (odds ratio 6.3)
		6. Radiation	
Embolic disorders		7. Rheumatoid arthritis	
I. Air embolism		8. Sarcoidosis	
II. Amniotic fluid embolism		9. Scleroderma	
III. Parasitic diseases (e.g., schistosomiasis)		10. Systemic lupus erythematosis	
IV. Thromboembolism			
V. Tumor embolism			

2. Pulmonary vasoconstriction produces an acute elevation in pulmonary vascular pressures (pulmonary hypertension).

III. Causes of pulmonary vasoconstriction

    A. Hypoxia (most potent stimulus)

    B. Acidosis (synergistic with hypoxia)

    C. Genetic (primary pulmonary hypertension)

        1. Hypothesized endothelial overproduction of vasoconstrictors (thromboxane A_2 and endothelin 1)

            a. Smooth muscle cells depolarized and calcium overloaded due to reduced expression of potassium-gated channels

            b. Produces vasoconstriction

            c. May promote cell proliferation which adds to pulmonary hypertension in setting of vasoconstriction

            d. Excessive adventitial remodeling associated with excessive metalloproteinase and elastase activity, which results in increased production of extracellular matrix (collagen, elastin, fibronectin, tenascin)

        2. Newly hypothesized additional mechanism

            a. Increased levels of the nitric oxide synthase (NOS) inhibitor asymmetric dimethylarginine (ADMA) due to dysregulation of dimethylarginine dimethylaminohydrolase (DDAH), the enzyme which metabolizes ADMA

            b. Increased levels of ADMA and decreased levels of DDAH may contribute to pulmonary hypertension through the mechanism of competitive inhibition of pulmonary NOS enzymes.

        3. Continued pulmonary hypertension for even a few days associated with vascular changes

            a. Thickening of tunica media

            b. Endothelial swelling

            c. Muscular hypertrophy

            d. Proliferation of muscle fibers in peripheral pulmonary vessels (normally nonmuscularized)

        4. Continued insults (e.g., hypoxia) result in significant narrowing of pulmonary vessels and increase in RV mass

            a. May be due to blunted endothelium-related vasodilation responses

IV. Incidence: Most common in males over 40

    A. COPD most common etiology of hypoxic pulmonary hypertension and resultant cor pulmonale (incidence of COPD is 5 in 10,000)

        1. At autopsy one study found 40% of COPD patients had cor pulmonale

        2. COPD most common in elderly

        3. Cor pulmonale fairly common in COPD

            a. Cor pulmonale occurs mostly in older, male patients

    B. In setting of primary pulmonary hypertension, most common in women (median age of 35)

        1. Incidence of primary pulmonary hypertension is 8 in 100,000

        2. Women affected five times more often than men

V. Considerations across the life span
   A. Pediatric
      1. Cystic fibrosis associated with cor pulmonale
      2. Pulmonary hypertension commonly associated with many congenital heart defects
         a. Transposition of great vessels with or without patent ductus or ventricular septal defect
         b. Single ventricle without pulmonic stenosis
         c. Double outlet right ventricle
         d. Truncus arteriosus
      3. Pulmonary vascular obstructive disease
         a. Cause unknown
         b. Progresses rapidly
            i. Large ventricular septal defect
           ii. Unilateral absence of pulmonary artery (less common)
          iii. Left to right shunts in a high altitude environment
          iv. Double outlet right ventricle
            v. Truncus arteriosus
          vi. Down's syndrome
         vii. Complete atrioventricular canal defects
      4. Heart failure symptoms in infants
         a. DOE (feeding problems)
         b. Respiratory distress (predominantly tachypnea)
         c. Decreased urine output
      5. Heart failure symptoms in children
         a. Rapid heart rate (160–180)
            i. Little variability at rest
           ii. Summation gallops to auscultation
         b. Color—ashen pale to faintly cyanotic
         c. DOE
         d. Excessive perspiration
         e. Decreased urine output
   B. Pregnancy
      1. Primary pulmonary hypertension is predominant etiology of cor pulmonale in this population
         a. Right ventricular ischemia and failure
         b. Cardiac arrhythmias common
      2. Pulmonary embolism most likely mechanism of death
      3. Anesthetics with negative inotropic effects to be avoided due to right ventricular dysfunction
      4. Deterioration occurs in second trimester
         a. Fatigue
         b. Dyspnea
         c. Syncope
         d. Chest pain
         e. Right ventricular failure

C. Elderly
   1. Cor pulmonale complicated by age-related changes
   2. Increased matrix remodeling leading to increased myocardial stiffness
      a. Impaired diastolic relaxation
      b. Impaired systolic ejection
   3 Preload must be maintained to fill stiff right ventricle and maintain cardiac output
   4. Threats
      a. Fluid volume deficits
      b. Hypotension

VI. Complications/sequelae
   A. Right ventricular failure
   B. Left ventricular diastolic tamponade (reduced cardiac output due to reduced ventricular chamber size associated with pressure from hypertrophied right ventricle and bulging of the interventricular septum into the left ventricle)
   C. Tricuspid insufficiency (valve fails to close properly due to annular dilation secondary to right ventricular hypertrophy and failure of leaflet coaptation)
   D. Development of thrombi in pulmonary circulation due to changes in walls of pulmonary vasculature
   E. Hepatic congestion and failure
      1. Failure to properly metabolize drugs
      2. Impaired liver function/synthesis of clotting factors, proteins, etc.
   F. Renal hypoperfusion and failure
   G. Gastrointestinal edema and absorption failures
   H. Peripheral edema and development of stasis ulcers

Assessment

I. History
   A. Patients tend to develop symptoms gradually (2 to 5 years of symptoms prior to diagnosis)
      1. Dyspnea
         a. Early symptom increasing in severity over time
         b. Universally present with development of hypoxemia, pulmonary hypertension, right ventricular failure
      2. Increasing fatigue
      3. Chest pain common—may be difficult to distinguish from angina
      4. Orthopnea may or may not be associated with worsening cardiac function in setting of COPD
      5. Reduced appetite and eating (increased hepatic congestion)
      6. Increasing lower extremity edema
      7. Fluid overload
      8. Presyncope and syncope (dizziness) with exertion

II. Physical exam
   A. Typically not sensitive, especially in patients with COPD and chest hyperinflation
      1. Jugular pressure difficult to assess due to wide fluctuation of intrathoracic pressures
         a. Jugular venous distension (JVD)
         b. Prominent jugular v wave (tricuspid regurgitation)
   B. Peripheral edema may or may not be present
   C. Characteristic findings of cor pulmonale (may be obscured or modified by hyperinflation of COPD)
      1. Systolic parasternal or epigastric lift (right ventricular hypertrophy)
      2. Right ventricular S_3, S_4
      3. Murmur of tricuspid regurgitation (softer than that of mitral regurgitation)
      4. Murmur of pulmonic regurgitation (softer than that of aortic regurgitation)
      5. Accentuation of second heart sound (P_2)
         a. Loud and palpable valve closure
   D. May have dry crackles at lung bases
   E. Clubbing
   F. Peripheral or central cyanosis
   G. Hepatojugular reflux
   H. Hepatomegaly, may be pulsatile
   I. Lower extremity edema
   J. Ascites
   K. Anasarca
III. Diagnostic tests—Most important are echocardiography, right heart catheterization (pulmonary artery catheter), and 12 lead EKG
   A. EKG: Criteria are specific but not sensitive
      1. EKG criteria for cor pulmonale without COPD
         ▪ Presence of any one of first three criteria raises suspicion of right ventricular hypertrophy
         ▪ Diagnosis is more certain if two or more of these criteria are present
         ▪ Last four criteria common in cor pulmonale secondary to primary alveolar hypoventilation, interstitial pulmonary disease, or pulmonary vascular disease
         a. Right-axis deviation with mean QRS axis to right of +110 degrees
         b. R/S amplitude in V_1 >1
         c. R/S amplitude in V_6 >1
         d. Clockwise rotation of electrical axis
         e. P-pulmonale pattern (an increase in P wave amplitude in leads II, III, AVF)
         f. S_1Q_3 (McGinn-White pattern with tall S wave in lead I and deep Q wave in lead III) or $S_1S_2S_3$ (tall S waves in leads I, II, and III) pattern
         g. Normal voltage QRS

2. EKG criteria for cor pulmonale in COPD
   - First seven criteria nonspecific but suggest cor pulmonale
   - Last three criteria are characteristic of cor pulmonale in COPD
   a. Isoelectric P waves in lead I or right-axis deviation of the P vector
   b. P-pulmonale pattern
   c. Tendency for right axis deviation of the QRS
   d. R/S amplitude ratio in V_6 <1
   e. Low voltage QRS
   f. S_1Q_3 or $S_1S_2S_3$ pattern
   g. Incomplete right bundle branch block (rarely complete)
   h. Clockwise rotation of the electrical axis
   i. Occasional large Q wave or QS in inferior (II, III, AVF) or midprecordial leads (V_3, V_4) suggesting healed myocardial infarction
3. EKG findings of right ventricular hypertrophy late event in cor pulmonale
   a. Occurs only after prolonged dilatation of right ventricle
4. EKG evidence of right heart strain
   a. P pulmonale
   b. Right-axis deviation (30 degrees or more of QRS)
   c. Right ventricular hypertrophy
   d. Right ventricular strain pattern: appears in 80% of patients with primary pulmonary hypertension
   e. Rhythm disturbances
      i. Atrial ectopy
      ii. Atrial fibrillation
      iii. Atrial flutter
      iv. Atrial tachycardia

B. Chest X-ray: Important tool
   1. May appear normal in early disease
   2. Skeletal abnormalities responsible for right ventricular failure may be visible (kyphoscoliosis)
   3. Pulmonary parenchymal abnormalities associated with COPD may be evident
   4. Diameters of proximal pulmonary arteries that are indicative of pulmonary hypertension
      a. Right descending pulmonary artery >16 mm
      b. Left descending pulmonary artery >18 mm
   5. Advanced disease
      a. Counterclockwise rotation of heart
      b. Reduced prominence of aortic knob
      c. Lobular appearance of left heart

C. Pulmonary function testing
   1. May suggest presence of pulmonary vascular disease associated with cor pulmonale
   2. May be helpful in identifying etiology of pulmonary hypertension and right ventricular failure
      a. Gas exchange abnormalities

b. Obstructive abnormalities

c. Abnormalities of carbon monoxide diffusing capacity

d. Restrictive abnormalities

D. Echocardiography
1. Right ventricular hypertrophy defined as posterior free wall thickness of >5 mm (poor sensitivity)
2. Change in shape of right ventricle
   a. More concentric, less C-shaped—"left ventricularization" of the right ventricle
   b. D-shaped left ventricle
   c. Volume decreases in relationship to mass
3. Detection of other abnormalities
   a. Dilation of pulmonary artery
   b. Dilation and hypertrophy of right ventricle (even if posterior wall not visible)
   c. Diastolic flattening of interventricular septum (eventually becomes concave)
4. Helpful in determining secondary etiologies
   a. Left ventricular dysfunction
   b. Mitral valve abnormalities
   c. Congenital heart disease
5. Helpful for follow-up evaluation after treatment initiated

E. Nuclear imaging
1. Ventriculography
   a. Determination of right ventricular ejection fraction
2. Ventilation-perfusion (V/Q) scanning
   a. Useful in determining if etiology due to pulmonary thromboembolic disease
3. Pulmonary arteriography
   a. Useful in diagnosis of pulmonary thromboembolic disease if V/Q scan nondiagnostic
4. Right-heart catheterization: Gold standard for diagnosis of pulmonary hypertension
   a. Normal wedge pressure in primary pulmonary hypertension
   b. Abnormal wedge pressure requires left-heart catheterization
   c. Determination of right-to-left shunting

F. Magnetic resonance imaging (MRI)
1. Potentially useful in evaluation of ventricular volume and ejection fraction
2. Determination of wall stress
3. Evaluation of thromboembolic disease

Common Therapeutic Modalities

I. Right ventricular afterload reduction strategies
A. Supplemental oxygen
1. Reduction of hypoxic pulmonary vasoconstriction

2. Relief of tissue hypoxia
   a. May allow reversal of right ventricular dysfunction
B. Treatment of COPD to maximize pulmonary function may improve oxygenation, theoretically improving cor pulmonale
C. Vasodilator therapy to reduce resistance to blood flow in the pulmonary circulation (includes calcium channel blockers and other medications)
D. Calcium channel blockers—oral agents—first line medications
   1. Conventional therapy until 1990
      Remain treatment of choice in patients with favorable acute response to inhaled nitric oxide or adenosine
   2. Approximately 20% of patients will respond
   3. Optimum dosing uncertain
   4. Diltiazem: 120–900 mg/day
   5. Nifedipine: 30–240 mg/day
   6. Amlodipine: 5–20 mg/day
   7. Nicardipine: 60–240 mg/day
   8. Side effects
      a. Systemic hypotension
      b. Pulmonary edema
      c. Salt and water retention with peripheral edema
      d. Increasing areas of V/Q mismatch
      e. Right ventricular failure
E. Recommended treatments for nonresponders to calcium channel blockers (NYHA Class III heart failure)
   1. Bosentan
      a. Used as a first-line treatment
      b. Also used for NYHA Class IV heart failure
         i. May be used with IV epoprostenol for an enhanced effect
         ii. May allow reduction in epoprostenol dose and reduction in side effects
      c. Dosing
         i. 62.5 mg BID for 4 weeks
         ii. Increased to maintenance dose of 125 mg bid after 4 weeks
      d. Side effects
         i. headache, flushing, nasopharyngitis
         ii. nausea, vomiting
         iii. abnormal hepatic function
         iv. leg edema, anemia (dose-related)
      e. If patient deteriorates further while on Bosentan, consider switching to IV prostacylin or inhaled iloprost
   2. Iloprost aerosol
      a. May be better tolerated by patients with systemic hypotension
      b. Critical that aerosol delivery system is capable of delivering aerosol particles of 3.0–5.0 micrometers to insure alveolar deposition

    c. Dosing

        i. 100 to 150 micrograms daily dose

        ii. Typically dosed every 2–3 hours

        iii. May require as much as 200 micrograms per day

    d. Side effects

        i. flushing, headache, jaw pain

        ii. fluctuations in exercise capacity—best immediately after inhalation and then declines slowly over 2–3 hours

    e. If patient fails to improve with aerosol iloprost, IV prostacyclin, or iloprost must be started without delay

  3. Treprostinil

    a. Should not be considered in NYHA Class IV heart failure patients

    b. Administered as subcutaneous infusion (similar to insulin pump)

    c. Dosing

        i. 1.25 ng/kg/minute for 4 weeks

        ii. 2.5 ng/kg/minute dose may be titrated to maximum of 40 ng/kg/minute

        iii. infusion sites should be rotated every 3 days

    d. Side effects

        i. jaw pain, headache, diarrhea

        ii. flushing, foot pain

        iii. infusion site pain (can be severe) and erythema

  4. Beraprost oral (investigational)

    a. First stable and orally active prostacyclin analogue

    b. An "orphan" drug

    c. Should not be considered in NYHA Class IV heart failure patients

    d. Dosing

        i. 60 mcg per day in 4 divided doses

        ii. Increased by 60 mcg/day over 1–2 weeks to patient tolerance

    e. Side effects

        i. Headache, flushing, jaw pain

        ii. Diarrhea, leg pain, nausea

E. Preferential pulmonary vasodilators—agents used for NYHA Class IV heart failure

  1. Prostacyclin (Epoprostenol, PGI_2, Flolan)

    a. Remains gold standard treatment for advanced pulmonary artery hypertension and cor pulmonale

    b. Used as a bridge to transplantation

    c. Started at 2 ng/kg/minute IV

    d. Increased by 1 to 2 ng/kg/minute every 10–15 minutes

    e. Optimal dosing remains undefined

    f. Side effects determine dose limit

        i. Severe nausea/vomiting, diarrhea, headache, systemic hypotension

        ii. Flushing, chest pain, anxiety, dizziness

        iii. Abdominal pain, musculoskeletal pain, tachycardia

      g. Dosage adjusted as tolerance develops, disease worsens or dose-limiting side effects appear

      h. Continued indefinitely until lung transplantation or death

  2. Iloprost (investigational)

      a. Unlike epoprostenol, stable at room temperature

      b. Dosing

        i. 1 to 5 ng/kg/minute IV

        ii. Maximum dose 10 ng/kg/minute

      c. Side effects and limitations similar to epoprostenol

      d. Not approved for use in the United States

  3. Adenosine

      a. Diagnostic short-term infusion to evaluate vasodilator reserve: identifies patients who will potentially respond to calcium channel blockers

      b. 0.001–0.05 mg/kg/minute

      c. Increased by 0.01–0.02 mg/kg/minute

      d. Side effects

        i. Chest pain, chest pressure

        ii. Flushing, headache

        ii. Nausea

        iv. Ankle swelling

  4. Inhaled nitric oxide (investigational)

      a. 5–80 ppm

      b. Administered using special gas delivery equipment: nitrogen dioxide scavengers and detectors

      c. Side effects

        i. Suppression of endogenous nitric oxide production

        ii. May interfere with platelet function resulting in bleeding

        iii. Nitric oxide binds to hemoglobin producing methemoglobin, which is incapable of carrying oxygen. Methemoglobin levels must be closely monitored.

II. Other agents/treatment approaches

  A. Anticoagulants

    1. Warfarin drug of choice

    2. Target INR 2.0–3.0

  B. Diuretics

    1. To reduce increased intravascular volume and hepatic congestion

    2. Used judiciously as right ventricle is preload dependent

  C. Surgical approaches (NYHA Class IV heart failure)

    1. Atrial septostomy

    2. Lung transplantation or heart-lung transplantation

  D. Digitalis

    1. Utilized in past to strengthen force of cardiac contraction

    2. No evidence concerning the efficacy of digitalis in cor pulmonale

III. Promising pharmacological approaches

  A. L-Arginine supplementation

    1. Can enhance nitric oxide levels

2. Oral L-arginine has been shown to reduce pulmonary pressures by approximately 15 mm Hg.
   3. Clinical trials underway in Europe as of 2003
   B. Sildenafil
      1. Primarily used in treatment of erectile dysfunction
      2. Selective cGMP inhibition
      3. Appears most effective in combination with a prostacyclin analog (iloprost)
      4. Trials underway to determine appropriate dosing
IV. Home care considerations
   A. Supplemental oxygen therapy
      1. Physician will order
         a. Goal: SaO_2 90%–95%
         b. May be required only for activity
      2. Oxygen required for altitudes above 2,500 feet
         a. Consultation with physician and airlines prior to travel
   B. Epoprostenol home therapy
      1. Must be reconstituted from powder
      2. Unstable at
         a. pH less than 10.2
         b. Room temperature longer than 8 hours
      3. Storage of reconstituted drug
         a. Chilled ice packs increase stability up to 24 hours
         b. Refrigeration increases stability up to 48 hours
         c. Must be protected from light
      4. Drug delivery
         a. Ambulatory pump
         b. Ice packs kept in pouch around pump
         c. Long-term central venous catheterization required
      5. Back-up supplies required
         a. Reconstituted drug (refrigerated)
         b. Batteries
         c. Space pump
      6. Recommended that a companion or significant other be available to assist in preparing and administering epoprostenol at home
      7. Patient must be taught that once the drug is started, it cannot be abruptly discontinued due to risk of death or rebound pulmonary hypertension
   C. Financial considerations
      1. Epoprostenol $60,000–$120,000 per year
      2. Bosentan $30,000 per year
      3. Treprostinil $50,000–$90,000 per year

WEB SITES

www.vh.org/Providers/TeachingFiles/PulmonaryCoreCurric/COPD/Pulm HypertensionExcellent peer-reviewed paper, "Diagnosis of pulmonary hypertension and cor pulmonale," by Peterson, Kline, Dayton, and Beltz on University of Iowa's Web site.

www.umdnj.edu/rspthweb/bibs/cor_pulm.htm—Cor pulmonale and pulmonary hypertension bibliography.

www.pulmonary-hypertension-treatments.com—Attorney-operated Web site with readable information concerning pulmonary hypertension/cor pulmonale for patients. Focus is new treatments, research, and patient rights.

www.emedicine.com/med/topic449.htm—Well written, in-depth review article concerning diagnosis and treatment of cor pulmonale.

www.nlm.nih.gov/medlineplus/ency/article/000129.htm—Comprehensive patient education article published by the National Institutes of Health.

www.medscape.com/viewarticle/404385—Article by Hurst detailing EKG findings of cor pulmonale associated with chronic obstructive pulmonary disease.

REFERENCES

Ricciardi, M. J., & Rubenfire, M. (1999). How to manage primary pulmonary hypertension: Giving hope to patients with a life-threatening illness. *Postgraduate Medicine, 105*(3), 45–54.

Wiedemann, H. P., & Matthay, R. A. (1997). Cor pulmonale. In Braunwald, E. (Ed.), *Heart disease: A textbook of cardiovascular medicine Vol. 2* (pp. 1604–1625). Philadelphia: W. B. Saunders.

ADDITIONAL READINGS

Archer, S., & Rich, S. (2000). Primary pulmonary hypertension: A vascular biology and translational research "work in progress." *Circulation, 102*(22), 2781–2791.

Coe, P. F. (2000). Managing pulmonary hypertension in heart transplantation: Meeting the challenge. *Critical Care Nurse, 20*(2), 22–28.

Galie, N., Manes, A., & Branzi, A. (2002). Emerging medical therapies for pulmonary arterial hypertension. *Progress in Cardiovascular Diseases 45*(3), 213–224.

Hoeper, M. M., Schwarze, M., Ehlerding, S., Adler-Schuermeyer, A., Spiekerkotten, E., Niedermyer, J., et al. (2000). Long-term treatment of primary pulmonary hypertension with aerosolized iloprost, a prostacyclin analogue. *New England Journal of Medicine, 342,* 1866–1870.

Hoeper, M. M., Galie, N, Simmonneau, G., & Rubin, L. J. (2002). New treatments for pulmonary arterial hypertension. *American Journal of Respiratory and Critical Care Medicine, 165,* 1209–1216.

MacNee, W. (1994). Pathophysiology of cor pulmonale in chronic obstructive pulmonary disease (Part One). *American Journal of Respiratory and Critical Care Medicine, 150*(3), 833–852.

Millat, L. J., Whitly, G. S. J., Li, D., Leiper, J. M., Siragy, H. M., Carey, R. M., et al. (2003). Evidence for dysregulation of dimethylarginine dimethylaminohydrolase I in chronic hypoxia-induced pulmonary hypertension. *Circulation, 108*, 1493–1498.

Mori, M., & Gotoh, T. (2000). Regulation of nitric oxide production by arginine metabolic Enzymes. *Biochemical and Biophysiological Research Communications, 275*, 715–719.

Restrepo, C. I., & Tapson, V. F. (1998). Pulmonary hypertension and cor pulmonale. In E. Topol (Ed.), *Comprehensive cardiovascular medicine Vol. 1* (pp. 737–755). Philadelphia, PA: Lippincott–Raven.

Rubin, L. J., Badesch, D. B., Barst, R. J., Galie, N., Black, C. M., Keogh, A., et al. (2002). Bosentan therapy for pulmonary arterial hypertension. *New England Journal of Medicine, 346*(12), 896–903.

Sabo, J. A., & Nord, P. (2000). Intravenous epoprostenol: A new therapy for primary pulmonary hypertension. *Critical Care Nurse, 20*(6), 31–40.

Wiedemann, H. P., & Matthay, R. A. (1997). Cor pulmonale. In E. Braunwald (Ed.), *Heart disease: A textbook of cardiovascular medicine Vol. 2* (pp. 1604–1625). Philadelphia: W. B. Saunders.

Pulmonary Complications of Human Immunodeficiency Virus (HIV)

28

Ann Peterson

INTRODUCTION

CD4 counts in HIV positive patients influence susceptibility to opportunistic infections (OIs) including pulmonary infections.

I. Overview of Human Immunodeficiency Virus (HIV)
    A. Definitions
        HIV is an RNA retrovirus causing infection in human hosts that will ultimately lead to severe immunosuppression resulting in complications of opportunistic infections and cancers.
        1. Acquired Immune Deficiency Syndrome (AIDS) is a late-stage condition caused by HIV. AIDS defining is often utilized for epidemiological reasons and for seeking funding. Refer to the table "Indicator Conditions in Case Definition of AIDS (Adults) –1997" for a list of conditions that meet the criteria for case definition of AIDS. (http://www.hopkinsaids. edu/publications/book/ch1_table1_4.html#t14)
        2. Examples of pulmonary opportunistic infections from the case definition table include Pneumocystis pneumonia and pulmonary Mycobacterium tuberculosis.
        3. Other respiratory conditions from the case definition table include Cytomegalovirus (CMV), and recurrent pneumonia (≥ 2 episodes in 12 months; Bartlett & Gallant, 2003).

B. Incidence

In late 2003 it was estimated that the global number of persons living with HIV was 40 million (34.6–42.3 million). The estimate of the number of cumulative deaths due to HIV/AIDS for 2003 was 3 million in data from UNAIDS. In the last 20 years it is estimated that 20 million have died due to HIV. In some countries such as in Africa, HIV/AIDS is the leading cause of death (Quinn, 2001; http://www.unaids.org/epdemic_update/report_dec01/index.htlm).

C. Considerations across the life span

1. Pediatric

a. The etiology and pathogenesis of HIV/AIDS are similar in children compared to adults. However, in children the interval between virus acquisition and appearance of disease is often shorter and the progression of the disease is faster. Also, pediatric patients are more likely to have central nervous system involvement in the early phases of HIV infection.

b. Lymphocytic infiltrative disease to the lungs resulting in pneumonia is more common in children (Shelhamer et al., 1991).

c. Primary prophylaxis refers to preventing a first episode of disease. Secondary prophylaxis is the prevention of relapse or disease recurrence. Primary TMP-SMX prophylaxis of HIV exposed newborns for PCP begins by age 4–6 weeks because the peak incidence of PCP occurs at age 4 months.

II. Pneumocystis Pneumonia (PCP)

A. Definition

1. PCP is the acronym for a disease known as Pneumocystis jiroviceci pneumonia or Pneumocystis pneumonia. In PCP a fungus organism causes pneumonia. Although for years the causative organism for PCP was thought to be a protozoan analysis of rRNA indicates the fungal nature of the agent (Kovacs, Gill, Meschnick, & Masur, 2001; Stringer, Beard, Miller, & Wakefield, 2002; Walzer, 2000).

2. The organism that causes PCP in humans was formerly called *P. carinii formae specialis hominis*. Now the preferred name is *Pneumocystis jiroveci*. Because much of the review of the literature refers to *P. carinii*, the organism will be referred to as *Pneumocystis organism* and the disease as *PCP* for most of the discussion below except for direct quotations from authors.

3. The risk of PCP increases with a CD4 count of <200/mm^3, prior PCP infection, or HIV-associated thrush. Recommended PCP prophylaxis agents are

a. TMP-SMX

b. Dapsone

c. Dapsone plus pyrimethamine plus leucovorin

d. Aerosolized pentamidine

e. Atovaquone (Bartlett & Gallant, 2003)

B. Etiology: PCP is caused by a fungus leading to pulmonary infection in an immune suppressed host (Walzer, 2000).

C. Transmission

1. There is some debate about transmission of PCP. Some of the literature reflects possible transmission modes from contact with another person versus reactivation of latent virus in the setting of an immune suppressed host. It is not known which mechanism is more common as the cause of acute disease (Girard, 2004).

2. Morris, Swanson, Ha, and Huang state that the transmission of Pneumocystis organisms by airborne mechanisms from animal to animal clearly occurs but not cross species. They suggest that "active acquisition of P. carinii from environmental exposure or person-to-person transmission may play a role in the development of the disease" (Morris et al., 2000, p. 1622). Molecular epidemiologic studies suggest that new infections of PCP may not be reactivation of latent infection (Kovacs et al., 2001.) Supporting this theory is the work of Dohn and associates who explored geographic clustering of PCP through the review of hospital outbreaks associated with patient contacts (Dohn et al., 2000).

3. Although the Center for Disease Control and Prevention Guidelines do not indicate that respiratory isolation is required for patients with PCP, some hospitals recommend that patients with PCP should not share a room with an immunosuppressed patient (Masur, 1999).

D. Pathophysiology

1. The immune suppression of HIV/AIDS can lead to decreased function of the normal defense mechanisms of the lower airways leading to an increased risk of pneumonia such as PCP (Wilkins & Dexter, 1998). *P. jiroveci* is first inhaled and then later reaches the alveoli.

2. The cysts of *P. jiroveci* deposit in pulmonary secretions and lung tissues. The organisms and byproducts are found in the intra-alveolar spaces.

3. There are several stages of the infection. A diploid zygote gives rise to a 4–6 μm sized sporozoite also referred to as a *pre-cyst*. An intracystic body or spore develops. The infection alters normal lung epithelial cell function causing lung damage, altered surfactant function, and inflammation associated with cytokine response (Walzer, 2000).

4. Infection in the lung can be bilateral and eventually spread throughout the lungs. However, unilateral lung involvement is possible. Changes in the lung can be severe involving hypoxia, increased alveolar-arterial oxygen gradient, respiratory alkalosis, impaired diffusing capacity, and changes in lung capacities similar to those seen in adult respiratory distress syndrome (Walzer, 2000).

E. Incidence

1. The most common occurrence of PCP is in individuals with CD4 counts between 0 and $100/mm^3$.

2. The risk of PCP increases with prior PCP infection and HIV-associated thrush.

3. Prior to 1991, PCP was the most common AIDS defining infection with an incidence of 65%–85% for pulmonary disorders associated with HIV infection (Shellhamer et al., 1991). Today, PCP is considered the most common life-threatening OI for HIV+ individuals (Kovacs et al., 2001).

4. PCP is preventable but even today with the development of antiretroviral therapy (ART) and knowledge about PCP prophylaxis there are still too many HIV+ individuals becoming infected with PCP. Some of the reasons for the occurrence of PCP include lack of treatment for HIV, noncompliance with treatment, PCP prophylaxis not prescribed, and illness despite prophylaxis (Masur, 2002).

5. An analysis of ICU admissions in HIV+ patients revealed that from 11% to 22% of these patients had PCP. Mortality rates have improved with time due to PCP prophylaxis, improved ART, and corticosteroid therapy for PCP. However, PCP still remains a common complication of HIV infection and the most common cause of respiratory failure for HIV patients in the ICU (Afessa & Green, 2000).

F. Considerations across the life span
1. Pediatric
   a. PCP may be the first presenting clinical sign of AIDS in children.
   b. Risk factors for PCP in children are higher when CD4 counts are low.
   c. Treatment usually involves glucocorticoids, trimethoprim-sulfamethoxazole TMP-SMX, or Pentamidine (Pizzo & Mueller, 1993).
2. Pregnancy
   Follow management guidelines as in adults and treatment strategies should take into consideration potential teratogenic and mutagenic effects of drug therapy.
3. Elderly
   Poly-pharmacy and co-morbid conditions such as hypertension and diabetes may complicate clinical management.

G. Complications/sequelae
1. Untreated PCP results in interstitial fibrosis. Mild fibrosis may occur even with successful treatment (Girard, 2004).
2. In PCP, bullae and cavities can form and potentially lead to a pneumothorax. Spontaneous pneumothorax is also associated with HIV+ patients with PCP on mechanical ventilation in the ICU (Afessa, 2000). Noncaseating granulomatous inflammation and alveolar and interstitial edema can form in the setting of PCP (Girard, 2004).
3. The development of drug resistance of *P. jiroveci* to therapy with sulfonamides (such as trimethoprim-sulfamethoxazole [TMP-SMX]) may occur due to widespread use of these agents. HIV+ individuals who break through sulfonamide prophylaxis are more likely to be either experiencing a deteriorating immune response and/or non-compliance

with drug prophylaxis rather than developing drug resistance (Masur, 1999).

4. Most of the patients who break through sulfonamide prophylaxis will respond to high dose IV Bactrim therapy for PCP. TMP-SMX is the drug of choice for most patients unless they have experienced a life-threatening hypersensitivity reaction to the agent in the past (Masur, 1999).

5. The atypical radiographic patterns seen more frequently with HIV+ patients include: asymmetrical pulmonary disease, upper lobe involvement mimicking TB, pleural effusions, and enlarged hilar and mediastinal nodes (Shelhamer, Pizzo, Parrillo, & Mazur, 1991).

6. Respiratory failure sometimes occurs even in the setting of therapy. Treatments may include supplemental oxygen therapy, intubation, and mechanical ventilation.

H. Assessment
   1. History: PCP is characterized by one or more of the following
      a. Exercise intolerance
      b. Fever (≥38.0° C)
      c. Chest pain (sometimes substernal)
      d. Persistent and escalating non-productive cough
      e. Dyspnea
      f. Substernal "catching" (Masur, 1999)
   2. Physical exam
      a. Rales are detected in about 33% of adults
      b. Chills
      c. Hypoxia (may be severe) with an increased alveolar-arterial oxygen gradient and respiratory alkalosis
      d. Anxiety
      e. Tachypnea
      f. Tachycardia
      g. Cyanosis, nasal flaring, and intercostal retractions in some children

I. Diagnosis
   1. Diagnosis is based on detection of cysts in sputum or pulmonary secretions. Induced sputum or bronchoscopy and bronchial alveolar lavage (BAL) may be indicated to obtain specimens.
   2. Lung biopsy is done if unable to obtain diagnosis, if the BAL is not diagnostic, and if the patient is not improving on treatment for PCP.
   3. Chest X-ray, often the first diagnostic test, can demonstrate bilateral interstitial abnormalities, upper lobe disease, lobar infiltrates, or nodules.
   4. Computerized tomography (CT) scan patterns in PCP may have a ground glass appearance.
   5. Arterial blood gases with arterial oxygen tensions A-a gradient.
   6. Laboratory blood tests: LDH, serum albumin, and CBC with a differential are commonly ordered (Shelhamer et al., 1991).

J. Common therapeutic modalities
  1. Prophylaxis
    Recommended PCP prophylaxis agents are: TMP-SMX, Dapsone, Aero-solized pentamidine, or Atovaquone. Prophylaxis is indicated by vary-ing criteria such as in the setting of CD4 counts <200/mm³, previous history of PCP or any type of pneumonia, and wasting (Masur, 1999).
  2. Treatment
    a. Oxygen and respiratory support
    b. Trimethoprim (TMP) + sulfamethoxazole (SMX) IV or PO: first choice therapy
    c. Trimethoprim + dapsone PO
    d. Atovaquone PO: well tolerated for mild disease (Masur, 1999)
    e. Clindamycin IV or PO + primaquine PO
    f. Pentamidine IV: used for severe cases (Bartlett & Gallant, 2003)
    g. Steroids are administered to patients in respiratory failure. Pred-nisone is prescribed for individuals with an initial presentation of a pO_2 < 70 mm Hg or A-a gradient > 35 mm Hg on room air. The schedule for prednisone is 40 mg BID for 5 days, then 40 mg QD for 5 days, then 20 mg QD until completion (Bartlett & Gallant, 2003).
    h. Symptom management drugs such as anti-emetics for nausea and vomiting secondary to treatment medications
K. Home care considerations
  1. Home health care workers (HCWs) who suspect that their patients are presenting with increasing dyspnea and cough should consult with the physician to work-up the possibility of respiratory infections. Hospital admission is often warranted.
  2. HCWs are in a key position to reinforce teaching for medication ad-herence for OI prophylaxis.
III. Kaposi's Sarcoma
  A. Definition
    1. Kaposi's Sarcoma (KS) is a malignancy or neoplastic disease that can occur with HIV infection. Moritz Kaposi defined KS in 1872. Prior to the HIV epidemic, KS was considered an indolent disease of elderly Mid-dle Eastern and Eastern European males. The condition was uncom-monly seen in the 1970s associated with immunosuppressed allograft recipients (Trubowitz & Volberding, 2000). The form of KS associated with HIV appears to be more virulent than the form seen in the past.
  B. Etiology
    1. The causative agent of KS is a human herpes virus type 8 (HHV-8). It is a gamma herpes virus like the Epstein-Barr virus. The virus has been detected in secretions such as saliva, semen, and prostate tis-sues (Rosen & Schneider, 1998; Strauss, 2000).
  C. Transmission
    1. Transmission is not fully known but thought to occur through sexual contact (Osmond, et al., 2002; Rosen & Schneider, 1998; Trubowitz & Volberding, 2000). Transmission of HHV-8 is associated with a history

of sexually transmitted diseases and number of male sexual partners (Tirelli & Vaccher, 2004)

D. Pathophysiology

1. KS can affect several types of tissues including skin, bowel, airways, parenchyma, pleurae, and intrathoracic lymph nodes (Rosen & Schneider, 1998).

2. Herpes viruses can cause a primary infection with subsequent latency in the immune system. Later the virus can reactivate and be transmitted to others.

3. KS pathophysiology includes "angiogenesis, endothelial spindle cell growth (KS cells), inflammatory cell infiltration and edema" (Tirelli & Vaccher, 2004, p. 1313). Immune dysregulation and angiogenic factors contribute to pathology of KS lesions with triggers or escalation by the HHV-8 infection. Immunologic factors associated with KS include CD8+ T-cells, interferon-γ, interleukin 1 β, interlekin-6, and tumor necrosis factor $-\alpha$ as well as other factors. The HIV Tat protein plays a role in progression of KS (Tirelli & Vaccher, 2004).

E. Incidence

1. In the early 1980s in the United States, the incidence of KS associated with AIDS was between 47%–50%. In 1991, it was reported that KS occurs in 4%–6% of HIV+ individuals and in about 25% of AIDS patients. Between 1996 to 1997, the average incidence of KS was reported to have decreased to 7.5 per 1,000 patient years (Trubowitz & Volberding, 2000). The declining incidence is thought to be due to the use of ART.

2. Although the incidence of pulmonary KS is considered rare for HIV+ women, a series of 7 women was studied by Haramati and Wong. Their research identified missed diagnoses for KS in 3 patients. The HIV+ women with pulmonary KS had associated risk factors of heterosexual contacts, IV drug use or both IV drug use and heterosexual contacts (Cannon et al., 2001; Haramati & Wong, 2000).

3. Considerations Across the Life Span: Pediatric

   1. Children have a lower incidence of KS compared to white homosexual or bisexual males.

   2. In one report to CDC of children with AIDS, of 3,431 children under 13 evaluated, only 20 children were diagnosed with KS.

F. Complications/sequelae

1. The incidence of KS is increased with CD4 counts less than 200/mm^3.

2. Pulmonary KS is associated with an increased risk of respiratory failure and death.

3. Pulmonary KS in the setting of HIV can lead to pleural effusions. About half of the patients with pulmonary KS experienced this complication as described in a 3-year retrospective review of hospital admissions in Florida (Afessa, 2000; Bartlett & Gallant, 2003).

4. Hemorrhage of the tracheobronchial tree or airway has been reported and is usually managed by treatment of any coagulation abnormalities.

G. Assessment
  1. History
     a. Asymptomatic in many cases of airway lesions
     b. Airway obstruction
     c. Mild hemoptysis (Feinberg & Baughman, 1999)
     d. Skin and oral cavity lesions
     e. Chest pain
  2. Physical exam
     a. Hoarseness
     b. Cough ("barking" quality)
     c. Fever (>38.3° C)
     d. Dyspnea
     e. Shortness of breath
     f. Hypoxia
     g. Bronchospasm
     h. Multiple cutaneous lesions (often but not always)
  3. Diagnostic tests
     a. Chest X-ray: Pulmonary opportunistic infections may look similar to KS by radiographic evaluation. KS is associated with hilar and mediastinal adenopathy, lymph node enlargement, pleural effusions, and a diffuse interstitial appearance (Bartlett & Gallant, 2003; Shelhamer et al., 1991; Trubowitz & Volberding, 2000).
     b. Chest CT may help define abnormalities (Haramati & Wong, 2000; Masur, 1999). CT scans may demonstrate parenchymal and subpleural nodules, bronchovascular thickening, parenchymal masses, and pleural effusions (Feinberg & Baughman, 1999).
     c. Bronchoscopy may be used to identify lesions of KS or establish the presence of other OIs of the lungs.
     d. Transbronchial lung biopsy to diagnose KS is controversial because hemorrhage can result. Open lung biopsy or VATS procedures result in a high diagnostic yield. CT guided procedures are sometimes used to obtain tissue specimens for diagnosis of pulmonary KS (Haramati & Wong, 2000).
     e. KS has a gallium-negative and thallium-positive pattern while infections have the opposite pattern (Gale & Gale, 1998; Krown, 1999).
     f. Diagnosis of KS of the lungs may be inferred in the setting of a patient with KS of the skin with a serosanguinous pleural effusion (Rosen & Schneider, 1998).

H. Common therapeutic modalities
   Treatments are either local, systemic, or both including
  1. Chemotherapies (Prevention and Treatment)
     a. Prevention and treatment of KS is best achieved through use of ART to maintain a high CD4 count and a low viral load. ART may help to limit the progression of KS (Bartlett & Gallant, 2003).
     b. Examples of some of the best chemotherapeutic agents used for KS include: liposomal doxorubicin (Doxil) and liposomal daunorubin

(DaunoXome). Refractory KS is treated with paclitaxel (Taxol). Other agents used are bleomycin, vinblastine, etoposide (VP-16), and vincristine. "Combinations such as Adriamycin, bleomycin, and vincristine have resulted in response rates up to 60% in patients with pulmonary KS" (Bartlett & Gallant, 2003; Krown, 1999; Trubowitz & Volberding, 2000, p. 1440).

    c. Interferon (IFN)-alpha (α) has been successfully used with some patients however due to the time that it takes to have drug action, it is not used in those patients presenting with acute respiratory distress. Dose limiting side effects of IFN-α are flu-like symptoms, neutropenia, and depression (Krown, 1999).

2. Although KS is caused by a virus the use of antiviral agents such as foscarnet or ganciclovir have not been shown effective for acute or chronic care management.

3. Radiation can be used if indicated for symptomatic airway obstruction or parenchymal lesions.

4. Symptom management or palliative care is sometimes warranted in advanced cases based on the wishes of the individual.

I. Home care considerations

1. For patients with adequate insurance and family supports consider HCW home visits intermittently between therapies such as chemotherapy and radiation.

2. Individuals without adequate health care insurance and funding may qualify for community, state, or federal programs for home health care visits, Ryan White funding (for hospice care, medications, and other services).

WEB SITES

Centers for Disease Control and Prevention, National Center for HIV, STD, and TB Prevention, Division of HIV/AIDS Prevention
    http://www.cdc.gov/hiv/pubs/facts.htm
    http://www.cdc.gov/hiv/stats.htm
    http://www.cdc.gov/hiv/pubs/brochure.htm
    http://www.cdc.gov/hiv/pubs/faqs.htm
    http://www.cdc.gov/hiv/hivinfo/cdcfax.htm
    http://www.cdc.gov/hiv/hivinfo.htm
    http://www.cdc.gov/hiv/conferen.htm
    http://www.cdc.gov/hiv/stats/cumulati.htm
National Institute of Allergy and Infectious Diseases, National Institutes of Health, Division of Acquired Immunodeficiency Syndrome.
    http://www.niaid.nih.gov/default.htm
    http://www.niaid.nih.gov/daids/
United States Public Health Service (USPHS) and Infectious Diseases Society of America (IDSA), USPHS/IDSA Prevention of Opportunistic Infections

Working Group. Masur, H., Kaplan, J. E., & Holmes, K. K. (Co-Chairs) (2001). 2001 *USPHS/IDSA Guidelines for the Prevention of Opportunistic Infections in Persons Infected with Human Immunodeficiency Virus.* AIDS Treatment Information Service (ATIS): Current Treatment Guidelines.
http://www.hivatis.org/trtgdins.html#Opportunistic

United States Department of Health and Human Services, National Aging Information Center
http://www.hhs.gov/
http://www.aoa.dhhs.gov/NAIC/Notes/hivaging.html

The Surgeon General's HIV/AIDS Web site
http://www.surgeongeneral.gov/aids/

Federal Drug Administration, HIV and AIDS Activities
http://www/fda.gov/oashi/aids/hiv.html

National Pediatric and Family HIV Resource Center, University of Medicine and Dentistry of New Jersey
http://www.pedhivaids.org

HIV/AIDS Treatment Information Service, A U.S. Department of Health and Human Services Project Managed by the National Library of Medicine, Panel on Clinical Practices for the Treatment of HIV Infection
http://www.hiv.hivatis.org

Johns Hopkins AIDS Service
http://www.hopkins-aids.edu/

The Body: An AIDS and HIV Information Resource
http://www.thebody.com/hivatis/pediatric/ped1.html
http://www.thebody.com/jh/jh.html

REFERENCES

Afessa, F. (2000). Pleural effusion and pneumothorax in hospitalized patients with HIV Infection. *Chest, 117*(4), 1031–1037.

Afessa, B., & Green, B. (2000). Clinical course, prognostic factors, and outcome prediction for HIV Patients in the ICU, *Chest, 118*(1), 138–145.

Bartlett, J. G., & Gallant, J. E. (2003). *Medical management of HIV infection (2003 Edition).* Baltimore, MD: Johns Hopkins University.

Cannon, M. J., Dollard, S. C., Smith, D. K., Klein, R. S., Schuman, P., Rich, J. D., et al. (2001). Blood-born and sexual transmission of human herpes virus 8 in women with or at risk for Human Immunodeficiency Virus Infection, *The New England Journal of Medicine, 344*(9), 637–643.

Dohn, M. N., White, M. L., Vigdorth, E. M., Buncher, C. R., Hertzberg, V. S., Baughman, R. P. et al. (2000). Geographic clustering of *Pneumocystis carinii* pneumonia in patients with HIV Infection. *American Journal of Respiratory and Critical Care Medicine, 162*(5), 1617–1621.

Feinberg, J. & Baughman, R. P. (1999). Pulmonary disease. In R. Dolin, H. Masur, & M. S. Saag (Eds.), *AIDS therapy* (pp. 699–711). Philadelphia, PA: Churchill Livingstone.

Gale, D. R. & Gale, M. E., (1998). Pulmonary imaging. In G. L. Baum, J. D. Crapo, B. R. Celli, & J. B. Karlinsky (Eds.), *Textbook of pulmonary diseases* (Vol. 1, pp. 181–188). Philadelphia, PA: Lippincott-Raven.

Girard, P. M., (2004). Pneumocystis carinii Pneumonia. In Cohen, J. & Powderly, W. G. (Eds.), *Infectious diseases* (Vol. 2, 2nd ed., pp. 1313–1314). Philadelphia, PA: Mosby.

Haramati, L. B., & Wong, J. (2000). Intrathoracic Kaposi's Sarcoma in women with AIDS. *Chest, 117,* 410–414.

Kovacs, J. A., Gill, V. J., Meschnick, S., & Masur, H. (2001). New insights into transmission, diagnosis, and drug treatment of Pneumocystis carinii Pneumonia. *Journal of the American Medical Association, 286*(19), 2450–2460.

Krown, S. E. (1999). Kaposi Sarcoma. In R. Dolin, H. Masur, & M. S. Saag (Eds.), *AIDS therapy* (pp. 307–321). Philadelphia, PA: Churchill Livingstone.

Masur, H. (1999). Pneumocystosis, In R. Dolin, H. Masur, & M. S. Saag (Eds.), *AIDS therapy* (pp. 291–306). Philadelphia, PA: Churchill Livingstone.

Masur, H. (2002). Abstract 586. In J. G. Bartlett, Report from ICACC: Update on Opportunistic Infections. *The Hopkins HIV Report, 14*(1), 5. The 41st Interscience Conference on Antimicrobial Agents and Chemotherapy (ICACC).

Masur, H., Kaplan, J. E., & Holmes, K. K. (Co-Chairs) (2001). 2001 *USPHS/IDSA Guidelines for the Prevention of Opportunistic Infections in Persons Infected with Human Immunodeficiency Virus.* AIDS Treatment Information Service (ATIS): Current Treatment Guidelines.

Morris, A. M., Swanson, M., Ha, H., & Huang, L. (2000). Geographic distribution of Human Immunodeficiency Virus-associated Pneumocystis carinii Pneumonia in San Francisco. *American Journal of Respiratory and Critical Care Medicine, 162*(5), 1622–1626.

Osmond, D. H., Buchbinder, S., Cheng, A., Graves, A., Vittinghoff, E., Cossen, C. K., et al. (2002). Prevalence of Kaposi Sarcoma-Associated Herpes virus Infection in homosexual men at beginning of and during the HIV Epidemic, *Journal of the American Medical Association, 287*(2), 221–225.

Pizzo, P. A., & Mueller, F. U. (1993). Pediatric AIDS: What the pediatric oncologist needs to know. In P. A. Pizzo, & D. G. Poplick (Eds.). *Principles and practice of pediatric oncology* (2nd ed., pp. 945–946). Philadelphia, PA: J. B. Lippincott.

Quinn, T. C. (2001, March). HIV in the New Millennium (Presenter) *Clinical Care of the Patient with HIV infection.* Symposium conducted at the meeting of the 11th Johns Hopkins Department of Medicine Annual Course on HIV, Baltimore, Maryland.

Rosen, M. J., & Schneider, R. F. (1998) Pulmonary Complications of HIV Infection. In G. L. Baum, J. D. Crapo, B. R. Celli, & J. B. Karlinsky (Eds.), *Textbook of pulmonary diseases* (Vol. 1, pp. 561–575). Philadelphia, PA: Lippincott-Raven.

Shelhamer, J., Pizzo, P., Parrillo, J., & Masur, H. (1991). *Respiratory diseases in the immunosuppressed host.* Philadelphia, PA: J. B. Lippincott Co.

Strauss, S. E., (2000), Human Herpesvirus Type 8 (Kaposi's Sarcoma-Associated Herpes Virus). In G. L. Mandell, J. E. Bennett, & R. Dolin (Eds.), *Principles and*

Practice of Infectious Diseases. (Vol. 2, 5th ed., pp. 1618–1621). Philadelphia, PA: Churchill Livingstone.

Stringer, J. R., Beard, C. B., Miller, R. F., & Wakefield, A. E. (2002). A new name (Pneumocystis jiroveci) for Pneumocystis from humans. *Emerging Infectious Diseases, 8*(9), 891–896.

Tirelli, U. & Vaccher, E., (2004). Neoplastic Disease. In Cohen, J. & Powderly, W. G. (Eds.), *Infectious Diseases* (Vol. 2, 2nd ed., pp. 1313–1314). Philadelphia, PA: Mosby.

Trubowitz, P. R., & Volberding, P. A. (2000). Malignancies in Human Immuno- deficiency Virus Infection. In G. L. Mandell, J. E. Bennett, & R. Dolin (Eds.), *Principles and practice of infectious diseases.* (Vol. 2., 5th ed., pp. 1439–1442). Philadelphia, PA: Churchill Livingstone.

Walzer, P. D. (2000). Pneumocystis carinii. In G. L. Mandell, J. E. Bennett, & R. Dolin (Eds.), *Principles and practice of infectious diseases* (Vol. 2, 5th ed., pp. 2781–2795). Philadelphia, PA: Churchill Livingstone.

Wilkins, R., & Dexter, J. (1998). Bacterial Pneumonia. In Wilkens, R., Dexter, J. & Gold, P. (Eds.), *Respiratory disease, a case study approach to patient care* (2nd ed., pp. 323–338). Philadelphia, PA: F. A. Davis Company.

SUGGESTED READINGS

Afessa, F. (2000). Pleural effusion and pneumothorax in hospitalized patients with HIV Infection. *Chest, 117*(4), 1031–1037.

Bartlett, J. G., & Gallant, J. E. (2000). *Medical Management of HIV Infection (2000–2001 Edition)*. Baltimore: Port City Press.

Bartlett, J. G., & Gallant, J. E. (2001). *Medical Management of HIV Infection (2001–2002 Edition)*. Timonium, MD: H & N Printing & Graphics.

Chernecky, C. C., & Berger, G. J. (2001). *Laboratory tests and diagnostic proce- dures* (3rd ed.). Philadelphia, PA: W. B. Saunders Co.

Cohen, O., Cicala, C., Vaccarezza, M., & Fauci, A. (2000). The immunology of human immunodeficiency virus infection. In G. L. Mandell, J. E. Bennett, & R. Dolin (Eds.), *Principles and practices of infectious diseases* (Vol. 1, 25th ed., pp. 1374–1387). Philadelphia, PA: Churchill Livingstone.

Del Rio, C., & Curran, J. W. (2000). Epidemiology and prevention of Acquired Im- munodeficiency Syndrome and Human Immunodeficiency Virus Infection. In G. L. Mandell, J. E. Bennett, & R. Dolin (Eds.), *Principles and practices of in- fectious diseases* (Vol. 1, 25th ed., pp. 1340–1344). Philadelphia, PA: Churchill Livingstone.

Kovacs, J. A., & Masur, H. (2000). Prophylaxis against opportunistic infections in patients with Human Immunodeficiency Virus Infection. *The New England Journal of Medicine, 342*(19), 1416–1429.

Masur, H. (2000). Management of opportunistic infections associated with Human Immunodeficiency Virus Infection. In G. L. Mandell, J. E. Bennett, & R. Dolin (Eds.), *Principles and practices of infectious diseases* (Vol. 1, 25th ed., pp. 1500–1519). Philadelphia, PA: Churchill Livingstone.

Masur, H. (1991). Pneumocystis carinii Pneumonia. In J. Shelhamer, P. A. Pizzo, J. E. Parilb, & H. Masur (Eds.), *Respiratory disease in the immunosuppressed host* (pp. 409–427). Philadelphia, PA: J. B. Lippincott.

Nduati, R., John, G., Mbori-Ngaetia, D., Richardson, B., Overbaugh, J., Mwatha, A. et al. (2000). Effect of breastfeeding and formula feeding on transmission of HIV-1. *Journal of the American Medical Association, 283*(9), 1167–1174.

Panel on Clinical Practices for the Treatment of HIV Infection. (2001). *Guidelines for the use of antiretroviral agents in HIV-infected Adults and Adolescents* (Booklet). Menlo Park, CA: Department of Health and Human Services/ Henry J. Kaiser Family Foundation.

Schoub, B. D. (1999). *AIDS and HIV in perspective: A guide to understanding the virus and its consequences* (2nd ed.). Cambridge: Cambridge University Press.

Sprecht, N. L. (1993). Pneumonia in the immunocompromised patient. In R. L. Wilkins & J. R. Dexter (Eds), *Respiratory disease: A case study approach to patient care* (2nd ed., pp. 339–356). Philadelphia, PA: F. A. Davis.

Suffredini, A. F. & Shellhamer, J. H. (1991). Pulmonary disease in the HIV-infected patient. In J. Shelhamer, P. A. Pizzo, J. E. Parilb, & H. Masur (Eds.), *Respiratory diseases in the immunosuppressed host* (pp. 537–566). Philadelphia, PA: J. B. Lippincott Co.

Watts, D. H. (1999). Managing pregnant patients. In R. Dolin, H. Masur, & M. S. Saag (Eds.), *AIDS therapy* (pp. 279–287). Philadelphia: PA Churchill Livingstone.

Wood, B. J., & Wood, S. D. (1998). HIV imaging. In Wood, B. J. & Wood, S. D. (Eds.), *Radiology* (pp. 185–189). Baltimore, MD: Williams & Wilkins.

Pulmonary Hypertension

Christine Archer-Chicko

INTRODUCTION

Pulmonary hypertension is a serious, progressive disease in which there are pathologic changes in the small vessels of the pulmonary vascular bed. This disease is confirmed at cardiac catheterization and without appropriate therapeutic intervention, cor pulmonale and eventual death would ensue. Since the prognosis for patients is improved and changing with the advent of newer therapies, health care providers need to be aware of the early symptoms and the patient populations at risk to facilitate a prompt referral to a pulmonary hypertension center.

I. Overview

This chapter will focus on pulmonary arterial hypertension, including pathophysiology, classification, clinical presentation, diagnostic evaluation, and therapeutic interventions.

  A. Definition

Pulmonary arterial hypertension is an elevation of pressure in the main pulmonary artery at rest or with exercise. More specifically, pulmonary arterial hypertension exists when the mean pulmonary artery pressure is >25 mm Hg at rest or >30 mm Hg during exercise at catheterization with a normal capillary wedge pressure.

  B. Etiology

Although the exact etiology of pulmonary hypertension is unknown, there are risk factors and medical conditions that are associated with the disease.

    1. Drugs and toxic agents

      a. Anorectic agents: Aminorex, Fenfluramine, Dexfenfluramine

      b. Rapeseed oil

      c. Amphetamines

      d. L-tryptophan

       e. Other possible agents: Meta-amphetamines, Cocaine, Chemo-
          therapeutic agents

  2. Demographics
     a. Female gender

  3. Medical conditions
     a. Pregnancy
     b. Systemic hypertension
     c. HIV infection
     d. Liver disease/Portal hypertension
     e. Collagen vascular disease
     f. Congenital systemic-pulmonary cardiac shunts
     g. Other possible condition: Thyroid disease

  4. The exact cause of pulmonary hypertension varies from patient to patient and it appears that multiple factors may play a role. The main focus of research regarding the pathogenesis is related to the vascular endothelium and its role in control of the pulmonary vascular bed. It is believed to be metabolically active tissue that responds to changes in oxygen partial pressure, blood flow, and transmural pressure. Different forms of pulmonary hypertension may exhibit particular patterns of endothelial cell dysfunction that may correspond to the specific type of injury. Although there are a variety of stimuli that may be responsible, there is new evidence that a genetic component may make an individual susceptible to a particular stimulus.

C. Pathophysiology

  1. Under normal conditions, the pulmonary vascular bed is a low-pressure system (or circuit) with a mean pressure approximately one-sixth of the systemic arterial pressure. It has a large capacity to compensate for an increase in blood flow without elevating the circuit's pressure. The pulmonary vascular bed achieves this compensation by dilation of blood vessels and by recruiting pulmonary vessels that are not usually perfused at rest.

  2. Pulmonary hypertension is present when there is an elevation in the pulmonary vascular pressures. It may be an acute or chronic elevation of pressures depending on the etiology.

  3. On a cellular level, this disease process occurs as a result of several types of pathologic changes that occur in the pulmonary vessels, which alters their structure and ultimately, their function.

  4. Although the pathologic abnormalities in the pulmonary vascular bed may differ slightly depending upon the etiology of the hypertension, there are common changes seen in precapillary pulmonary hypertension conditions. These changes are collectively referred to as *plexogenic pulmonary arteriopathy*. Common features of plexogenic pulmonary arteriopathy include
     a. Dilated main pulmonary arteries (may become larger than the aorta and/or may create a localized aneurysm)
     b. Pulmonary arterial atherosclerosis involving the larger vessels

    c. Intimal fibrosis of the larger elastic and muscular arteries (scars the vessel wall and may obliterate the lumen)

    d. Thickening of the media of small muscular arteries caused by a combination of muscle hypertrophy and hyperplasia (Although there are variations, the degree of medial thickening may indicate the severity of the pulmonary hypertension.)

    e. Cellular intimal proliferation and fibrosis of medium sized and small vessels

    f. In situ thrombosis

    g. Plexiform lesions that appear as a vascular dilation with a plexus of numerous slit-like vascular channels separated by small amounts of connective tissue and fibroblast-like cells

5. In some cases, in the early stages, the elevated pulmonary artery pressures are largely caused by vasoconstriction (such as by hypoxemia) and therefore, may be somewhat reversible. In other cases, the elevated pressures are a result of structural changes in the pulmonary vascular bed (such as by emboli) and therefore, are most likely irreversible.

6. Over time, cellular proliferation and the development of fibrosis within the media and intimal layers of the small pulmonary arteries and arterioles leads to increasing pulmonary vascular resistance and a loss of vasodilator responsiveness.

7. Clinically, as patients develop elevated pulmonary artery pressures and increased pulmonary vascular resistance, the heart becomes strained from the added workload. These cardiac changes can be seen in the right ventricular (RV) wall as concentric hypertrophy. The magnitude of the RV wall changes is related to the severity and the chronicity of the pulmonary hypertension. Eventually, the right ventricle will fail (known as *cor pulmonale*) because of the excessive workload and RV dilatation will be seen.

D. Incidence

  1. Genetic predisposition

    The estimated prevalence of familial primary pulmonary hypertension (PPH) worldwide is at least 6% but is probably higher.

  2. Familial PPH has unique characteristics

    a. The age of onset of PPH is variable and the penetrance is incomplete.

    b. Genetic anticipation has been seen; in each subsequent generation the age of presentation becomes younger.

    c. Many individuals in families with PPH inherit the gene yet never develop PPH themselves.

    d. Fewer males are born into PPH families as compared to the general population, which may suggest that the PPH gene may effect fertilization or influence fetal loss.

  3. Patients with familial PPH have a similar gender ratio, age of onset, and natural history of the disease as those with so-called sporadic PPH.

4. Documenting familial PPH is difficult because the disease may appear to have involved distant family members or have skipped generations (as a result of incomplete penetrance or variable expression of the PPH gene) and therefore been thought of as sporadic PPH.

5. Both familial PPH and sporadic PPH have essentially identical pathologic and clinical features, and it is believed that the same gene(s) may be responsible for the development of both forms of the disease.

6. Transmission of the PPH gene has been seen in as many as five generations in one family and is believed to represent a single autosomal dominant gene.

7. The low penetrance of this gene translates into a 10%–20% chance of developing the disease.

8. The locus of a gene linked to familial PPH has been identified on chromosome 2q31–32. This appears to be a mutation in the bone morphogenetic protein receptor II (BMPR II). Alterations in this gene appear to result in uncontrolled cellular proliferation in response to stimuli.

9. Because little information is known regarding the PPH gene and its relationship to the disease, genetic testing is not recommended at this time.

II. Types/classification of pulmonary hypertension (World Health Organization [WHO] meeting held in Evian, France in September 1998)

   A. Pulmonary arterial hypertension

      1. Primary pulmonary hypertension (PPH)

         a. Types of PPH

            i. Sporadic

            ii. Familial

         b. Specific features of PPH

            i. Incidence is 1–2 per million population per year.

            ii. Typically affects young woman age 21–51 with a female to male predominance of at least 1.7 to 1.

            iii. In most cases the etiology is unknown and cases appear to occur in a sporadic fashion, however, there is a small subset of patients in which the PPH is familial.

            iv. The prognosis for patients with PPH is somewhat improved and changing with the availability of new treatment options. Patients may remain relatively stable on oral agents or other therapies, such as continuous intravenous Epoprostenol (Flolan), for several years. Furthermore, lung transplantation is another available treatment option. In the past, patients could only expect progressive dyspnea, right heart failure, and death within a few years.

      2. As related to collagen vascular disease

         a. Pulmonary arterial hypertension is most commonly seen in the Scleroderma spectrum of diseases, although it has been observed in all types of collagen vascular disease.

         b. These patients frequently have Raynaud's phenomenon supporting the concept that the pulmonary hypertension is a part of a generalized vasculopathy.

3. As related to congenital systemic-to-pulmonary shunts
   a. Pulmonary arterial flow may have been increased for a long time before the patient develops pulmonary hypertension. Eventually, the persistent left-to-right shunting creates irreversible, pathologic changes in the pulmonary vascular bed.
   b. Clinically, most patients are fairly asymptomatic although may complain of fatigue, palpitations, and dyspnea on exertion. If the shunt is large, patients may be underdeveloped and susceptible to recurrent respiratory infections.
   c. In addition, patients may demonstrate cyanosis, clubbing, and cachexia.
   d. Physical exam is consistent with the particular type of congenital abnormality.
   e. Survival and prognosis in these patients is better than those with PPH.
4. As related to portal hypertension
   a. Overall the incidence of pulmonary hypertension in patients with cirrhosis is low; however, in severe cases of liver disease, it may be more prevalent.
   b. There are two theories regarding the pathogenesis of pulmonary hypertension in liver disease
      i. There may be vasoactive or vasotoxic substances produced in the gastrointestinal tract that are normally metabolized by the liver but instead reach the pulmonary vasculature in patients with cirrhosis, portal hypertension, and portosystemic shunts.
      ii. There may be a relationship between pulmonary hypertension and the altered hemodynamics in liver disease.
5. Human immunodeficiency virus (HIV) infection
   a. Clinical presentation is identical to PPH, yet the age of onset is earlier (32 +/− 5 years).
   b. The natural history of this type of pulmonary hypertension is rapidly progressive with one study documenting a 1-year survival rate at 50%.
6. Drugs/toxins
   a. Anorexigens
   b. Other
   c. A variety of drugs and toxins have been responsible for causing pulmonary hypertension:
      i. Appetite suppressants: fenfluramine and dexfenfluramine
      ii. Contaminated rapeseed oil
      iii. Medicinal preparations containing large quantity of L-tryptophan
      iv. Various plant alkaloids such as *C. fulva* found in bush tea
      v. Amphetamines
      vi. Cocaine
7. Persistent pulmonary hypertension of the newborn

B. Pulmonary venous hypertension
   1. Left-sided atrial or ventricular heart disease
   2. Left-sided valvular heart disease
   3. Extrinsic compression of central pulmonary veins
      a. Fibrosing mediastinitis
      b. Adenopathy/tumors
   4. Pulmonary veno-occlusive disease
   5. Other
      a. Pulmonary venous hypertension has a different pathophysiology and clinical course than pulmonary arterial hypertension. It occurs as a result of any disease/condition that significantly increases the pulmonary venous pressure.
      b. Because the primary site of the pulmonary hypertension is postcapillary, the veins and venules reflect the pathologic changes prior to irreversible, secondary changes to the arterial side of the pulmonary vascular bed.
      c. Patients present with complaints of orthopnea and paroxysmal nocturnal dyspnea as initial symptoms rather than dyspnea on exertion. They may have a history of episodes of chronic congestive heart failure with pulmonary edema.
C. Pulmonary hypertension associated with disorders of the respiratory system or hypoxemia
   1. Chronic obstructive pulmonary disease (COPD)
   2. Interstitial lung disease
   3. Sleep-disordered breathing
   4. Alveolar hypoventilation disorders
   5. Chronic exposure to high altitude
   6. Neonatal lung disease
   7. Alveolar-capillary dysplasia
   8. Other
      a. It is believed that hypoxemia is the main cause of pulmonary hypertension in this group of diseases. Pulmonary artery pressures do not increase as dramatically as in primary vascular disease. In addition, the histologic features of plexogenic arteriopathy are not present.
      b. Emphysema patients have pulmonary hypertension as a result of both hypoxemia and destruction of the microvasculature. The pulmonary hypertension can acutely worsen during periods of exacerbation or respiratory insufficiency.
      c. Supplemental oxygen usually provides significant clinical improvement.
      d. Patients who have had a pulmonary resection may later develop pulmonary hypertension as a result of increased blood flow through the reduced pulmonary vascular bed creating sclerotic changes in the pulmonary vasculature.
D. Pulmonary hypertension caused by chronic thrombotic or embolic disease

1. Thromboembolic obstruction of proximal pulmonary arteries
2. Obstruction of distal pulmonary arteries
    a. Pulmonary embolism (thrombus, tumor, ova or parasites, foreign material)
    b. In situ thrombosis
    c. Sickle cell disease: Pulmonary hypertension can occur as a consequence of either acute pulmonary emboli or of chronic unresolved pulmonary emboli.
    d. For management of acute pulmonary emboli, refer to chapter 23, "Pulmonary Thromboembolism."
    e. The treatment of chronic unresolved pulmonary emboli includes anticoagulation, pulmonary vasodilators, and consideration of surgery to remove the chronic organized emboli material. (See Thromboendarterectomy section below.)
  E. Pulmonary hypertension caused by disorders directly affecting the pulmonary vasculature
    1. Inflammatory
        a. Schistosomiasis
        b. Sarcoidosis
        c. Other
    2. Pulmonary capillary hemangiomatosis
III. Considerations across the life span
  A. Pediatrics
    1. Children are usually diagnosed earlier when they have WHO Functional Class II symptoms. This is probably because children are more active than adults and their symptoms are picked up more quickly.
    2. Unfortunately, if pulmonary hypertension is not treated, it will worsen more quickly in children as compared to adults.
    3. Overall, the prognosis for children with treatment is better than for adults. There are a few possible reasons for this.
        a. Children have more vasoreactivity to their pulmonary vascular bed and therefore will respond more readily to vasodilator therapies.
        b. Because children are not fully grown, there is some capacity to develop more blood vessels in the pulmonary vascular bed.
        c. Being diagnosed early is beneficial.
  B. Pregnancy
    1. A subset of young women will be diagnosed with pulmonary hypertension following a pregnancy and childbirth. It is not yet known what influence hormones may have in this instance.
    2. Young women of child-bearing age with pulmonary hypertension are counseled to avoid pregnancy because of high risk of maternal mortality.
  C. Elderly
    1. Older patients with pulmonary hypertension are typically those with an underlying and advanced medical condition such as Scleroderma, Idiopathic pulmonary fibrosis, or Emphysema, and so forth.

2. Ten percent of PPH patients present after the age of 60; in these patients the female to male ratio is more equal than in younger patients.

IV. Complications/sequelae
  A. Progression of pulmonary hypertension/failure of therapy leading to right heart failure and death
  B. Progression of secondary disease process (Liver disease, HIV disease, Scleroderma, etc.)
  C. Hypoxemia
  D. Intolerance of oral vasodilator therapy
    1. Hypotension
    2. Tachycardia
    3. Weakness
  E. Problems of fluid balance
    1. Overdiuresis
    2. Fluid overload
  F. Electrolyte imbalance related to use of diuretics
  G. Non-therapeutic anticoagulation
    1. Excessive anticoagulation leading to bleeding
    2. Insufficient anticoagulation
  H. Problems related to continuous intravenous Epoprostenol therapy
    1. Failure to respond to therapy
    2. Mechanical failure
      a. Loss of Hickman catheter function—hole or leak in the catheter, line misplacement (catheter falls out or is pulled out accidentally)
      b. Malfunction of infusion pump
      c. Defective tubing or medication cassette
    3. Patient error
      a. Incorrectly setting infusion pump
      b. Incorrectly mixing medication
      c. Lack of sterile technique
    4. Hickman catheter infection
      a. Cellulitis at site
      b. Hickman catheter tract infection
      c. Bloodstream infection (sepsis)

V. Assessment
  A. History
    1. Current functional status including experience of dyspnea, dizziness, syncope or fatigue, degree of functional impairment and development of central or peripheral edema
    2. Past medical history including disease processes or risk factors associated with pulmonary hypertension such as
      a. Liver disease
      b. Collagen vascular disease
      c. Thromboembolic disease
      d. Lung disease
      e. Valvular heart disease
      f. Congenital heart disease

g. Disordered breathing or snoring

h. HIV disease

i. Thyroid dysfunction

3. Substance abuse including illicit drugs or ingestion of diet pills and duration of use

4. Family history of cardiac, pulmonary, or thromboembolic disease

B. Physical exam

■ The clinical presentation is dependent upon the underlying disease process.

■ Typically, patients initially present with complaints of dyspnea, fatigue, and a decline in exercise capacity. Some may report having experienced a syncopal episode or periods of dizziness. Chest pain is often very difficult to differentiate from angina.

1. Common signs and symptoms

a. Dyspnea with exercise or rest

b. Fatigue

c. Decline in exercise capacity

d. Edema

e. Chest pain (angina-like)

f. Palpitations

g. Syncope or presyncope

h. Cough

i. Hoarseness

j. Hypotension

k. Hypoxemia

2. Physical exam findings

a. Vitals: normal or low BP

b. General: pale or cyanotic

c. Head eyes ears nose throat (HEENT): increased jugular venous distension

d. Respiratory

i. depends upon presence of lung disease

ii. usually clear (adventitious sounds are possible)

iii. If a pleural effusion is present, decreased sounds at affected base(s)

e. Cardiac: RV lift, RV third and/or fourth heart sound increased split of second heart sound with increased pulmonic component systolic murmur at 2nd Left intercoastal space (ICS) increasing with inspiration (Tricuspid regurgitation) soft diastolic murmur at 3rd Left ICS close to sternum (Pulmonic regurgitation)

f. Abdomen

i. hepatomegaly

ii. ascites

g. Extremities

i. peripheral edema, especially in lower extremities

ii. pale, cool extremities

iii. pale or dusky nailbeds

C. Diagnostic tests/screening

1. May allow early diagnosis in minimally symptomatic patients or in symptomatic patients whom were not suspected as having pulmonary hypertension and initiation of timely treatment when reversible pathogenic mechanisms are present.

2. Includes a comprehensive patient interview to elicit clear or subtle symptoms that developed and/or progressed over time. Some patients choose to ignore the early symptoms or ascribe them to stress, aging, and lack of exercise or overwork. An astute care provider recognizes populations at risk, early symptoms and promptly refers the patient for screening.

3. A transthoracic echocardiogram is currently the preferred diagnostic study used for pulmonary hypertension screening (noninvasive, low risk, and has a relatively high sensitivity and specificity). In patients who have exertional symptomatology and a relatively normal resting echocardiogram, performing an echocardiogram immediately after maximal exercise may aid in the detection of early pulmonary vascular disease.

4. Patient populations who should be screened for pulmonary hypertension include

   a. Connective tissue diseases

      i. Scleroderma

         It is recommended that these patients have an echocardiogram annually due to the high prevalence of pulmonary hypertension in this group.

      ii. Systemic lupus, rheumatoid arthritis, and other connective tissues diseases

         There is a low occurrence of pulmonary hypertension in this group; therefore, only patients who are symptomatic should be screened.

   b. Families with PPH

      An echocardiogram may be considered for first-degree relatives at the time of diagnosis or at any time symptoms consistent with pulmonary hypertension develop. Otherwise, an echocardiogram may be performed every 3–5 years in asymptomatic individuals.

   c. Liver disease/portal hypertension

      All patients who are being evaluated for liver transplantation should be evaluated for pulmonary hypertension before listing because pulmonary hypertension places them at high risk for transplantation and because there are therapeutic options available.

   d. HIV infection

      There is low prevalence in this group so only symptomatic individuals require screening.

   e. Patients with a history of diet drug use

      Because of the low prevalence in this population, only symptomatic individuals require an echocardiogram to screen for pulmonary hypertension.

f. Patients with a history of intravenous drug use

An echocardiogram is recommended only for symptomatic patients because the prevalence of pulmonary hypertension in this group is uncertain.

D. Diagnostic tests/evaluation

1. Chest X-ray

Reveals evidence of pulmonary hypertension in more than 90% of advanced cases. Prominence of the main pulmonary artery and hilar vessel enlargement are frequently seen. Cardiomegaly is present with an enlarged RV on the posteroanterior view and increased retrosternal filling on the lateral view. Pruning of the vessels with hyperlucent lung periphery may also be seen.

2. Electrocardiogram (EKG)

Patients with PH usually have normal sinus rhythm with evidence of right atrial (RA) and right ventricular (RV) enlargement. RA enlargement is seen when P waves are greater than 2.5 mm in leads II, III, and aVF. RV hypertrophy is present when a tall R wave and a small S wave in lead V_1, a tall S wave with small R wave in lead V_5 or V_6 and right axis deviation (QRS axis > 90').

3. Transthoracic echocardiogram with doppler

a. A two-dimensional echocardiogram can detect abnormalities of the RV such as hypertrophy, dilatation, and global hypokinesis. It can also assess for structural and functional problems involving left ventricular function, valvular abnormalities and provide information regarding intracardiac shunts.

b. Measurement of the tricuspid regurgitant jet provides an estimate of the pressure gradient between the RV and the RA. It is useful in determining the RV systolic pressure, which is a close estimate of the pulmonary artery pressure.

c. May be used as a noninvasive method to follow patients and monitor the progression of their disease and their response to therapy.

4. Ventilation perfusion scan

Must be performed to rule out chronic thromboembolic pulmonary hypertension. A negative or low probability scan rules out chronic emboli as the cause of the elevated pulmonary pressures.

5. Pulmonary angiogram

If the lung scan shows one or more segmental or larger ventilation-perfusion mismatches, an angiogram should be performed in evaluating for thromboendarterectomy. This should be done at centers experienced in performing angiograms in patients with pulmonary hypertension and with experience in interpreting studies for chronic pulmonary emboli.

6. Computed tomography (CT) of the chest

a. A high-resolution scan may also be performed to assess lung parenchyma for fibrosis and emphysema and to detect pulmonary veno-occlusive disease.

b. The value of serial CT scans has not been documented.

7. Magnetic resonance imaging (MRI) of the chest
    a. MR imaging can be used to provide detailed images of cardio-vascular structure and may be useful in the setting of congenital heart disease.
    b. The usefulness of serial MRI studies has not been established.
8. Pulmonary function studies
    a. Patients with PPH may have the following functional abnormalities on pulmonary function tests (PFTs): mild restriction, small airways dysfunction, reduced carbon monoxide diffusing capacity, and impaired gas exchange as evidenced by hypoxemia. If more severe restrictive or obstructive abnormalities are seen, an additional pulmonary disease should be considered.
    b. In patients with unexplained dyspnea, an isolated decrease in diffusing capacity on PFTs should raise the possibility of pulmonary vascular disease.
9. Exercise testing
    Six-minute walk tests or cardiopulmonary exercise tests are helpful at the time of diagnosis and as serial studies to evaluate and trend the functional status of patients with pulmonary hypertension.
10. Connective tissue serologies
    No specific pattern of serologic titers is associated with pulmonary hypertension.
11. Lung biopsy
    a. Performance is limited to establish a diagnosis in a complicated case, since treatment options are sometimes only diagnosis specific.
    b. Transbronchial biopsy is not helpful as the specimens are typically inadequate and the procedure may be risky due to elevated pulmonary pressures.
    c. Open lung biopsy with thoracoscopy is the preferred method.
    d. Biopsy specimens should be referred to a pathologist with expertise in pulmonary vascular disease.
12. Right heart catheterization and pulmonary vasodilator testing
    a. The right heart catheterization is required to accurately confirm the diagnosis of pulmonary hypertension. It is also used to assess the severity of the disease and to guide therapy.
    b. The following hemodynamic parameters should be measured as part of the catheterization
        i. right atrial pressure
        ii. right ventricular systolic and end-diastolic pressure
        iii. pulmonary artery systolic, diastolic and mean pressure
        iv. pulmonary capillary wedge pressure
        v. systemic and pulmonary arterial oxygen saturation
        vi. cardiac output
    c. It is recommended that all patients should have acute testing with a short-acting vasodilator to determine the vasoreactivity

of their pulmonary vascular bed. The following vasodilators are recommended.

    i. Inhaled nitric oxide

    ii. Intravenous or inhaled epoprostenol sodium (Flolan)

    iii. Intravenous adenosine (Adenocard)

  d. Patients who appear to respond to the acute vasodilator testing may also have a favorable response to oral calcium channel blockers. Although there is no consensus about what constitutes a positive vasodilator response, a minimum acceptable response would be a reduction in the pulmonary vascular resistance of 20% associated with either no change or an increase in the cardiac output.

  e. Patients who do not demonstrate vasoreactivity to the acute vasodilator testing are unlikely to demonstrate a clinical improvement with oral calcium channel blocker therapy.

  f. The right heart catheterization may be repeated at serial intervals (i.e., annually) or when the physician needs to re-evaluate the patient's hemodynamic status in order to optimize medical therapy.

VI. Common therapeutic modalities

  A. Medical management of pulmonary hypertension

    1. Anticoagulation

    Action: prevents the formation of in situ thrombi in the small pulmonary arteries in patients with all forms of pulmonary hypertension. Additional risk factors for clot formation include a sedentary lifestyle, dilated right heart chambers, sluggish blood flow, and venous insufficiency.

    Agents: Warfarin (Coumadin)

    Dosing: recommended range is an INR 1.5 to 2.5, however, may be individualized depending on clinical situation

    Side Effects: hemorrhagic episodes

    Effectiveness: has been shown to be effective in improving patient survival.

    2. Oxygen

    Action: prevents hypoxemia and reduces hypoxic vasoconstriction

    Dosing: maintain acceptable PaO_2 and oxygen saturations above 90% at rest, during activity and while sleeping

    Effectiveness: has been shown to reduce mortality and improve function and quality of life for patients with chronic obstructive pulmonary disease.

    3. Inotropic agents

    Action: improves right ventricular performance

    Agents: Digoxin (Lanoxin)

    Dosing: to maintain therapeutic drug levels

    Side Effects: toxicity (arrhythmias, weakness, nausea, vomiting, diarrhea, blurred vision, halos, dizziness, chest pain, palpitations, anxiety)

Effectiveness: there is data to support the benefits of chronic inotropic therapy in right heart failure.

4. Diuretics

Action: reduces intravascular volume, hepatic congestion, peripheral edema

Agents: Furosemide (Lasix), Spironolactone (Aldactone), Metolazone (Zaroxolyn), Bumetanide (Bumex), Torsemide (Demadex)

Dosing: individualized

Side effects: electrolyte imbalance, overdiuresis

Effectiveness: has been shown to be effective in managing heart failure and in improving dyspnea.

5. Vasodilator agents (Oral agents)

The goal of vasodilator therapy is to reduce the pulmonary artery pressure and to increase the cardiac output without producing systemic hypotension.

a. Calcium channel blockers

Action: inhibit calcium influx through the channel into cardiac and smooth muscle cells causing vasodilation of the pulmonary vascular smooth muscle. They also may have negative inotropic effects.

Agents: Nifedipine (Procardia), Diltiazem (Cardizem), Amlodipine (Norvasc)

Dosing: most patients require high doses; however, dosing is very individualized

Side effects: peripheral edema, systemic hypotension, pulmonary edema, right heart failure, death

Effectiveness: approximately only 20% of patients respond to calcium channel blockers. Patients who do not demonstrate an acute vasodilator response are unlikely to benefit from chronic therapy. However, patients who do respond to calcium channel blockers have demonstrated a 95% survival at 5 years in contrast to a 36% survival in nonresponders.

b. Angiotensin II receptor antagonist

Action: blocks the vasoconstrictor and aldosterone-secreting effects of angiotensin II to receptor sites on vascular smooth muscle

Agents: Losarten (Cozaar), Enalapril (Vasotec), Captopril (Capoten), and others

Dosing: individualized

Side effects: hypotension, tachycardia

Effectiveness: individual patients may respond to these agents, but they are generally less effective than calcium channel blockers

6. Endothelin receptor–A & B antagonist

The vascular endothelium or blood vessel wall lining is comprised of endothelial cells. These endothelial cells produce a number of substances that may promote or impede blood flow through the blood vessel. Endothelin is one such substance that is a potent vasoconstrictor and causes smooth muscle proliferation that can lead to increased pressure in the blood vessel and chronic changes in the vascular wall. In patients with PPH or PH and Scleroderma, there are high concentrations of endothelin in their blood, which are believed to be responsible for the pathologic effects.

a. Bosentan (Tracleer)

Action: blocks both endothelin receptor subtypes (ET_A and ET_B) thereby preventing the pathogenic effects of endothelin, which includes pulmonary vasoconstriction, inflammation, proliferation, and fibrosis

Dosing: 62.5 mg BID or 125 mg BID

Side effects: may elevate hepatic enzymes (reversible with lower dose or cessation of therapy); likely to cause major birth defects

Note(s): It is required that liver function tests be monitored on a monthly basis in all patients. In addition, patients are counseled to avoid pregnancy while taking Bosentan and to utilize a barrier method of birth control.

Effectiveness: a new drug class for chronic oral therapy; has improved exercise capacity and hemodynamics in patients with PPH and PH due to Scleroderma; long-term effectiveness, improved survival, and long-term safety of Bosentan has been documented.

7. Prostaglandins: Intravenous agents

a. Epoprostenol sodium (Flolan)

Action: potent systemic and pulmonary vasodilator inhibits platelet aggregation and smooth muscle proliferation; has a short half-life of 3–5 minutes and is chemically unstable at room temperature

Dosing: administered as a continuous intravenous infusion with a small ambulatory infusion pump through a central venous access (i.e., Hickman catheter). Patients are usually initiated on a low dose 2 ng/kg/min and titrated up as tolerated. The method of dosing is very individualized. Patients develop a tolerance and usually require increased doses on a periodic basis.

Side effects: flushing, hypotension, jaw discomfort, diarrhea/ soft stools, headache, nausea/vomiting, musculoskeletal pain, thrombocytopenia.

Note: There are additional adverse effects that may occur as a result of the delivery system: Hickman site infections, sepsis, pump malfunction/failure, catheter dislodgment, or loss of function. Patients are cautioned that an inadvertent interruption in therapy could result in a rebound effect due to the short half-life of the drug. Patients must receive extensive education on how to be prepared to handle an emergency situation.

Effectiveness: Has been shown to improve exercise tolerance, quality of life, hemodynamics, and survival in patients with WHO Functional Class III and IV symptoms. Clinically, it lowers the pulmonary artery pressure, increases the cardiac output, improves oxygen transport, and possibly reverses pulmonary vascular remodeling. It has been successfully used for patients who did not demonstrate any vasoreactivity at the time of acute vasodilator testing. In addition, some patients have remained stable with an epoprostenol infusion and have been able to defer the timing of lung transplantation.

8. Prostaglandins: Subcutaneous agents
   a. Treprostinil (Remodulin)

   Action: vasodilation of the systemic and pulmonary vascular beds and inhibition of platelet aggregation (same as Epoprostenol sodium); has a half-life of 3 hours; stable at room temperature

   Dosing: administered as an infusion via a subcutaneous needle and tubing with a small ambulatory infusion pump. Patients are typically started on a low dose of 1.25 ng/kg/min and then increased gradually over time. The method of dosing is very individualized.

   Side effects: headache, flushing, stomachache, diarrhea, jaw pain, and skin reaction/pain at the site of infusion. (Skin reactions include: erythema, rash, and induration. Approximately 85% of patients experience significant pain at the infusion site necessitating the use of oral pain killers, non-steroidal anti-inflammatory agents, or topical agents for pain relief.)

   Effectiveness: improves exercise tolerance (increasing 6-minute walk distances), hemodynamics, and symptoms of pulmonary hypertension similar to Epoprostenol sodium.

9. Investigational agents: Prostacyclin analogues
   a. Beraprost

   Action: an oral agent that has similar pharmacological properties to Epoprostenol but has a longer half-life (35–40 minutes)

   Effectiveness: studies have shown patients treated with Beraprost experience an improvement in 6-minute walk distances at 3 and 6 months, but the beneficial effect did not last as the dose could not be titrated up as needed.

   b. Iloprost

   Action: an inhaled agent which has been approved in Europe and appears to support beneficial effects (pulmonary vasodilation and improved exercise capacity) on both a short- and long-term basis. Note: the pulmonary selectivity of inhaled Iloprost reduces systemic effects, such as hypotension, making this therapy a safer choice.

   Dosing: has a short duration of action (30–90 minutes), which requires frequent inhalation treatments (6–12 treatments per 24-hour period) in order to maintain the beneficial effect

   Effectiveness: effective in reducing mean pulmonary artery pressure (MPAP) by 10%–20% after a single inhalation; may be superior to Nitric oxide in reducing pulmonary vascular resistance

   Note: Inhaled Iloprost has been shown to be even more beneficial in combination with Sildenafil (studies are ongoing). In addition, when both agents are used together, the frequency of Iloprost treatments can be reduced to 4–5 treatments per 24 hours.

10. Investigational agents: Endothelin receptor-A antagonists
    a. Sitaxsentan
       Action: an oral endothelin receptor-A antagonist currently under study; believed to have the advantage of blocking the vasoconstrictive effects of ET-A on the pulmonary vascular bed while maintaining the vasodilating and endothelin 1 clearance functions of ET-B.
       Dosing: 100 mg–500 mg twice daily (based on body weight for doses 4–6 mg/kg)
       Side effects: nasal congestion, flushing, increased PT/INR levels
       Effectiveness: appears to have its greatest effect on lowering pulmonary artery pressures, rather than improving cardiac output; also improved exercise capacity
    b. Ambrisentan
       Also an oral endothelin receptor-A antagonist undergoing clinical testing. May have lees hepatic effects than other endothelin receptor blockers.
11. Investigational agents: Phosphodiesterase type 5 (PDE-5) inhibitors
    a. Sildenafil (Viagra)
       Action: an oral agent that acts by blocking PDE-5 thereby increasing cyclic GMP levels (the intracellular mediator which regulates vascular tone).
       Dosing: currently under study—published case reports utilized doses ranging from 25 mg 2 times a day to 100 mg 5 times a day
       Side effects: headaches
       Effectiveness: appears to reduce pulmonary vascular resistance without significantly reducing systemic blood pressure; seems well-tolerated although studies of side effects of daily dosing are underway
12. Investigational agents: Nitric oxide
    Action: improves arterial oxygenation and decreases pulmonary hypertension by selectively dilating the pulmonary vasculature; functions as endothelium derived (vascular smooth muscle) relaxing factor (EDRF)
    Dosing: administered as inhaled gas in small increments (up to 80 parts per million) to evaluate the vasoreactivity of the pulmonary vascular bed during acute vasodilator trials; not yet available for use on a chronic basis
    Side Effects: may inhibit platelet function
    Effectiveness: There is a substantial amount of evidence supporting the use of nitric oxide as short-term therapy for the treatment of pulmonary hypertension; however the use of nitric oxide chronically remains investigational.
B. Surgical management of pulmonary hypertension
    1. Atrial septostomy
       a. The creation of an intra-atrial opening which allows right to left shunting in the setting of severe right heart failure. Physiologically,

this procedure decompresses the right atrium and right ventricle alleviating signs of heart failure; however, the creation of this type of shunt reduces systemic arterial oxygen saturation.
  b. Considered investigational
  c. Indications
    i. Recurrent syncope and/or right heart failure despite maximal medical therapy
    ii. As a bridge to transplant when maximal medical therapy is failing
    iii. When all other therapeutic options are exhausted
  d. Patient selection
    Systemic arterial oxygen saturation > 90% on room air
  e. During the procedure patients should have the following support
    i. Mild sedation to control anxiety
    ii. Supplemental oxygen
    iii. Hemodynamic monitoring with special attention to systemic arterial oxygen saturation
  f. This procedure should only be attempted in institutions that have experience in caring for patients with advanced pulmonary hypertension and experience in performing atrial septostomy.
  g. Atrial septostomy should not be performed in patients with impending death on maximal cardiopulmonary support.
  h. Predictors of procedure failure and/or death
    i. Mean right atrial pressure > 20 mm Hg
    ii. PVR index > 55 U.M^2
    iii. Predicted one year survival less than 40%
    iv. The procedure should be performed in a stepwise fashion so that the smallest atrial septal defect is created that effectively causes beneficial hemodynamic results.
    v. The acute hemodynamic effect of an atrial septostomy is an increase in systemic oxygen transport by increasing cardiac output. In addition, the reduced right atrial pressure lessens systemic venous congestion, which improves right heart failure.
    vi. With exercise, the right to left shunting increases with increased oxygen transport although the systemic arterial oxygen saturation will be further reduced.
    vii. The endpoint of an atrial septostomy is a 5%–10% reduction of the systemic arterial oxygen saturation.
    viii. Management following septostomy includes transfusion of packed red cells or the use of erythropoietin to increase oxygen delivery. Chronic anticoagulation is also recommended.
2. Pulmonary thromboendarterectomy (refer to chapter 23 "Pulmonary Thromboembolism" for specific details)
  a. A surgical treatment option for patients with chronic thromboembolic pulmonary hypertension (CTEPH).

b. The procedure involves removal of chronic embolic material from the pulmonary vasculature, which reduces pulmonary vascular resistance and pulmonary hypertension, improves right heart failure, and the function of the lung.

c. Patient selection is an important process to achieve a successful outcome. Ideal candidates have organized thrombotic material in the proximal pulmonary vascular bed from the main pulmonary arteries to the segmental branches.

d. The surgery is more complex than conventional cardiac surgery involving a median sternotomy incision, cardiopulmonary bypass, induced hypothermia, and circulatory arrest.

e. Postoperative complications include reperfusion pulmonary edema and right heart failure.

f. Mortality is about 10% at experienced institutions.

3. Lung transplantation (refer to chapter 38 "Lung Transplantation")

a. Transplantation is an effective treatment for patients with severe pulmonary hypertension.

b. PPH patients who receive a single lung transplant have a higher mortality rate than others who have bilateral or heart-lung transplant.

c. One-year survival is approximately 70%–75%, 3-year survival is 55%–60%, and 5-year survival is 40%–45%.

d. Medical therapies, such as Epoprostenol, have become available and successful in deferring the timing of lung transplantation.

e. Transplantation should be considered when patients experience progression of the pulmonary hypertension to WHO Functional Class III or IV despite advanced medical therapy.

f. Patients should be referred to a transplant center at the appropriate time with consideration to the following

  i. The patient's prognosis with optimal medical management

  ii. Anticipated waiting time in the geographic region

  iii. Expected survival after transplantation

g. While there are several transplant options available including bilateral sequential, single, and heart-lung, there is no consensus regarding the best procedure.

VII. Outcomes and interventions

A. Outcomes

1. Despite advances, pulmonary hypertension remains a serious medical condition that warrants care from a physician with expertise in the field of pulmonary vascular disease.

2. Early statistics have reported a survival of 2–3 years. With the advent of newer therapies, the survival rate has improved.

3. Patients who respond to calcium channel blocker agents have demonstrated a >90% survival at 4 years.

4. Patients (WHO Functional Class III and IV) treated with intravenous Epoprostenol therapy have demonstrated the following survival

a. >1 year   85%

b. >2 years   70%

c. >3 years   63%

d. >5 years   55%

5. Medical conditions that predict poor prognosis

　a. Higher pulmonary vascular resistance and pressure: The higher pressure imposes an excessive workload on the right ventricle resulting in right heart failure and death

　b. Absence of a favorable response to vasodilator therapy

　c. Advanced functional heart classification: Patients who are more symptomatic are presumed to be experiencing severe right heart failure and hemodynamic dysfunction.

　d. Elevated right atrial pressure: A mean right atrial pressure >20 mm Hg indicates advanced right heart failure and is predictive of an early mortality.

　e. Low pulmonary artery (mixed venous) saturation: A pulmonary artery saturation <63% reflects hypoxemia and low cardiac output and indicates a higher risk of early death.

　f. Failure to use anticoagulation

　g. Pericardial effusion—moderate or large in size

B. Future directions

1. To gain a better understanding of the vascular endothelium and its role in the control of the pulmonary vascular bed.

2. To identify what triggers the vascular endothelium to develop pathologic changes and to understand the common pathways for pulmonary hypertensive diseases.

3. To learn more about the gene(s) responsible for sporadic and familial PPH and to begin to develop therapies that are effective in protecting patients from developing pulmonary hypertension.

4. To develop biochemical and physiologic tests to diagnose and monitor the disease.

5. To develop new treatment options based on established pathobiologic mechanisms.

6. To understand which combinations of pharmacologic agents are most effective at targeting the pathophysiologic pathways.

VIII. Home care considerations

A. Patient education

1. Disease process

　a. Signs/symptoms of worsening disease

　b. When and how to call for medical attention

　c. Over-the-counter medications to avoid

　　Vasoconstricting agents such as decongestants

　d. Use of effective contraception

2. Therapeutic medications

3. Fluid management, dietary restrictions, and nutritional management

4. Anticoagulation therapy

5. Oxygen therapy
6. Physical activity, maintenance of strength, and energy conservation
7. Routine self-care/good health practices
8. Stress management

WEB SITES

National Registry for Familial Primary Pulmonary Hypertension: http://www.mc.vanderbilt.edu/vumcdept/pulmonary/fpph.html

National Organization for Rare Disorders (NORD): www.rarediseases.org

PPH Cure Foundation: http://www.pphcure.org

Pulmonary Hypertension Association: http://www.phassociation.org

Pulmonary Hypertension Central: http://www.phcentral.org/index.shtml

Scleroderma Foundation: http://www.scleroderma.org/

SUGGESTED READINGS

Bach, D. S. (1997). Stress echocardiography for evaluation of hemodynamics: Valvular heart disease, prosthetic valve function, and pulmonary hypertension. *Progress in Cardiovascular Diseases, 39*(6), 543–554.

Badesch, D. B., Tapson, V. F., McGoon, M. D., Brundage, B. H., Rubin, L. J., Wigley, F. M., et al. (2000). Continuous intravenous epoprostenol for pulmonary hypertension due to the scleroderma spectrum of diseases: A randomized, controlled study. *Annals of Internal Medicine, 132,* 425–434.

Barst, R. J. (2000). Role of atrial septostomy in the treatment of pulmonary vascular disease. *Thorax, 55*(2), 95–96.

Barst, R. J., McGoon, M., McLaughlin, V., et al. (2003). Beraprost therapy for pulmonary hypertension. *Journal of the American College of Cardiology, 41,* 2119–2125.

Barst, R. J., Rich, S., Widlitz, A., et al. (2002). Clinical efficacy of sitaxsentan, an endothelin-A receptor antagonist, in patients with pulmonary arterial hypertension. *Chest, 121,* 1860–1868.

Barst, R. J., Rubin, L. J., Long, W. A., et al. (1996). A comparison of continuous intravenous epoprostenol (prostacyclin) with conventional therapy for primary pulmonary hypertension. *New England Journal of Medicine, 334,* 296–301.

Barst, R. J., Rubin, L. J., McGoon, M. D., et al. (1994). Survival in primary pulmonary hypertension with long-term continuous intravenous prostacyclin. *Annals of Internal Medicine, 121,* 409–415.

Channick, R. N., & Rubin, L. J. (2002). Endothelin receptor antagonism: a new era in the treatment of pulmonary arterial hypertension. *Advances in Pulmonary Hypertension, 1*(1), 13–17.

Channick, R. N., Simmonneau, G., Sitbon, O., et al. (2001). Effects of the dual endothelin-receptor antagonist bosentan in patients with pulmonary hypertension: A randomised placebo-controlled study. *The Lancet, 358,* 1119–1123.

Conte, J. V., Gaine, S. P., Orens, J. B., Harris, T., & Rubin, L. J. (1998). The influence of continuous intravenous prostacyclin therapy for primary pulmonary hypertension on the timing and outcome of transplantation. *Journal of Heart and Lung Transplantation, 17,* 679–685.

Cooper, C. B., Waterhouse, J., & Howard, P. (1987). Twelve year clinical study of patients with hypoxic cor pulmonale given long-term domiciliary oxygen therapy. *Thorax, 42,* 105–110.

Deng, Z., Morse, J. H., Slager, S. L., et al. (2000). Familial primary pulmonary hypertension (gene PPH-1) is caused by mutations in the bone morphogenetic protein receptor–II gene. *American Journal of Human Genetics, 67,* 737–744.

Eells, P. L. (2004). Advances in prostacyclin therapy for pulmonary arterial hypertension. *Critical Care Nurse, 24*(2) 42–54.

Fishman, A. P. (2001). Clinical classification of pulmonary hypertension. *Clinics in Chest Medicine, 22*(3), 385–391.

Fraser, R. S., Muller, N. L., Colman, N., & Pare, P. D. (1999). Pulmonary hypertension. In R. S. Fraser & P. D. Pare (Eds.), *Diagnosis of diseases of the chest* (4th ed., pp. 1879–1945). Philadelphia, PA: W. B. Saunders Co.

Frazier, S. K. (1999). Diagnosing and treating pulmonary hypertension. *Nurse Practitioner, 24*(9), 18–26.

Gaine, S. (2000). Grand Rounds: Pulmonary hypertension. *Journal of the American Medical Association, 284,* 3160–3168.

Galie, N., Hinderliter, A. L., Torbicki, A., et. al. (2003). Effects of the oral endothelin-receptor antagonist Bosentan on echocardiographic and Doppler measures in patients with pulmonary arterial hypertension. *Journal of the American College of Cardiology, 41,* 1380–1386.

Galie, N., Manes, A., & Branzi, A. (2001). Medical therapy of pulmonary hypertension—The prostacyclins. *Clinics in Chest Medicine, 22*(3), 529–537.

Galie, N., Manes, A., & Branzi, A. (2002). The new clinical trials on pharmacological treatment in pulmonary arterial hypertension. *European Respiratory Journal, 20,* 1037–1049.

Gildea, T. R., Arroliga, A. C., & Minai, O. A. (2003). Treatments and strategies to optimize the comprehensive management of patients with pulmonary arterial hypertension. *Cleveland Clinic Journal of Medicine, 70*(Suppl 1), S18–S27.

Hoeper, M. M., Schwarze, M., Ehlerding, S., et al. (2000). Long-term treatment of primary pulmonary hypertension with aerosolized iloprost, a prostacyclin analogue. *New England Journal of Medicine, 342*(25), 1866–1870.

Hopkins, W. E., Ochoa, L. L., Richardson, G. W., & Trulock, E. P. (1996). Comparison of the hemodynamics and survival of adults with severe primary pulmonary hypertension or Eisenmenger syndrome. *Journal of Heart and Lung Transplantation, 15,* 100–105.

Krowka, M. J. (2000). Pulmonary hypertension: Diagnostics and therapeutics. *Mayo Clinic Proceedings, 75*(6), 625–630.

McKane, C. L. (1998). Pulmonary thromboendarterectomy: An advance in the treatment of chronic thromboembolic pulmonary hypertension. *Heart & Lung, 27*(5), 293–296.

McLaughlin, V. V., Gaine, S. P., Barst, R. J., et al. (2003). Efficacy and safety of tre-postinil: An epoprostenol analog for primary pulmonary hypertension. *Journal of Cardiovascular Pharmacology, 41*(2), 293–299.

McLaughlin, V. V., Genthner, D. E., Panella, M. M., & Rich, S. (1998). Reduction in pulmonary vascular resistance with long-term epoprostenol (prostacyclin) therapy in primary pulmonary hypertension. *New England Journal of Medicine, 338,* 273–277.

McLaughlin, V. V., & Rich, S. (1998). Pulmonary hypertension-Advances in medical and surgical treatment options. *Journal of Heart and Lung Transplantation, 17,* 739–743

McLaughlin, V. V., Shillington, A., & Rich, S. (2002). Survival in primary pulmonary hypertension. The impact of epoprostenol therapy. *Circulation, 106,* 1477–1482.

Mesa, R. A., Edell, E. S., Dunn, W. F., et al. (1998). Human immunodeficiency virus infection and pulmonary hypertension: Two new cases and a review of 86 reported cases. *Mayo Clinic Proceedings, 73,* 37–45.

Olschewski, H. (2002). Inhaled iloprost for treatment of pulmonary arterial hypertension. *Advances in Pulmonary Hypertension, 1*(3), 16–21.

Olschewski, H., Simonneau, G., Galie, N., et al. (2002). Inhaled iloprost for severe pulmonary hypertension. *New England Journal of Medicine, 347*(5), 322–329.

Ouidz, R. J. (2002). Cardiac catheterization in pulmonary arterial hypertension: A guide to proper use. *Advances in Pulmonary Hypertension, 1*(2), 17–21.

Palevsky, H. I. (1997). Therapeutic options for severe pulmonary hypertension. *Clinics in Chest Medicine, 18,* 595–609.

Rich, S. (Ed.). (1998). Primary pulmonary hypertension: Executive Summary from the World Symposium-Primary Pulmonary Hypertension 1998. The World Health Organization. Retrieved from http://www.who.int/ncd/cvd/pph.html

Rich, S., Dantzker, D. R., Ayres, S. M., et al. (1987). Primary pulmonary hypertension: A national prospective study. *Annals of Internal Medicine, 107,* 216–226.

Rich, S., Kaufmann, E. & Levy, P. S. (1992). The effect of high doses of calcium channel blockers on survival in primary pulmonary hypertension. *New England Journal of Medicine, 327,* 76–81.

Rich, S., & Levy, P. S. (1984). Characteristics of surviving and nonsurviving patients with primary pulmonary hypertension. *American Journal of Medicine, 76,* 573–578.

Rich, S., Seidlitz, M., Dodin, E., et al. (1998). The short-term effects of digoxin in patients with right ventricular dysfunction from pulmonary hypertension. *Chest, 114,* 787–792.

Rubin, L. J., Badesch, D. B., Barst, R. J. et al. (2002). Bosentan therapy for pulmonary arterial hypertension, *New England Journal of Medicine, 346,* 896–903.

Rubin, L. J. (1995). Pathology and pathophysiology of primary pulmonary hypertension. *American Journal of Cardiology, 75,* 51A–54A.

Rubin, L. J., Barst, R. J., Kaiser, L. R., et al. (1993). Primary pulmonary hypertension. *Chest, 104,* 236–250.

Sandoval, J., Rothman, A., & Pulido, T. (2001). Atrial septostomy for pulmonary hypertension. *Clinics in Chest Medicine, 22*(3), 547–560.

Severson, C. J., & McGoon, M. D. (2002). Continuous intravenous epoprostenol for pulmonary arterial hypertension: highlighting practical issues, special considerations. *Advances in Pulmonary Hypertension, 1*(3), 4–8.

Simonneau, G., Barst, R. J., Galie, N., et al. (2002). Continuous subcutaneous infusion of treprostinil, a prostacyclin analogue, in patients with pulmonary arterial hypertension. *American Journal of Respiratory and Critical Care Medicine, 165,* 800–804.

Simonneau, G., Fartoukh, M., Sitbon, O., et al. (1998). Primary pulmonary hypertension associated with the use of fenfluramine derivatives. *Chest, 114,* 195S–199S.

Sitbon, O., Badesch, D. B., Channick, R. N., et al. (2003). Effects of the dual endothelin receptor antagonist Bosentan in patients with pulmonary hypertension. *Chest, 124,* 247–254.

Sitbon, O., Humbert, M., Nunes, H., et al. (2002). Long-term intravenous epoprostenol infusion in primary pulmonary hypertension. *Journal of the American College of Cardiology, 40,* 780–788.

Steudel, W., Hurford, W. E., & Zapol, W. (1999). Inhaled nitric oxide: Basic biology and clinical applications. *Anesthesiology, 91*(4), 1090–1121.

Thomas, A. Q., Gaddipati, R., Newman, J. H., & Lloyd, J. E. (2001). Genetics of Primary Pulmonary Hypertension. *Clinics in Chest Medicine, 22*(3), 477–491.

Weinberger, S. E. (1992). Pulmonary hypertension. In Weinberger, S. E. (Ed.), *Principles of pulmonary medicine* (pp. 174–181). Philadelphia: W. B. Saunders.

Wensel, R., Opitz, C. F., Ewert, R., et al. (2000). Effects of iloprost inhalation on exercise capacity and ventilatory efficiency in patients with primary pulmonary hypertension. *Circulation, 101*(20), 2388–2392.

Williamson, D. J., Wallman, L. L., Jones, R., et al. (2000). Hemodynamic effects of bosentan, an endothelin receptor antagonist, in patients with pulmonary hypertension. *Circulation, 102*(4), 411–418.

Tobacco and Other Substance Abuse

Kathleen O. Lindell and Mary L. Wilby

INTRODUCTION

Tobacco use is the leading cause of preventable death and disability in the United States. Greater than 3,000 youth under the age of 18 begin use of tobacco on a daily basis in the United States, causing this to be a major public health concern in the United States and in the world. Other substances of abuse, including marijuana and cocaine, are also associated with serious health risks.

I. Overview

Tobacco use is the number one cause of preventable death, disability, and premature death in the United States. Other substances of abuse (marijuana and cocaine in this forum) are also associated with serious health risks. This chapter will review the effects of use of these drugs.

A. Definitions

1. Tobacco use refers to any one of the following: smoking cigarettes, pipes, or cigars and/or using smokeless tobacco, such as chew, snuff, or dip.

2. Other substance abuse in this forum applies to marijuana and cocaine, both of which may be inhaled or cocaine used intravenously.

B. Etiology

1. Components

a. The principal addictive component of tobacco, nicotine, accounts for much of the compulsive behavior surrounding tobacco usage.

b. Delta-9-tetrahydrocannabinol (THC) and other cannabinoids are responsible for the psychoactive effects of marijuana.

c. Cocaine has potent sympathomimetic and central nervous system (CNS) stimulant effects that users of the drug seek.

2. Mechanisms of action: Tobacco
   a. When nicotine is smoked, nicotine readily enters the bloodstream through the lungs. When it is sniffed or chewed, nicotine passes through the mucous membranes of the mouth or nose to enter the circulation. Nicotine can also enter the bloodstream by passing through the skin.
   b. Once nicotine reaches the circulation, it is distributed throughout the body and brain where it activates specific types of receptors known as cholinergic receptors, present in many brain structures, as well as in muscles, adrenal glands, the heart, and other organs. These receptors are normally activated by the acetylcholine. Acetylcholine and its receptors are involved in many activities, including respiration, maintenance of heart rate, memory, alertness, and muscle movement.
   c. Because the chemical structure of nicotine is similar to that of acetylcholine, nicotine is also able to activate cholinergic receptors. Unlike acetylcholine, nicotine can disrupt the normal functioning of the brain. Regular nicotine use causes changes in both the number of cholinergic receptors and the sensitivity of these receptors to nicotine and acetylcholine. These changes may be responsible for the development of tolerance to nicotine.
   d. Once tolerance has developed, a nicotine user must regularly supply the brain with nicotine to maintain normal brain functioning. When nicotine levels drop, the nicotine user will begin to feel uncomfortable withdrawal symptoms.
   e. Nicotine also stimulates the release of dopamine in the nucleus accumbens. The release of dopamine is similar to that seen for other drugs of abuse, including cocaine. This is thought to underlie the pleasurable sensations experienced by many smokers.
   f. Cigarette smoking causes a dramatic decrease in the levels of monoamine-oxidase-A (MAO-A) resulting in an increase in dopamine levels. This effect is not by nicotine, but another unknown compound in cigarette smoke. Thus, there may be multiple routes by which smoking affects dopamine levels to produce feelings of pleasure and reward.
   g. The addictive nature of tobacco accounts for its persistent use in spite of the serious health risks such use poses. Cessation of tobacco use, even among patients with the strong desire to quit, may be very difficult due to this addictive quality.
3. Mechanisms of action: Marijuana
   a. THC and other cannabinoids are readily absorbed through the lungs, thus the most common route of administration is smoking, either as a cigarette or with a pipe. It can be taken orally, which delays the onset of action but prolongs its duration.
   b. The cannabinoids bind to endogenous receptors in the CNS and are responsible for the psychoactive effects. Two endogenous cannabinoid receptors have been identified.

  c. Impaired concentration and motor performance may last for up to 24 hours after use. Changes in cognition, coordination, and judgment may last after the feeling of the "high" has ended. Accumulation of marijuana in fatty tissue, with slow release of THC into the enterohepatic circulation is responsible for this delay.

 4. Cocaine

  a. Cocaine is a local anesthetic with marked CNS stimulant effects due to its ability to interfere with reuptake of serotonin and catecholamines.

  b. Cocaine may be inhaled nasally or injected intravenously. Crack may be smoked, either through a pipe, or mixed with marijuana or tobacco in cigarettes. It is rapidly absorbed through the pulmonary circulation and reaches the CNS in seconds.

  c. Cocaine hydrochloride is a heat-sensitive white powder. When boiled with baking soda and water, the resultant precipitate yields a lipid soluble, heat-stable free base form commonly known as crack.

C. Pathophysiology

 1. Tobacco

  a. In addition to nicotine, cigarette smoke contains more than 4,000 substances, many of which may cause cancer or damage the lungs. A partial list of these substances includes acetone, ammonia, arsenic, carbon monoxide, cyanide, formaldehyde, methane, tar, and toluene.

  b. Cigarette smoke is a heterogeneous aerosol produced by the combustion of both the tobacco leaf and the additive substances used in the manufacturing of cigarettes. Most of cigarette smoke is composed of a gas that is inhaled through the mouthpiece of the cigarette.

  c. Tissue response to these elements are multiple and complex and have not been fully investigated. Most research has centered on those elements believed to be particularly harmful, including nicotine, carbon monoxide, and identified carcinogens such as polynuclear aromatic hydrocarbons, aromatic amines, and nitrosamines.

  d. Symptoms often are absent, and patients find it difficult to visualize themselves living with a chronic illness not yet present. Therefore, it may be useful to discuss the short-term symptoms of tobacco use affecting smokers.

  e. When a person smokes, the following physiological processes occur

   i. An increased heart rate of 15–25 bpm (can present with tachycardia and chest palpitations)

   ii. Increased blood pressure of 10–20 mm Hg

   iii. Corrosion of the lip and palate mucous membranes

   iv. Sensation of choking in the airways and shortness of breath

   v. Decreased energy level and exercise intolerance (carbon monoxide enters the system, depriving tissues of oxygen)

      vi. A morning cough

     vii. Increased gastric acid flow, which may lead to gastric ulcers

    viii. Increase in nervousness or anxiety

     ix. Impotence and infertility

      x. Exacerbations of asthma

     xi. Premature skin aging

2. Marijuana

   a. Marijuana smoke contains approximately four times more tar and 50% more carcinogens than tobacco. Marijuana is smoked without filters so the amounts of irritants inhaled into the lining of the upper airway are markedly increased.

   b. Acute marijuana intoxication causes the following physical and psychological signs and symptoms: tachycardia, increased blood pressure, conjunctival injection, dry mouth, increased appetite, impaired reaction time, euphoria, time distortion, depression and anxiety, impaired short-term memory, paranoia, and mystical thinking.

   c. Chronic use of marijuana may result in reduction in activities and relationships not involved in use of the drug. In addition the following have been reported in chronic users: decreased concentration and analytic skills, impaired cognitive skills, decreased ability to establish and attain goals. This has been referred to as amotivational or chronic cannabis syndrome. Chronic health problems associated with marijuana are similar to those associated with tobacco.

   d. Long-term use results in decreased pulmonary function, chronic cough, bronchitis, and decreased exercise tolerance. Data from several studies suggest that marijuana smoke probably increases risk for lung cancer as well as squamous cell carcinomas of the head and neck. Studies showing histological changes, chronic cough, and increased sputum production suggest that marijuana is also linked to development of COPD.

3. Cocaine

   a. Mechanisms of lung injury include barotrauma, inflammation, ischemia, and direct cellular toxicity. Crack smoking accounts for most pulmonary toxicity, but intravenous use, snorting, and ingestion can also result in lung damage.

   b. Acute pulmonary toxicity within 1–48 hours after smoking cocaine may cause a syndrome of diffuse alveolar infiltrates, eosinophilia, and fever, frequently referred to as "crack lung."

   c. Common practices among some crack smokers, which may cause barotrauma, include performing a Valsalva maneuver after inhalation and forcefully inhaling into the mouths of their smoking partners. Chronic lung toxicity may cause a number of histiopathologic changes, including diffuse alveolar damage, alveolar hemorrhage, bronchiolitis obliterans with organizing pneumonia, interstitial pneumonitis, noncardiac pulmonary edema, pulmonary infarction, hypertrophy of the pulmonary arteries, and interstitial pulmonary fibrosis. It is believed that these tissue alterations result from several mechanisms, including, direct cellular toxicity, constriction of the pulmonary vasculature with ischemia, and inflammatory and hypersensitivity responses.

  d. Acute cocaine intoxication may cause the following signs and symptoms: tachycardia, arrhythmia, chest pain, increased blood pressure, hot flashes or chills, reduced appetite, muscle weakness, seizures, changes in affect, agitation or irritability, hypervigilance, paranoia, and impaired judgment. Signs and symptoms of cocaine-induced lung injury may include fever; chest or back pain (frequently pleuritic); hyperpnea and dyspnea, often with minimal exertion; cough; wheezing; hemoptysis; and melanoptysis (black sputum) as a result of inhaling the carbon residue from materials used to light crack.

D. Incidence
  1. Tobacco
    a. In 2004, an estimated, 22.5% of all adults (46 million people) smoke cigarettes in the United States. This makes nicotine, the addictive component of tobacco, one of the most heavily used addictive drugs in the United States.
    b. Cigarette smoking estimates by age are as follows: 18–24 years (28.5%), 25–44 years (25.7%), 45–64 years (22.7%), and 65 years or older (9.3%).
    c. Cigarette smoking is more common among men (25.2%) than women (20.0%).
    d. Prevalence of cigarette smoking is highest among American Indians/Alaska Natives (40.8%), followed by whites (23.6%), African Americans (22.4%), Hispanics (16.7%), and Asians [excluding Native Hawaiians and other Pacific Islanders] (13.3%).
    e. Cigarette smoking estimates are highest for adults with a General Education Development (GED) diploma (42.3%) or 9–11 years of education (34.1%), and lowest for adults with an undergraduate college degree (12.1%) or a graduate college degree (7.2%).
    f. Cigarette smoking is more common among adults who live below the poverty level (32.9%) than among those living at or above the poverty level (22.2%).
    g. More than 3,000 adolescents under the age of 18 start to smoke every day. Cigarette use is increasing on college campuses nationwide with 28.5% of all college students smoking tobacco.
  2. Marijuana
    a. Marijuana is the most frequently used illicit drug in the United States. Its use is rising, particularly among junior high and high school students. Use is frequent in all social strata. NIDA's 1996 Monitoring the Future study showed increased use among 8th and

10th graders with patterns of use for other illicit drugs unchanged. The survey revealed that the majority of teens believed marijuana isn't harmful.

b. A number of factors contribute to the increased use of marijuana including: increased availability at relatively low cost, marijuana is often considered "less risky" than other drugs, law enforcement may focus more attention on other drugs, more potent marijuana is available, it is easier to sell because of high profit margins and low risks for penalties, it may be used as a vehicle for delivery of other drugs such as crack or PCP.

3. Cocaine

a. Despite restrictions on its availability, cocaine is abused throughout the world.

b. The 1997 National Survey on Drug Abuse estimated that 1.5 million Americans 12 years and older are chronic cocaine users with 40% of these using crack.

c. It is the leading cause of illicit drug–related visits to emergency rooms in the United States. Several studies have linked increasing crack cocaine use with an increase in asthma morbidity and mortality, particularly in urban populations.

E. Considerations across the life span

1. Pediatric

a. Between 8,000 and 26,000 children are diagnosed with asthma every year in the United States. The odds of developing asthma are twice as high among children whose mothers smoke at least 10 cigarettes/day.

b. Children are also at increased risk of developing ear infections.

c. Use of marijuana by adolescents has been associated with decreased likelihood of finishing high school, an increase in violence, high-risk sexual behaviors, and impaired functioning at school.

2. Reproductive

a. Women who smoke during pregnancy subject themselves and their developing fetus and newborn to special risks, including pregnancy complication, premature birth, low-birth weight infants, stillbirth, and infant mortality.

b. Research also suggests that intrauterine exposure and passive exposure to secondhand smoke after pregnancy are associated with increased rate of SIDS.

c. Smoking has a damaging effect on women's reproductive health and is associated with reduced fertility and early menopause.

d. Smoking marijuana has been shown to lower testosterone levels in males as well as lowering sperm counts and decreasing sperm motility.

e. In females there may be short menstrual cycles and increased prolactin levels with associated galactorrhea. THC accumulates in breast milk and crosses into the placenta. This may cause low birth weight and abnormal responses in the new born.

    f. Cocaine use during pregnancy increases risk of complications of pregnancy, including placenta previa, placenta abruptio, retarded intrauterine growth, premature labor, and stillbirth.

    g. Cocaine use during pregnancy has also been associated with many birth defects as well as impaired neuropsychological development in children.

  3. Elderly

    a. Smoking cessation at any age halts the progression of smoking-related health effects.

    b. There is an accelerated rate at which obstructive lung disease progresses as one continues to smoke.

F. Complications/sequelae

  1. Tobacco use accounts for approximately 432,000 premature deaths each year, including 50,000 deaths in non-smokers due to second-hand smoke, or environmental tobacco smoke (ETS). While nicotine may produce addiction to tobacco products, it is the thousands of other chemicals in tobacco that are responsible for its many adverse health effects.

  2. Children exposed to cigarette smoke are found to have increased respiratory infections and more ear infections, a greater risk of asthma and Sudden Infant Death Syndrome (SIDS). Coronary artery disease, stroke, ulcers, and an increased incidence of respiratory infections are associated with cigarette smoking.

  3. Smoking either cigarettes or cigars is the major cause of lung cancer and is also associated with cancers of the larynx, esophagus, bladder, kidney, pancreas, stomach, and uterine cervix. Smoking is also the major cause of chronic bronchitis and emphysema.

  4. The use of smokeless tobacco is also associated with serious health problems. Chewing tobacco can cause cancers of the oral cavity, pharynx, larynx, and esophagus. It also causes damage to gums that may lead to the loss of teeth.

  5. Smoking any substance—tobacco, marijuana, or crack—increases a smoker's risk of developing bacterial pneumonia and other infections of the lungs. Smoking anything appears to damage or paralyze the cilia, the respiratory system's first line of defense, and weakens the ability of the lungs to remove inhaled particles, making the lungs more vulnerable to infection. Pulmonary alveolar macrophages are exposed to the highest concentrations of cocaine.

II. Assessment

A. History

  1. The 5th Vital Sign refers to asking the patient about history of current or past tobacco use, along with blood pressure, weight, pulse, and temperature. Use of the 5th Vital Sign is recommended when obtaining vital signs on all patients at all health provider visits. The patient

should also be asked about use of other substances of abuse during the initial encounter with the health care provider.

2. The Fagerstrom Scale is a tool to measure nicotine dependence. A score greater than 7 suggests that an individual is highly addicted to nicotine.

3. Past medical history in those who use cocaine and marijuana may include frequent urinary tract infections. Those who use cocaine frequently report frequent sinus infections, nasal congestion, upper respiratory infections, rhinitis, nosebleeds, and burns. Weight loss is common in cocaine users. Abstinence from cocaine frequently causes anxiety, fatigue, irritability, and sleep disturbances. Marijuana use may produce fatigue, decreased motivation, panic attacks, and paranoia.

B. Physical exam

1. Often the first indicator that an individual smokes tobacco is the presence of a smoking odor on the individual or items (X-rays) they might carry with them. This odor is the result of the effect of burning tobacco. One of the byproducts of tobacco is tar, which when exposed to room air which is cooler than the smoker's inhalation, changes from a vapor state to a solid state. The tar becomes tenacious in character and adheres to all that it comes in contact with. This results in tobacco stains commonly associated with tobacco use; such as, on fingers and teeth, the yellowing of walls in rooms, film on the inside of car windows, and the smell that lingers on the clothes of those exposed to tobacco smoke.

2. The marijuana user may appear to be in a dreamlike state. There is frequently the appearance of conjunctival injection. Tachycardia and hypertension along with nonspecific ST-T wave changes on the electrocardiogram may be present.

3. Examination of the cocaine abuser frequently reveals nasal bleeding, erythematous nasal mucosa, nasal septal atrophy with perforation. Tachycardia, hypertension, and cardiac arrhythmias are frequent with cocaine use.

C. Diagnostic tests

1. There are several tests to measure the biological markers of tobacco use. These include carbon monoxide in exhaled air, serum, saliva, or urine cotinine levels, cotinine (main nicotine metabolite with 18–20 hour half-life), and thiocyanate.

2. Cannabinoid metabolites can be measured in the urine and are present for several weeks in chronic marijuana users.

3. Benzoylecognine, a metabolite of cocaine is also measurable in urine and may be present for 5–10 days after cessation in chronic users.

III. Common therapeutic modalities treatment

A. Successful treatment of any addiction begins with willingness to accept treatment. Assessment of the individual's readiness and motivation for change is a key factor. A therapeutic relationship with a consistent provider, the support of caring others, education about their condition to demystify and inform the patient and instill hope for successful treatment, and cognitive and behavioral strategies to decrease the risk of relapse are all essential.

B. Prochaska and DiClemente (1983) have developed the transtheoretical model of change and theorizes that there are five stages of change.

1. *Pre-contemplation*—the stage in which there is no intention to change behavior in the foreseeable future. Many individuals in this stage are unaware of underaware of their problems.

2. *Contemplation*—the stage in which people are aware that a problem exists and are seriously thinking about overcoming it but have not yet made a commitment to take action.

3. *Preparation*—the stage that combines intention and behavioral criteria; individuals here are planning to take action in the next month.

4. *Action*—the stage in which individuals modify their behavior, experiences, or environment in order to overcome their problems.

5. *Maintenance*—the stage in which people work to prevent relapse and consolidate the gains attained during action.

C. The "5 A's" for brief intervention—Agency for healthcare research and quality (AHRQ) Guideline recommends these practical tips for incorporation into daily practice.

1. Ask about tobacco use
2. Advise to quit
3. Assess willingness to make a quit attempt
4. Assist in quit attempt
5. Arrange follow-up

D. Tobacco cessation—Like addiction to heroin or cocaine, addiction to nicotine is a chronic, relapsing disorder. A cigarette smoker may require several attempts over many years before that person is able to permanently give up smoking. In addition to nicotine withdrawal, the patient will also need to be aware of his/her triggers associated with tobacco use and continued presence of these triggers during nicotine withdrawal. Interventions that involve both medications and behavioral treatments show the most promise. Common triggers include: coffee, alcohol, completion of a meal, work breaks, smoking buddies, and all the other behaviors associated with tobacco use. Approaches for tobacco cessation include

1. Cold turkey
   a. Quitting cold turkey involves selecting a quit date, and complete cessation of any and all sources of tobacco on that date.
   b. With removal of the nicotine source, the patient needs to be aware that nicotine withdrawal symptoms will occur for a few days up to 2 weeks (i.e., irritability, fatigue, dizziness, difficulty concentrating, and cravings for cigarettes).
   c. Encouraging patient to drink plenty of water is a strategy that may also be helpful.

2. Nicotine replacement therapy (NRT)
   a. NRT helps to reduce the physical withdrawal symptoms that occur when the patient stops nicotine use. Over time, proper use of nicotine replacement therapy will help to wean the patient off nicotine.
   b. Nicotine replacement therapy is available in the following forms: gum, patch, oral inhaler, lozenge, and nasal spray.
   c. NRT should be started on the quit date and only after the patient has completely stopped the tobacco source.
   d. Gum and patches are available over the counter, and oral inhaler and nasal spray are available by prescription.
   e. The AHRQ guideline cautions the use of nicotine replacement therapy in patients within 4 weeks of a myocardial infarction.
3. Bupropion hydrochloride
   a. Another medication approved by the FDA as an aid for quitting smoking is the antidepressant bupropion, or Zyban.
   b. Bupropion hydrochloride has been available for years as an antidepressant and found to be effective in reducing the cravings smokers experience when they stop smoking.
   c. The manner of action is unknown but thought to work on certain pathways in the brain that are involved in nicotine addiction and withdrawal.
   d. Bupropion hydrochloride is available by prescription only and should be started 1 week prior to the patient's quit date to achieve adequate drug levels in the bloodstream to prevent craving.
   e. This medication is taken once daily for 3 days and then increased to twice a day dosing for the duration of therapy, which is usually 3 months. Research on duration of therapy is underway.
   f. A patient may also use this therapy along with nicotine replacement therapy for additional relief from nicotine withdrawal symptoms.
   g. It is contraindicated in patients with a history of seizures or disorders that promote seizure activity (e.g., alcoholism, unstable diabetes, or altered metabolic state, such as in eating disorders), and also for patients currently taking MAO inhibitors or one of the other bupropion hydrochloride preparations, such as Wellbutrin SR.
   h. Smokers with comorbid psychiatric conditions may present special challenges. Psychiatric disorders are more common among smokers than in the general population.
   i. Smoking cessation or withdrawal from nicotine may exacerbate symptoms of other conditions. They may also be at higher risk for return to smoking after a quit attempt.
   j. Bupropion may be useful in assisting with delay in weight gain after tobacco cessation.
E. Marijuana and cocaine cessation—Treatment of abuse most often includes detoxification along with intensive psychosocial support.

Medications can be used to reduce the reinforcing effects of the abused substance. A comprehensive approach with attention to cognitive, behavioral, emotional, physical, social, and spiritual needs provides the best chance for recovery.

1. Medications often used to reduce drug craving include clonidine and bromocriptine. Other pharmacologic agents are under investigation.

2. Those who maintain physical and psychological abstinence are said to be in recovery. Relapse is always possible and preventive strategies are crucial to assist the individual in stressful times, which may precipitate relapse.

IV. Home care considerations

A. Nurses working with patients in the home should be aware of symptoms of withdrawal from nicotine and other substances and provide education for patients and their caregivers. Recognition of withdrawal symptoms and communication with other health care providers to provide treatment as needed for relief of withdrawal symptoms is important for successful withdrawal/detoxification.

B. Obsessive thinking about the substance is the hallmark of psychological dependence. Remembrances of the desired effects of the substance may compel the patient to re-initiate use of the substance.

C. Relapse is always possible. Relapse prevention is an important part of treatment especially during periods of stress. Nurses can teach cognitive and behavioral strategies to assist patients to identify high-risk situations and behaviors, develop activities to replace substance use behaviors.

D. Teach patient and family members that substance abuse treatment is a lifelong process that requires abstinence and changes in lifestyle, which are facilitated by the support of family and concerned others.

WEB SITES

AHRQ 2000: www.surgeongeneral.gov/tobacco
Centers for Disease Control and Prevention: http://www.cdc.gov/tobacco
Join Together Online: http://www.quitnet.org
National Cancer Institute: http://wwww.nci.nhi.gov
NCADI: http://www.health.org
NicNet: http://tobacco.arizona.edu
NIDA: http://www.nida.nih.gov
Nursing Center for Tobacco Intervention: http://www.con.ohio-state.edu/tobacco
The Robert Wood Johnson Foundation: http://www/rwjf.org
Society for Research on Nicotine and Tobacco: http://www.srnt.org/
Tobacco Free Nurses: www.tobaccofreenurses.org

REFERENCE

Prochaska, J. O., & DiClemente, C. C. (1983). Stages and processes of self change of smoking: toward an integrated model of change. *Journal of Clinical Psychology, 51,* 390–395.

SUGGESTED READINGS

Agency for Health Care Policy and Research. (1997). Smoking cessation: Implementing the Agency for Health Care Policy and Research guidelines in clinical practice. Based on Smoking cessation, clinical practice guideline no. 18. Rockville, MD: Author.

Bachman, J. G., Johnson, L. D., & O'Malley, D. (1998). Explaining recent increases in students' marijuana use; Impacts of perceived risks and disapproval, 1976–1996. *American Journal of Public Health, 88,* 887–892.

Benowitz, N. L. (1991). Pharmacodynamics of nicotine: Implications for rational treatment of nicotine addiction. *British Journal of Addiction, 86,* 495–499.

Carpenito, L. J. (2000). *Nursing diagnosis applications for practice* (8th ed.) Philadelphia, PA: Lippincott.

Centers for Disease Control and Prevention. (1994). CDC Surveillance Summaries, for selected tobacco use behaviors in United States. MMWR 43 (No.SS-3). Atlanta, GA: Author.

Centers for Disease Control: National Centers for Health Statistics. (1998). *Targeting tobacco use: The nation's leading cause of death at-a-glance.* Atlanta, GA: Author.

Centers for Disease Control. (2004). Cigarette smoking among adults-United States, 2002. *Morbidity and Mortality Weekly Report, 53*(20), 428–431.

Crits-Christoph, P., et al. (1999). Psychosocial treatments for cocaine dependence: NIDA collaborative cocaine treatment study. *Archives of General Psychiatry, 56,* 493–502.

Cunnington, D., et al. (2000). Necrotizing granulomata in a marijuana smoker. *Chest, 117,* 1511–1514.

Fiore, M. C. (2000). Treating tobacco use and dependence: an introduction to the USHS clinical practice guideline. *Respiratory Care, 45,* 1196–1261.

Fiore, M. C., Jorenby, D. E., Schensky, A. E., Smith S. S., Bauer, R. R., & Baker, T. B. (1995). Smoking status as the new vital sign: Effect on assessment and intervention in patients who smoke. *Mayo Clinic Proceedings, 70,* 209–213.

Fiore, M. C., Smith, S. S, Jorenby, D. E., & Baker, T. B. (1994). The effectiveness of the nicotine patch for smoking cessation: A meta-analysis. *Journal of the American Medical Association, 271*(24), 1940–1947.

Fliegel, S. E., et al. (1997). Tracheobronchial histopathology in habitual smokers of cocaine, marijuana, and/or tobacco. *Chest, 112,* 319–326.

Heath, J., Andrews, J., & Balkstra, C. R. (2004). Potential reduction exposure products and FDA tobacco and regulation: A CNS call to action. *Clinical Nurse Specialist, 18*(1), 40–48; quiz 49–50.

Heatherton, T. F., Kozlowski, L. T., Frecker, R. C., & Fagerstrom, K. O. (1991). The Fagerstrom Test for nicotine dependence: a revision of the Fagerstrom Tolerance Questionnaire. *British Journal of Addiction, 86,* 1119–1127.

Hurt, R. D., Sachs, D. P., Glover, E. D., Offord, K. P., Johnston, J. A., Dale, L. C., et al. (1997). A comparison of sustained-release Bupropion and placebo for smoking cessation. *New England Journal of Medicine, 337*(17), 1195–1202.

Institute of Medicine. (1994). *Growing up tobacco free: Preventing nicotine addiction in children and youths.* Washington, DC: National Academy Press.

Johnson, M. K., et al. (2000). Large bullae in marijuana smokers. *Thorax, 55,* 340–342.

Klebanoff, N. A., & Smith, N. M. (1997). *Behavior management in home care.* Philadelphia, PA: Lippincott.

Lindell, K. O., & Reinke, L. F. (1999). Nursing strategies for smoking cessation. *Heart & Lung, 28,* 295–302.

Rome, L., et al. (2000). Prevalence of cocaine use and its impact on asthma exacerbation in an urban population. *Chest, 117,* 1324–1329.

Shiffman, S. M., Jarvik, M. E. (1976). Smoking withdrawal symptoms in two weeks of abstinence. *Psychopharmacology, 50,* 35–39.

U.S. Department of Health and Human Services. (1989). Reducing the health consequences of smoking: 25 years of progress. A report of the Surgeon General. DHHS Publication # 89–8411. Atlanta, GA: Office of Smoking and Health, Centers for Disease Control & Prevention.

U.S. Department of Health and Human Services. (1991). Healthy People 2000: National health promotion and disease prevention objectives. Washington, DC: DHHS Publication No. 91-50212.

U.S. Environmental Protection Agency. (1986). Respiratory health effects of passive smoking: Lung Cancer and other disorders. Washington, DC: Office of Research and Development.

Wechsler, H., Rigotti, N. A., Gledhill-Hoyt, J., & Lee, H. (1998). Increased levels of cigarette use among college students: A cause for national concern. *Journal of the American Medical Association, 280*(19), 1673–1678.

Wewers, M. E., Ahijevych, K. L., & Sarna L. (1998). Smoking cessation interventions in nursing practice. *Nursing Clinics of North America, 33*(1), 61–74.

Pediatric Specific Disorders

V

Newborn Respiratory Disorders

31

Rosalie O. Mainous

INTRODUCTION

Neonatal respiratory disease or dysfunction is the most frequent diagnosis seen in the newborn in the first 28 days of life. Many respiratory disorders can quickly become life threatening. Anatomically, neonates are at risk for respiratory dysfunction due to increased compliance of the thorax, weak intercostal muscles, a short neck, and an increased airway resistance due to smaller nares and a decreased peripheral airway diameter (Blackburn & Loper, 1992). Additionally, neonates are obligate nose breathers.

Respiratory Distress Syndrome

I. Overview
    A. *Definition.* Formerly known as Hyaline Membrane Disease, Respiratory Distress Syndrome (RDS) is primarily a disease of the preterm infant but has been seen in the term infant. It is the absence or reduction of surfactant supported by clinical (tachypnea [more than 60/min], chest retractions, and cyanosis) and roentgenographic evidence (reticulogranular pattern and bronchograms). Without biochemical evidence of a lack of surfactant, some centers term the respiratory distress seen in preterms as Respiratory Insufficiency of Prematurity (Martin & Fanaroff, 1997).
    B. *Etiology.* A lack or reduction of pulmonary surfactant that may be intensified by risk factors such as maternal diabetes, low gestational age, and asphyxia.
    C. Pathophysiology
        1. Surfactant production, which normally occurs in the Type II Alveolar cells, is diminished.

2. Deficiency of surfactant leads to a decrease in lung compliance. Alveolar hypoventilation and a V/Q mismatch follow (Martin & Fanaroff, 1997).

3. Atelectasis, a hallmark of RDS occurs along with edema and cell injury (Casey, 1999).

4. Barotrauma, cold stress, and acidosis may accelerate this process (Martin & Fanaroff, 1997).

D. Incidence

1. Males outnumber females 2:1 (Hagedorn, Gardner, & Abman, 1998).

2. The younger the infant, the more likely to be affected.

3. Occurs principally in infants less than 1,200 grams and 30 weeks gestation (Hagedorn et al., 1998).

4. Each year in the United States, approximately 4,000 infants are diagnosed (Moise & Hansen, 1998).

E. Complications/sequelae

1. Pulmonary edema

2. Sodium imbalance

3. Fluid intolerance

4. Oliguria

5. Acidosis

6. Marked V/Q abnormalities

7. Air leak following introduction of assisted ventilation

8. Bronchopulmonary dysplasia

9. Infection

10. Patent ductus arteriosus

II. Assessment

A. History

1. Immaturity

2. Maternal diabetes

3. Cesarean section without labor (Casey, 1999)

4. Asphyxia at birth

5. L/S ratio less than 2:1

6. Multiple gestations

B. Physical

1. Fine inspiratory rales (Ariagno, 1995)

2. Cyanosis on room air

3. Nasal flaring

4. Tachypnea

5. Expiratory grunting

6. Retractions

7. Hypothermia

8. Hypotension

C. Diagnostic tests

1. Blood gas sampling: Oxygen is required to maintain; PaO_2 should be maintained between 50–80 mm Hg, $PaCO_2$ in the 40–50 mm Hg, and pH at least 7.25 (Martin & Fanaroff, 1997). Trancutaneous monitors, carbon dioxide monitors, and pulse oximetry will all provide

minute-to-minute diagnostic information (Gomella, Cunningham, Eyal, & Zenk, 1999) that should be correlated with blood gases.

2. Chest X-ray: A-P film will have a classic reticulogranular pattern often referred to as *ground glass* as well as prominent air bronchograms. This pattern usually develops in the first 6 hours of life (Hansen & Corbett, 1998a). Many have a larger thymic silhouette (Martin & Fanaroff, 1997).

3. Septic work up: Blood cultures and complete blood cell count. Any infant that presents with respiratory distress in the first 24 hours must be considered as a possible Group B Streptococcus infection due to a similar radiographic presentation (Casey, 1999). The hematocrit may also be used to rule out anemia or polycythemia (Hagedorn et al., 1998).

III. Common therapeutic modalities

    A. *Surfactant therapy.* Numerous surfactant therapy trials have taken place in the last several years. Infants less than 1,000 grams should be treated prophalactically (in the delivery room) and larger infants prior to 6 hours of life. A mammalian surfactant is preferred (Hansen & Corbett, 1998a). The types available are Natural Surfactants (Survanta, Curosurf, Surfacten, Infasurf, and Aveofact) and Synthetic Surfactants (ALEC and Exosurf). Surfactant therapy offers the greatest benefit when antenatal corticosteroids have also been used. Surfactant administration requires the use of an endotracheal tube. After the administration of surfactant, infants should be closely monitored and ventilator settings reduced to prevent overdistension of the lung and hyperoxemia (Halliday, 1997).

    B. Respiratory support

        1. Intubation and mechanical ventilation

            a. Correct blood gas abnormalities with as little lung injury as possible.

            b. Clinical trials show that there is an advantage to ventilating at a rate of 60 breaths/min with a short inspiratory time compared with 30 breaths/min (Hansen & Corbett, 1998a).

            c. Flow synchronized patient-triggered ventilation allows for more rapid weaning and shorter time to extubation (Donn, Nicks, & Becker, 1994).

            d. Conventional ventilation or high frequency ventilation may be instituted.

            e. An increase in PIP or V_T will increase CO_2 elimination and decrease $PaCO_2$. PEEP increases may lead to an increase in tidal volume and an increase in $PaCO_2$ (Carlo, Martin, & Fanaroff, 1997).

    C. Closure of the patent ductus arteriosus

        1. Assess with echocardiography.

        2. If still present at DOL 3–4, institute indomethacin therapy or surgically close.

IV. Nursing diagnoses, outcomes, and interventions

    A. Impaired gas exchange

      Goal: To decrease work of breathing and promote adequate gas exchange (decrease acidosis, decrease cyanosis, eliminate adventitious breath sounds)

1. Supplemental oxygen
2. Use assisted ventilation for PaO_2 < 50 mm Hg and/or $PaCO_2$ greater than 60 mm Hg (Casey, 1999).
3. A new clinical strategy is permissive hypercapnia (PHC) in surfactant-treated neonates. In a study with 49 preterm infants, infants with permissive hypercapnia had significantly less days of assisted ventilation than did a normocapnic group. The PHC group had a higher $PaCO_2$, and lower PIP, MAP, and respiratory rate (Mariani, Cifuentes, & Carlo, 1999).
4. May need a blood transfusion to maintain hematocrit at 40% (Martin & Fanaroff, 1997).
5. Restore acid base-balance with administration of $NaHCO_3^-$ (only if adequate ventilation).
6. Follow ABGs, pulse oximetry, breath sounds, and assess for a murmur.
7. Fluid restrict if possible to decrease pulmonary edema in the first 48 hours of life.
8. Judicious use of chest physiotherapy for the prevention of atelectasis due to the potential for an acute deterioration in blood gases.
9. Provide sedation (Phenobarbital, etc.) if needed, such as infants that fight the ventilator.
10. Daily chest X-rays (CXRs) to observe for air leaks and disease progression
11. Preoxygenate by increasing O_2 15% prior to suctioning (Peters, 1992).
12. Infants placed prone have higher PaO_2s than those supine (Bancalari & Sinclair, 1992).

B. Ineffection thermoregulation
   Goal: Attain a neutral thermal environment and stabilization of temperature.
   1. Assess humidity and temperature of inspired air (Martin & Fanaroff, 1997).
   2. Place in neutral thermal environment.

C. Decreased cardiac output
   Goal: Promote normalization of blood pressure and diminish shunting.
   1. Monitor blood pressure, if possible with an arterial line
   2. Provide Dopamine/Dobutamine as indicated
   3. Volume replacement
   4. Adequate fluid and electrolytes

D. High risk for less than body requirement, nutrition
   Goal: Promote a positive nitrogen balance
   1. Start on TPN by 2nd day of life
   2. Make sure adequate calories for energy expenditure

Meconium Aspiration Syndrome

I. Overview
   A. *Definition.* Meconium is the first stool of the newborn and is composed of epithelial cells, mucus, and bile. In the event the infant passes this

stool prior to or during delivery, it may be present in the amniotic fluid. If asphyxia is the cause of the meconium passing, gasping may occur in utero. The infant is born having aspirated meconium in utero or during labor and delivery. Meconium must be found below the cords to constitute MAS (Whittsett, Pryhuber, Rice, Warner, & Wert, 1994).

  B. Etiology
1. Physical obstruction of the glottis, trachea, or smaller airways (Hagedorn et al., 1998)
2. Thick meconium as opposed to thin meconium
3. Post-term delivery
4. Decreased Ph (marker of acute intrauterine asphyxia) and concentrations of blood erythropoieten (marker of chronic asphyxia) (Hansen & Corbett, 1998a) are risk factors.
5. Intrauterine gasping in response to asphyxia
6. Fetal tachycardia puts the infant at high risk (Miller, Fanaroff, & Martin, 1997).

  C. Pathophysiology
1. Particulate meconium causes a partial or complete obstruction.
2. In areas of total obstruction, atelectasis occurs.
3. In areas of partial obstruction, a ball-valve phenomena occurs, which leads to air trapping and hyperexpansion (Gomella et al., 1999).
4. A chemical pneunonitis occurs.
5. Alveolar edema and surfactant dysfunction occur, leading to hypoxia.

  D. Incidence
1. MAS occurs in 35% of those infants with meconium fluid staining or in 4% of all live births (Whittsett et al., 1994).
2. Meconium staining of amniotic fluid occurs in anywhere from 10% (Blackburn & Loper, 1992) to 26% of all deliveries (Hansen & Corbett, 1998a).

  E. Complications/sequelae
1. Pulmonary air leaks due to overinflation (pneumothorax, pneumomediastinum, pulmonary interstitial emphysema)
2. Persistent pulmonary hypertension of the newborn
3. Pneumonia
4. Pleural effusion (Hagedorn et al., 1998)
5. Polycythemia
6. Acidosis

II. Assessment
  A. History
1. Intrauterine growth restriction (IUGR)
2. Post-term
3. Meconium stained fluid
4. Asphyxia
5. Usually 34 weeks or greater

  B. Physical
1. Respiratory distress from mild to severe
2. Diffuse rales and rhonchi

3. Expiration phase of respiration prolonged
4. Barrel chest
5. Decreased muscle tone if significant asphyxia
6. Nail beds and skin stained green/brown

C. Diagnostic tests
1. CXR reveals coarse, irregular densities (Miller et al., 1997), patchy areas of atelectasis, and over inflation including flattened diaphragm (Gomella et al., 1999).
2. Cardiomegaly may be seen on CXR.
3. ABGs show hypoxemia and evidence of right to left shunting (low PaO_2 with high O_2 administration).

III. Common therapeutic modalities
A. Correction of hypoxemia and acidosis.
B. O_2 therapy and mechanical ventilation may be required.
C. Lengthening the expiratory time may limit hyperinflation (Whittsett et al., 1994).
D. Role of antibiotics is controversial. MAS may resemble bacterial pneumonia. Treat with antibiotics until culture negative (Hansen & Corbett, 1998a).
E. Because of evidence of surfactant inactivation, there is some support for surfactant therapy to decrease the incidence of air leaks and increase oxygenation (Hansen & Corbett, 1998a). MAS infants treated with surfactant lavage have been shown to have significantly improved mean oxygen indices, MAP, FiO_2, and arterial/alveolar oxygen tension ratios (Lam & Yeung, 1999).
F. Avoid positive pressure ventilation, if possible.
G. Nitric oxide (iNO) or extracorporeal membrane oxygenation (ECMO) may be required.

IV. Nursing diagnosis, outcomes, and intervention
A. High risk for, and ineffective airway clearance.
   Goal: Removal of all particulate matter
   1. During delivery: suction mouth and nose on perineum with DeLee Suction catheter.
   2. Suction airway below the cords under direct visualization in the delivery room if thick meconium.
   3. May require repeated entubations and tracheal suctioning in delivery room.
   4. Leave endotracheal tube in place on third pass (Blackburn & Loper, 1992).
   5. Frequent pulmonary hygiene; suctioning with saline lavage.
   6. Chest physiotherapy unless pulmonary hypertension is worsening.

B. Impaired gas exchange
   Goal: Prevention or reduction in atelectasis; normalization of ABGs
   1. Since many term infants fight the ventilator, sedation and/or paralysis may be necessary.
   2. Provide warmed, humidified oxygen.
   3. Progress to assisted ventilation if ABGs dictate

4. May want to use a lower PEEP because of the ball-valve phenomena and to avoid inadvertent PEEP.

5. Use high rates to ensure alkalosis.

6. High frequency ventilation may be necessary; have ventilator on standby.

Bronchopulmonary Dysphasia

I. Overview

A. *Definition:* Bronchopulmonary dysphasia (BPD), a chronic lung disease, does not have an agreed upon definition or standard diagnostic criteria. Northway, in 1967, developed the first definitions and diagnostic criteria; while useful, they do not cover all the cases of BPD seen today (Northway, Rosan, & Porter, 1967). Bancalari (1997) proposed that many cases today are milder than what has been seen in past and that these cases be referred to as chronic lung disease (CLD). BPD should be reserved for the original stage IV described by Northway. Stage IV occurs after 20 days of life and includes massive fibrosis of the lung, hyperinflation on X-ray, and hypertrophy of pulmonary arterioles and capillaries (Hansen & Corbet, 1998b). A commonly held definition of CLD is all infants following mechanical ventilation that remain in oxygen therapy for >28 days with X-rays showing atelectasis and overinflation, or infants with a persistent requirement of oxygen at 36 weeks post-conceptual age.

B. *Etiology*
   1. Low gestational age
   2. Barotrauma from positive pressure ventilation
   3. Prolonged hyperoxia
   4. PDA—increased shunting left to right
   5. Acute lung injury
   6. Pulmonary edema (may be related to excessive fluid intake)
   7. Pulmonary structural immaturity and/or severe surfactant deficiency
   8. Family history of reactive airway disease puts infant at risk (Hansen & Corbet, 1998b)
   9. Inflammatory process
   10. Poor nutrition

C. Pathophysiology
   1. Injury (prematurity of the lung, oxygen injury, barotrauma) associated with
      a. Edema
      b. Cell necrosis
      c. Airlessness from atelectasis (failure to expand) consolidation or collapse (deMello & Reid, 1995)
      d. Increased permeability of vessels
      e. Smooth muscle hypertrophy
   2. Resolution and healing (deMello & Reid, 1995)
      a. Phagocytosis and absorption of products of inflammation

        b. Condensation of lung into scar

        c. Overexpansion of intervening aerated lung

    3. Catch-up growth. In the surviving lung alveolar multiplication and vascular remodeling (deMello & Reid, 1995)

  D. Incidence

    1. 35%–40% of infants in the 750 gram to 1500 gram weight range. May or may not have been treated with surfactant (Davis & Rosenfeld, 1994).

    2. Figures vary because of the discrepancy in definitions and diagnostic criteria.

    3. May be confused with Wilson-Mikity because of similar X-ray presentation. May distinguish by comparing histories.

    4. Incidence is related to gestational age and birthweight.

    5. Mortality rate after discharge with BPD is approximately 10% (Hansen & Corbett, 1998b).

  E. Complications/sequelae

    1. Congestive heart failure from cor pulmonale (Casey, 1999)

    2. V/Q mismatch

    3. Pulmonary hypertension

    4. Recurrent infection

    5. Progressive respiratory failure

    6. Weight gain below normal curve

    7. Decreased number of alveoli

    8. BPD "spells"—possibly related to bronchospasm and manifested by irritability, cyanosis, hypoxia and hypercapnia (Casey, 1999)

    9. Home oxygen therapy

    10. Pulmonary Interstitial Emphysema

    11. Airway damage (bronchomalasia)

II. Assessment

  A. History

    1. Moderate to severe RDS

    2. Prolonged mechanical ventilation

        a. High peak inspiratory pressures

        b. Continual endotracheal intubation

    3. PDA

    4. Excessive fluid intake prior to diuretic phase in the first days of life

  B. Physical

    1. Bronchospasm

    2. Tachypnea

    3. Oxygen dependence

    4. Rales in bases of lung fields, rhonchi, and wheezing

    5. Retractions

    6. Barrel chest

    7. Prolonged expiratory time

    8. Increased secretions

    9. Liver may be enlarged secondary to right heart failure

C. Diagnostic tests
1. Pulmonary Function Tests show increased airway resistance and decreased tidal volume (Hansen & Corbet, 1998b).
2. CXR shows pulmonary edema and strands of density alternating with hyperlucency bilaterally (Bancalari, 1997). A scoring system for radiographic changes was developed by Toce, Farrell, Leavitt, Samuels, and Edwards (1984) and examines five prominent findings: lung expansion, emphysema, fibrosis, cardiovascular abnormalities, and a subjective assessment. A score of 10 is worst, 0 the best.

III. Common therapeutic modalities
A. Respiratory support
1. MAP to prevent atelectasis and maintain $FiO_2 < 0.5$ (Davis & Rosenfeld, 1994).
2. Inspiratory time of 0.3 to 0.5 seconds.
3. May increase PEEP to 5–8 cm H_2O to reduce expiratory airway resistance (Bancalari, 1997).
4. Wean to a rate of 5–15 and extubate—do not wean to CPAP.
5. Provide methylxanthines (theophylline) prior to extubation.
6. May wean to an N/C.
7. End-tidal CO_2 does not correlate well in BPD.
8. May tolerate $PaCO_2$ to 60s as long as Ph is acceptable; permissive hypercapnia has been associated with a decreased incidence of BPD (Barrington & Finer, 1998).
9. It is thought by some that since a synchronized ventilatory pattern will reduce the incidence of pnuemothoraces, that SIMV will also reduce the incidence of BPD (Barrington & Finer, 1998).
B. Pharmacologic therapy
1. Diuretics
a. Furosemide (lasix)
b. Chlorathiazide (diuril)
c. Hydrochlorthiazide (hydrodiuril)
d. Spironolactone (aldactone)—K+ sparing
2. Methylxanthines
a. Aminophylline
b. Caffeine
3. Albuterol: B_2-agonist: improves pulmonary resistance and lung compliance
4. Systemic corticosteroids: reduces inflammation and improves pulmonary mechanisms
a. Dexamethasone appears to shorten the time to extubation (Hansen & Corbet, 1998b).
i. Side effects include hyperglycemia, neutrophilia, and hypertension. Vitamin E is an antioxident but a randomized blinded trial did not show benefit (Watts et al., 1991).
5. Vitamin A has demonstrated a reduction in BPD in some studies but not in others (Barrington & Finer, 1998).

C. Nutrition
1. Promote high intake of calories while restricting fluid intake.
2. Assess for fractures on X-ray, particularly rib, as a sign of rickets. Provide calcium and vitamin D.
3. Provide early lipid administration with TPN.
4. Aggressive anti reflux measures if gastroesophageal reflux is present.
D. Preventative therapies
1. Antenatal steroids are associated with a significantly lower rate of mortality and a lower incidence of CLD (Wells, Papile, Gardner, Hartenberger & Merker, 1999).
2. Surfactant replacement therapy
3. Limit barotrauma
4. Antioxidant therapy. Current studies using superoxide dismutase show promise in decreasing the clinical signs of BPD (Kenner, 1998).
IV. Nursing diagnoses, outcomes, and interventions
A. Impaired gas exchange
Goal: Maintain PaO$_2$ at >55 mm Hg
1. Oxygen to maintain SaO$_2$ > 90% as determined by pulse oximetry
2. Carefully manage infant to avoid hyperoxia
3. Suctioning to remove excess secretions and prevent plugs.
4. Inhaled brochodilators; if systemic brochodilators, obtain levels
5. Evaluate need for a tracheostomy if still requiring intubation after 6 weeks
6. Chest physiotherapy may be required but use special caution since infant will be at risk for rib fractures.
B. Alt in nutrition, less than body requirements
Goal: Growth in the 50th percentile.
1. Use growth charts and plot length, weight, and head circumference.
2. Anti reflux positioning.
3. Provide calories for increased work of breathing and to compensate decreased fluid intake.
4. Monitor for osteopenia.
C. Alt in fluid management: fluid sensitive
Goal: Maintain fluid balance to prevent pulmonary edema and right sided heart failure.
1. Strict intake and output (I & O).
2. Assess lung sounds for fluid retention.
3. Administer diuretics.
4. Follow serum electrolytes, particularly if on diuretic therapy.
5. Watch for a hypochloremic alkalosis with long-term use of diuretics (Casey, 1999)
D. High risk for infection (secondary to fluid retention, corticosteroids, invasion into airway [ETT])
Goal: Does not acquire RSV or bacterial pathogen
1. Good hand washing
2. Treat any suspected infection.
3. Be aware that corticosteroid therapy will mask signs of infection.

Home Care Considerations

Many more sick infants survive today to be discharged home with a chronic health care condition or possibly an acute exacerbation that can be managed at home in a more cost efficient manner than in-patient care. Successful home care of the newborn with a respiratory disorder is dependent upon a favorable transition to home plan and active participation on the part of the caregiver (Forsythe, 1999). The ideal scenario would involve an interdisciplinary team and meaningful parental involvement as discharge criteria and outcomes are identified jointly. Sometimes case managers are utilized or a neonatal nurse practitioner may serve in this capacity.

A. Numerous factors should be assessed in order to develop the transition plan.
1. Reimbursement mechanisms for durable medical equipment such as home monitors and skilled home health nursing care must be determined.
2. Details related to the home environment such as siblings, household members that smoke, the presence of pets, availability of heat or air conditioning, type of bedding, and sleeping arrangements should be elicited.
3. Identify the need for social service involvement.
4. If the infant has been hospitalized for an extended period of time, determine if any immunizations are needed prior to discharge.
5. The care plan developed should be multidisciplinary and well coordinated between different services and departments.
6. Identify community services for follow up and eligibility of patient and family.
7. A developmental assessment should be done prior to discharge and at intervals during home care for the respiratory condition, particularly if the infant is on home ventilator.
8. Respite care for the family may be an issue depending on the severity of the disorder.
9. Assess barriers to learning and provide resources to alleviate (Forsythe, 1999).
10. Set time to teach parents CPR and to do monitor training if required.
11. Complete all screening for hearing and metabolic disorders prior to discharge.
12. Provide a list of emergency phone numbers.
B. Once the infant is in the home, evaluate the transition plan based on predetermined outcomes. Look at the readmission rate and the comfort level of the parent. More than 50% of infants with BPD are readmitted to the hospital in the first 2 years for a respiratory illness (Chye & Gray, 1995). Determine if resources have been adequate to meet needs of both infant and family.
C. These children are at risk for significant developmental delays and adverse neurological outcomes. They also demonstrate more significant

hearing and vision impairments. Screen for sensory deficits, learning disorders, and behavior problems.

WEB SITES

The Cochrane Neonatal Collaborative Review Group: http://www.nichd.nih. gov/cochraneneonatal/
Hot Neonatology Web sites: http://members.home.net/cotton/neoweb.html
Neonatology on the Web: http://www.neonatology.org/
NICU Web: http://depts.washington.edu/nicuweb/
Pediatric Points of Interest: http://ww2.med.jhu.edu/peds/neonatology/poi.html
Pediatric Pulmonary On-Line Children's Hospital Oakland: http://www.pedi resp-pulm.com/profresouce.html
The R.A.L.E. Repository: http://www.rale.ca/
Vermont Oxford Network: http://www.vtoxford.org/

REFERENCES

Ariagno, R. L. (1995). Respiratory problems in the pre-term infant. In G. B. Reed, A. E. Clareaux, & F. Cochburn (Eds.), *Diseases of the fetus and newborn: Pathology, imaging, genetics and management* (Vol. 2, 2nd ed., pp. 1387–1397). London: Chapman & Hall Medical.

Bancalari, E. (1997). Neonatal chronic lung disease. In H. A. Fanaroff & R. J. Martin (Eds.), *Neonatal-perinatal medicine: Diseases of the fetus and infant* (6th ed., pp. 1074–1089). St. Louis: Mosby.

Bancalari, E., & Sinclair, J. C. (1992). Mechanical ventilation. In J. C. Sinclair & M. B. Bracken (Eds.), *Effective care of the newborn infant* (pp. 200–220). Oxford: Oxford University Press.

Barrington, K. J., & Finer, N. N. (1998). Treatment of bronchopulmonary dysplasia. *Clinics in Perinatology, 25*(1), 177–202.

Blackburn, S. T., & Loper, D. L. (1992). *Maternal, fetal and neonatal physiology.* Philadelphia: W. B. Saunders.

Carlo, W. A., Martin, R. J., & Fanaroff, A. A. (1997). Assisted ventilation and complications of respiratory distress. In A. A. Fanaroff & R. J. Martin (Eds.), *Neonatal-perinatal medicine: Diseases of the fetus and neonate* (Vol. 2, 6th ed., pp. 1028–1040). St. Louis: Mosby.

Casey, P. M. (1999). Respiratory distress. In J. Deacon & P. O'Neill (Eds.), *Core curriculum for neonatal intensive care nursing* (2nd ed., pp. 118–150). Philadelphia: W. B. Saunders.

Chye, J. D., & Gray, P. H. (1995). Rehospitalization and growth of infants with bronchopulmonary dysplasia: A matched control study. *Journal of Pediatric Child Health, 31*, 105–111.

Davis, J. M., & Rosenfeld, W. N. (1994). Chronic lung disease. In G. B. Avery, M. A. Fletcher, & M. G. MacDonald (Eds.), *Neonatalogy: Pathophysiology and management of the newborn* (4th ed., pp. 453–477). Philadelphia: Lippincott.

deMello, D. E., & Reid, L. M. (1995). Respiratory tract and lungs. In G. B. Reed, A. E. Claireaux, & F. Cockburn (Eds.), *Diseases of the fetus and newborn: Pathology, imaging, genetics and management* (Vol. 1, 2nd ed., pp. 523–560). London: Chapman and Hall Medical.

Donn, S. M., Nicks, J. J., & Becker, M. A. (1994). Flow synchronized ventilation of preterm infants with respiratory distress syndrome. *Journal of Perinatology, 14*(2), 90–94.

Forsythe, P. L. (1999). Transition of the high-risk neonate to home care. In J. Deacon & P. O'Neill (Eds.), *Core curriculum for neonatal intensive care nursing* (2nd ed., pp. 772–780). Philadelphia: W. B. Saunders.

Gomella, T. L., Cunningham, M. D., Eyal, F. G., & Zenk, K. E. (Eds.). (1999). *Neonatology: Management, procedures, on-call problems, diseases and drugs* (4th ed.). Stamford, CN: Appleton & Lange.

Hagedorn, M. I., Gardner, S. L., & Abman, S. H. (1998). Respiratory diseases. In G. B. Merenstein & S. L. Gardner (Eds.), *Handbook of neonatal intensive care* (4th ed., pp. 437–499). St. Louis: Mosby.

Halliday, H. L. (1997). Surfactant therapy: Questions and answers. *Journal of Neonatal Nursing, 3*(3), 30, 32, 34–36.

Hansen, T., & Corbett, A. (1998a). Disorders of the transition. In H. W. Taeusch & R. A. Ballard (Eds.), *Avery's diseases of the newborn* (7th ed., pp. 602–629). Philadelphia: W. B. Saunders.

Hansen, T., & Corbett. A. (1998b). Chronic lung disease. In H. W. Taeusch, & R. A. Ballard (Eds.), *Avery's diseases of the newborn* (7th ed., pp. 634–647). Philadelphia: W. B. Saunders.

Kenner, C. (1998). Complications of respiratory management. In C. Kenner, J. W. Lott, & A. A. Flandermeyer (Eds.), *Comprehensive neonatal nursing: A physiologic perspective* (2nd ed., pp. 290–305). Philadelphia: W. B. Saunders.

Lam, B. C. C., & Yeung, C. Y. (1999). Surfactant lavage for meconium aspiration syndrome: A pilot study. *Pediatrics, 103*(5), 1014–1018.

Mariani, G., Cifuentes, J., & Carlo, W. A. (1999). Randomized trial of permissive hypercapnia in preterm infants. *Pediatrics, 104*(5), 1082–1088.

Martin, R. J., & Fanaroff, A. A. (1997). The respiratory distress syndrome and its management. In A. A. Fanaroff & R. J. Martin (Eds.), *Neonatal-perinatal medicine: Diseases of the fetus and infant* (Vol. 2, 6th ed., pp. 1018–1028). St. Louis: Mosby.

Miller, M. J., Fanaroff, A. A., & Martin, R. J. (1997). Respiratory disorders in pre-term and term infants. In A. A. Fanaroff & R. J. Martin (Eds.), *Neonatal-perinatal medicine: Diseases of the fetus and infant* (Vol. 2, 6th ed., pp. 1040–1065). St. Louis: Mosby.

Moise, A. A., & Hansen, T. N. (1998). Acute acquired parechymal lung disease. In T. N. Hansen, T. R. Cooper, & L. E. Weisman (Eds.), *Contemporary diagnosis and management of neonatal and respiratory diseases* (2nd ed., pp. 79–95). Newton, PA: Handbooks in Healthcare (Division of AMM Co.).

Northway, W. H., Rosan, R. C., & Porter, D. Y. (1967). Pulmonary disease following respirator therapy of hyaline-membrane disease: Bronchopulmonary dysplasia. *New England Journal of Medicine, 276*(7), 357–368.

Peters, K. L. (1992). Does routine nursing care complicate the physiologic status of the premature neonate with respiratory distress syndrome? *Journal of Perinatal-Neonatal Nursing, 6*(2), 67–84.

Toce, S. S., Farrell, P. M., Leavitt, L. A., Samuels, D. P., & Edwards, D. K. (1984). Clinical and radiographic scoring systems for assessing bronchopulmonary dysphasia. *American Journal Diseases in Children, 138,* 581.

Watts, J. L., Milner, R., Zipursky, A., Paes, B., Gill, G., Fletcher, B., et al. (1991). Failure of supplementation with vitamin E to prevent bronchopulmonary dysplasia in infants less than 1500 g birth weight. *European Respiratory Journal, 4*(2) 188–190.

Wells, L. R., Papile, L. A., Gardner, M. O., Hartenberger, C. R., & Merker, L. (1999). Impact of antenatal corticosteroid therapy in very low birth weight infants on chronic lung disease and other morbidities of prematurity. *Journal of Perinatology, 19*(8), 578–581.

Whittsett, J. A., Pryhuber, G. S., Rice, W. R., Warner, B. B., & Subert, S. E. (1994). Acute respiratory disorders. In G. B. Avery, M. A. Fletcher, & M. G. MacDonald (Eds.), *Neonatology: Pathophysiology and management of the newborn* (4th ed., pp. 429–477). Philadelphia: Lippincott.

SUGGESTED READING

Gomella, T. L., Cunningham, M. D., Eyal, F. G., & Zenk, K. E. (Eds.) (1999). *Neonatology: Management, procedures, on-call problems, diseases and drugs* (4th ed.). Stamford, CT: Appleton & Lange.

Bronchiolitis

32

Becky E. Tribby

INTRODUCTION

I. Overview
   A. Definition
      1. Acute lower respiratory tract viral induced infection of the small bronchi and bronchioles in children less than 3 years of age (Andersen, 1998). The most critical stage of illness is 48–72 hours after the cough starts. In most cases, recovery is complete within a few days (Orenstein, 2000).
   B. Etiology including physical and psychosocial risk factors
      1. Respiratory syncytial virus is major cause of bronchiolitis (45%–75%); parainfluenza (15%–30%); and adenovirus, rhinovirus, and influenza virus each account for 3%–10%. *M. pneumoniae* has been found in a small percentage of cases (Andersen, 1998).
      2. Most common in nonbreastfeeding male infants between 3 and 6 months of age who live in crowded conditions.
      3. Risk factors include smoking mothers and attendance at day care centers (Orenstein, 2000).
      4. Highly seasonal with hospitalizations occurring between November to April with peak activity in January and February (Shay et al., 1999).
   C. Pathophysiology
      Bronchiolitis is an upper respiratory tract infection with viruses replicating in the epithelium of the upper respiratory airways and spreading down the epithelium of the airway by cell to cell transfer (Andersen, 1998). Edema, mucus, and cellular debris obstruct the infant's very small bronchioles. This increases airway resistance leading to constriction of the airways and hyperinflation of the lungs. If obstruction is complete,

trapped air is absorbed resulting in atelectasis. This can impair gas exchange resulting in hypoxia. Metabolic acidosis and respiratory alkalosis can develop (McKinney et al., 2000).

D. Incidence
   1. Most common lower respiratory tract illness.
   2. Approximately 10% of babies develop bronchiolitis in first year of life.
   3. Hospitalization is needed for about 2% to 3% of all cases of bronchiolitis, but approximately 17% of hospitalizations of infants are due to bronchiolitis (Perlstein et al., 1999).
   4. From 1980 through 1996 it is estimated that 1,648,281 children less than 5 years of age were admitted to the hospital for bronchiolitis. Fifty-seven percent were children younger than 6 months of age and 81% were younger than 1 year of age (Shay et al., 1999).
   5. Hospitalization rates increased from 1.3 per 1,000 children aged 1 through 4 years in 1980 to 2.3 per 1,000 in 1996. Rates for children less than 1 year of age increased from 12.9 to 31.2 during this time.
   6. Males were 1.6 times more likely to be hospitalized than females.
   7. Increase in hospitalization in the last 15 years is attributed to trends in childcare practices, changes in the criteria for hospitalization due to increased use of pulse oximetry, and decreasing mortality among premature and medically complex infants (Shay et al., 1999).

E. Complications/sequelae
   1. One percent of children younger than 1 year of age receive intubation for mechanical ventilation (Shay et al., 1999).
   2. The fatality rate is less than 1% and may be due to prolonged apneic episodes, respiratory acidosis that is not compensated, or severe dehydration. Children with congenital heart disease, bronchopulmonary dysplasia, immunodeficiency, or cystic fibrosis have higher rates of morbidity and mortality (Orenstein, 2000).
   3. Bacterial acute otitis media is a complication for approximately 60% of children with bronchiolitis. They require typical antimicrobial therapy for acute otitis media (Andrade, Hoberman, Glustein, Paradise, & Wald, 1998).
   4. Adenovirus may be associated with long-term complications, including bronchiolitis obliterans and unilateral hyperlucent lung syndrome (Swyer-James syndrome; Orenstein, 2000).
   5. The prevalence of wheezing in children 9 to 10 years after hospitalization for bronchiolitis was three times greater than for a control group of children. Overall lung growth was not affected, but airway abnormalities were increased in the children with bronchiolitis (Noble et al., 1997).

II. Assessment
   A. History
      1. Two- to 3-day course of rhinorrhea with serous nasal drainage, sneezing, cough, irritability, and none to low grade (<39° C) fever.
      2. Respiratory distress can develop with paroxysmal wheezy cough, tachypnea (respiratory rate 60–80 breaths/min) dyspnea, and irritability.

    3. Infant may be refusing to take food or liquids or may vomit during or after feedings due to cough (McKinney et al., 2000).

  B. Physical

    1. Nasal flaring, intercostal and subcostal retractions, increased respiratory rate (>60 per minute).

    2. Prominent expiratory wheezes and occasionally inspiratory wheeze, diffuse fine crackles, transmitted upper airway sounds and prolonged expiratory phase.

    3. Liver and spleen may be palpable due to hyperinflation of the lungs.

    4. Severe air hunger and cyanosis may be present (Orenstein, 2000).

  C. Diagnostic tests

    1. Routine nasopharyngeal washing for RSV antigen is not recommended.

    2. Chest X-ray is not routinely needed. Blood gases are obtained if clinically indicated (Perlstein et al., 1999).

    3. The risk of bacteremia, urinary tract infection, and meningitis is extremely low.

    4. Blood cultures, white cell counts, urinalysis and cultures, and cultures of cerebrospinal fluid are often obtained, but are usually not necessary (Greenes & Harper, 1999; Liebelt, Qu & Harvey, 1999).

III. Common therapeutic modalities

  A. Mild disease

    1. Treatment is supportive and can be done at home.

    2. Offer small frequent feedings to provide adequate fluid intake.

    3. Provide humidification, bulb suctioning of nose, and rest (McKinney et al., 2000).

  B. Respiratory distress

    1. The basic management goals during hospitalization are to maintain adequate oxygenation and hydration.

    2. These include cool mist therapy, aerosol therapy with saline, bronchodilators or steroids (Perlstein et al., 1999).

    3. While there is no increase in respiratory distress in infants treated with chest physical therapy, there is also no benefit to the management of acute viral bronchiolitis if there is no other pathogenesis (Nicholas, Dhouieb, Marshall, Edmunds, & Grant, 1999).

    4. Inhalations using epinephrine may be tried in selected patients. If significant improvement is not seen within 60 minutes, the therapy should not be continued (Perlstein et al., 1999).

    5. A 6-week course of nebulilzed budesonide did not show a significant difference in the reduction of symptoms of acute bronchiolitis, nor the prevention of wheezing after 6 months (Richter & Seddon, 1998).

    6. Nasogastric feedings or parenteral fluids may be needed to prevent dehydration from tachypnea.

    7. Infants should be isolated in a single room and good handwashing is a must (McKinney et al., 2000).

IV. Nursing diagnoses, outcomes, and interventions
   A. Impaired gas exchange related to edema and mucus.
   B. Ineffective airway clearance related to increased secretions.
      1. Expected outcome
         a. Clear breath sounds with normal respiratory rate, depth, and rhythm.
         b. Secretions will be cleared from the airway.
         c. Improved gas exchange with oxygen > 95% on room air.
      2. Interventions
         a. Monitor and document vital signs and respiratory status including rate.
         b. Auscultate for adventitious breath sounds.
         c. Observe for the presence of retractions every 2 hours during the acute phase and as needed as the infant improves.
         d. Cardio respiratory monitoring with appropriate alarms set.
         e. Use either continuous or spot-check pulse oximetry.
         f. Administer humidified oxygen to keep saturations > 95%.
         g. Position head at a 30° to 40° upright angle to maintain airway and decrease pressure on the diaphragm.
         h. Instill normal saline nose drops and suction with bulb syringe as needed for blockage of nasal passages with mucus.
         i. Provide periods of uninterrupted rest between care.
   C. Fluid volume deficit related to decreased intake and insensible loss
      1. Expected outcome: Adequate hydration with moist mucus membranes, flat fontanel, normal urine output and stable weight
      2. Interventions
         a. Monitor and document hydration status (skin turgor, fontanel, and mucus membranes).
         b. Monitor intake and output.
         c. Obtain daily weights and electrolyte values.
         d. Encourage frequent oral intake of clear fluids. IV fluids or ng feedings are indicated if respiratory distress limits oral intake or puts the infant at risk for aspiration.
   D. Ineffective thermoregulation related to infectious illness
      1. Expected outcome: Body temperature within normal limits
      2. Intervention
         a. Monitor and document temperature every 2 to 4 hours and as needed.
         b. Control environmental temperature and dress infant in light clothing.
         c. Administer acetaminophen or ibuprofen as ordered to reduce fever.
   E. Anxiety related to hospitalization and dyspnea
      1. Expected outcomes
         a. Infant will be content with adequate sleep and stable vital signs.
         b. Parents will participate appropriately in infant's cares and verbalize understanding of their infant's condition.

2. Interventions
   a. Explain hospital routines and procedures to parents and encourage them to stay with and care for infant as much as possible.
   b. Maintain a calm environment and allow parents to voice their concerns (McKinney et al., 2000).
V. Home care considerations
   A. Mild disease—no need for hospitalization
      1. Providing adequate fluids and rest can treat infants with mild disease at home.
      2. Educate parents to monitor for signs of respiratory distress.
      3. Avoid exposure to cigarette smoke.
   B. Post-discharge care
      1. Symptoms will be resolved by time of discharge.
      2. Resume normal infant cares.
      3. Avoid exposure to cigarette smoke (McKinney et al., 2000).

WEB SITES

Link to Common Pediatric Problems to Bronchitis/Bronchiolitis
http://www.wrongdiagnosis.com/sym/bronchitis.htm
http://www.mayoclinic.com/health/bronchiolitis
1. Family Practice Handbook
2. Bronchiolitis
3. Bronchiolitis: Information for Parents and Patients
KidsHealth: http://www.KidsHealth.org (search for bronchiolitis)
American Medical Association: http://www.ama-assn.org (link to Consumer Health Information—KidsHealth—Infections and Immunizations—Bronchiolitis)

REFERENCES

Andersen, P. (1998). Pathogenesis of lower respiratory tract infections due to Chlamydia, Mycoplasma, Legionella and viruses. *Thorax, 53*(4), 302–307.

Andrade, M. A., Hoberman, A., Glustein, J., Paradise, J. L., & Wald, E. R. (1998). Acute otitis media in children with bronchiolitis. *Pediatrics, 101*(4), 617–619.

Greenes, D. S., & Harper, M. B. (1999). Low risk of bacteremia in febrile children with recognizable viral syndromes. *Pediatric Infectious Disease Journal, 18*(3), 258–261.

Liebelt, E., Qu, K., & Harvey, K. (1999). Diagnostic testing for serious bacterial infections in infants aged 90 day or younger with bronchiolitis. *Archives of Pediatrics & Adolescent Medicine, 153*(5), 525–530.

McKinney, E. S., Ashwill, J. W., Murray, S. S., James, S. R., Gorrie, T. M., & Droske, S. C. (Eds.). (2000). *Maternal-child nursing* (pp. 1217–1222). Philadelphia, PA: W. B. Saunders Company.

Nicholas, K. J., Dhouieb, M. O., Marshall, T. G., Edmunds, A. T., & Grant, M. B. (1999). An evaluation of chest physiotherapy in the management of acute bronchiolitis: changing clinical practice. *Physiotherapy, 85*(12), 669–674.

Noble, V., Murray, M., Webb, M. S. C., Alexander, J., Swarbrick, A. S., & Milner, A. D. (1997). Respiratory status and allergy nine to 10 years after acute bronchiolitis. *Archives of Disease in Childhood, 76*(4), 315–319.

Orenstein, D. M. (2000). Bronchiolitis. In R. E. Behrman, R. M. Kliegman, & H. B. Jenson, (Eds.), *Nelson Textbook of Pediatrics* (16th ed., pp. 1285–1287). Philadelphia, PA: W. B. Saunders Company.

Perlstein, P. H., Kotagal, U. R., Bolling, C., Steele, R., Schoettker, P. J., Atherton, H. D., et al. (1999). Evaluation of an evidence-based guidelines for bronchiolitis. *Pediatrics, 104*(6), 1334–1341.

Richter, H., & Seddon, P. (1998). Early nebulized budesonide in the treatment of bronchiolitis and the prevention of postbroncholitic wheezing. *The Journal of Pediatrics, 132*(5), 849–853.

Shay, D. K, Holman, R. C., Newman, R. D., Liu, L. L., Stout, J. W., & Anderson, L. J. (1999). Bronchiolitis-associated hospitalizations among U.S. children, 1980–1996. *Journal of the American Medical Association, 282*(15), 1440–1446.

Respiratory Syncytial Virus {33}

Pamela K. DeWitt

INTRODUCTION

I. Overview
   A. Respiratory syncytial virus (RSV) was first isolated in 1956 and is the most common cause of lower respiratory tract infection in infants and young children. It accounts for approximately 90,000 hospitalizations and 4,500 deaths in the United States each year (Wilkins & Dexter, 1998). Most hospitalizations occur in infants less than 6 months old. Nearly all children have been infected with RSV by 2 years of age (Glezen, Taber, Frank, & Kasel, 1996). The primary infection with RSV is usually the most severe and re-infection throughout life is common. While RSV infections can occur year round, temperate climates primarily have annual outbreaks, which peak in winter months (American Academy of Pediatrics [AAP], 1998).
   B. Epidemiology
      1. The only source of infection is humans and transmission is by direct or close contact with contaminated secretions (AAP, 1997). Infection does not cause immunity; reinfection occurs throughout the life span. Viral shedding usually lasts from 3 to 8 days and can last up to 4 weeks in young infants (AAP, 1997).
      2. Those children most at risk for severe or fatal RSV infection have a history of
         a. Prematurity
         b. Cyanotic or complicated congenital heart disease
         c. Chronic lung disease
         d. Immunodeficiency
         e. Therapy causing immunosuppression
         f. Exposure to cigarette smoke (Raza et al., 1999)

C. Pathophysiology
   1. The virus affects the entire respiratory tract. Lung pathology of the small airways includes epithelial necrosis, sloughing of tissue into the airways, edema, increased mucous production, and eventual airway plugging. After plugging occurs, lung hyperinflation and atelectasis develop.
   2. Hypoxemia and increased work of breathing may develop in the more severe instances.

II. Assessment
   A. History
      1. RSV infection should be suspected when young children and infants have cold or flu symptoms during the season or local outbreak.
   B. Physical findings
      1. Tachypnea
      2. Retractions
      3. Nasal flaring
      4. Grunting respirations
      5. Poor appetite
      6. Apneic episodes
      7. Cardiac dysrythmias (Olesch & Bullock, 1998)
      8. Expiratory wheezing, crackles, or diminished respirations
      9. Low PaO_2, elevated $PaCO_2$ as demonstrated with an ABG
      10. Hyperinflation and interstitial pneumonitis on chest X-ray
      11. Otitis media (Andrade Hoberman, Glustein, Paradise, & Wald, 1998)
   C. Diagnosis
      1. Direct, rapid diagnosis can be made with an enzyme immunoassay or immunoflourescent technique. Nasal or nasopharyngeal washes are used to collect specimens.
      2. Isolation from cell cultures takes 3 to 5 days. Serology testing of young infants does not reliably demonstrate the presence of the virus (AAP, 1997).

III. Common therapeutic modalities
   A. Treatment for RSV is most often supportive in nature.
      1. Supplemental oxygen and adequate hydration are often used.
      2. Bronchodilators (Goh, Chay, Foo, & Ong, 1997) and dexamethosone (DeBoeck, Van der Aa, Van Lierde, Corbeel, & Eeckels, 1997) have not been found to be effective in treating RSV.
   B. Ribavirin
      1. Controversial and less frequently used.
      2. It is often restricted to the treatment of the most severely ill, young children.
      3. Ribavirin therapy is delivered by aerosol to the lower airways via oxygen hood, tent or directly into a ventilator circuit. The treatments are given for 12 to 20 hours a day and 1 to 7 days (AAP, 1997).
   C. Long-term effects
      1. Changes in pulmonary function tests have been noted in children who had severe RSV infections (Stein et al., 1999).

2. Recurrent or chronic wheezing for several years has also been described in children who had severe RSV infections (Stein et al., 1999).

D. Prevention

1. Reducing exposure and training parents and caregivers about transmission are critical aspects of RSV prevention (AAP, 1998). Prevention measures include
   a. Eliminate exposure to cigarette smoke
   b. Limit exposure to contagious settings
   c. Good hand washing

2. A vaccine is being developed to give to infants in the first few weeks of life, but it is not available at this time (Crowe, 1998).

3. Respiratory syncytial virus immune globulin intravenous (RSV-IGIV) has been used since early 1996 to prevent RSV infection for children younger than 24 months with chronic lung disease or a history of prematurity.
   a. RSV-IGIV is given intravenously over 4 hours on a monthly basis throughout the RSV season.
   b. RSV-IGIV may decrease non-RSV respiratory infections.
   c. It is not recommended for children with cyanotic congenital heart disease and MMR and Varicella vaccinations must be deferred for 9 months after the last dose of RSV-IGIV (AAP, 1998).

4. Palivizumab, a monoclonal antibody, was approved by the FDA in June 1998 to prevent RSV infections in high-risk infants.
   a. Palivizumab is not a human blood product and is given IM, once a month, during the RSV season.
   b. It does not interfere with vaccination administration and is less expensive than RSV-IGIV.
   c. It too is not recommended for children with congenital heart disease (AAP, 1998).

IV. Nursing diagnosis, outcomes, and interventions

A. Nursing diagnosis: Ineffective breathing related to inflammatory process.

1. *Goal:* Establish normal respiratory function
   a. Expected outcomes
      i. Respirations within normal limits
      ii. Respirations are unlabored
   b. Nursing interventions
      i. Maintain open airway and maximum lung expansion with positioning
      ii. Reposition as needed to maintain optimum position
      iii. Promote rest and sleep

2. *Goal:* Optimize oxygenation
   a. Expected outcomes
      i. Oxygen saturation remains above 95%
      ii. Arterial blood gases (ABGs) remain within normal limits

   b. Nursing interventions
    i. Monitor oxygen saturation
    ii. Provide humidified oxygen.
  B. Nursing diagnosis: Ineffective airway clearance related to mechanical obstruction, inflammation, and increased secretions.
   1. *Goal:* Maintain patient airway
    a. Expected outcome: Airways remain clear
    b. Nursing interventions
     i. Maintain adequate hydration
     ii. Perform chest physiotherapy
     iii. Suction secretions as needed
     iv. Have emergency intubation equipment available
  C. Nursing diagnosis: High risk for fluid volume deficit related to difficulty taking fluids, insensible losses from suctioning and hyperventilation
   1. *Goal:* Will exhibit adequate hydration
    a. Expected outcomes
     i. Appropriate fluid balance
     ii. Balanced intake and output
     iii. Serum electrolytes within normal limits
    b. Nursing interventions
     i. Maintain intravenous infusion at appropriate rate
     ii. Offer oral fluids as tolerated
     iii. Measure intake and output
  D. Nursing diagnosis: Potential for impaired gas exchange related to immature neurologic development and severe viral infection
   1. *Goal:* Will maintain adequate respiratory pattern
    a. Expected outcomes
     i. Appropriate respiratory pattern
     ii. Arterial blood gases within normal limits
     iii. Serum glucose within normal limits
    b. Nursing interventions
     i. Assess respiratory pattern regularly
     ii. Check for thermal stability
     iii. Prevent hypoglycemia
     iv. Monitor continuously
     v. Have emergency intubation equipment available
  E. Nursing diagnosis: Altered family processes related to illness and hospitalization of infant
   1. *Goal:* Will exhibit ability to cope
    a. Expected outcomes
     i. Family will ask appropriate questions
     ii. Family appropriately involved in care
    b. Nursing interventions
     i. Provide family with information and support
     ii. Explain procedures and therapy

      iii. Reinforce information as needed

      iv. Encourage family involvement in child's care

V. Home care

    A. Post hospitalization will include family education and procedures to prevent re-infection.

    B. Supplemental home oxygen may be required until the lower respiratory tract infection subsides.

    C. Keep the child well hydrated to prevent plugging of the airways.

    D. Premature infants or those who developed apnea may need home monitoring.

    E. This is usually continued until symptoms are gone and off home oxygen.

REFERENCES

American Academy of Pediatrics. (1997). Respiratory Syncytial Virus. In Peter, G. (Ed.), *Red book: Report of the committee on infectious disease* (24th ed.). Elk Grove Village, IL: American Academy of Pediatrics.

American Academy of Pediatrics, Committee on Infectious Diseases and Committee on Fetus and Newborn. (1998). Prevention of respiratory syncytial virus infections: Indications for these of Palivizumab and update on the use of RSV-IGIV (RE9839). *Pediatrics, 102*(5), 1211–1216.

Andrade, M. A., Hoberman, A., Glustein, J., Paradise, J. L., & Wald, E. R. (1998). Acute otitis media in children with bronchiolitis. *Pediatrics, 101*(4 Pt. 1), 617–619.

Crowe, J. E., Jr. (1998). Immune responses of infants to infection with respiratory viruses and live attenuated respiratory virus candidate vaccines. *Vaccine, 16*(14–15), 1423–1432.

DeBoeck, K., Van der Aa, N., Van Lierde, S., Corbeel, L., & Eeckels, R. (1997). Respiratory syncytial virus bronchiolitis: A double-blind dexamethosone efficacy study. *Journal of Pediatrics, 131*(6), 919–921.

Glezen, W. P., Taber, L. H., Frank, A. L., & Kasel, J. A. (1996). Risk of primary infection and reinfection with respiratory syncytial virus. *American Journal of Diseases in Children, 140*, 543–546.

Goh, A., Chay, O. M., Foo, A. L., & Ong, E. K. (1997). Efficacy of bronchodilators in the treatment of bronchiolitis. *Singapore Medical Journal, 38*(8), 326–328.

Olesch, C. A., & Bullock, A. M. (1998). Bradyarrhythmia and supraventricular tachycardia in a neonate with RSV. *Journal of Paediatric Child Health, 34*(2), 199–201.

Raza, M. W., Essery, S. D., Elton, R. A., Weir, D. M., Busuttil, A., & Blackwell, C. (1999). Exposure to cigarette smoke, a major risk factor for sudden infant death syndrome: Effects of cigarette smoke on inflammatory responses to viral infection and bacterial toxins. *FEMS Immunology and Medical Microbiology, 25*(1–2), 145–154.

Stein, R. T., Sherrill, D., Morgan, W. J., Holberg, C. J., Halonen, M., Taussig, L. M., et al. (1999). Respiratory syncytial virus in early life and risk of wheeze and allergy by age 13 years. *Lancet, 354*(9178), 541–545.

Wilkins, R. L., & Dexter, J. R. (Eds.). (1998). *Respiratory disease: A case study approach to patient care* (2nd ed.). Philadelphia, PA: F. A. Davis Company.

SUGGESTED READING

Dudas, R. A., & Karron, R. A. (1998). Respiratory syncytial virus vaccines. *Clinical Microbiology Review, 11*(3), 430–439.

Croup

Joyce J. LoChiatto and Mary Horn

INTRODUCTION

Two causes of potential upper airway obstruction in children are croup and epiglottitis. This chapter describes the differences between croup and epiglottitis.

I. Overview
  A. Definition
     The term *croup* describes a syndrome characterized by the abrupt onset of a barky cough, inspiratory or expiratory stridor, hoarseness, and or respiratory distress of varying severity resulting from obstruction in the region of the larynx. The term was once used exclusively to describe diphtheria; it is now used primarily to describe viral laryngotracheobronchitis. Croup may be caused by mechanical, infectious, and non-infectious reasons as outlined in tables 34.1 and 34.2. It is specifically subglottic inflammation and resultant swelling that compromises the airway in croup (Fitzgerald & Kilham, 2004).
  B. Etiology
     Infectious croup usually viral in origin is presented under the subheadings of laryngitis, laryngotracheitis, spasmodic croup, laryngotracheobronchitis (bacterial tracheitis/diptheria), laryngotracheobronchopneumonitis (Cherry, 1998). Multiple organisms contribute to croup (Table 34.1).
  C. Pathophysiology
     Croup is an airway obstruction caused by inflammation of the larynx and the subglottic area. The respiratory route, either via direct droplet spread or hand-to-mucosa inoculation, transmits the causative virus. The cells of the local respiratory epithelium become infected after inhalation of the virus. There is marked edema of the fibrous connective tissue that

Table 34.1 Infectious Organisms Causing Croup

Most common organisms	Mild cases	Infrequent cases	Other causes
Parainfluenza viruses (50% caused by Type 1) Season: Winter	Associated with Croup: Rhinoviruses, enteroviruses, herpes simplex virus, and Myocoplasma pneumonia	Parainfluenza type 2 and type 3	Influenza A and B, respiratory syncytial virus (RSV), parainfluenza 2, adenoviruses, and herpes simplex virus, human metapneumovirus
Enteroviruses (coxsackievirus A and B and echovirus parainfluenza type 3) Season: Summer		Moribilli (measles) virus may cause upper airway obstruction from bacterial tracheitis. Diphtheria must be considered if the child has not been immunized. This organism may cause a membranous obstruction (Asher, 1999; Wald, 1999). Recently, 20% of previously virus negative lower respiratory tract illnesses were attributed to human metapneumovirus (Williams et al, 2004).	Noninfectious Laryngotracheobronchitis (Bacterial Tracheitis, secondary bacterial infection of viral laryngotracheitis) Causative organism: *Staphylococcus aureus*, *Haemophilus influenza* type B and nontypable *Haemophilus*, *Streptococcus pneumoniae*, *Klebsiella pnemoniae*, *Streptococcus pyogenes* group A (Wald, 1999). Prior to the Hib B vaccine, studies indicated an 89% incidence of croup, 8% incidence of epiglottitis, and 2% incidence of bacterial tracheitis (Al-Jundi, 1997).

		Congenital abnormalities exacerbated by respiratory
Mechanical Croup	**Trauma**	**infections**
Gastroesophageal reflux	Blunt external trauma	Immunologic (hereditary)
Foreign body aspiration		Laryngotracheomalacia
Allergic: Acute	Thermal injuries	Vascular ring
Angioneurotic edema		
Epiglottitis		
Neurogenic reflex	Chemical injuries	Congenital subglottic stenosis,
laryngospasm	(ingestions)	vocal cord paralysis
Tumors	Secondary to extubation	
Retropharyngeal abscess	Neurological	Subglottic hemangiomas
Vocal cord paralysis		Cysts and laryngoceles

Table 34.2 Differential Diagnoses: Noninfectious Croup/Airway Obstruction

lies under the surface of the epithelium of the mucous membranes, submucosa, and is accompanied by cellular infiltration with histocytes, lymphocytes, plasma cells, and polymorphonuclear leukocytes (Geelhoed, 1997). There is redness and swelling of the nasopharynx, most marked in the lateral walls of the trachea just below the vocal cords. Unfortunately, since a fixed cricoid cartilage surrounds the trachea, any inflammatory swelling that occurs creates encroachment on the internal airway lumen, narrowing it to a slit. The infant's glottis and subglottic region are normally narrow, and a small decrease in diameter results in a large increase in airway resistance and a decrease in airflow. As the airway enlarges with age, the impact of the swelling of the subglottic area is proportionally less obstructive (Geelhoed, 1997).

Obstruction to airflow through the upper airway results in stridor and difficulty breathing and may progress to hypoxia when stridor is severe. Hypoxia with mild obstruction indicates lower airway involvement from lower airway obstruction or lung parenchymal infection or fluid accumulation. Hypercapnia occurs as a late change as hypoventilation increases and progresses with secretion accumulation creating obstruction (Asher, 1999; Persing, 2000; Slota, 1997).

D. Incidence

The incidence of croup is 1.5/100 children under 6 years of age but it is seen in children of any age (Al-Jundi, 1997). It usually occurs between 1 and 3 years of age; boys are affected more often than girls. Peak incidence occurs at 2 years of age. The youngest reported patient is 3 months of age. A peak in autumn is associated with parainfluenza virus. Viral croup is rare after 10 years of age (Asher, 1999; Shepherd, 2004).

E. Complications of croup
    1. Epiglottitis (see below for further discussion).
    2. Occurrence of otitis media may occur simultaneously.
    3. Severe respiratory distress, decreased air entry, airway obstruction, muscle fatigue altered level of consciousness, hypoventilation, and potential of a cardiac arrest (Fisher, 2004).
    4. Hypoxemia and hypercapnea
    5. Because of pain with swallowing, dehydration may occur due to decreased fluid intake (Rosekrans, 1998).
    6. Bacterial tracheitis (secondary bacterial infection of viral laryngotracheitis) is a relatively uncommon condition. Endotracheal intubation is necessary due to potential cardiac arrest and airway obstruction.
    7. Stenosis and narrowing of the trachea from scarring is usually a result of a long-term complication. In instances of severe sloughing of the tissue in the airway, a tracheostomy may be necessary to maintain airway patency (Al-Jundi, 1997).

II. Common therapeutic modalities
    A. Outpatient: Office Treatment (including the Emergency Department)
        Emergency management of croup begins with the assessment of the severity of airway obstruction (Jaffe, 1998). Croup Score is an assessment scale that may be utilized in the patient with croup symptoms. It includes level of consciousness, desaturation, stridor, air entry, and retractions (range of 0–5 points used for the presence of certain signs; Rosekrans, 1998; see Appendix "A Croup Scoring System Based on Four Clinical Signs"). A recent report showed where two children had been recently seen by an experienced pediatrician, diagnosed with viral croup, and managed with outpatient glucocorticoids; both had a respiratory arrest out of hospital. The cases emphasize the need for careful assessment and close follow-up of patients with croup (Fisher, 2004). Treatments are managed according to the degree of airway severity.
    B. Office treatment for mild croup
        Aerosolized cool mist humidification applied while the child sits on the parent's lap.
        1. Aerosolized cool mist may be preferred over using a croupette to deliver the mist because the dense mist may obscure the vision of the caretaker in observing the respiratory distress in the child. It may also provoke anxiety in the child, therefore increasing respiratory distress due to anxiety from separation from their parent (Rosekrans, 1998). Children with cyanosis or hypoxemia should receive supplemental oxygen (Jaffe, 1998). Advantage of mist is controversial (Jamshidi et al., 2001).
        2. Children with wheezing may trial cool mist; however, if the cool mist is contributing to the wheezing, the treatment should be discontinued (Jaffe, 1998).
        3. A study involving children with mild croup who received oral dexamethasone treatment concluded that they are less likely to seek subsequent medical care and demonstrated more rapid symptom

resolution compared with children who receive nebulized dexamethasone or placebo treatment (Luria et al., 2001).

C. Office treatment for moderate/severe croup

1. Racemic epinephrine, in use since 1971, is a 1:1 mixture of the *d* (dextrorotatory) and *l* (levorotatory) isomers of epinephrine. The *l* isomer causes vasoconstriction of the precapillary arterioles via stimulation of the alpha-receptors and thereby decreases capillary hydrostatic pressure (Malhotra & Leonard, 2001). The final result is fluid reabsorption from the interstitial space and resolution or improvement of the laryngeal mucosal edema. Therefore, the airway diameter increases.

2. Racemic epinephrine dosage: 0.5–0.75 ml of 2.25% solution diluted with 3.5 ml of water (1:8), via a nebulizer with a mouthpiece held in front of the child's face. This can be repeated every 20 minutes if the child is monitored closely. Peak effect is observed in 2 hours. Initially racemic epinephrine was used in preference to the *l* isomer of epinephrine because it was thought to be associated with fewer side effects (tachycardia, hypertension) than l-epinephrine (Malhotra & Leonard, 2001).

3. Note: Aerosolized epinephrine should be reserved for children who have moderate to severe respiratory distress in conjunction with retractions, and if symptoms of stridor do not respond to cool mist and analgesics.

4. In the 1980s, if a child received nebulized epinephrine for croup in the emergency department, it became an indication for admission into the hospital.

5. The current recommendations are to discharge a child from the emergency department after 3–4 hours of observation with the following treatment outcomes.

   a. No symptoms of stridor at rest.

   b. Normal airway entry.

   c. Normal color.

   d. Normal level of consciousness.

   e. Received one dose of dexamethasone 0.6 mg/kg, orally or intramuscularly (Kaditis & Wald, 1998).

   f. If these outcomes are not met, admit to acute care.

D. Admission to acute care: Severe croup

Administration of racemic epinephrine is recommended as it provides some relief and comfort until the appropriate personnel arrive to intubate. There is a decrease in tracheostomies since the use of racemic epinephrine possibly due to the general relief it provides, which then allows time for the steroids to work. Two percent of hospitalized children need endotracheal intubations and mechanical ventilation (Malhotra & Leonard, 2001).

1. Systemic corticosteroids are recommended when patients present with severe, moderate, or even mild croup symptoms.

2. Corticosteroids: Decreases edema of the laryngeal mucosa via anti-inflammatory action and reduced capillary permeability. Data supports clinical improvement at 12 and 24 hours after treatment with a significant reduction of the need for endotracheal intubations. A further study indicated a decreased successful extubation period without need for reintubation when steroids were administered (Asher, 1999; Stannard & O'Callaghan, 2002).

   a. Dosage: dexamethasone 0.3–0.6 mg/kg, intramuscularly or orally as a single dose.

   b. Adverse effects: One case study of a child developing laryngotracheitis caused by *Candida albicans*, after an 8-day course of (1 mg/kg/day) in addition to antibiotics.

   c. Contraindications: Children with varicella or tuberculosis (unless the child is receiving appropriate antituberculosis therapy), laryngotracheobronchitis, laryngotracheobronchopneumonitis, or epiglottis (Cherry, 1998).

   d. Considerations: Steroids may mask the disease process with airway hemangiomas.

3. Nebulized budesonide glucocorticoid reaches inflamed tissue rapidly, with no apparent systemic effects. One study indicated that when nebulized budesonide (2 mg) was given initially and then (1 mg) every 12 hours to children with moderate to severe croup, significant improvement and hospital shorter stays were noted, in comparison to the children who received a placebo (Kaditis & Wald, 1998). As concluded from clinical trials, when nebulized budesonide is given in conjunction with oral dexamethasone in the outpatient setting; patient recovery is enhanced.

4. Heliox, a mixture of Helium and O_2, has been used for management of severe croup (Rosekrans, 1998) and is administered via aerosol continuously in pediatric intensive care setting.

E. Home treatment: Mild croup symptoms

1. Keep the child calm and quiet. Have the parent or caregiver hold the child to offer comfort and reassurance.

2. Increase environmental humidity: The child should sit in a steamy bathroom by running hot water in the shower or bath, for 10–15 minutes (Fox, 1997). If breathing does not improve then the child should be brought to the outside cool air and the air will help shrink the upper airway mucosa and further abate the symptoms (Allen, 1991). Cool mist humidifier should be continued for four to five nights. The physician should be notified if no improvement of symptoms.

3. Cool mist moistens secretions (facilitating clearance) and soothes inflamed mucosa. In addition, humidity decreases the viscosity of tracheal secretions. The mist may activate mechanoreceptors in the larynx that produce a reflex slowing of respiratory flow rate. As the child is exposed to the mist, the act of holding the child and offering reassurance may prevent anxiety and therefore hyperventilation. In

some instances cool mist must be discontinued because the use creates bronchospasm and wheezing (Kaditis & Wald, 1998).

4. Encourage clear fluids or popsicles. Offer small amounts of favorite drinks frequently.

5. Acetaminophen 10–15 mg/kg every 4–6 hours or ibuprofen, 10 mg/kg for fever and irritability (Kaditis & Wald, 1998).

6. Do not administer medications that may depress the respiratory system, induce drowsiness, and mask anxiety or restlessness (e.g., antihistamines, cough syrups with codeine).

7. Visit your primary care facility for oral or intramuscular dose of steroids in the office for further treatment, if symptoms persist (Fox, 1997; Johnson et al., 1998; Paton, 2002).

III. Clinical presentation of croup (Variability depends on severity of illness)

A. Respirations: Increased respiratory rate, with prolonged inspiratory phase, tachypnea-labored respirations with (supraclavicular) and intercostals retractions may use accessory muscles, may have wheezing and rhonchi on expiration (croup scores are usually utilized for research purposes rather than clinical evaluation purposes).

B. Activity: In sitting position experiencing restlessness, irritability, or agitation. Level of consciousness may range from alert to lethargy to unconsciousness.

C. Harsh, barking cough

D. Hoarse voice

E. Mild infection of nasopharynx, mild edema of mucous membranes

F. Inspiratory stridor with activity or if severe when at rest

G. Possible low-grade fever

IV. Assessment

A. History

1. Croup (viral)

a. General appearance: Gradual onset of symptoms of a progressive upper respiratory infection (URI). Symptoms of rhinorrhea, coryza, and low-grade fever vary over days or up to a week. Usually the child looks nontoxic or nonseptic. Assess skin color, activity level, and level of consciousness.

b. Degree of respiratory distress: Assess skin color: cyanosis or pallor, and need for oxygen. Usually progresses to a barking cough and hoarseness. Symptoms include stridor on inspiration, and increasing symptoms at night.

c. Oxygen desaturation (indicated by oximetry) is usually a late and unreliable sign of severity of croup (Fitzgerald & Kilham, 2004; Stoney & Chakrabarti, 1991). Occasionally, decreased oxygen saturation may be present in less severe croup.

2. Spasmodic croup

a. Symptoms are similar to viral croup in which the patient experiences acute attacks of inspiratory stridor at night, then subsides quickly and reoccurs in subsequent nights (may be related to reactive airway disease, allergic, and psychological factors). Develops 2–3 days after URI (Asher, 1999).

  b. Children are usually between 1 and 3 years of age.

3. Bacterial tracheitis (secondary bacterial infection of viral larygnotracheitis)

  a. Child may have viral croup for several days with mucopurulent discharge (Al-Jundi, 1997).

  b. Child has history of fever above 38.5° C.

B. Diagnostic tests

1. Diagnostic tests will vary for airway obstruction depending on history and physical and age of the child.

2. Chest X-ray is done to rule out foreign body aspiration (air trapping or atelectasis may suggest this or infectious process; Wohl, 1999).

3. A lateral neck X-ray examination is obtained to rule out upper airway obstruction for the classic Steeple sign, which is a narrowed air column in the subglottic area seen on the posterior anterior view. (For a pictorial view refer to the Web site, www.virtualpediatrichospital.org.) The hypopharynx may be overdistended on the lateral view. These findings are only present in 50% of cases of croup and many children with croup have normal signs on X-ray (Rosekrans, 1998).

Epiglottitis

I. Overview

A. Definition: Inflammation of the epiglottis that appears more commonly in young children. If not treated it may result in death. The epiglottis is a thin leaf structure located immediately posterior to the root of the tongue. It covers the entrance of the larynx when the individual swallows.

B. Etiology: Acute epiglottitis is usually a manifestation of *Haemophalus influenza* type b (Hib) infection, a bacterial infection. The epiglottis swells and turns red very quickly obstructing the airway. The involvement is supraglottic because it involves the larynx above the cords. Epiglottitis represents a true upper airway emergency with life-threatening complications if handled incorrectly (Al-Jundi, 1997; American College of Emergency Physicians [ACEP], 1998a). Causative organisms: *Haemophilus influenza* type b (Hib) causes 98% of cases (Al-Jundi, 1997). Other pathogens are *Streptococcus pneumoniae*, and low frequency of *Streptococcus pyogenes, Staphylococcus aureus, Haemophilus parainfluenza* and group A *Streptococcus*. Recent findings have shown Group B streptococcal infection (Young, Finn, & Powell, 1996) and other pathogens such as *Candida albicans* especially in immunocompromised patients are increasing (Al-Jundi, 1997). Prior to the Hib B Vaccine, studies indicated an 89% incidence of croup, 8% incidence of epiglottitis, and 2% incidence of bacterial tracheitis (Al-Jundi, 1997).

C. Pathophysiology: Epiglottitis is a medical emergency characterized by severe airway obstruction caused by swelling and inflammation of epiglottis, false cords, and aryeiglottic folds (Garpenholt, Huggosson, Fredlund, Bodin, & Olcen, 1999). Pharynx is often colonized with potentially dangerous pathogenic organisms. Bacteria penetrate the mucosal barrier and invade the bloodstream. Edema then leads to reduction in the caliber of the airway, which leads to turbulent air flow on inspiration and stridor.

D. Incidence: It occurs usually in older children with a peak incidence at 2–7 years of age. It may occur at any age or any season (ACEP, 1998b; Bodin & Olcen, 1999; Young et al., 1996). The incidence of epiglottitis has declined since the Hib B vaccine from 10.9/10,000 to 1.8/10,000 efficacies of 85% (Al-Jundi, 1997).

E. Complications: Laryngospasm with total airway obstruction (due to the normally narrower airway, any swelling causes increased airway resistance and decrease airflow). It is a surgical emergency because of the potential for rapid airway obstruction and potential cardiac arrest resulting in a life-threatening situation (Fisher, 2004; Persing, 2000).

II. Physical exam/clinical presentation

1. Do not attempt to visualize the epiglottis. Keep the patient calm and in preferred position of comfort (Al-Jundi, 1997; Chiocca, 1996).

   a. Immediately notify MD or refer to hospital protocols for management of epiglottitis that are listed in most children's hospitals.

   b. Sudden and progressive onset, no previous illness, gravely ill.

   c. Physical appearance: sitting forward, mouth open, tripod position, thrusting chin forward to breathe, drooling, toxic appearance, agitated, and restless.

   d. May present with mild to high fever, rapid pulse, difficulty swallowing, and dysphagia.

   e. Rapid respirations with stridorous inspirations, use of accessory muscles or both on inspiration and expiration, inspiratory retractions and cyanosis.

   f. Severe respiratory distress, decreased air entry, restlessness, and irritability.

   g. Gasping for air; sternal and intercostal retractions.

   h. Muffled voice, absence of coughing.

   i. Decreased O_2 saturations.

   j. Sore throat, drooling, beefy red swollen epiglottis upon direct visualization in the operating room (i.e., anesthesiologist present in the OR with intubation and tracheostomy equipment present).

   k. Do not place in supine position (Al-Jundi, 1997).

III. Assessment

A. History: Diagnostic tests

1. Labs/X-ray may be obtained only after the airway is secured! With epiglottitis, the X-ray will appear abnormal before it is clinically seen as respiratory compromise.

2. CBC: elevated WBC with bandemia.

3. Blood cultures are positive 80%–90% of the time.

4. Obtain a rapid strep and throat culture *only* if epiglottitis is ruled out (Rosekrans, 1998).

5. Do not disturb the child by drawing arterial blood gases (ABGs). If obtained, it would reveal hypoxemia with respiratory alkalosis. If hypoxemia were not reversed, the patient's condition would progress to respiratory acidosis.

IV. Common therapeutic modalities

    A. Outpatient and office treatment: Transfer into an acute care facility

    B. Epiglottitis: Emergency Department (ED) or Pediatric Intensive Care Unit (PICU)

      1. Treatment

        a. Deliver 100% O_2.

        b. Remain calm.

        c. Let the child stay in a comfortable position, but do not lie the child down.

        d. Do not examine the throat with a tongue blade.

        e. The ED generally has protocols for managing epiglottitis. The exam should be completed in the operating room with the child breathing spontaneously, or in the ED or PICU if all emergency arrangements are made for intubation.

        f. The airway anatomy may be so distorted from inflammation and edema that the glottis structures may be unidentifiable. Once an appropriate level of inhalation anesthetic is given, an IV line is placed and visualization of the glottis and intubation is possible. In the event that the exam causes laryngospasm and an acute airway obstruction, a tracheostomy will be necessary. Extubation cannot occur until there is an air leak around the endotracheal tube and swelling has decreased.

        g. Laryngeal and blood cultures are obtained before initiating antibiotic therapy; third-generation cephalosporins (e.g., cefotaxime) are antibiotics of choice for epiglottitis. There is no evidence that corticosteroids are helpful in the treatment of epiglottitis.

        h. The vaccine against *Haemophilus influenza* type B (*HIB*) may be warranted in the event that it is the causative organism (Al-Jundi, 1997; Bodin & Olcen, 1999; Curley & Moloney-Harmon, 2001).

        i. Recommended antibiotics: Cefuroxime 150 mg/kg/day IV divided q 8 hours.

        j. Cefotaxime 200 mg/kg/day IV divided q 8 hours, or Ceftriaxone 100 mg/kg/day IV divided every 12–24 hours (Cherry, 1998). First dose stat in OR. If bacterial tracheitis is suspected, see below.

    C. Laryngotracheobronchitis (bacterial tracheitis)

      1. Antibiotic therapy: (usually antibiotics that cover staphylococcus, since it is the most common organism cultured) initial treatment with oxacillin (150 mg/kg/day every 6 hours intravenously) and a third-generation cephalosporin, such as cefotaxime (150 mg/kg/day every 6 hours IV) (Cherry, 1998).

2. Severe infections: vancomycin (40 mg/kg/day intravenously every 6 hours) may be used instead of oxacillin (Cherry, 1998).

APPENDIX A: AN ADAPTED CROUP SCORING SYSTEM BASED ON FIVE CLINICAL SIGNS

Zero represents the normal state or absence of the sign; the highest number represents the most severe distress. The range for each sign is weighted to reflect the clinical implications of the most severe form of that sign (Grant & Curley, 2001).

Adapted with permission from Westley, C. R., Cotton, E. K., Brooks, J. G. (1978). Nebulized racemic epinephrine by IPPB for the treatment of croup. *American Journal of Diseases of Children, 132*, 486. Copyright 1978, American Medical Association.

WEB SITES

http://www.uihealthcare.com/vh/
www.virtualpediatrichospital.org
http://kidshealth.org
http://www.pcc.com/lists/pedtalk.archive/9702/threads.html

REFERENCES

Al-Jundi, S. (1997). Acute upper airway obstruction: croup, epiglottitis, bacterial tracheitis, and retropharyngeal abscess. In D. L. Levin & F. C. Morris (Eds.), *Essentials of pediatric intensive care: Vol. 1.* (2nd ed., pp. 121–127). New York: Churchill Livingston, Quality Medical Publishing.

Allen, C. L. (1991). Home management of the child with viral croup (laryngo-tracheobronchitis). *Journal of the American Academy of Nurse Practitioners, 3*(2), 59–63.

American College of Emergency Physicians and American Academy of Pediatrics (AAP) (Eds.). (1998a). Advanced pediatric life support (*APLS*). *The Pediatric Emergency Medicine Course,* 3–11.

American College of Emergency Physicians and American Academy of Pediatrics (AAP) (Eds.). (1998b). *The pediatric emergency medicine course.* Elk Grove Village, IL: American Academy of Publishers.

Asher, M. I. (1999). Infections of the respiratory tract. In L. M. Taussig, L. I. Landau, P. N. Le Souef, W. J. Morgan, F. D. Martinez, & P. D. Sly (Eds.), *Pediatric respiratory medicine* (pp. 539–545). St. Louis, MO: Mosby.

Bodin, L., & Olcen, P. (1999). Epiglottitis in Sweden before and after introduction of vaccination against Haemophalus Influenza Type B. *Pediatric Infectious Disease Journal, 18*(6), 490–493.

Cherry, J. D. (1998). Croup. In R. D. Feigin & J. D. Cherry, *Textbook of pediatric infectious diseases* (Vol. 2, 4th ed., pp. 228–239). Philadelphia: Saunders.

Chiocca, E. (1996). Actionstat. *Nursing, 96*, 9–25.

Curley, M., & Moloney-Harmon, P. (2001). *Critical care nursing of infants and children* (2nd ed.). Philadelphia: W. B. Saunders.

Fisher, J. (2004). Out-of-hospital cardiopulmonary arrest in children with croup. *Pediatric Emergency Care, 20*(1), 35–36.

Fitzgerald, D. A., & Kilham, H. A. (2003). Croup: Assessment and evidence-based management [Review]. *Medical Journal of Australia, 179*(7), 372–377.

Fox, J. (1997). *Respiratory system in primary health care of children.* St. Louis, MO: Mosby.

Garpenholt, O., Huggosson, S., Fredlund, H., Bodin, L., & Olcen, P. (1999). Epiglottitis in Sweden before and after introduction of vaccination against haemophilus influenza type b. *Pediatric Infectious Disease Journal, 18*(6), 90–93.

Geelhoed, G. C. (1997). Croup. *Pediatric Pulmonology, 23*(5), 370–374.

Grant, M. J. C., & Curley, M. A. Q. (2001). Pulmonary critical care problems. Chapter 19 in M. A. Q. Curley & P. A. Moloney-Harmon (Eds.), *Critical care nursing of infants and children* (2nd ed., pp. 655–662). Philadelphia: W. B. Saunders.

Jaffe, D. (1998) Editorial: The treatment of croup with glucocorticoids. *New England Journal of Medicine, 339*(8), 553–555.

Jamshidi, P. B., Kemp, J. S., & Peter, J. R. (2001). The effect of humidified air in mild to moderate croup: Evaluation using croup scores and respiratory inductance plethysmorgraphy. *Academic Emergency Medicine, 8*(5), 417.

Johnson, D., Jacobson, S., Edney, P., Hadfield, P., Mundy, M., & Schuk, S. (1998). A comparison of nebulized budesonide, intramuscular dexamethasone and placebo for modereately severe croup. *New England Journal of Medicine, 339*(8), 498–503.

Kaditis, A. G., & Wald, E. R. (1998). Viral croup: Current diagnosis and treatment. *Pediatric Infectious Disease, 17*(9), 827–833.

Luria, J. W., Gonzalez-del-Rey, J. A., DiGiulio, G. A., McAneney, C. M., Olson, J. J., & Ruddy, R. M. (2001). Effectiveness of oral or nebulized dexamethasone for children with mild croup. *Archives of Pediatrics & Adolescent Medicine, 155*(12), 1340–1346.

Malhotra, A., & Krilov, L. (2001). Viral croup. *Pediatrics in Review, 22*, 5–12.

Paton, J. Y. (2002). Oral dexamethasone led to fewer treatment failures than did nebulized dexamethasone or placebo in children with mild croup. *ACP Journal Club, 137*(1), 31.

Persing, G. (2000). *Respiratory care exam review.* Philadelphia: W. B. Saunders Company.

Rosekrans, J. A. (1998). Viral croup: Current diagnosis and treatment. *Mayo Clinic Proceedings, 73*(11), 1102–1107.

Slota, M. C. (Ed.). (1997). *Core curriculum for pediatric critical care nursing ACCN critical care.* Philadelphia: W. B. Saunders.

Stannard, W., & O'Callaghan, C. (2002). Management of croup. *Pediatric Drugs, 4*(4), 23–40.

Stoney, P. J., & Chakrabarti, M. K. (1991). Experience of pulse oximetry in children with croup. *Journal Laryngology & Otology, 105*, 295–298.

Wald, E. (1999). Croup. In J. McMillan, C. DeAngelis, R. Feigin, & J. Warshaw, (Eds.), *Oski pediatrics* (3rd ed., pp. 1307–1309). Philadelphia: Lippincott, Williams and Wilkins.

Westley, C. R., Cotton, E. K., & Brooks, J. G. (1978). Nebulized racemic epinephrine by IPPB for the treatment of croup. *American Journal of Diseases of Children, 132*, 486.

Williams, J., Harris, P., Tollefson, S., Halburnt-Rush, R., Pingsterhaus, J., Edwards, K. M., et al. (2004). Human Metapneumovirus and lower respiratory tract disease in otherwise healthy infants and children. *New England Journal of Medicine, 350*(5), 443–450.

Wohl, D. L., & Farmer, T. L. (1999). A child has recurrent croup: But what's the real diagnosis? *The Journal of Respiratory Diseases, 20*(3), 243–258.

Young, N., Finn, A., & Powell, C. (1996). Group B streptococcal epiglottitis. *The Pediatric Infectious Disease Journal, 15*(1), 9.

SUGGESTED READINGS

Ausejo, M., Sainz, A., Phen, Ba', Kellner, J. D., Johnson, D. W., Moher, D., et al. (1999). The effectiveness of glucocorticoids in treating croup: Meta-analysis. *BMJ, 319*(4), 595–600.

Brown, J. C. (2002). The management of croup. *British Medical Bulletin, 61*, 189–202.

Harmon, P. (2001). *Critical care nursing of infants and children* (2nd ed.). Philadelphia: W. B. Saunders Co.

Hopkins, A., Lahiri, T., Salerno, R., & Heath, B. (2006). Changing epidemiology of life-threatening upper airway infections: The reemergence of bacterial tracheitis. *Pediatrics, 118*, 1418–1421.

Landau, L. I., & Geelhoed, G. C. (1994). Aerosolized steroids for croup: Editorial. *New England Journal of Medicine, 331*(5), 322–323.

Wong, D., & Whaley, A. (1990). *Clinical manual of pediatric nursing* (3rd ed.). New York: Mosby.

Therapeutic Modalities

Respiratory Pharmacology

Christine V. Champagne and Richard Champagne

INTRODUCTION

The use of respiratory medications has been shown to reduce the frequency and severity of exacerbations and may improve quality of life. Knowledge of the purpose of each medication and the expected side effects is necessary for the nurse to assist patients in improving control over their symptoms.

1. Inhaled medications are specific to the respiratory system and require knowledge of the nurse and patient to ensure correct technique so that the medication can reach the site where it can be effective.
2. Bronchodilators and anti-inflammatory medications are utilized with the goal of opening the airway for improved breathing.
3. Anti-microbial medications should be utilized correctly and only when necessary in order to control problems with growing bacterial resistance.

I. Bronchodilators
   A. Beta-adrenergic agonists (Beta2-agonists)—Short acting
      1. Generic (trade) names
         a. Inhaled: albuterol (Proventil, Proventil HFA, Ventolin, Ventolin HFA), bitolterol (Tornalate), pirbuterol (Maxair), levalbuterol (Xopenex).
         b. Oral: albuterol (Proventil Repetabs, Volmax)
      2. Indication—short-term relief of bronchoconstriction. The inhaled preparations are the treatment of choice for acute exacerbations of asthma. No effect on the inflammatory response.
      3. Mechanism of action—relaxation of bronchial smooth muscles by increasing cAMP

4. Onset/duration of action—onset of action for the inhaled preparations are within minutes and are effective for 4–8 hours. Oral preparations have an onset of 30–45 minutes and are effective for 6–8 hours.

5. Dosage and methods of delivery—Inhaled: recommended dosage 2 puffs every 4–6 hours as needed per metered dose inhaler (MDI), not to exceed 12 puffs per day. Or nebulized albuterol: 2.5 mg mixed in 2.5 ml saline or levalbuterol 0.63–1.25 mg per nebulizer every 4–6 hours.

   a. Higher doses are utilized in some clinical settings.

   b. In asthma, recommended on an as needed basis for treatment of acute symptoms.

   c. In COPD, usually given as maintenance therapy and given on a routine schedule rather than as needed for acute symptoms.

6. Combination therapy—Combined albuterol and ipratropium bromide are available (Combivent) in an MDI and DuoNeb for nebulization. Dosing guidelines are the same as individual delivery.

7. Key side effects—tremors, anxiety, tachycardia, palpitations. Frequently described as "the feeling you get when you drink too much coffee." Increased side effects with oral administration (systemic effect).

8. Nursing highlights

   a. Medications given by inhalation are only effective if correct inhaler or nebulizer technique is utilized. Patient must be instructed on proper technique with return demonstration and periodic review of technique. See Table 35.1.

   b. In asthma, used as RESCUE therapy. If using bronchodilator rescue medication > twice weekly, maintenance steroid therapy recommended. See Table 35.2.

   c. Instruct patient that increased use of RESCUE bronchodilator is a signal of poor symptomatic control and to contact his/her health care provider.
   Do not increase dose unless directed to do so.

   d. Immediate hypersensitivity reactions to inhalation aerosol may occur in patients who are sensitive to soybeans or peanuts.

B. Beta adrenergic agonists (Beta2-agonists)—Long acting

   1. Generic/trade names—salmeterol (Serevent), formoterol (Foradil)

   2. Indication—used for long-term bronchodilitation: maintenance therapy for asthma and COPD, nocturnal asthma, and exercise-induced asthma. No effect on the inflammatory response.

   3. Mechanism of action—relaxation of bronchial smooth muscles by stimulating cAMP.

   4. Onset/duration of action—salmeterol: onset of action 1 hour and duration is 8–12 hours. Formoterol: onset occurs within minutes and duration is 12–24 hours.

   5. Dosage and methods of delivery—Salmeterol dosage is 2 puffs every 12 hours by metered dose inhaler (MDI) or one inhalation every 12 hours by dry powder inhaler (DPI). Formoterol is available as a

METERED DOSE INHALERS (MDI)

Rx Manufacturer	Product Available	Technique	Highlights

Boehringer
Glaxo
 	
3M
Schering
Generic Co.
Forest
Aventis
	Atrovent,
	Combivent
	Ventolin (HFA),
	Flovent, Serevent
	Q-Var
	Proventil (HFA)
	Albuterol
	Aerobid
	Azmacort
		1. Remove lid of delivery device
		2. Hold canister with thumb on bottom & 1–2 fingers on top of canister. Shake well.
		3. Breathe out fully
		4. Place inhaler at opening of mouth.
		5. Choose open or closed mouth technique.
		   Open–leave mouth open around mouthpiece
		   Closed–seal your lips tightly around mouthpiece
		6. While inhaling deeply with a steady force, fully depress the top of the canister
		7. **Hold this breath for 10 seconds**—at least 5 secs, if unable
		8. Repeat steps 2–7 for additional puffs as pre-scribed, waiting in between puffs (ideally a minute or longer)
		9. After completion, replace lid
			Open technique–it has been suggested that the air coming in the sides may carry the medicine further into the lungs rather than lodging at the back of the throat.
			Holding devices are recommended because they increase the distance of medication
			Azmacort is manufactured with a built-in spacer
			See manufacturer's recommendations for cleaning

3M	Maxair	1. Remove lid of delivery device 2. "Trigger" device by holding upright & lift-ing lever up until it snaps into place & stays 3. Shake inhaler	Priming spray (initial use or >48 hrs) Trigger as directed. Release the spray by pressing the white test fire slide on the bottom of the mouthpiece in the direction marked. Do this twice.

(continued)

Table 35.1 MDI and DPI Instructions for Use (*continued*)

METERED DOSE INHALERS (MDI)

Rx Manufacturer	Product Available	Technique	Highlights
		4. Breathe out fully. Seal lips around mouthpiece 5. Inhale deeply with a steady force. You will hear a click when medicine is released. Do not stop breathing in when the click is heard 6. Remove inhaler from mouth at maximal inspiration 7. **Hold this breath for 10 seconds**—at least 5 secs, if unable 8. While holding device upright, lower the lever 9. Repeat steps 2–8 for additional puffs as prescribed, waiting in between puffs (ideally a minute or longer) 10. After completion, make sure lever is down & lid is replaced	Do not block airvents at bottom Must be held upright while raising lever See manufacturer's recommendations for cleaning

DRY POWDERED INHALERS (DPI)

Rx Manufacturer	Product Available	Technique	Highlights
Astra Zeneca	Pulmicort Turbuhaler	1. Remove lid by twisting white top from brown base	Each time a **new** inhaler is opened it must be primed. Prime by holding upright & twist brown grip fully to right, then fully to left until click is heard. Repeat to inhale first dose.

	Instructions	Notes
	2. Hold upright. Load by twisting brown grip fully to the right & then to left until a click is heard	Never blow into the delivery device. It is not necessary to wait between puffs Window on side: red at top indicates 20 doses remaining, red at bottom—empty
	3. Breathe out fully. Seal lips around mouthpiece	
	4. Inhale deeply with a steady force	
	5. Remove inhaler from mouth at maximal inspiration	
	6. **Hold this breath for 10 seconds**—at least 5 secs, if unable	
	7. If repeated doses are prescribed, repeat steps 2–6	
	8. After completion, make sure lever is down & lid is replaced	
Glaxo Serevent Diskus, Advair	1. While holding diskus in one hand, place thumb of other hand on the thumb grip and push away until mouthpiece appears & snaps into position	Counter located on side will count remaining doses. Each time lever is slid into position, will count as a dose. Never blow into the delivery device.
	2. Hold the diskus in a level position, slide the lever away—as far as it will go until it clicks.	
	3. Breathe out fully. Seal lips around mouthpiece	
	4. Inhale deeply with a steady force	
	5. Remove inhaler from mouth at maximal inspiration	
	6. **Hold this breath for 10 seconds**—at least 5 secs, if unable	
	7. After completion, close the diskus using thumb grip.	

(continued)

Table 35.1 | MDI and DPI Instructions for Use (continued)

DRY POWDERED INHALERS (DPI)

Rx Manufacturer	Product Available	Technique	Highlights
Novartis	Foradil	1. Peel paper back from blister card & push capsule through remaining foil immediately before use 2. Pull off inhaler cover & twist open shaft in direction indicated by arrow on the side of the shaft. 3. Put capsule in chamber & twist mouthpiece closed 4. Press both side buttons, once only, while holding inhaler upright to puncture capsule. Release buttons. 5. Place lips around mouthpiece after exhaling. Blue buttons should be on the side. 6. Inhale deeply with a steady force. Note a whirling noise 7. Remove inhaler from mouth at maximal inspiration 8. **Hold this breath for 10 seconds**—at least 5 secs, if unable 9. Check capsule, if remaining medication, close & inhale again 10. Discard empty capsule. Close & replace lid.	If sweet taste & whirling noise not noted on inspiration, instruct patient to tap the inhaler on the side to loosen the capsule & inhale again. Capsule is less likely to shatter if punctured only once. Built-in screen should catch any pieces. Never blow into the delivery device.

Boehringer	Spiriva	1. Pull open the dust cap by pushing down on the green projection & pulling upward on the cap. Open mouthpiece	If an additional capsule is exposed when opening, it must be discarded. Capsules should be used immediately upon opening.
		2. Remove 1 capsule from blister card by pulling foil to first STOP line immediately before use.	Never blow into the delivery device. Theoretically, residue on opened capsule could dilate pupil for 24 hours if eye was
		3. Place capsule in central chamber.	mistakenly touched after contact with the capsule.
		4. Close the mouthpiece until you hear a click.	
		5. While mouthpiece is pointed up, push the green button in to pierce the capsule & release	
		6. Breathe out fully. Seal lips around mouthpiece	
		7. Inhale deeply with a steady force. The capsule will vibrate	
		8. Remove inhaler from mouth at maximal inspiration	
		9. **Hold this breath for 10 seconds**—at least 5 secs, if unable	
		10. Repeat steps 6–9 to be sure full dose is inhaled	
		11. Open inhaler. Dump capsule into trash without touching it & close mouthpiece & cap	

Table 35.2	Common Respiratory Pathogens

Infection	Most Common Pathogens
Sinusitis	
Acute	S. pneumoniae, H. influenzae, M. catarrhalis
Chronic	H. influenzae, S. pneumoniae, M. catarrhalis
Avoid macrolides, treat for full 2 weeks for acute and 4 weeks for chronic	
Pharyngitis	Group A strep
Rare in adults >30, differentiate viral vs bacterial	
AECB	S. pneumoniae, H. influenzae, M. catarrhalis, C. pneumoniae

Community Acquired Pneumonia	Typical:
	  S. pneumoniae, H. influenzae, M. catarrhalis
	Atypical:
	  Legionella, Mycoplasma

Nosocomial Pneumonia	Gram neg:
	  P. aeruginosa, E. coli, K. pneumoniae, S. marcescens
	Gram pos:
	  S. aureus: methicillin sensitive (MSSA), methicillin resistant (MRSA)

Tuberculosis	
Bronchiectasis	P. aeruginosa
Cystic Fibrosis	
Important to select antibiotics with low resistance potential that have good penetration into respiratory secretions	

capsule delivered by the manufacturer's delivery device, dose is one capsule every 12 hours.

6. Combination therapy: Combined fluticasone and salmeterol are available (Advair) in a DPI with dosage of one puff BID of 500/50, 250/50, and 100/50 (fluticasone/salmeterol).

7. Key side effects—tremors, anxiety, tachycardia, palpitations.

8. Nursing highlights

a. Medications given by inhalation are only effective if correct inhaler or nebulizer technique is utilized. Patient must be instructed on proper technique with return demonstration and periodic review of technique. See Table 35.1.

      b. Stress that salmeterol is not helpful as RESCUE therapy because of its delayed onset of action.

      c. Instruct patient to continue to carry RESCUE bronchodilator for quick relief.

C. Anticholinergics—Short acting

  1. Generic/trade names—Ipratropium bromide (Atrovent)

  2. Indication—short-term relief of bronchoconstriction. Effective in the treatment of COPD either in combination with B-agonists (most common) or alone.

  3. Mechanism of action—Inhibits the component of bronchoconstriction regulated by the parasympathetic nervous system with primary effect on the larger airways (unlike B-agonists that act primarily on smaller airways).

      a. Airway diameter is predominantly controlled by the parasympathetic division of the autonomic nervous system.

      b. Blocks the effects of acetylcholine on the airways. Acetylcholine causes increased mucus secretion and smooth muscle contraction, resulting in bronchoconstriction.

  4. Onset/duration of action—onset 15 minutes, duration 4–6 hours.

  5. Dosage and methods of delivery—Inhaled: recommended dosage 2 puffs every 4–6 hours per metered dose inhaler (MDI), not to exceed 12 puffs per day. Or nebulized: 0.5 mg mixed in 2.5 ml saline per nebulizer every 4–6 hours.

      a. Higher doses are utilized in some clinical settings.

      b. Usually given as maintenance therapy and given on a routine schedule rather than as treatment for acute symptoms.

  6. Combination—Combined albuterol and ipratropium bromide are available (Combivent) in an MDI and DuoNeb for nebulization.

  7. Key side effects—cough, bad taste, dryness of oral mucosa, nervousness. Temporary blurred vision will occur if sprayed in eyes. Systemic effects of inhaled anticholinergics are uncommon because they are poorly absorbed.

  8. Nursing highlights

      a. Medications given by inhalation are only effective if correct inhaler or nebulizer technique is utilized. Patient must be instructed on proper technique with return demonstration and periodic review of technique. See Table 35.1.

      b. Instruct patient that increased use of RESCUE bronchodilator is a signal of poor symptomatic control and to contact his/her health care provider.

        Do not increase dose unless directed to do so.

      c. Immediate hypersensitivity reactions to inhalation aerosol of MDI may occur in patients who are sensitive to soybeans or peanuts.

D. Anticholinergic—Long acting

  1. Generic/trade names—tiotropium (Spiriva)

2. Indication—used for long-term bronchodilitation: maintenance therapy for COPD. Thought to have an accumulative effect and improve exercise tolerance by reducing air trapping.
3. No effect on the inflammatory response.
4. Mechanism of action—same as short acting.
5. Dosage and method of delivery—is available as a capsule delivered by the manufacturer's delivery device, dose is one capsule every 24 hours.
6. Onset and duration—onset occurs within minutes and duration is 24 hours.
7. Key side effects—same as ipratropium bromide.
8. Nursing highlights
    a. Medications given by inhalation are only effective if correct inhaler or nebulizer technique is utilized. Patient must be instructed on proper technique with return demonstration and periodic review of technique. See Table 35.1.
    b. Capsules must be used immediately after removal from foil packet.
    c. Instruct patient to continue to carry RESCUE bronchodilator for quick relief.

E. Methylxanthine derivatives
1. Generic/trade names—theophylline (Theodur, Uniphyl, Choledyl, Slo-bid, Unidur, Theo 24).
2. Indication—Treatment of symptoms and reversible airflow obstruction.
3. Mechanism of action—Relaxation of smooth muscle of the bronchial airways and pulmonary blood vessels. However, they are less effective bronchodilators than inhaled Beta2 agonists with a much greater incidence of serious side effects. May have a positive effect on diaphragmatic contractility and may decrease fatigability of the diaphragm.
4. Dosage and methods of delivery—Dosage based on maintaining serum theophylline levels at a safe and effective level (10–20 mcg/ml) Most oral preparations are sustained release. Intravenous use of aminophylline in the hospital is now rarely utilized.
5. Key side effects—relatively high incidence of side effects, which include nausea, headache, gastrointestinal (GI) distress, tachycardia, cardiac dysryhythmias, seizures. Death has been reported.
6. Nursing highlights
    a. Long-acting theophylline products administered at bedtime may be indicated for treatment of patients with nocturnal asthma. Instruct patient not to crush sustained release preparations.
    b. Prior to inhaled bronchodilators, theophylline was the only available maintenance medication for use in patients with lung disease. Limited use currently.
    c. Many foods, drugs, and pathophysiologic conditions can alter the metabolism of theophylline. This can result in subtherapeutic or toxic levels with previously appropriate doses.

    d. Instruct patients that if they alter their smoking status while on theophylline, levels will need to be closely monitored. Many potential drug interactions; check use of any medication used concomitantly with theophylline.

    e. Routine monitoring of theophylline levels is necessary. Levels of 5–10 mcg/ml are associated with less side effects while levels >20 are associated with severe reactions.

II. Anti-inflammatory

  A. Steroids—Oral

Corticosteroids, which suppress the inflammatory response, are the most potent and effective anti-inflammatory medication currently available for adults and children. Systemic gluco-corticosteroids are used to gain prompt control of inflammation. Long-term use is avoided whenever possible because of the risks of serious side effects.

    1. Generic/trade names—prednisone (Deltasone), prednisolone (Prelone), methylprednisolone (Medrol).

    2. Indication—Respiratory: conditions of inflammation of airway or tissue, such as asthma, sarcoidosis, pneumonitis.

    3. Mechanism of action—Inhibition of the release of mediators from macrophages and eosinophils, reducing the microvascular leakage in the airways, inhibiting the influx of inflammatory cells into the reactive site and decreasing peripheral blood eosinophilia.

    4. Onset—onset occurs within 6–24 hours

    5. Dosage

      a. Bolus and taper—indicated for exacerbation due to inflammation. Bolus initiated (Prednisone: 5–60 mg) and then followed by a gradual weaning in even increments to usual maintenance dosage or discontinuation. Taper is associated with fewer side effects (i.e., Prednisone: 40 mg daily for 2 days, 30 mg daily for 2 days, 20 mg daily for 2 days, etc.). A Medrol Dose Pack is also available with twenty-one 4 mg tabs for gradual taper for more convenient dosing when cost is not a factor.

      b. Maintenance—minimum dosage to achieve symptom-control given as a daily dose. Alternate-day dosing is associated with fewer side effects.

      c. Dose given in the morning to coincide with endogenous cortisol production and mimic the normal circadian rhythm.

    6. Key side effects

      a. Dose/duration dependent: osteoporosis, glaucoma, cataracts, elevated blood sugar, electrolyte imbalances, insomnia, heartburn, mood swings, blurry vision, headache, increased appetite, fluid retention, impaired healing, weight gain.

      b. Rapid withdrawal can cause adrenal insufficiency. Symptoms include fatigue, muscular weakness, joint pain, fever, anorexia, nausea, dyspnea, dizziness, fainting.

    c. Inhaled steroids have been shown to have no long-term effect on suppression of growth in children. This is still a concern with oral steroids.

  7. Nursing highlights

    a. Instruct patient on taper schedule. Ideally patient should be given a calendar with tapering schedule.

    b. Monitor for side effects. Instruct patient of possible side effects.

    c. Instruct patient not to discontinue abruptly.

    d. Consider Vitamin D and/or calcium supplement if on long-term therapy.

    e. Consider periodic ophthalmic examination if on long-term therapy.

    f. Instruct patient to notify all health care providers when taking oral steroids.

    g. If discontinuation of oral steroid is planned after 3 or more months of maintenance dosing, consider cortisol testing to determine if adrenal glands are functioning adequately.

B. Steroids—Inhaled/intranasal

Inhaled and intranasal steroids are indicated for the long-term control of inflammation.

  1. Generic/trade names

    a. Inhaled—triamcinolone (Azmacort), flunisolide (Aerobid, Aerobid-M), beclomethasone (Qvar 40, Qvar 80), fluticasone (Flovent 44 mcg, 110 mcg, & 220 mcg), budesonide (Pulmicort Turbohaler and spansules)

    b. Intranasal—beclomethasone (Beconase, Vancenase), triamcinolone (Nasacort), budesonide (Rhinocort), fluticasone (Flonase), mometasone (Nasonex)

  2. Indication—same as oral, however these products act locally and can control the disease with minimal systemic side effects related to adrenal suppression.

  3. Onset/duration of action—minimum of 4–5 days before therapeutic effect can be seen.

  4. Dosage and methods of delivery

    a. Inhaled—44–1250 mcg based on symptom control. The greater the dose the greater the risk of systemic absorption and associated side effects (see oral steroid side effects). Administered as metered dose inhalers (MDI) or dry powder inhalers (DPI), or by nebulizer, usually twice per day.

    b. Intranasal—50–200 mcg daily delivered in once per day or twice daily dosing.

  5. Combination: Combined fluticasone and salmeterol is available (Advair) in a DPI. Three varying dosages of fluticasone are available with the same strength of salmeterol in each preparation for twice a day dosing.

6. Key side effects
   a. Inhaled—oropharyngeal candidiasis, hoarseness, and dry cough. Incidence of these can be decreased by rinsing mouth after use and the use of a spacer/holding chamber with MDIs.
   b. Intranasal—mild, transient local irritation, dryness, epistaxis, headache
7. Nursing highlights
   a. Medications given by inhalation are only effective if correct inhaler or nebulizer technique is utilized. Patient must be instructed on proper technique with return demonstration and periodic review of technique. See Table 35.1.
   b. There is no immediate relief from use of these inhaled products as there is with bronchodilators. Symptom control results from the treatment of the underlying problem—inflammation—and may not be noticeable for 2–4 weeks.
   c. Patients sometimes self-discontinue when symptoms resolve. They should be instructed to continue use even if symptom free.

C. Leukotriene modifiers
   1. Generic/trade names—Leukotriene D4 receptor antagonists: montelukast (Singulair), zafirlukast (Accolate).
   2. Indication—leukotrienes are potent bronchoconstrictors, and some also cause edema and inflammation. These medications may be useful in decreasing the dosage of oral steroids and controlling symptoms in patients with severe persistent asthma. Montelukast (Singulair) is also approved for usage with sinusitis and allergic rhinitis.
   3. Dosage and methods of delivery—given orally
      a. Montelukast—adults: 10 mg each evening, pediatrics: 4–5 mg chewable tab each evening
      b. Zafirlukast—adults: 20 mg twice daily on empty stomach
   4. Key side effects—dizziness, gastrointestinal upset, Churg-Strauss syndrome has been reported. Elevated liver enzymes are possible with inhibitors and liver profile should be monitored.
   5. Nursing highlights
      a. Instruct patient not for use in an acute asthma attack.
      b. Zafirlukast has possible drug interactions with aspirin, erythromycin, theophylline, and warfarin.

D. Mast cell stabilizer
   1. Generic/trade names—Cromolyn sodium (Intal), nedocromil sodium (Tilade)
   2. Indication—Prevention of bronchoconstriction before exposure to known trigger.
   3. Mechanism of action—Inhibits the immediate response from exercise and allergens and prevents the late-phase response. It is the inflammatory drug of choice in children with mild, persistent asthma (inhaled steroids are first-line with moderate to severe persistent asthma). It is particularly effective in exercise-induced asthma.

4. Dosage and methods of delivery—initial dose is 20 mg, four times daily per nebulizer or 2 puffs QID from a metered dose inhaler (MDI). For the prevention of exercise-induced bronchospasm, use 2 puffs from MDI 20–30 minutes before exercise.

5. Key side effects—transient, mild, unpleasant taste and rhinitis

6. Nursing highlights
   a. Medications given by inhalation are only effective if correct technique for the inhaler or nebulizer is utilized. Patient must be instructed on proper technique with return demonstration and periodic review of technique.
   b. Instruct patient that the MDI should be used 20–30 minutes *before* exercise for the prevention of exercise induced bronchospasm.

III. Upper respiratory medications
   A. Nasal decongestants
      1. Generic/trade names—pseudoephedrine (various: Sudafed, Triaminic AM), phenylephrine (various: Neo-synephrine), oxymetazoline (Afrin, Dristan, Vicks Sinex).
      2. Indication—for temporary relief of nasal congestion due to viral infections (common cold), sinusitis, hay fever, or other allergens. May have some effect on Eustachian tube congestion thus may provide some relief of ear blockage and ear pressure.
      3. Dosage and methods of delivery
         a. Oral—15–240 mg daily. Immediate acting and sustained release available
         b. Intranasal—1–2 sprays each nostril, one to two times daily
      4. Key side effects—nervousness, dizziness, dryness, irregular heartbeat, sleepiness, or insomnia. Use in caution with patients with known hypertension and/or cardiovascular disease due to possible added vasoconstriction. Rebound congestion may occur with intranasal use, causing increased use by patient and resultant increased congestion. May cause increased urinary difficulties in patients with benign prostatic hypertrophy.
      5. Nursing highlights
         a. Caution for use in patients with hypertension, cardiovascular disease, hyperthyroidism, diabetes, or prostatic hypertrophy.
         b. Intranasal use should not be greater than 3–5 days.
         c. Do not crush sustained released medications.
         d. Phenylpropanolamine, previously available in multiple preparations was recalled by the FDA due to increased incidence of vascular accidents, especially in the elderly.
      6. Combined decongestants and anti-histamine/decongestant combinations are available (i.e., Claritin D, Allegra D, Zyrtec D, Astelin Nasal Spray).
   B. Antihistamines
      1. Generic/trade names
         a. Nonselective—dexchlorpheniramine (various), brompheniramine (various: Dimetapp), diphenhydramine (various: Benadryl),

clemastine (various: Tavist), promethazine (various: Phenergan), cyproheptadine (Periactin).

    b. Selective—cetirizine (Zyrtec), loratadine (Claritin), fexofenadine (Allegra), desloratidine (Clarinex).

  2. Indication—Used for the temporary relief of sneezing, itchy, watery eyes, itchy throat, and runny nose due to hay fever and other allergens. They have varying degrees of anticholinergic and antihistaminic effects, which make them useful as sedatives (nonselective) and antitussives, and for use against allergy and itching, and for the prevention of motion sickness.

  3. Mechanism of action—Reduce or prevent the physiologic effects of histamine. Dosage—based on preparation and desired effect—see manufacturer recommendations. Immediate acting and sustained release preparations available.

  4. Key side effects

    a. Nonselective—drowsiness, sedation, dizziness, hypotension, headache, dryness: mouth, nose or throat, and gastrointestinal upset.

    b. Selective—headache, dryness: mouth, nose or throat, gastrointestinal upset, comparatively low incidence of drowsiness, fatigue.

  5. Nursing highlights

    a. Must discontinue approximately 3–4 days prior to skin testing for allergens.

    b. Use with caution in patients with COPD because the anti-cholinergic (drying) effects may thicken secretions and impair expectoration (Cada, 2001).

    c. Warn patient of possible sedating effects and possible disturbed coordination, which could be exaggerated with alcohol consumption.

  6. Combined anti-histamines and anti-histamine/decongestant combinations are available (i.e., Claritin D, Allegra D, Zyrtec D, Astelin Nasal Spray).

  C. Anti-inflammatory RX—see steroids—intra-nasal and leukotriene inhibitors

IV. Cough preparations

  A. Antitussives

    1. Generic/trade names

      a. Narcotic—codeine, oxycodone, hydrocodone

      b. Non-narcotic—diphenhydramine (various), benzonatate (various: Tessalon Perles), dextromethorphan (various)

    2. Indication—for suppression of cough induced by chemical irritation or mechanical respiratory tract infections

    3. Mechanism of action—depression of the cough reflex

    4. Dosage and methods of delivery—oral and topical (lozenges). Dosage based on preparation and desired effect—see manufacturer recommendations. Immediate acting and sustained release preparations available.

5. Key side effects
   a. Narcotic—potential for abuse and dependence with narcotics. Uncommon but monitor in high-risk patients. Constipation, gastrointestinal upset, headache, drowsiness, dry mouth
   b. Non-narcotic—sedation, headache, dizziness, gastrointestinal upset
6. Nursing highlights
   a. Caution patients that syrup preparations may contain varying amounts of sugar, alcohol, and/or dyes.
   b. Monitor patients who may be high risk for problems with dependence or abuse.
   c. Instruct patients with lung disease (asthma, COPD) that a cough effective in moving secretions should not be suppressed. Health care provider should be notified if medication not effective or cough continues long term.
7. Combined preparations with expectorant, antihistamine, decongestant, anticholinergic, xanthines, and/or analgesics, are available in both immediate acting and sustained release formulas. They are available in liquid, capsule, tablets, and drops for all ages.

B. Expectorants
1. Generic/trade names—guaifenesin (various: -tuss, Humabid, Organidin)
2. Indication—for the symptomatic relief of a dry, nonproductive cough or in the presence of mucous in the respiratory tract. However, there is a lack of convincing studies to document efficacy (Cada, 2001).
3. Dosage and methods of delivery—600–1200 mg every 12 hours as needed for cough. (Short-acting preparations are also available.)
4. Key side effects—gastrointestinal upset, dizziness, headache
5. Nursing highlights
   a. Instruct patient to contact their health care provider if cough persists for more than one week or is accompanied by other symptoms.
   b. Encourage patient to take with a glass of water; increasing oral intake, unless contraindicated, is beneficial in liquefying secretions.
6. Combined preparations with antitussive, antihistamine, decongestant, anticholinergic, xanthines, and/or analgesics are available in both immediate acting and sustained release formulas. They are available in liquid, capsule, tablets, and drops for all ages.

V. Vaccines/immunizations
A. Influenza
1. Generic—Influenza vaccine (various): developed annually based on the currently circulating A and B viruses.
2. Indication—for the production of immunity to influenza virus. Recommended annually for those who are thought to be at high risk for the complications of influenzae.

a. Greater than 65 years of age

b. Adults and children with chronic respiratory, cardiovascular, metabolic, renal, or immuno-suppressant disease or therapy.

c. Women who will be in the second or third trimester of pregnancy during the flu season.

d. Groups that can transmit influenzae to high-risk patients, such as health care workers.

3. Onset/duration—Antibody reaches therapeutic level approximately 2 weeks after injection and lasts 4–6 months

4. Dosage and method of delivery

a. Adults—0.5 ml intramuscularly annually, October to March year. It is suggested that health care providers may begin to immunize their at-risk patients if they are already being seen as early as Labor Day.

b. Pediatrics—divided doses (2) are recommended for children under the age of nine receiving for the first time. <3 years—0.25 ml, >3 years—0.5 ml

5. Key side effects—side effects are generally inconsequential in adults and occur at a low frequency

a. Local—soreness at injection site lasting <2 days

b. Systemic—more frequently in children: fever, malaise, and myalgia begins 6–12 hours later and lasts <2 days, temporary CNS disturbances

7. Nursing highlights

a. Do not vaccinate if allergy to eggs or thimerosal (found in contact solution also)

b. Steroid therapy—delay immunization for 2 weeks after cessation of short-term immuno-suppressant therapy—will interfere with their production of antibodies. Patients on chronic maintenance steroids can be vaccinated.

c. Instruct patient that receiving vaccine does not eliminate the possibility of illness from influenzae. Rather, if exposed to influenza, antibodies are already developed and should decrease the severity and the incidence of hospitalization or death.

d. Influenzae does not prevent other viral infections that the patient sometimes develops around the same time as the immunization (and then incorrectly blames on the vaccine).

B. Pneumonia

1. Generic/trade names—pneumococcal vaccine, 23 valent (Pneumovax).

2. Indication—for immunization against *pneumococcal pneumonia* and *bacteremia*. Recommended for those who are at high risk for the complications of pneumonia (same risk groups as influenzae except during pregnancy—see above). These recommendations are subject to change yearly.

3. Onset/duration—current recommendation is to repeat the pneumonia vaccination in 5 years if the patient received the first vaccination at age 65 or younger.

4. Dosage and method of delivery—>2 years of age: 0.5 ml intra-muscularly.

5. Key side effects—soreness at injection site lasting <2 days, increased if patient has received prior pneumococcal vaccine within 2 years.

6. Nursing highlights
   a. Steroid therapy—delay immunization for 2 weeks after cessation of short-term immuno-suppressant therapy—will interfere with their production of antibodies. Patients on maintenance steroid therapy should receive the immunization.
   b. Instruct patient that vaccine does not prevent all types of pneumonia.
   c. Patients who received 14 valent pneumoccocal vaccine should have re-vaccination with 23 valent.

VI. Smoking cessation (see chapter 30 "Tobacco and Other Substance Abuse")
   A. Nicotine Replacement
      1. Generic/trade names—various
      2. Indications—aid to smoking cessation
      3. Dosage and method of delivery—see chart
         a. Transdermal
         b. Chewing gum
         c. Inhaler
         d. Nasal spray
      4. Key side effects—general: nervousness, gastrointestinal upset, tachy-arrhythmias, potential for addiction, local irritation
      5. Nursing highlights
         a. Instruct patient it is most effective when used with a comprehensive behavioral smoking cessation program.
         b. Warn patient of dangers of smoking while on nicotine replacement.
         c. Advise patient to keep used and unused systems out of the reach of children.
         d. Nicotine replacement should not be used greater than 6 months.
         e. No smoking cessation program will be successful unless the patient *wants* to quit smoking.
   B. Non-nicotine
      1. Generic/trade name—bupropion (Zyban, Wellbutrin SR)
      2. Indication—aid to smoking cessation. Research studies done on bupropion as an antidepressant revealed an increased rate of smoking cessation in the treated group. Subsequent studies for smoking cessation validated this effect.
      3. Dosage and method of delivery—initially 150 mg once daily for 3 days, then increase to BID at least 8 hours apart.
      4. Key side effects—dry mouth, insomnia, tremors, agitation, gastrointestinal upset, constipation, seizures.
      5. Nursing highlights
         a. Patients experiencing side effects should discontinue bedtime dosing.

b. Patients should set a "quit date" for smoking approximately 2 weeks after starting bupropion.

c. May be used with nicotine replacement therapy.

VII. Antibiotics

A detailed list of antibiotics and indications for their use would be unmanageable for this type of publication. A review for general anti-microbial therapy is provided but the reader is encouraged to look for more detailed handling of the subject in individual chapters, such as pneumonia, cystic fibrosis, tuberculosis, and so forth.

A. Classifications

1. Class: Penicillins, cephalosporins, macrolides, fluoroquinolones, (see Table 35.3)

2. Indications (respiratory): Bacterial sinusitis, bacterial pharyngitis, acute bronchitis, acute exacerbation of chronic bronchitis, pneumonia, tuberculosis, bronchiectasis, acute exacerbation of cystic fibrosis.

3. Dosage and method of delivery IV, oral, and inhaled. Dosage dependent on chosen antiobiotics (ABX) and concomitant diseases.

4. Key side effects—allergic reaction, diarrhea, nausea and vomiting, skin rash. Others specific to ABX.

5. Nursing highlights

a. Approximately 10% of patients with penicillin allergy will have a cross-reaction to cephalosporins.

b. Yeast infections (oral or vaginal) are a possible complication of antibiotic therapy and may require treatment.

c. *Clostridium difficile,* which causes persistent and possibly severe diarrhea, may result from use of antibiotics.

d. Antibiotic overuse and misuse will promote bacterial resistance.

B. Considerations

1. Factors in selection—therapeutic recommendations are based on most likely pathogens, drug allergy history, anti-microbial effectiveness (which may change by region of the country, from year-to-year), possible side effects, ease of dosing, cost, and safety.

a. Minimum inhibitory concentration (MIC)—minimum amount of drug in blood effective for eradication of bacteria

b. Resistance—may be natural or developed over time

i. MRSA

ii. Pseudomonas

iii. Pneumococcus

c. Cost considerations

i. IV to PO: switching early from IV to PO antibiotics reduces cost, early hospital discharge, less need for home IV therapy, and elimination of IV line related infections.

ii. Monotherapy is possible for most infections: cost savings, less chance of medication error/drug interaction, increased compliance.

Table 35.3 — Commonly Used Oral Antibiotics by Classification for Pulmonary Infections

Penicillins

Amoxicillin (Amoxil)
Amoxicillin/clavulanic acid (Augmentin)

Cephalosporins

Cefuroxime axetil (Ceftin)
Cefprozil (Cefzil)
Cefaclor (Ceclor)
Cephalixin (Keflex)
Cefixime (Suprax)
Cefpodoxime (Vantin)
Cefdinir (Omnicef)

Sulfonamides

Trimethoprim/Sulfamethoxazole (Bactrim DS)

Macrolides

Azithromycin (Z-pak)
Clarithromycin (Biaxin)
Erythromycin (EES)
Pediazole

Fluoroquinolones

Ciprofloxacin (Cipro)
Levofloxacin (Levaquin)
Gatifloxacin (Tequin)
Moxifloxacin (Avelox)

Others

Vibramycin (Doxycyline)

      iii. Combination therapy increases cost and potential for side effects but may be more effective in certain cases.

      iv. Generic vs. nongeneric

      v. Antibiotic adverse reactions requiring change in therapy.

  2. Factors in dosing

    a. Duration—most bacterial infections in normal hosts are treated with antibiotics 5–10 days. This may need to be adjusted for concomitant illnesses or immuno-compromised patients.

    b. Concomitant illness—dosage must be adjusted for most antibiotics with renal and/or hepatic insufficiency

  3. Empiric antibiotic therapy—microbiology susceptibility data are not ordinarily available prior to initial treatment with antibiotics. Patients who

are mildly ill may be started on oral antibiotic most likely to treat the presumed infection and only cultured if this empiric treatment fails.

    4. Inappropriate therapy

        a. Use of antibiotics to treat nonbacterial infections (i.e., viral infections) or colonization

        b. Overuse of combination therapy

        c. Failure to switch to oral antibiotics when indicated

        d. Inadequate allergy history

        e. Drug interactions—i.e., warfarin (Coumadin)

VIII. Other

    A. Influenzae

        1. Generic/trade name—oseltamivir (Tamiflu), zanamivir (Relenza), symmetrel (Amantadine)

        2. Indication—indicated for the treatment of uncomplicated acute illness due to influenza infection, type A and B. (Used to decrease duration and severity and/or reduce incidence of complications.)

        3. Amantadine—Influenza Type A only

            a. Dosage and method of delivery—Tamiflu—oral, one 75 mg capsule twice daily for 5 days. Relenza—inhaled, 10 mg twice daily for 5 days. Amantadine—200 mg daily in one dose for adults, 4.4–8.8 mg/kg/day for pediatrics

            b. Key side effects—mild nausea, insomnia, vertigo

            c. Nursing highlights

                i. Inhaled method must be taught.

    B. Respiratory enzyme—alpha-1 proteinase inhibitor (Prolastin, Aralast) Used in the treatment of alpha-1 antitrypsin deficiency, "genetic emphysema." Replacement gene therapy given by weekly, bi-weekly, or monthly intravenous infusion. Very expensive but the only known treatment for this deficiency.

    C. Investigational

        1. Phosphodiesterase inhibitors (PDE4) and neurocrine receptor antagonists—several medications under study that interrupt the inflammatory process at varying points. Hoped to be an effective alternative to corticosteroids without their side effects.

        2. ATRA Trial—all-trans retinoic acid—under study to determine if it will regenerate lung tissue in patients with emphysema.

WEB SITES

American Academy of Asthma Allergy and Immunology http://www.aaaai.org
American Thoracic Society http://www.thoracic.org
Asthma and Allergy Foundation of America http://www.aafa.org
Infectious Disease Society of America http://www.idsociety.org
National Heart/Lung/Blood Institute http://www.nhlbi.nih.gov

REFERENCE

Cada, D. J. (Ed.). (2001). *Facts and comparisons.* St. Louis: Wolters Kluwer.

SUGGESTED READINGS

Bartlett, J. G. (1999). *Respiratory tract infections* (2nd ed.). Pennsylvania: Lippincott Williams & Wilkins.

Bartlett, J. G., Dowell, S. F., Mandell, L. A., File, T. M., Musher, D. M., & Fine, M. J. (2000). Practice guidelines for the management of community-acquired pneumonia in adults. *Clinical Infectious Diseases, 31*, 347–382.

Bisno, A. L., Gerber, M. A., Gwaltney, J. M., Kaplan, E. L., & Schwartz, R. H. (2002). Practice guidelines for the diagnosis and management of group a streptococcal pharyngitis. *Clinical Infectious Diseases, 35*, 113–125.

Cunha, B. A. (2002). *Antibiotic essentials.* Royal Oak, MI: Physicians Press

Dean-Barr, S. L., Geiger-Bronsky, M., Gift, A., & Hagarty, E. (Eds.). (1994). *Standards and scope of respiratory nursing practice.* Washington, DC: American Nurses Publishing.

Murphy, J. L. (Ed.). (1999). *Physician assistants' prescribing reference.* New York: Prescribing Reference.

National Institutes of Health. (2001). Global Initiative for Chronic Obstructive Lung Disease (GOLD). NIH Publication No. 2701A.

National Institutes of Health. (2002). Expert Panel Report–2002: Guidelines for the Diagnosis and Management of Asthma–Update on Selected Topics. NIH Publication.

Niederman, M. S., Mandell, L. A., Anzueto, A., Bass, J. B., Broughton, W. A., Campbell, G. D. et al. (2001). American Thoracic Society: Guidelines for the Management of Adults with Community-acquired Pneumonia, *American Journal of Respiratory Critical Care Medicine, 7*(163), 1730–1754.

Mechanical Ventilation

36

Irene Grossbach

INTRODUCTION

1. The overall goal of mechanical ventilation is to restore and maintain gas exchange in the patient with oxygenation and/or ventilatory failure until the underlying problem resolves or to maintain support of the patient with chronic ventilatory problems. These goals may be achieved by noninvasive ventilation techniques (negative and positive pressure support) or invasive methods.

2. Although various physiological measurements have been proposed to determine need for mechanical ventilation, the patient's clinical status is the most important criterion.

3. The purposes of noninvasive ventilation techniques are to decrease the work of breathing and respiratory distress, provide ventilatory muscle rest; improve oxygenation, sleep fragmentation, respiratory muscle strength and endurance; improve daytime hypoxemia and hypercapnia; and decrease the frequency and episodes of respiratory failure.

4. Fundamental differences between volume and pressure-targeted modes of positive pressure ventilation are
   a. Volume-controlled (volume-targeted, volume-limited) modes guarantee volume at the expense of letting airway pressure vary.
   b. Pressure-controlled (pressure-targeted, pressure-limited) modes guarantee pressure at the expense of letting tidal volume vary.

5. Successful outcomes for ventilator dependent patients is dependant upon the application of sound principles of mechanical ventilation, making accurate assessments, identifying various potential patient/ventilator related problems and implementing appropriate interventions to prevent or resolve problems.

6. Failure to successfully be discontinued from ventilator support may be due to
   a. Various physiological problems, conditions including disorders of drive to breathe, impaired respiratory muscle function (neuromuscular diseases, etc.), chest bellow dysfunction, structural abnormalities of thorax and rib cage that alter mechanics of breathing (obesity, pleural effusion, chest hyperinflation, etc.), increased work of breathing and load on respiratory pump, conditions that cause increased minute ventilation and respiratory drive and cardiac problems.
   b. Health care team knowledge, assessment skills, ability to synthesize and evaluate information.
   c. Equipment factors
   d. Psychological factors: commonly not the initial cause for failure but may become the major issue due to repeated failures resulting from physiological problems or conditions and inappropriate attempts to discontinue mechanical ventilation support.

Overview

Providing mechanical ventilation support is a common practice in acute and long-term care settings. This chapter reviews noninvasive ventilation techniques, invasive mechanical ventilation, common modes and control dials on mechanical ventilators. It outlines patient/ventilator-related problems, causes, and management, and summarizes management to achieve successful discontinuation from mechanical ventilation.

I. Noninvasive ventilation techniques: Negative and positive pressure support
   A. Negative pressure support
      1. Devices: poncho, chest shell or cuirass, iron lung, body suit.
      2. Purpose: ventilatory muscle rest; improve oxygenation, sleep fragmentation, respiratory muscle strength, and endurance; improve daytime hypoxemia, hypercapnia; and decrease frequency of episodes of respiratory failure.
      3. How it works: Ventilator controls pressure at body surface. Negative pressure generated on chest pulls chest wall out improving ventilation and decreasing $PaCO_2$.
      4. Indications
         a. Insufficient ventilatory reserve to sustain ventilation off device for some period of time for daily cares.
         b. Chronic conditions rather than unpredictable and rapidly changing conditions, such as Guillain-Barré Syndrome and Myasthenia Gravis, or stable improvement expected such as post polio syndrome.
      5. Contraindications
         a. Upper airway obstruction
         b. Unable to clear airway of secretions, protect airway. Poor candidates include patients with CNS depression, recurrent vomiting, risk of aspiration due to bulbar dysfunction.

6. Limitations/problems
   a. Inhibits nursing access to patient as device must cover chest or abdomen up to neck.
   b. May not be able to use if patient is claustrophobic.
   c. Patient must be in supine or semi-supine position.
   d. May produce upper airway obstruction when not triggered by patient, particularly during sleep. (Normally the dilating muscles of pharynx are activated prior to diaphragm contraction in order to reduce upper airway resistance.)
   e. If device cycles asynchronously with spontaneous breathing effort it may produce upper airway narrowing or occlusion.

B. Postural devices
   1. Devices
      a. Rocking bed: cyclical tilting from supine to upright during inspiration; tidal volume dependent on angle of bed tilt.
      b. Abdominal binder: assists ventilation by deflation of air bag over abdominal area during inspiration; may only be used in sitting position during wakefulness.
   2. Purpose: same as negative pressure devices.
   3. How it works: gravity pulls on abdominal viscera to move air in, upright position increases tidal volume; device requires absolute timing control by patient rather than device.
   4. Limitations/problems: less effective than other negative pressure devices or nasal CPAP; use is limited to patients with low mechanical impedance (e.g., neuromuscular patient with no secretion problems).

C. Noninvasive positive pressure ventilation (NPPV) support
   1. Definitions/methods of support
   NPPV: alternative method of ventilating the lung via a nasal or face mask or mouthpiece; application of positive pressure during inspiration via upper airway for purpose of augmenting alveolar ventilation.

   Methods of support are
   a. Mask CPAP (continuous positive airway pressure): application of constant positive airway pressure throughout the ventilatory cycle via use of full face mask with positive end expiratory pressure (PEEP) application; *does not* provide additional inspiratory assistance and may be successful in hypoventilation cases where inspiratory assistance (ventilation support) is needed.
   b. Positive pressure ventilator provides additional inspiratory assistance (ventilation support); achieved by various commercial brand positive pressure ventilators.
   c. Bi-level positive airway pressure machines can be set to deliver inspiratory positive airway pressure (synonymous to pressure support mode) and an expiratory pressure (PEEP setting).

d. BiPAP: trade name for ventilator made by specific manufacturer. Various manufacturers make ventilators to provide bi-level positive airway pressure support.

2. Purpose/goals: same as conventional intubation and mechanical ventilation
   a. Rest fatigued inspiratory muscles.
   b. Decrease $PaCO_2$ by improved ventilation, decreasing deadspace.
   c. Decrease left ventricular afterload in pulmonary edema.

3. Appropriate candidates: Selection guidelines
   a. NPPV can support patients in acute respiratory failure and avert intubation in 50%–75% of cases and can lower mortality and shorten hospital stay.
   b. Hypoxemic and/or hypercapnic respiratory failure, e.g., due to COPD exacerbation, pneumonia, congestive heart failure, asthma, post-extubation and post-operative respiratory failure, cystic fibrosis, acute decompensation in neuromuscular disease, cardiogenic pulmonary edema.
   c. Chronic respiratory failure (COPD, neuromuscular disease)
   d. Patients who do not want endotracheal intubation but may need short- or long-term ventilatory support.

4. Contraindications
   a. Excessive secretions or unable to clear airway.
   b. Upper airway obstruction problems.
   c. High risk for gastric aspiration.
   d. Hemodynamic instability.
   e. Facial surgery.
   f. May be difficult to ventilate if abnormal facial anatomy.
   g. Worsening respiratory failure with decreased lung compliance and/or increased airway resistance problems.
   h. Note: Technique may be successful with uncooperative patient with appropriate interventions including optimum ventilator setting and/or mask adjustments to improve breathing comfort, positive communications that foster cooperation and allow patient participation and control.

5. Procedure for optimal NPPV support
   a. Set up machine, mask ready for use.
   b. Position patient with head of bed elevated to comfort, usually about 45 degrees, may use reverse trendelenberg position at 45 degrees if obese, abdominal distention.
   c. Explain in a calm, reassuring, and simple manner that the mask can help breathing feel more comfortable and can decrease shortness of breath, and encourage patient to try it. Maintain calm, confident, reassuring approach.
   d. Turn on ventilator, apply face mask.
   e. Place mask firmly on the face to obtain a good seal; hold mask in place with hand until patient becomes more comfortable and in

synchrony with ventilator, then apply straps. Allow patient participation if desired.

f. Immediately after mask is in place, adjust ventilator settings as necessary to achieve improved breathing comfort as soon as possible with resulting patient compliance with therapy.

g. Secure mask. Avoid applying straps too tight, which decreases patient compliance, increases skin breakdown, and may increase or cause leak problems.

h. Monitor and prevent excess moisture condensation in mask. Turn off humidifier, wipe condensation from mask as necessary, and ask patient regarding comfort of air temperature.

i. Resolve excessive air leaks: may include strap adjustment, different mask size, style, brand; adding or deleting air if mask is air cushioned, may put in dentures, skin padding to facial area.

j. Prevent skin breakdown: monitor for skin pressure areas from mask, may require mask readjustment or different mask, skin protection with padding.

k. May initiate other measures to improve ventilation, breathing comfort, and decrease work of breathing including medications to decrease anxiety, pain, and correct underlying acute lung problem, fan directed on face, etc.

6. Clinical monitoring, response goals
   a. Keep SpO_2 > 90%. Adjust FIO_2 as needed.
   b. Patient appears more comfortable, conveys improved breathing comfort.
      Note: improvement may be immediate or within first 10–20 minutes.
   c. Respiratory rate less than 30; decreased work of breathing signs and symptoms including neck muscle and abdominal muscle contraction.
   d. ABGs improve within 30 to 60 minutes.

7. Complications, risk factors
   a. Nasal bridge, chin, facial abrasion, necrosis: Properly fitted mask and use of skin protection dressing can prevent complications and minimize air leaks. Avoid nasal gastric tube placement unless needed to release gastric distention.
   b. Gastric distention: Few problems have been noted with inflation pressures less than 25 cm (below the opening pressure of the gastroesophageal junction).
   c. Aspiration.
   d. Inability to clear secretions.
   e. Conjunctivitis due to air leaks; may be prevented with properly fitted mask.
   f. Dry nose/mouth: Humidify inspired air. Maintain water at refill line and regulate temperature.
   g. Moisture condensation in mask: may try turning off humidifier.

II. Mechanical ventilator modes and function
  A. Classification of mechanical ventilators
    1. Volume controlled (volume targeted, volume-cycled) ventilation
      a. Terminates inspiration when a preset volume of gas is delivered.
      b. Preset volume is delivered unless a specified pressure limit is exceeded (upper airway pressure alarm is set) or air leak in system.
      c. Peak airway pressure required to deliver the volume varies with changes in airway resistance, lung compliance. As airway resistance increases or lung compliance decreases, the peak pressure rises to deliver the prescribed volume.
    2. Pressure controlled (pressure targeted, pressure-limited) ventilation
      a. Relies on a preset pressure to determine the volume of gas delivered and maintains a targeted amount of pressure at the airway opening until a specified time (pressure control) or flow (pressure support) cycling criteria is met.
      b. Volume delivered is variable and depends upon various factors that increase airway resistance (e.g., secretions, bronchospasm) and decrease lung compliance (e.g., pulmonary edema, pleural effusion, abdominal distention) (see Figure 36.1).
    3. Fundamental differences between volume- and pressure-controlled ventilation
      a. Volume-controlled modes guarantee volume at the expense of letting airway pressure vary.
      b. Pressure-controlled modes guarantee pressure at the expense of letting tidal volume vary.
    4. Definition of mode: how the machine ventilates the patient; describes whether breaths are volume constant (volume-controlled) or pressure constant (pressure-controlled), whether breaths are mandatory, spontaneous or a combination of the two, and which conditional variables determine a change in ventilator function.
  B. Modes of positive pressure ventilation operation
    Note: Many modes or techniques are emerging to improve the efficiency of mechanical ventilation. Various authors and manufacturers use different terms to describe the same mode and this may cause some confusion. Following are basic concepts and terms to explain mechanical ventilator modes.
    1. Continuous mandatory ventilation (CMV)
      a. Other names listed in literature-control mode, assist/control, volume control, continuous mechanical ventilation, controlled mechanical ventilation, controlled mandatory ventilation, volume-controlled ventilation, control ventilation.
      b. All breaths are mandatory (machine triggered and/or cycled) and delivered at preset frequency, volume or pressure and inspiratory time.
      c. Mandatory breaths could be volume- or pressure-controlled, patient or machine triggered, pressure, volume or flows limited depending on type of ventilation and hospital practice.

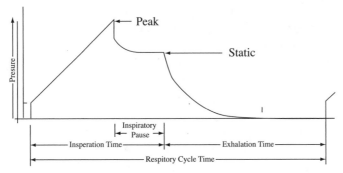

Figure 36.1. Peak-status pressure.

    d. Includes all modes that deliver only mandatory (ventilator triggered) or a combination of mandatory and assisted breaths (patient triggers the assisted breath).

    e. Controlled mode: On some ventilators, the sensitivity or trigger level setting can be adjusted so that significant negativity must be generated in order to provide a ventilator-assisted breath or a predetermined time adjustment is made on some ventilators without regard to patient effort. This controlled "lockout" mode is not used because the patient capable of assisting will increase work of breathing, be agitated, and fight the ventilator. Sedation and/or paralysis would likely be necessary for toleration of mode in the assisting patient.

2. Assist-control (A/C)

    a. Other names listed in literature: CMV with assist, assisted mechanical ventilation (AMV), assisted ventilation.

    b. Mandatory breaths are delivered at a set frequency, volume or pressure and flow rate. With minimal inspiratory effort (sensitivity setting adjusted –1 to –2 cm), the patient can trigger additional breaths as desired at the preset tidal volume or pressure.

    c. A/C implies only that there are both patient and machine triggering of breaths. It is important to state the control variable as many ventilators can be set for either volume-controlled or pressure-controlled ventilation breath types. Some ventilators are only capable of providing volume-controlled ventilation on the A/C mode.

3. Synchronized intermittent mandatory ventilation (SIMV)

    a. Patient receives a preset number of mandatory breaths (patient on machine triggered) at a set volume or pressure. The patient can breathe spontaneously between machine breaths from a continuous flow of gas or demand system or the addition of pressure support (PS). Ventilator breaths are synchronized so they do not interfere with patient's respiratory efforts.

    b. SIMV + PS: Combining of two modes: volume-controlled mandatory breaths plus pressure supported spontaneous breaths. PS is routinely used to overcome circuit, tube resistance and prevent increased work of breathing on spontaneous breaths. Volume on the spontaneous, pressure-supported breaths is variable and determined by the patient's effort or drive, preset pressure level and various airway resistance and lung compliance factors.

4. Pressure support ventilation (PSV)
   a. Other names listed in literature: Inspiratory pressure support (IPS), inspiratory assist (IA), inspiratory flow assist (IFA).
   b. Form of ventilatory support that is patient-triggered and augments patient's spontaneous inspiratory effort with a preset amount of positive inspiratory pressure. The higher the set inspiratory pressure level, the more gas flows to the patient and the greater the tidal volume delivered. Tidal volume, respiratory rate, inspiratory time and flow rate are variable and regulated by the patient. Factors altering tidal volume and respiratory rate include set pressure level, changes in airway resistance, lung compliance and patient effort or drive. For example, tidal volume decreases if the patient develops bronchospasm or obstruction from secretions because more pressure is required and PS is a pressure-limited mechanical breath. Expiration begins when the set inspiratory pressure level or a low terminal flow is achieved or due to other expiratory criteria depending on the ventilator.
   c. PSV was originally designed to overcome airway resistance and increased work of breathing caused by the endotracheal tube and other imposed ventilator resistances. Common practice is PS 5–10 cm depending on the ventilator.
   d. Mode contraindicated as primary mode of ventilation support if frequent airway resistance, lung compliance problems due to variable Vt, inadequate delivery of ventilation and related potential adverse effects. Mode nonfunctional if patient is apneic or inadequate respiratory drive (patient-triggered mode).

5. Pressure control mode (PCM)
   a. Similar to PSV except a machine rate, inspiratory time and pressure support level is set. The patient can be apneic and supported on PCM.
   b. Ventilator attempts to maintain a preset airway pressure waveform during inspiration.
   c. Pressure Control Inverse Ratio Ventilation (PCIRV): Version of PCM pressure controlled, time triggered, pressure limited and timed cycled. All breaths are mandatory. Parameters are adjusted to provide desired longer inspiratory to expiratory (I:E) ratio. Inverse ratio ventilation can also be provided with volume-controlled breaths.

6. Continuous positive airway pressure (CPAP)
   a. Description: application of constant positive airway pressure applied throughout the ventilatory cycle, which increases airway and alveolar pressure but does not provide additional inspiratory assistance (ventilation support). Varying levels of positive end expiratory pressure (PEEP) are used, commonly 5–10 cm.

      b. CPAP mode on some ventilators may increase work of breathing due to artificial airway, ventilator circuitry, and other factors that increase airway resistance. PS mode may be used instead.

C. Newer or specialized modes of ventilation

  1. Many newer ventilator options and modes exist that are not covered in this chapter. Refer to individual manufacturers or other text.

  2. Mandatory minute ventilation (MMV)

      a. Other names listed in literature: minimum minute volume, extended mandatory minute ventilation (EMMV), augmented minute volume (AMV).

      b. Description: mode of ventilator operation that ensures patient receives minimum, clinician-determined minute ventilation (V_E) and that also allows the patient to breathe spontaneously. When V_E falls below this target, PSV is provided on some ventilators or the ventilator automatically switches to volume-controlled breath to provide a safety net. May be useful with patients being discontinued from the ventilator or with unstable ventilatory drive (Branson & Campbell, 2001).

  3. Dual control modes: Capable of controlling either volume or pressure based on a desired tidal volume. Dual control may be within a breath or from breath to breath currently using two techniques

      a. Uses measured input to switch from pressure control to volume control in the middle of the breath.

      b. Uses measured input to manipulate the pressure level of the pressure-support or pressure-controlled mandatory breath-limited breath from breath to breath to achieve tidal volume.

  4. Advantages of limiting peak inspiratory pressure to avoid lung overdistention (pressure control) while maintaining constant volume even if there are changes in respiratory system resistance and compliance (Branson, 2001).

  5. Examples of dual control within a breath

      a. Terms by Manufacturer: Volume-assured pressure support (VAPS) Bird 8400 ST and Tbird, Bird Corp., Palm Springs, CA; Pressure Augmentation (PA)-Bear 1000, Bear Medical, Riverside, CA.

      b. Mode allows ventilator to deliver a pressure support breath (pressure control) or switch to volume-controlled breath within the breath.

      c. Rationale for use: During PS, VAPS, and PA can be considered a safety net that provides a minimum tidal volume. Meant to combine high variable flow of a pressure support breath with constant volume delivery of volume-limited breath.

  6. Dual control breath to breath

      a. Terms by Manufacturer: Volume support, Pressure-Regulated Volume Control (PRVC)-Siemens 300, Adaptive Pressure Ventilation (APV)-Hamilton Galileo, Variable Pressure Control-Venturi, Auto-flow-Evita 4.

      b. Volume support is pressure support ventilation that uses tidal volume as the feedback control for continuously adjusting the pressure support level. When compliance decreases, pressure increases until Vt is restored. If lung compliance increases, pressure support decreases to maintain constant Vt (Branson, 2001).

    c. Automatic tube compensation (ATC): Technique of ventilator operation that is capable of determining resistance characteristics of artificial airways and providing necessary pressure support to compensate for resistance.

    d. High frequency ventilation (HFV): High frequency jet ventilation (HFJV), high frequency oscillation (HFO)

       i. Mechanical ventilation support using breathing frequencies severalfold higher than normal (>100 breaths/min in adult and >300 breaths/min in neonate/pediatric patient).

       ii. Tidal volume may be less than anatomic dead space but product of tidal volume and rate is generally much higher than conventional ventilation.

       iii. Conventional ventilator not capable of this support. Must use specialized ventilator.

       iv. Rationale for use: Lung protective strategy—small Vt and pressure changes prevents alveolar overdistention and may improve ventilation-perfusion matching and gas exchange due to better alveolar recruitment, rapid flow pattern.

       v. Conclusions: Clinical data demonstrates improved outcomes for neonatal and some forms of pediatric respiratory failure. Convincing data does not exist for adults at present and further study is needed to determine its application. HFV should be limited to specific applications including select neonates and adult airway surgical procedures. Routine bronchopleural fistulas can be ventilated adequately with conventional mechanical ventilation. Skilled personnel are essential for delivering safe and proper support.

D. Common ventilator settings

  1. Tidal volume (Vt): volume of gas delivered in a normal inspiration. Vt during mechanical ventilation of patients with normal lungs is approximately 10–12 cc/kg ideal body weight. High Vt ventilation may produce volutrauma (alveolar overdistention) or barotrauma (alveolar disruption from excess pressure). Vt as low as 5–8 mL/Kg may be appropriate in patients with acute lung injury to prevent injury due to overdistention. Vt may be chosen based the peak alveolar pressures (plateau pressure) to maintain a plateau pressure <35 cm H_2O.

  2. Respiratory rate (RR): Number of respirations delivered by ventilator in one minute

  3. Minute volume (MV): Volume of gas expired in one minute (Vt × RR = MV).

  4. Peak flow: speed at which the tidal volume is delivered in liters per minute (LPM). A normal flowrate in the uncomplicated patient is

approximately 30–50 LPM. Patients with respiratory distress and/or high minute volumes need higher flowrates (60–100 plus LPM) in order to match inspiratory efforts, and to decrease work of breathing and related adverse effects.

5. Trigger sensitivity: amount of effort (negative inspiratory pressure or flow in LPM depending on ventilator) required by the patient to trigger the ventilator to deliver a breath; normally set so the patient requires minimal effort (–1 to –2 cm).

6. Positive end expiratory pressure (PEEP): increases the transalveolar pressure and volume, may recruit collapsed alveoli, and improve oxygenation. Common PEEP levels 5–15 cm.

7. Percent oxygen (% O_2): oxygen concentration.

8. Peak inspiratory pressure (PIP) or peak airway pressure: displays the total pressure required to inflate the lungs and includes various airway resistance and lung compliance factors. (See Figure 36.1.)

9. Plateau pressure (Pplat) or static pressure: clinical measurement used to reflect alveolar pressure and therefore lung compliance. Results suggest that plateau pressures in excess of 30–35 cm H_2O may increase the risk of barotrauma. Pplat is monitored with adjustments in tidal volume and PEEP settings in efforts to avoid aveolar overdistention as reflected by rising Pplat.

   a. Interpretation of PIP, Pplat
      i. When the PIP is high or rises, measurement of plateau pressure 2 may assist evaluating the cause of elevated PIP-airway resistance versus lung compliance problems.
      ii. The difference between the PIP and the plateau pressure (Pplat), generally about 10 cm H_2O, reflects pressure caused by airway resistance. If the difference is greater than 10 cm H_2O, the cause of the high PIP is an increase in resistance to gas flow. Rising PIP with no change in Pplat (lung) pressure suggests airway resistance problems (e.g., secretions, bronchospasm, narrowed endotracheal tube).
      iii. If the PIP increases and the difference between peak and plateau pressures remain approximately 10 cm H_2O or less, then the cause of elevated PIP is generally a reduction in lung compliance (e.g., lung overdistention due to high tidal volume, PEEP, pulmonary edema).

10. Clinical alarms are triggered by a ventilator setting or patient condition and can occur in the usual course of patient care. Some ventilators are capable of visually displaying the specific problem or condition causing the alarm and other ventilators only sound an audible alarm indicating a problem.

III. Management of patient/ventilator-related problems

   A. Following is a summary of common clinical alarm conditions and problems, causes and interventions to assure optimum management of the ventilator dependent patient. (See Table 36.1.)

| Table 36.1 | Management of Patient-/Ventilator-Related Problems |

Problem	Causes	Interventions
1. Increased Airway Pressure, Airway Pressure Alarm Sounds (HIGH PRESSURE ALARM)	Conditions causing increased airway resistance including: –Secretions –Coughing due to airway irritation from jarring of tubes, secretions –Displaced tube –Kinked tubing –Water obstructing tube	▢ Suction as needed. ▢ Avoid jarring, moving tube during turning, other interventions. Support tube properly on ventilator arm to avoid pulling, jarring, discomfort and to prevent interference with patient movement. ▢ Evaluate, drape tubing to avoid kinks; drain water prior to repositioning (to prevent water from going into trachea) and PRN. ▢ Obtain chest x-ray to evaluate for proper endotracheal tube (ETT) placement. ▢ Evaluate with MD whether patient is candidate for withdrawal from ventilator support, extubation, which will resolve problem of coughing, gagging from tube irritation.
	–Bronchospasm	▢ Bronchodilators as ordered; avoid interventions that increase airway irritation: suction only as needed, do not instill saline or allow tubing condensation to drain into airway; avoid jarring tube.
	Inadequate inspiratory flow-rate due to various factors that alter respiratory pattern, increase respiratory rate: anxiety, fear, pain, hypoxemia, CNS and metabolic disorders, etc.	▢ Readjust ventilator flow setting to meet inspiratory demands (patient "in synch," not fighting ventilator, delivery of breath is in correct timing with inspiratory effort, conveys breathing comfort). ▢ Provide calm, confident, reassuring approach.

Problem	Causes	Interventions
		■ Provide ventilation as needed with manual resuscitation bag (MRB) "in synch" with inspiratory efforts. Consult with expert prn.
		■ Evaluate for causes of increased ventilatory requirements, correct problems.
	Attempting to speak, alternative communication methods ineffective, inappropriate or not implemented.	■ Refer to Problem Number 5: Impaired Ability to Communicate
	Displacement of endotracheal tube with tip in vocal cord or against tracheal wall, coiled in mouth; Tracheostomy tube with tip against anterior or posterior tracheal wall (assessments: appears displaced, unable to pass catheter beyond distal end of tube).	■ Initiate emergency airway assistance with tube repositioning and/or reintubation. ■ Ventilate airway with MRB and 100% oxygen (tracheostomy or face mask) as needed
	Conditions causing decreased lung compliance including pneumonia, pulmonary edema, pneumothorax, Endotracheal tube (ETT) advanced into right mainstem bronchus.	■ Auscultate chest routinely to determine changes in breath sounds ■ Notify MD of unexplained higher airway pressures, changes in BS. ■ Verify correct ETT placement—obtain chest x-ray, reposition tube as needed.
	Biting on ETT.	■ Remind not to bite on ETT. ■ May reposition in area of mouth without teeth or use appropriate bite block system. ■ May need to sedate to achieve adequate oxygenation and ventilation if other nonpharmacologic interventions ineffective.
	Occlusion in breathing circuit, inspiratory or expiratory filters	■ Check ventilator breathing circuit for water, kinks. Empty excess water from tubing.

(continued)

| | **Table 36.1** | Management of Patient-/Ventilator-Related Problems (*continued*) |

Problem	Causes	Interventions
	Unusually high tidal volume (Vt), PEEP setting	▪ Change nebulizer filters per recommendation, PRN. ▪ Ventilate patient as needed with MRB. ▪ Evaluate, set appropriate Vt, PEEP to avoid alveolar overdistention, injury. Vt goals approximately 10 mL/kg, may be lower (5–8 mL/kg) to maintain safe alveolar pressures (plateau pressures <35 cm).
	High pressure alarm set too low	▪ Set appropriate high pressure alarm (commonly 10–20 cm higher than patient's peak airway pressure).
	High flow rate setting = generates higher resistance and pressure	▪ Evaluate flow rate setting, adjust to meet inspiratory demands; may need high setting.
2. Not Receiving Prescribed Tidal Volume (Vt) (LOW EXHALED TIDAL VOLUME ALARM, LOW INSPIRATORY PRESSURE ALARM)	Conditions which create air leaks: cuff leak, ventilator circuit/connections loose, cracked, torn, disconnected (including nebulizer attachment, temperature probe site, humidifier), blocked or kinked tube	▪ Ventilate with MRB if patient is in acute respiratory distress and you are unable to immediately correct problem. ▪ Check all tubing connections. Secure connections. Replace PRN. ▪ Evaluate cuff leak problem (not enough air in cuff, torn cuff, leak in one-way inflation port, head position, displaced ETT). Correct problem.
	Various airway resistance, lung compliance factors which increase peak pressure, set off upper pressure alarm limit causing the volume which is not delivered to be dumped from ventilator.	▪ Evaluate patient, correct problems causing high airway pressures (Refer to Problem No. 1).

Problem	Causes	Interventions
	Bronchopleural air leak (bubbling observed in chest drainage unit waterseal chamber), which results in passage of air from airways to pleural space	▪ Implement measures that minimize bronchopleural pressure gradient, maintain adequate oxygenation, ventilation (pH > 7.25–30) including low Vt, minimizing PEEP/CPAP and time spent in inspiration, matching inspiratory flowrate, lowest number of mechanical breaths compatible with adequate ventilation (spontaneous ventilation if possible), position differences to decrease leak, sedation if spontaneous movements worsen leaks; treat underlying problem.
3. Receiving No Volume (DISCONNECT ALARM)	Major air leaks (patient disconnected from ventilator, tubing circuit disconnected, large tube cuff leak, extubated self, loss of wall electrical or compressed air source	▪ Check patient, reattach airway adapter, connect circuit, correct cuff leak problem. ▪ Maintain adequate oxygenation and ventilation PRN with MRB. ▪ Obtain emergency assistance PRN.
4. APNEA ALARM	Patient has not triggered a breath within the apnea interval (usually 15–20 seconds, function operates in Spontaneous Mode-Pressure Support Ventilation)	▪ Evaluate patient, ventilate as needed with MRB. ▪ May need to switch to mode that provides more ventilation support.
5. Impaired Verbal Communication	Tracheostomy, endotracheal tube and need for ventilator support	▪ Explain reason for inability to communicate verbally. Evaluate, implement alternative effective method(s) to meet individualized needs: paper and pencil, lip reading, gestures, alphabet board, word or phrase board indicating major needs, specialized tracheostomy tube or one-way valve adapter, cuff deflation.

(continued)

Table 36.1 | Management of Patient-/Ventilator-Related Problems (*continued*)

Problem	Causes	Interventions
		▪ Ask "yes" or "no" type questions.
		▪ Anticipate usual needs related to comfort (reposition, suction, pain medication, etc.).
		▪ Maintain eye contact at patient's level. Be aware of cultural factors that may preclude eye contact.
		▪ Take time, be patient and work with patient frustration, anger, and feelings of insecurity at not being able to communicate.
		▪ Convey calm, confident, reassuring approach.
		▪ Involve family in plan of care as much as possible.
		▪ Obtain assistance PRN to determine what patient is trying to communicate.
		▪ Consult speech therapy PRN.
6. Pulling, Jarring of Tracheostomy, Endotracheal Tube Causing Discomfort	Insufficient attention to observing patient's airway, guiding tubing and providing extra tubing during turning or movement	▪ Guide and support airway and tubing in manner that prevents tube from pulling and jarring during activities.
		▪ Obtain necessary assistance with turning, transferring so one person can provide specific attention to preventing pulling and jarring tube.
	Tube not supported properly on ventilator arm	▪ Unclip ventilator tubing from ventilator support arm/reclip in manner that prevents tube pulling, jarring and maintains optimum tube alignment and support.
		▪ May disconnect from ventilator, turn, reconnect airway

Problem	Causes	Interventions
		adapter (may not be indicated in unstable patient).
		▣ Stabilize tracheostomy or ETT with one hand when reconnecting ventilator adapter or with airway suctioning.
	Inadequate securing of tube	▣ Properly secure tracheostomy, ETT to avoid displacement and prevent skin breakdown.
7. Thick Secretions	Inadequate humidification due to: Insufficient water in humidifier, heating unit not working properly, temperature set too low.	▣ Apply heated humidification. Add water to humidifier refill line prn; monitor, adjust temperature to manufacturer's specifications.
		▣ Change humidification system as needed to provide adequate heat, moisture.
	Inappropriate humidification system-passive acting device that collects patient's expired heat, moisture; referred to as artificial nose or heat and moisture exchanger (HME)	▣ Evaluate, maintain adequate fluid intake.
		▣ Monitor sputum for changes in color, amount, consistency. Notify MD for signs of infection or unusual changes in status. Monitor for improvements with antibiotic therapy
	Inadequate hydration Infection	▣ Drain water from tubing q. 1–2 hrs and prn. Drain into water traps or disconnect tubing and drain but do not drain back into humidifier
8. Anxiety, Agitation, Sets Off Upper Pressure Alarm, Exhibits Signs and Symptoms of Increased Work Breathing, Short of Breath	Airway irritation; Cough, secretions Tube irritation due to jarring, movement, displacement	**Non-Pharmacologic Management** **Physiological:** ▣ Prevent excess cough, irritation: –Suction only as necessary. –Do not instill saline. –Maintain thin secretions for better clearance. –Prevent jarring, moving tube.

(continued)

513

Table 36.1	Management of Patient-/Ventilator-Related Problems (*continued*)

Problem	Causes	Interventions
	Bronchospastic airways, need for better bronchodilator therapy, anti-inflammatory agents	–Evaluate for proper tube placement –Properly secure tube. –Avoid interventions that create shortness of breath.
	Pain	■ Provide bronchodilator, steroid, pain antibiotic therapy.
	Adverse drug effects, sleep deprivation causing agitation, confusion, uncooperative behavior	■ Evaluate for adverse drug effects causing agitation. ■ Reposition prn for comfort. ■ Assure adequate rest, sleep. **Psychological:**
	ICU environment (noises, unfamiliar people, procedures, fear of unknown, etc.)	■ Provide calm, confident, reassuring approach; consistent staffing ■ Explain interventions, orient to surroundings prn. ■ Avoid interventions that create SOB (weaning when not ready, inappropriate ventilator mode etc.). ■ Implement relaxation techniques: coaching, touch, music therapy, methods defined by patient. ■ Allow patient participation in decision making as capable. **Ventilator:**
	Inadequate flow rate resulting in feeling of not getting enough air and suffocating	■ Adjust ventilator flow rate setting to meet inspiratory demands. ■ Ventilate with MRB prn "in synch" with patient's inspiratory efforts. ■ Evaluate ventilator for appropriate mode, correct settings and delivery of prescribed volume.

Problem	Causes	Interventions
9. **Acute Respiratory Acidosis** (pH < 7.35 or may be normal if compensated; $PaCO_2$ > 45 mm Hg or greater than patient's usual $PaCO_2$ level)	Patient not receiving prescribed Vt due to air leaks Inadequate Vt to provide adequate gas exchange Insufficient respiratory rate COPD patient may have chronically elevated $PaCO_2$ levels High carbohydrate concentrations in TPN or enteral preparations which increase carbon dioxide production. (Glucose calories exceeding metabolic demands are converted to fat causing carbon dioxide production, increased $PaCO_2$. Patient may be unable to increase minute ventilation to maintain normal $PaCO_2$, particularly if on partial ventilator support, marginal ventilatory reserve or chronic lung disease.)	▪ Evaluate/correct air leaks (Refer to Problems 2–3). ▪ Increase Vt, switch to more supportive mode of ventilation. ▪ Increase respiratory rate setting. ▪ Maintain $PaCO_2$ at patient's normal baseline level. Do not overventilate to a normal $PaCO_2$ level if patient has chronic CO_2 retention. ▪ If major acidosis, make gradual changes to baseline $PaCO_2$, pH to avoid acute respiratory alkalosis with risk of cardiac arrhythmias, tetany, seizures. ▪ Monitor effects of nutrition therapy on respiration particularly if patient is on partial ventilator support, has normal lungs and developed compromised lung function or chronic lung disease. ▪ If increases in minute ventilation or carbon dioxide production noted, evaluate amount and source of non-protein calories. Consult with MD, dietitian for changes
10. **Acute Respiratory Alkalosis**	Factors that increase RR, minute ventilation including anxiety, restlessness, discomfort, pain, hypoxemia, central nervous system malfunction, metabolic acidosis, sensation of dyspnea caused by underlying lung pathology	▪ Decrease feelings of anxiety and fear through calm, confident, reassuring approach, providing explanations and other measures to decrease stress (relaxation/music therapy, touch, etc.). ▪ Evaluate ventilator for proper function (prescribed Vt, flow rate matches inspiratory demand) ▪ Provide adequate oxygenation.

(continued)

| Table 36.1 | Management of Patient-/Ventilator-Related Problems (continued) |

Problem	Causes	Interventions
		▪ Provide optimum pain medication.
		▪ Evaluate/treat metabolic problems.
		▪ Consider that hyper-ventilation may not be corrected by various interventions due to CNS dysfunction, hypermeta-bolic state. May allow respiratory alkalosis.
	High Vt, RR or minute vol-ume dialed on ventilator causing overventilation	▪ Evaluate, decrease Vt, RR (Note: Decreasing these settings while on volume control or assist/control mode may not correct the problem because the as-sisting patient triggers the ventilator at whatever rate desired in order to achieve desired minute ventilation.)
	Temporary therapy to cause cerebral vasoconstric-tion, decrease intracranial pressure (controversy on benefits, uses)	▪ Hyperventilate as pre-scribed limiting to short period (<24–48 hours), target $PaCO_2$ 25-30 mm Hg; Restore $PaCO_2$ gradually back to normal. Provide other measures to control intracranial hypertension.
		▪ Consider sedation.
	Too frequent or too many sighs	▪ Decrease or eliminate sighs.
	Ventilator self cycling: breath delivered without patient effort due to machine sensitivity setting incorrect or due to normal reset to positive side while patient on PEEP	▪ Maintain sensitivity dial at −1 to −2 cm.
		▪ Check airway pressure needle to make sure it rests at O point on airway pressure meter (machine will self cycle if needle becomes maladjusted to negative side).
		▪ Avoid air leaks in cuff/ventilator system

Problem	Causes	Interventions
		when patient is on PEEP therapy. On PEEP, sensitivity setting is automatically reset to positive side (i.e., for PEEP 5 cm, dial reset to +3 or 4 cm.). Air leaks = loss of PEEP = machine self-cycling = increased respiratory rate.
11. Low PaO$_2$, SpO$_2$	Inadequate oxygen percent Air leaks, volume loss causing inadequate oxygenation, ventilation, loss of PEEP, increased work of breathing ETT malposition, pneumothorax	▪ Increase FiO$_2$ ▪ Evaluate for air leaks, proper ventilator function. ▪ See Problems 1–4. ▪ Notify MD of unexplained changes. ▪ Evaluate for, correct tube malposition, pneumothorax. Obtain chest x-ray prn
	Secretions, increased lung consolidation, pulmonary edema, other abnormalities causing ventilation-perfusion (V/Q) disturbances, shunting	▪ Suction, pre/post oxygenate prn. ▪ Be aware of underlying pathophysiological problems causing abnormal oxygenation. ▪ Notifiy MD of unexplained changes.
	Position changes causing alveolar hypoventilation, V/Q disturbance	▪ Assess whether certain positions, activities cause deterioration in oxygenation status. ▪ Refrain from placing in positions that precipitate respiratory discomfort, unsafe drops in PaO$_2$ or obtain order to increase FiO$_2$ and/or Vt for goals of maintaining adequate oxygenation, ventilation.
12. High PaO$_2$	Oxygen concentration dialed in ventilator too high Improvement in clinical abnormalities causing V/Q disturbances	▪ Decrease FiO$_2$, regulate PEEP with goals of FiO$_2$ < .5, PaO$_2$ > 60 mm, adequate hemoglobin, cardiac output.

B. Additional potential problems associated with positive pressure ventilation support
1. Pulmonary damage from alveolar disruption due to excessive volumes (volutrauma) or pressures (barotrauma).
2. Decreased blood pressure, cardiac output (CO)
    a. Large lung volumes, PEEP (dialed on ventilator- or patient-related "air trapping, intrinsic, auto-PEEP" due to airflow obstruction) causes increased intrathoracic pressure and vascular pressures, reduces blood return to the heart. Impeded venous return causes lowering of right ventricular filling (preload) and right heart ventricular stroke volume.
    Note: Potential beneficial effect in patients with left ventricular dysfunction and elevated filling pressures due to reduced preload and afterload on heart causing improved contractility.
    b. Hypovolemia
    c. Significant stimulation (hypoxemia, acidemia, anxiety, and fear) of autonomic system cause arterial and venous constriction. Ventilator support usually relieves work of breathing, improves oxygenation and ventilation, produces relaxation. This combination plus drug effects often lead to profound and sudden decrease in sympathetic stimulation to cardiovascular system, arterial and venous relaxation, and a significant increase in vascular space.
3. Decreased renal blood flow, urine output.
4. Arrhythmias, vasovagal reactions during or after suctioning
    a. Arrhythmias related to hypoxemia due to suction induced arterial desaturation, bronchoconstriction.
    b. Vasovagal reactions (bradycardia, decreased blood pressure) due to increased intrathoracic pressure when coughing against obstruction of suction catheter and closed airway suction system, vomiting, lifting, act of defecation.
    c. During strain, venous return to the heart, systolic and pulse pressures decrease.
5. Pneumothorax/tension pneumothorax
    Positive pressure ventilation that causes pulmonary barotrauma including high tidal volume, pressure settings, PEEP, auto-PEEP.
    a. Underlying lung pathology (emphysematous blebs, lung surgery) may make some persons more susceptible to positive pressure effects.
C. Selected complications of endotracheal tube intubation: pain, discomfort, dental accidents, soft tissue trauma, retropharyngeal, hypopharyngeal perforation, esophageal intubation, aspiration, laryngospasm, right mainstem bronchus intubation, cardiac/respiratory arrest
V. Discontinuing mechanical ventilator support
A. Evaluation for determining readiness to be discontinued from ventilator
1. Is the underlying condition/problem(s) that required need for ventilator support reversed, stabilized, resolved: hemodynamically stable,

other organ function stable, patient with obstructive lung disease receiving optimum airway management.

   2. Failure to wean due to physiological problems/conditions including
      a. Disorders of drive to breathe (drug depression, head trauma, etc.)
      b. Impaired respiratory muscle function, decreased strength, endurance, contractility, paralysis (neuromuscular diseases, neuromuscular blocking agents, steroids, mineral and electrolyte deficiencies, sepsis, critical illness polyneuropathy, phrenic nerve paralysis, etc.)
      c. Chest bellow dysfunction, structural abnormalities of thorax and rib cage which alter mechanics of breathing (obesity, abdominal distention, pleural effusion, hyperinflation due to auto-PEEP, unstable chest wall due to trauma, surgery, etc.)
      d. Increased work of breathing and load on respiratory pump due to increased airway resistance, decreased lung compliance problems.
      e. Increased minute ventilation due to conditions which increase respiratory drive (neurogenic hyperventilation, metabolic acidosis due to sepsis, hypoxemia), CO_2 production (fever, pain, agitation, sepsis), increased deadspace ventilation (ARDS, pulmonary embolism, hypoxia, etc).
      f. Cardiac problems: Hypoxia, decreased CO = impaired oxygen delivery to respiratory muscles (acute ventricular dysfunction, hemodynamic instability, decreased CO, anemia).
   B. Health care team assessment, knowledge, skills, synthesis and evaluation: Pre-weaning evaluations to determine readiness, optimum procedure, accurate observations, decisions, evaluations.
   C. Equipment factors (malfunctions causing increased airway resistance, loose connections, cuff leaks causing inaccurate reading of volumes, hypoxemia due to inadequate FiO_2, etc.).
   D. Psychological: Commonly not the initial cause for failure but may become major issue due to repeated failures resulting from physiological problems, conditions, inappropriate attempts to wean.
   E. Weaning methods
      1. Variety of methods including T-tube (T-piece), CPAP, PSV, SIMV plus PS, combination of methods.
      2. Multicenter study supports use of PSV over SIMV and T-tube.
      3. Common simple and successful method for short-term mechanical ventilation is short PS trial (20–30 minutes) and extubate if stable.
      4. Multidisciplinary weaning team that uses coordinated and collaborative approach to weaning may have improved patient outcomes and decreased weaning times.
IV. Guidelines for weaning from mechanical ventilation
   A. Pre-wean evaluation
      1. Problems requiring ventilator support resolved, clinically stable.
      2. FiO_2 <50 %, PEEP < 5 cm.
      3. MV < 14 LPM.

 4. Spontaneous Vt (PS 5 cm > 5 ml/kg or >250–300 cc; RR < 30.
 5. Frequency to tidal volume ratio (f/Vt) < 100. (Not a measurement of endurance or ability to protect airway).
 6. Strong cough, likely will be able to clear airway of secretions (may be successful with moderate/large amounts if able to cough).
 7. If chronic carbon dioxide retainer: PCO_2 close to patient's baseline level.

B. Essential procedure for successful spontaneous ventilation includes
 1. Accurate evaluations to determine weaning readiness.
 2. Optimal position for breathing comfort.
 3. Maintain airway free of obstruction.
 4. Monitor for signs, symptoms indicating problems and make prompt, appropriate interventions including ventilator support as needed.

C. Weaning the difficult to wean patient
 1. Psychological factors: Anxiety and fear due to
  a. Premature weaning attempts. Is the underlying physiological condition/problem(s) that required need for ventilator support reversed, stabilized, resolved?
  b. Staff attitudes, skills, expertise.
  c. Incorrect procedure, techniques.
  d. Inadequate trust, confidence in staff.
  e. Sleep deprivation.
 2. Management for successful spontaneous ventilation
  a. Do not continue weaning trial if initial assessment (1–2 minutes) reveals respiratory distress (increased respiratory rate, increased heart rate, agitation, restlessness). Provide ventilator support with settings that provide breathing comfort, adequate rest and sleep. Reevaluate for physiological problems/conditions requiring correction.
  b. Monitor patient and prevent and/or immediately correct common problems including secretions, bronchospasm, water obstructing lines, kinked ventilator tubing or ET tube, suboptimal positioning, hypoxemia.
  c. May remind correct breathing pattern (full slow breath in, breath out longer) assuming patient is clinically stable. It is inappropriate to coach patient with physiological problems requiring correction to slow down breathing pattern.
  d. Maintain consistent personnel who can effectively intervene, especially during anxiety states, and who provide positive support, promote trust and confidence.
  e. Convey confidence and expertise in actions.
  f. Improve cooperation and trust, and prevent anxiety by allowing active patient participation and decision making in weaning decisions and providing ventilator support as necessary to prevent respiratory distress, discomfort.

Anxiety-Shortness of Breath Cycle

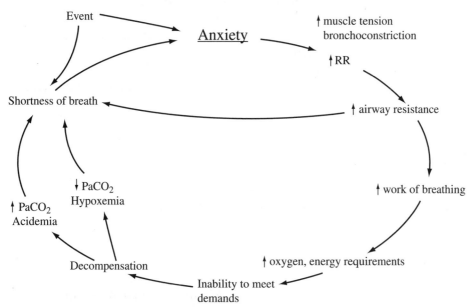

Figure 36.2. Anxiety-shortness of breath cycle.

      g. Assist patient in understanding effects of anxiety and fear on breathing pattern and intervene as necessary (see Figure 36.2).
         i. Event or trigger that causes anger, frustration, fear, anxiety, muscle tension, bronchospasm, increased work of breathing, more energy, oxygen requirements and breathing discomfort.
        ii. Attempt to break vicious cycle by alleviating cause(s).
      iii. Teach self-control and stress management through relaxation techniques; consult specialist as necessary.
      iv. Implementing relaxation techniques as appropriate including music therapy, biofeedback, various relaxation techniques, TV, radio.

VII. Long-term care, home care considerations for ventilator-dependent patients
  A. Can be cared for in designated long-term care facilities, skilled nursing facilities, or home when medically stable.
  B. Appropriate level of care and smooth transition to facility enhanced by working relationship between facilities, thorough communication of patient care needs, visit to facility and meeting with fellow residents and staff members to help develop trust and familiarity.
  C. Home discharge requires extensive evaluation and planning including
    1. Determining whether family support system is capable of providing care and desires responsibility,
    2. Evaluating home environment and determining needs for assuming care at home and preparing in advance to accommodate patient's needs.

3. Determining financial resources and mechanisms for reimbursement identified prior to discharge.
4. Providing extensive education to meet individual patient needs with demonstration of competencies. Skills include various aspects of airway management, troubleshooting patient and ventilator-related problems, care of enteral access or vascular devices.

D. Refer to literature for detailed assessments and planning for care at home or alternative care site.

WEB SITES

American Thoracic Society http://www.thoracic.org
Clinical Pulmonary Medicine http://www.clinpulm.com

REFERENCES

Branson, R. D. (2001). Preventing moisture loss from intubated patients. *Clinical Pulmonary Medicine, 7,* 187–198.

Branson, R. D., & Campbell, R. S. (2001). Modes of ventilator operation. In N. R. Macintyre & R. D. Branson (Eds.), *Mechanical ventilation* (pp. 51–84). Philadelphia: W. B. Saunders Company.

SUGGESTED READINGS

Chatburn, R. L., & Branson, R. D. (2001). Classification of mechanical ventilators. In N. R. MacIntyre & R. D. Branson, *Mechanical ventilation* (pp. 2–50). Philadelphia: W. B. Saunders Company.

Chatburn, R. L., & Scanlan, C. L. (1999). Ventilator modes and functions. In C. L. Scanlan, R. L. Wilkins, & J. K. Stoller (Eds.), *Egan's fundamentals of respiratory care* (7th ed., pp. 848–866). St. Louis: Mosby.

Esteban, A., Alia, I., Tobin, M. J., Gil, A., Gordo, F., Vallverdu, I., et al. (1999). Effect of spontaneous breathing trial duration on outcome of attempts to discontinue mechanical ventilation. Spanish Lung Failure Collaborative Group. *American Journal of Respiratory and Critical Care Medicine, 159,* 512–518.

Hill, N. S. (Ed.). (2000). *Long term mechanical ventilation.* New York: Marcel Dekker.

Hill, N. S., & Goldberg, A. E. (Eds.). (1998). ACCP statement on mechanical ventilation beyond the intensive care unit. *Chest, 113*(Suppl), 289S–344S.

MacIntyre, N. R. (2001). High-frequency ventilation. In N. R. MacIntyre & R. D. Branson, *Mechanical ventilation* (pp. 415–423). Philadelphia: W. B. Saunders Company.

Urden, L. D., Stacy, K. M., & Lough, M. E. (2002). Pulmonary disorders. *Thelan's critical care nursing: Diagnosis and Management* (4th ed.). St. Louis: Mosby.

Welsh, D. A., Summer, W. R., Boisblanc, B., & Thomas, D. (1999). Hemodynamic consequences of mechanical ventilation. *Clinical Pulmonary Medicine, 1,* 52–65.

Yang, K., & Tobin, M. J. (1991). A prospective study of indexes predicting outcome of trials of weaning from mechanical ventilation. *New England Journal of Medicine, 324,* 1445–1450.

Tracheostomy

Jo Ann Frey

I. Tracheostomy
   A. Definition
      1. A surgical procedure in which an artificial opening is made between the second and fourth tracheal rings.
      2. A surgical incision in the trachea is made for the purpose of establishing a patent airway.
      3. A tracheostomy (trach) tube is the preferred artificial airway.
         a. For patients requiring long-term mechanical ventilation.
         b. For those with inadequate secretion clearance.
      4. It is designed to get directly through the surgical opening.
      5. Its placement facilitates access to the lower respiratory tract to improve gas exchange.
   B. Indications
      1. To bypass an obstruction of the airway
      2. To prolong artificial ventilation
      3. To facilitate the removal of respiratory tract secretions
      4. To minimize a massive aspiration of oral or gastric contents
      5. To manage the airway on a long term basis, for example, patient in a comatose state or on long-term mechanical ventilation.
   C. Approach
      1. Complete evaluation of the airway should be performed.
      2. A thorough history, with a focus on
         a. Nutrition status
         b. Previous airway intervention, intubation, or tracheotomy
         c. Check for a history of sleep apnea, and head, neck, thoracic, or trauma surgery prior to surgery
      3. A focus on psychological factors such as anxiety, depression, and social support play an important role in adjustment to the tracheostomy.

4. The tracheal tube selection should fit the airway and the patient's needs.

5. The operating room traditionally has been the place for tracheostomy placement. However, the tracheostomy can be placed percutaneously at the bedside.

    a. The patient is placed in a supine position.

    b. Padding is sometimes placed below the shoulders to hyperextend the neck. The skeletal structure of the trachea is composed of C-shaped cartilage (trachea rungs).

    c. The surgical incision is made into the trachea, usually between the second and fourth tracheal rungs.

D. Preoperative

  1. Patient preparation

    a. An explanation of what to expect is given and the care that this will require, for example oxygen therapy, suctioning, and trach care.

    b. Preoperative teaching will vary, depending upon the illness of the patient and their basic needs.

    c. Teaching should focus on communication, nutrition, and care involved.

    d. An assessment of the patient and family's understanding of the technical aspects of the condition should be made.

    e. Teaching will guide the health care professional on the length of time needed for postoperative teaching in preparation for discharge.

E. Postoperative

  1. Assess patient for the following upon admission and throughout hospitalization

    a. Increased production of secretions

    b. Cardiopulmonary status

    c. Oxygen saturation

    d. Cardiac dysrhythmia (monitored patients)

    e. Bronchospasm

    f. Respiratory ease; respiratory distress

    g. Cyanosis

    h. Comfort, anxiety, agitation, or changes in level of consciousness

    i. Increased blood pressure or intracranial pressure

    j. Stoma condition: free of redness, swelling or purulent drainage

    k. Assess for signs and symptoms of respiratory infection:

      i. Increase in temperature

      ii. Changes in secretion: amount, color, odor

      iii. Malaise

      iv. Respiratory insufficiency secondary to secretions or inflammation

F. Troubleshooting tracheostomies

  1. Abnormal bleeding

    a. A small amount of bleeding from the tracheostomy stoma is not unusual for the first few days after surgery.

    b. Bleeding should subside after 24–48 hours.

    c. The physician should be notified if bleeding persists. Constant oozing is not expected and may be a sign that a bleeding vessel needs surgical intervention.

    d. Massive bleeding suggests a rupture of an artery and is considered life-threatening.

    e. Bleeding could also be the result of a stomal vein rupture. Contact the surgeon whenever there is constant bleeding that does not stop.

2. Obstructed airway

    a. Accumulation of secretions can obstruct the tracheostomy tube, limiting air flow.

    b. If not adequately removed, the tube may become occluded with dried or excessive secretions.

    c. Signs of inadequate airway clearance and impaired gas exchange:

        i. Dyspnea

        ii. Difficulty inserting the suction catheter

        iii. Pulse oximetry below 90%–92%

        iv. Increased heart rate and/or respiratory rate

        v. Rhonchi or very coarse crackles upon auscultation, if patient is able to move air

        vi. Restlessness or agitation

        vii. Cyanosis

    d. Humidification of inspired air, hydration, suctioning; installation of normal saline for humidification reasons; and teaching effective coughing and deep breathing will promote a patent airway.

    e. Pre-oxygenation (if on a ventilator) and suctioning to clear the airway of excessive secretions optimizes gas exchange, thereby improving the patient's subjective symptoms.

3. Tube dislodgement

    a. Accidental dislodgement by excessive manipulation, suctioning, or self-extubation may occur.

    b. Excessive manipulation or suctioning may also cause the patient to cough forcefully, causing the displacement of the tracheostomy tube from the stoma.

    c. Because the tracheostomy tract is not fully formed, dislodgement within 24–48 hours after surgery is a medical emergency.

    d. It takes about 5–7 days for the trach tract to mature.

    e. Prevention of accidental decannulation

        i. Use of twill ties (that are properly tied) or Velcro devices that secure the tube properly, only allowing about a finger breadth under the ties to adequately secure the ties.

        ii. Utilization of patient and family teaching regarding the importance of the tracheostomy to prevent self-extubation.

        iii. Evaluation of the need for medications to manage anxiety, depression, and agitation, considering the patient's clinical presentation.

iv. Maintaining sutures in place 5–7 days or longer to let the trach tract mature; especially for patients with increased neck circumference.

4. Infection
   a. The patient with a tracheostomy is at risk of infection.
   b. Infections may occur as a result of bypassing the protective airway mechanisms that filter, warm, and humidify inhaled air.
   c. Ineffective cough and immobilized secretions within the airway provide an excellent environment for bacterial growth.
   d. Prevention of infection
      i. Use of a sterile suctioning technique.
      ii. Support of ventilator circuits, if on a vent, can minimize mucosal damage and decrease the introduction of bacteria into the trachea and lower airways.
      iii. Soiled/wet tracheostomy dressings also provide a moist environment for bacterial growth, which can contribute to infection at the tracheal stoma. Soiled/wet tracheostomy dressings should be changed regularly.
      iv. A combination of meticulous handwashing and sterile technique, according to institutional policy and procedure, is considered prudent during suctioning and tracheostomy care.
      v. Continuous assessment for signs of infection, such as redness, drainage, pain, and swelling, is essential.
5. Subcutaneous emphysema
   a. Sometimes termed as "snap, crackle, pop"
   b. Generally related to inadvertent introduction of air into tissue
   c. Can often be seen as a smooth bulging of the skin
      i. Palpation of the skin produces an unusual crackling sensation as gas/air is displaced through the tissue.
      ii. Inspect and palpate the neck and upper chest for crepitus.
      iii. The crackling sensation upon palpation is the hallmark sign of subcutaneous emphysema.
   d. Subcutaneous emphysema may be alarming to the patient and family.

G. Complications
   1. Tissue damage can occur from mechanical causes, such as suctioning, increased intratracheal pressure, and scar formation.
   2. Complications from placement of artificial airways can be avoided by the maintenance of proper humidification, monitoring of cuff pressures and proper stabilization of the airway.
   3. Tracheosophageal fistula
      a. Also known as tracheal wall necrosis; results when an inflated cuff of the tracheostomy tube increases pressure on the tracheal mucosa.
      b. Increased pressure causes ischemia, which leads to necrosis and fistula formation.

    c. The fistula, an abnormal connection between the trachea and the esophagus, results from the erosion of the back wall of the trachea.

    d. The fistula allows air to escape into the stomach, causing aspiration of gastric contents.

    e. It is suspected if the patient coughs or chokes while eating and food particles are seen in tracheal secretions.

    f. If an increased amount of air is needed to maintain an adequate seal/tidal volume, while on mechanical ventilation, suspect a fistula.

    g. During mechanical ventilation, the presence of a low exhaled volume alarm suggests an inadequate seal and/or a decrease in the delivered tidal volume on the ventilator.

    h. Prevention

        i. The maintenance of proper cuff pressures will prevent damage of the tracheal mucosa.

        ii. Cuff pressures in excess of 25 cm/H_2O (18 mm Hg) may result in occlusion of tracheal capillaries and cause necrosis and tracheal stenosis.

        iii. The intent should be to inflate the cuff enough to achieve an adequate seal between the tracheostomy tube cuff and the tracheal wall. Minimal occlusive volume is a way to not overinflate the cuff.

        iv. The pressure exerted upon the tracheal wall by the tracheostomy cuff should not exceed the arterial blood pressure within the tracheal wall.

        v. The tracheal cuff pressure should be monitored according to institutional policy. This can be monitored by a respiratory therapist, but nursing should be mindful of these pressures.

        vi. Maintenance of appropriate cuff pressures will also help to minimize possible airway damage.

4. Tracheal stenosis

    a. Characterized by the narrowing of the tracheal lumen.

    b. Tracheal stenosis is a result of scar formation because of cuff-induced irritation of the tracheal mucosa.

    c. The most common cause of tracheal stenosis is trauma

        i. Internal trauma—caused by prolonged endotracheal intubation as a result of a tracheostomy, surgery, and irradiation.

        ii. External trauma—caused by blunt or penetrating neck traumas.

    d. Is usually assessed after the cuff is deflated or the tracheostomy tube is removed.

    e. Increased coughing, inability to expectorate secretions, shortness of breath, and/or difficulty talking may be noted in cases where stenosis has formed.

    f. Prevention

        i. Maintain proper cuff pressures.

        ii. Prevent infections.

          iii. Restrict tube movement and securing the tube in a midline position reduces irritation of the tracheal mucosa.

          iv. Tracheostomy ties should be taut enough to prevent accidental dislodgement, but not so tight as to cut off circulation, allowing just one fingerbreadth beneath the tie.

          v. Devices that use Velcro tabs allow the healthcare provider to reposition and stabililize the tracheostomy tube easily and quickly in emergent and nonemergent situations.

5. Tracheomalaica

    a. A weakness and/or floppiness of the walls of the trachea (main airway), which can lead to tracheal collapse, especially during time of increased airflow such as coughing, crying, or feeding.

    b. Breakdown of the cartilage in the trachea can also happen from prolonged intubation or chronic recurrent infections involving the trachea.

II. Minitracheostomy

  A. Definition

    Minitracheostomy tubes, are cuffless tubes, 3.5–4.0 mm diameter, inserted percutaneously between the thyroid and cricoid cartilage, into the cricothyroid membrane of the trachea, usually under local anesthesia.

  B. Indications

    1. Placement of a minitracheostomy is ideally an elective procedure.

    2. Uses include post-surgical intervention after major thoracic operations where excessive postoperative tracheobronchial secretions often occur and there may be difficulty with endotracheal suctioning.

    3. It is a minimally invasive method usually associated with few problems to facilitate endotracheal suction.

    4. With catheter insertion, it stimulates the trachea, enough to initiate cough and clear sections.

    5. It allows suction of lung secretions without the need for formal endotracheal intubation or tracheostomy.

    6. The tubes allow a size 10Fr catheter to pass down.

    7. It can also be placed in a life-threatening upper airway obstruction, where endotracheal intubation is not feasible and when there is insufficient time to perform tracheostomy.

  C. Approach

    1. Like a traditional tracheostomy the patient would be supine with a roll under the shoulders to extend the neck.

    2. After anesthetizing the upper airway, a vertical incision is made between the second and fourth cartilaginous rings and into the airway.

    3. An introducer is passed into the trachea. A small trach cannula is guided over the introducer and into the trachea. The introducer is then removed and the cannulas secured in place either with a cloth or sutured in place.

4. Aside from the standard chest X-ray, the passage of air through the cannula and aspiration of secretions are indications of intratracheal placement.

D. Preoperatively

1. As with placement of a traditional tracheostomy, patient preparation should include an explanation of what to expect.

2. An explanation about the altered breathing sensation, the care involved, for example oxygen therapy and suctioning, should be explained to the patient.

3. Temporary uses of this type of tube should be included in the teaching, if appropriate.

E. Postoperatively

1. See post-op notes with tracheostomy

2. Duration is anticipated as shorter than a traditional tracheostomy tube and is determined based upon an individual's clinical presentation

3. Frequent assessment is necessary.

   a. monitoring of vital signs and oxygen saturation
   b. assessing the amount, color, and quality of secretions
   c. signs and symptoms of respiratory distress or failure
   d. hemorrhage
   e. shock

5. Clinical indications for removal

   a. the reason for placement has been resolved
   b. decreased suctioning/tracheobronchial toilet
   c. effective cough
   d. psychological readiness

6. Removal can be done at bedside. An occlusive dressing is placed over the site, or according to institutional policy.

7. The tract site usually closes within 3 days

F. Complications (See trouble-shooting tracheostomies)

III. Types and uses of tracheostomy tubes

There are several different brands/types/manufacturers of tracheostomy tubes, but all have similar parts.

A. Double-lumen

1. Double-lumen or double cannula tube is the most common type of tracheostomy tube.

2. It has three parts

   a. Outer cannula with cuff or without a cuff and pilot tube: keeps the airway (trachea) open
   b. Inner cannula
      i. helps to keep the airway (outer cannula) patent and fits into the outer cannula
      ii. A universal adaptor (15 mm) for attachment to a ventilator and/or other respiratory equipment.
      iii. Some inner cannulas are disposable; others must be removed, cleaned, and reinserted.

    c. Obturator
      i. A solid plastic guide, which when placed inside the tube makes insertion of the outer cannula easier.
      ii. Used for trach changes or when a trach needs to be re-inserted.
      iii. Often kept at bedside for emergency reasons, check institutional policy.

B. Single cannula
    1. Has one hollow tube or cannula for both airflow and suctioning of secretions.
    2. *There is no inner cannula.*

C. Uncuffed single lumen tubes
    1. Are usually for neonates, infants, and young children
    2. May also be used in adults, especially if it is a larger and longer tube.
    3. This tube usually requires additional humidification to prevent the accumulation of secretions in the tube.

D. Cuffed tube
    1. A cuff is a soft balloon around the distal end of the tube that can be inflated to allow for mechanical ventilation in patients with respiratory failure
    2. When inflated, this cuff seals the airway and prevents a massive aspiration of oral or gastric secretions.
    3. The cuff creates a seal that directs air through but not around the tube.

E. Cuffless tube
    1. Used for the long-term management of patients.
    2. Can be single (no inner cannula) and double lumen tubes (inner cannula present).
    3. The patient should be able to support/protect their airway (effective cough and swallow) and not have a chance of returning to mechanical ventilation.

F. Fenestrated trach
    1. It is similar to other trach tubes but has one added feature.
    2. There is a hold or several holds in the outer cannula.
    3. The hole (fenestration) allows air to pass by the trach tube and through the hole up through the vocal cords and up through the mouth and nose.
    4. It allows the patient to breathe close to normal, when the trach is plugged/capped with either removal of the inner cannula that is non-fenestrated or with an inner cannula that is fenestrated.
    5. The fenestration allows the patient to speak and cough out secretions through their mouth and nose, if there is enough space around the tube and if the fenestration is not blocked by the back wall of the trachea.
    6. Fenestrated trachs may be used as a step before removal of a trach tube (decannulation). Different institutions use different devices, check with your institutional policy.
    7. Some surgeons use this as a trial to see how the patient is able to breathe while plugged, and to see if they can support their upper airway.

G. Tracheostomy plug
   1. Used in the process of decannulation mainly with fenestrated tubes, allowing patients to speak.
   2. There are cuffless nonfenestrated tubes that can also be plugged. Check manufacturers' guidelines and institutional policy.
H. Tracheostomy button
   1. The trach button is a small plastic or rubber button that keeps the trach stoma open.
   2. This allows for ready access to the trachea if needed.
I. Passy Muir valve
   1. An alternative to the use of a fenestrated tube, a Passy-Muir tracheostomy speaking valve, allows a patient with a tracheostomy tube to speak more normally.
   2. This one-way valve attaches to the inner cannula of the tracheostomy tube.
   3. It allows air to pass into the tracheostomy.
   4. A thin diaphragm, or valve, opens when the patient breathes in.
   5. When the patient breathes out, the diaphragm closes and air flow goes up around the tracheostomy tube, up through the vocal cords allowing voicing/sounds to be made.
   6. The patient breathes out through the mouth and nose instead of the tracheostomy.
   7. Advantages of the speaking valve
      a. Improves speech
      b. Improves swallowing
      c. Decreases secretions; requires less suctioning
      d. Improves smell; increases appetite
      e. Improves quality of life
      f. Directs air flow through the mouth and nose; patients can blow their nose and spit up secretions
      g. Can be used with oxygen, humidity, and ventilators
   8. Considerations
      a. Humidity and oxygen can be used with the valve in place
      b. The valve should be removed when administering aerosol treatments
      c. The valve should be removed and rinsed to remove any medications that could cause the valve to stick or not work well, if left on during breathing treatments.
   9. Speech pathology evaluation
      a. Roles
         i. Evaluation
         ii. Assessment
         iii. Adjusting treatment for swallowing and communication needs
         iv. Provides direct intervention to patients and their families, to include coordination of speech, language, and oral motor feeding interventions

533

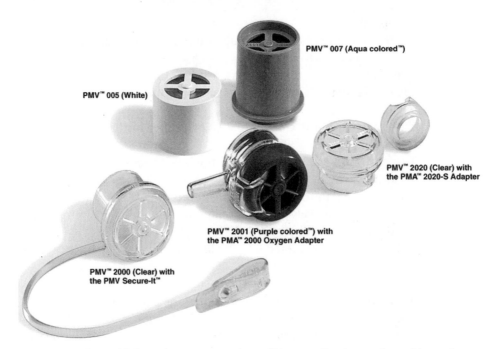

Figure 37.1. Passy-Muir tracheostomy and ventillator swallowing and speaking valves.

    10. Expected outcomes
        a. Improved speech and dexterity, less contamination risk (when valve is used in place of finger occlusion).
        b. Improved swallow, less aspiration risk, return of olfaction (smell)
        c. Enhanced appetite/weight gain
        d. Reduction of oral secretions, return of a stronger cough, and less suctioning needs
        e. Improved pulmonary function and energy.

SUGGESTED READINGS

Clarke, L. (1995). A critical event in tracheostomy care. *British Journal of Nursing, 4*(12), 676–681.

Dixon, L. (1998). Tracheostomy: Postoperative recovery. *Perspectives: Recovery Strategies From the OR to Home, 1*(1), 1, 4–7.

Hauck, K. A. (1999). Communication and swallowing issues in tracheostomized/ventilator-dependent geriatric patients. *Topics in Geriatric Rehabilitation, 15*(2), 56–70.

Heffner, J. E. (1999). Tracheotomy: Indications and timing. *Respiratory Care, 44*(7), 807–819.

Hess, D. R. (1999). Managing the artificial airway. *Respiratory Care, 44*(7), 759–770.

Hudak, M. B., & Bond-Domb, A. (1996). Postoperative head and neck cancer patients with artificial airways: The effects of saline lavage on tracheal mucus evacuation and oxygen saturation. *ORL–Head and Neck Nursing, 14*(1), 17.

Inwood, H. (1998). Advanced airway management. *Professional Nurse, 13*(8), 509–513.

Mason, M. F. (1993). *Speech pathology for tracheostomized and ventilator dependent patients.* Newport Beach, CA: Voicing, Inc.

Mehta, A. K., & Sing, V. K. (1999). Minitracheostomy in ventilatory insufficiency. *Medical Journal Armed Forces India, 55*(3), 217–219.

Murray, K. A., & Brzozowski, L. A. (1998). Swallowing in patients with tracheotomies. *AACN Clinical Issues, 9*(3), 416–426.

Parry, G. W., Batrick, N. C., Lan, O. J., & Cameron, C. R. (1995). Modification of minitracheostomy technique to limit bleeding complications. *European Journal of Cardiothoracic Surgery,* (9), 659–660.

Pate, M. F., & Zupata, T. (2002). Ask the experts. *Critical Care Nurse, 22*(2), 130–131.

Reibel, J. F. (1999). Decannulation: How and where. *Respiratory Care, 44*(7), 856–860.

Sievers, A., & Adams, J. (2000). Spotlight on research. *ORL–Head and Neck Nursing, 18*(2), 22.

St. John, R. E. (1999). Protocols for practice: Applying research at the bedside: Airway management. *Critical Care Nurse, 19*(4), 79–83.

Tamburri, L. M. (2000). Care of the patient with a tracheostomy. *Orthopaedic Nursing, 19*(2), 49–60.

Traver, G. A., Mitchell, J. T., & Flodquist-Priestly, G. (1991). *Respiratory care: A clinical approach.* Gaithersburg, MD: Aspen Publisher.

Weilitz, P. B., & Dettenmeier, P. A. (1994). Back to basics: Test your knowledge of tracheostomy tubes. *American Journal of Nursing, 94*(2), 46–50.

Wilson, D. J. (2004). Airway appliances. In H. C. Grillo (Ed.), *Surgery of the trachea and bronchi.* Hamilton, Ontario, Canada: BC Decker.

Wright, C. D. (2003). Minitracheostomy. *Clinical Chest Medicine, 24*(3), 431–435.

Lung Transplantation

38

Christine Archer-Chicko

INTRODUCTION

I. Historical perspective
   A. First human lung transplant was performed in 1963 by Dr. James Hardy at the University of Mississippi.
   B. Subsequent lung transplants failed as a result of dehiscence of the bronchial anastomosis related to bronchial ischemia and impaired healing from the use of high-dose steroids for immunosuppression.
   C. Introduction of cyclosporine in the early 1980s made solid organ transplantation more feasible.
   D. In 1983, Dr. Joel Cooper and colleagues performed the first successful single lung transplant at the University of Toronto. The same team also performed the first successful bilateral lung transplant in 1989.
   E. Recent technical advances include
      1. Development of bilateral sequential lung transplantation to replace en bloc double lung transplantation
      2. Development of a "telescoping" bronchial anastomosis technique to replace the omental wrap procedure, which required an abdominal incision.
   F. Despite advances and acceptance as a therapeutic option, the number of lung transplants performed annually worldwide is limited because of a scarcity of donors.
II. Patient selection
   A. General considerations
      1. Candidates have chronic, advanced lung disease with a life expectancy of less than 2–3 years.
      2. Because of the scarcity of donor lungs, candidates must have advanced disease to warrant the risks of transplant but must not be so

debilitated that they are unlikely to survive or regain an acceptable quality of life after the transplant.

3. Older patients have less successful outcomes. Each transplant center determines its specific age criterion; however, the American Thoracic Society (ATS) has recommended
   a. Single lung transplants—under 65 years
   b. Bilateral lung transplants—under 60 years
   c. Heart/lung transplants—under 55 years

4. Lung transplantation is not an option for acutely, critically ill patients. There is a waiting time of 12–24 months at most transplant centers and no emergency status on the waiting list.

5. Comorbid medical conditions must be optimally treated; some, such as diabetes with end-organ complications, are contraindications to transplant.

6. Patients must be ambulatory and able to participate in a pulmonary rehabilitation program. Many programs require patients to be able to achieve a specific distance (i.e., 600 feet) on a 6-minute walk test to ensure a minimum level of physical conditioning.

7. Patients must want the transplant because they are dissatisfied with their quality of life. They must be motivated to get through the often unpredictable postoperative course. In addition, patients must be willing to make a lifelong commitment to care for their transplanted organ, including taking immunosuppressive medications, monitoring themselves for complications (infection, rejection, etc.), and to remain compliant with follow-up care at the transplant center.

8. Ideal candidates should be within 20% of their ideal body weight (IBW).

9. Candidates should have no active psychiatric illness.

10. Patients must have family or significant other(s) whom are committed to assisting the patient through the transplant process.

11. Patients must be free of all substance abuse prior to transplant. Most centers require periodic screening while the patient is actively listed.

12. Adequate financial support (including medical insurance and prescription coverage) prior to transplant. The annual cost of immunosuppression following transplant is expensive.

13. Each lung transplant program bases their specific selection criterion on their own experience and capabilities.

B. Diseases amenable to transplantation (adapted from ATS statement)
   1. Chronic Obstructive Pulmonary Disease (COPD) includes Emphysema, Alpha-1 Antitrypsin Deficiency, Chronic Bronchitis, and Bronchiolitis Obliternans
      a. $FEV_1 < 25\%$ of predicted (without reversibility)
      b. $PaCO_2 > 55$ mm Hg and/or elevated pulmonary artery pressures
      c. Patients with elevated $PaCO_2$ on long-term oxygen therapy who continue to deteriorate

2. Cystic fibrosis (CF) and bronchiectasis
   a. FEV_1 < 30% predicted or rapidly progressive clinical deterioration with FEV_1 > 30% predicted
   b. Room air arterial blood gases (ABG) with $PaCO_2$ > 50 mm Hg; PaO_2 < 55 mm Hg
   c. The microbiology of sputum from these patients presents specific challenges. Patients colonized with multiple drug resistant organisms (i.e., *Pseudomonas aeruginosa* and *Burkholderia cepacia*) may be turned down by some centers because of concern about long-term survival.

3. Idiopathic Pulmonary Fibrosis (IPF) and Pulmonary Fibrosis of other etiologies
   a. Patients who exhibit symptoms at rest or with exercise; progressive decline in pulmonary function despite treatment with steroids or immunosuppressive therapy.
   b. Most patients become symptomatic when the vital capacity falls below 60%–70% predicted and/or the diffusing capacity falls below 50%–60% predicted.
   c. Due to the progressive nature of this disease and the high mortality, early referral to a transplant center is essential.

4. Systemic disease with Pulmonary Fibrosis includes Scleroderma, Rheumatoid Arthritis, Sarcoidosis, and post-chemotherapy
   Because of the varied nature of these diseases, each patient should be considered on an individual basis. As a general rule, the systemic disease should be quiescent.

5. Pulmonary hypertension without congenital heart disease includes Primary Pulmonary Hypertension or Secondary Pulmonary Hypertension (i.e., Thromboembolic Disease, Veno-occlusive Disease, Collagen Vascular Disease, etc.)
   a. Patients who are symptomatic with progressive disease despite aggressive medical and/or surgical interventions. These patients should be in NYHA Class III or IV.
   b. Hemodynamics that indicate failure of pre-transplant therapy are a cardiac index <2 $L/min/m^2$, a right atrial pressure >15 mm Hg, and a mean pulmonary artery pressure >55 mm Hg.

6. Pulmonary hypertension with congenital heart disease (Eisenmenger's Syndrome)
   a. Patients who are functionally at NYHA Class III or IV and have progressive symptoms despite advanced medical therapy.
   b. Patients whose congenital heart defect can be repaired at the time of transplant are candidates for bilateral lung transplantation; other patients will require heart-lung transplantation.

7. Advanced pulmonary disease and other organ failure
   a. Patients with more than one organ failure may be considered for multiorgan transplantation. As a general rule, they should meet selection criteria for each individual organ. Policies regarding

multiple organ transplantation are determined by each individual center.

C. Relative contraindications

1. Patients with advanced lung disease frequently have comorbid medical conditions that may affect their long-term outcome after lung transplant. As part of the transplant evaluation, patients should be thoroughly assessed for end organ dysfunction. Optimal candidates have well-controlled medical conditions and no evidence of end organ damage. The following are examples of comorbid conditions that may exclude patients from transplantation.

   a. Osteoporosis
   b. Systemic hypertension
   c. Diabetes mellitus
   d. Coronary artery disease
   e. Hyperlipidemia

2. It is recommended that patients not take steroids chronically. If patients require chronic steroids, a dose less than 15 mg daily is preferred.

3. Colonization with fungi or atypical mycobacterium

4. Although patients on mechanical ventilation have been successfully transplanted, their mortality rate is higher.

5. Prior chest surgery or pleurodesis

6. Collagen vascular disease without significant extrapulmonary manifestations

D. Absolute contraindications

1. Significant organ dysfunction (heart, liver, kidney)

2. HIV infection

3. Colonization with *Burkholderia cepacia* for CF patients as it typically causes a postoperative infection that is fatal

4. Malignancy within the past 5 years (other than uncomplicated skin cancer)

5. Hepatitis B antigen positivity

6. Hepatitis C with liver disease based on biopsy

III. Diagnostic studies

A. Pulmonary studies

1. Pulmonary function studies (including spirometry before and after bronchodilators, lung volumes, diffusing capacity of carbon monoxide)

2. Chest X-ray, posteroanterior and lateral

3. Arterial blood gas (ABG)

4. Ventilation-perfusion lung scan

5. High resolution CT scan

6. Six-minute walk test

7. Full or desaturation exercise test

B. Cardiac studies

1. Electrocardiogram (EKG)

2. Echocardiogram with pulse Doppler imaging

      3. Cardiac catheterization (left and right hemodynamics and coronary angiography)

  C. Laboratory studies

      1. Chemistry battery (including electrolytes, blood urea nitrogen, creatinine, liver function studies, nutritional indices), CBC with differential, platelet count, prothrombin time, partial thromboplastin time

      2. Blood type and crossmatch

      3. HLA typing

      4. Serologies: HIV, hepatitis screen (Hepatitis B & C), cytomegalovirus (CMV) titer, herpes simplex virus (HSV) titer, varicella-zoster (VZV) titer, Epstein-Barr virus (EBV) titer

      5. Urinalysis and 24 hour urine for creatinine clearance

  D. Other

      1. Skin testing—PPD and anergy panel (Mumps, Candida, Tetanus)

      2. Gynecologic exam

      3. Mammogram (for women over 40 years of age)

  E. Consultations

      1. Nutrition evaluation

      2. Social work evaluation

      3. Psychiatric evaluation (if indicated)

      4. Financial evaluation

IV. Preoperative considerations

  A. Patients need to remain as physically active as possible. Participation in a formal pulmonary rehabilitation program benefits patients through pulmonary conditioning and muscle strengthening.

  B. They need to continually work toward any goals identified from their evaluation such as weight loss or weight gain.

  C. Patients are encouraged to stay healthy and to adopt preventative health practices

      1. Avoid exposure to people with colds or infections.

      2. Perform routine handwashing.

      3. Take medications as prescribed.

      4. Obtain recommended vaccinations (Influenza, Pneumovax).

      5. Take daily multivitamins.

      6. Get adequate rest.

      7. Eat a healthy diet.

      8. Exercise regularly.

  D. Being emotionally prepared for the transplant is also very important. There are several ways patients can ready themselves for transplant and maintain control over anxiety and/or depression.

      1. Enlist the support of family and friends.

      2. Educate themselves by reading about the transplant process and attending educational activities such as support groups and seminars.

      3. Network with other patients to reduce social isolation.

      4. Maintain a structured daily routine.

      5. Learn stress management techniques.

6. Take anti-anxiety and/or anti-depression medications as prescribed.
7. Seek professional counseling sessions (if needed).

V. Allocation issues

A. There is no priority status on the active waiting list for lung transplantation. Patients must wait until their name rises to the top of the list. The only modification is for Idiopathic Pulmonary Fibrosis (IPF) patients who receive a 90-day credit when listed because of the rapidly progressive nature of that disease.

B. The lung is a very fragile organ and vulnerable to numerous insults at the time of transplant. In a brain-dead donor, the lungs are subject to neurogenic pulmonary edema, aspiration, pneumonia, excessive fluid administration, or damage from prior tobacco abuse. Of all potential donor lungs, less than 20% are suitable for transplantation.

C. The lung can tolerate a lack of perfusion for a very short time (less than 6 hours). This is known as *ischemic time*. Consequently, geographic distribution and routine prospective HLA crossmatching are limited.

D. Lungs are matched by size, blood type, and, at some centers, by CMV status.

VI. Operative considerations

A. Single lung transplantation

1. Most commonly performed lung transplant procedure
2. Technically easiest—involves posterolateral thoracotomy incision and three anastomoses: mainstem bronchus, pulmonary artery, and left atrial cuff (for the pulmonary veins)
3. Able to utilize one pair of lungs for two recipients
4. Not used for CF patients or those with bronchiectasis because the new lung would become infected from secretions of the native lung

B. Bilateral sequential lung transplantation

1. Involves performing two single lung transplants in a sequential fashion. A bilateral thoracotomy with transverse sternotomy ("clamshell" incision) is used to provide optimal exposure to the chest.
2. Able to perform the surgery ventilating the contralateral lung thereby avoiding the use of cardiopulmonary bypass reducing perioperative complications
3. Used for CF and bronchiectasis patients as well as for patients with pulmonary hypertension. (These patients normally require cardiopulmonary bypass.)
4. May be used for younger COPD patients as they have demonstrated superior function and survival as compared to single lung transplants

C. Heart-lung transplantation

1. The first lung transplantation procedure successfully performed (in 1981).
2. Currently, not as commonly performed because replacing the lung(s) alone has become a successful option for most patients.
3. The technique involves a median sternotomy approach and three anastomoses: tracheal, aortic, and right atrial.

      4. Has inherent disadvantages, including limited availability of heart-lung bloc because of preference given to status 1 patients on heart transplant waiting lists and mandatory use of cardiopulmonary bypass with increased perioperative bleeding risks.

      5. Used for patients with Eisemenger's syndrome and irreparable cardiac defects and in patients with advanced lung disease who have left ventricle dysfunction or extensive coronary artery disease.

  D. Lobar transplantation from living donors

      1. The newest form of bilateral lung transplantation

      2. Involves transplanting lower lobes from two blood group compatible living donors

      3. Used almost exclusively for CF patients (children or small stature adults), however, the indications are broadening to include other diagnoses.

      4. Donors should be significantly larger than the recipient so that the donor lower lobes fill each hemithorax of the recipient to avoid pleural space complications

      5. Survival is comparable to cadaveric lung transplantation

      6. Postoperatively the donors have a less than 20% decline in FVC, FEV_1, and TLC compared to preoperative values. These reductions in spirometry values have not resulted in any functional impairment.

VII. Immediate postoperative management

Goals include: caring for the newly transplanted lung(s), keeping the patient comfortable, and observing for complications

  A. Hemodynamic management

      1. Monitor vital signs

        a. Assess for changes in vital signs. Most patients enter the ICU hypothermic and require rewarming, especially if they were on cardiopulmonary bypass.

      2. Monitor hemodynamic status with Swan Ganz catheter

        a. Assess for hemodynamic instability. Patients may be hypotensive from anesthesia, changes in microvascular permeability, or from products of ischemia. Consider treating hypotension with vasoactives (epinephrine, dopamine, etc.); avoid administering large volumes of intravenous fluids.

        b. Assess for volume status. The lungs are prone to pulmonary edema because of alterations in microvascular permeability and severed lymphatic channels that are responsible for fluid clearance. If the patient is hypovolemic, it is advisable to replace fluids conservatively. For patients with a low blood count, transfusing cross-matched packed red cells (CMV matched) is recommended.

      3. Monitor EKG rhythm: Assess for cardiac arrythmias. Many patients experience atrial arrythmias, such as atrial fibrillation because the transplant involves the atria.

  B. Pulmonary management

      1. Monitor mechanical ventilation

        a. Assess for respiratory distress and/or asynchrony with ventilator.

      b. Assess for elevated airway pressures. If a patient develops elevated airway pressures, they may need to switch to an alternate ventilatory mode to reduce the pressures and protect the new anastomoses.

      c. Assess the patient's breathing effort and progression of weaning. Every effort should be made to assist the patient to wean as quickly as tolerated. Patients with prolonged intubations following transplant are at high risk for pneumonia.

      d. Assess for airway secretions. As with every intubated patient, it is very important to maintain a clear airway.

      e. Administer bronchodilator therapy every 4 hours.

  2. Monitor chest tubes

      a. Assess chest tube drainage. The drainage should reduce in amount and become more serous over subsequent days. (Chest tubes are usually removed when the drainage is less than 200 ml/24 hrs.)

      b. Assess the amount of the air leak. An air leak should also reduce over time. An increase in the air leak may signify an airway dehiscence and requires immediate evaluation.

  3. Monitor ABG

      a. Assess for hypoxemia or hypercapnia. Adjust ventilator settings accordingly.

      b. Assess acid-base balance. Adjust ventilator settings accordingly.

  4. Monitor chest X-ray

      a. Assess for barotrauma, infiltrates, edema, or diaphragm injury. Intervene as necessary.

      b. Assess for endotracheal tube position

  5. Monitor pulse oximetry: Assess for desaturations either at rest or with activity. These changes may signify an episode of acute rejection.

  6. Adjunct therapies: Chest PT, incentive spirometry, and turning/repositioning every 2–4 hours are important pulmonary toilet measures to facilitate bronchial hygiene. Patients have an altered cough reflex as a result of denervation.

C. Pain management

  1. Monitor patient's pain control: Assess for adequate pain control. Analgesia may be provided with an epidural catheter or intravenous catheter (may be patient controlled or continuous infusion). The patient controlled epidural catheter is the preferred method. Avoid excessive narcotic use that would result in oversedation.

D. Fluid and electrolytes

  1. Monitor laboratory work

      a. Assess for electrolyte abnormalities

      b. Assess nutritional status

  2. Monitor I & O, weights: Assess fluid balance. Administer diuretics as needed.

E. Infection

  1. Administer empiric antibiotic coverage.

2. Monitor bronchoscopic cultures.
   a. Assess culture results from both the donor and the recipient at the time of transplant.
   b. Reassess recipient prior to extubation and at any change in clinical status.
3. Place patient in reverse isolation precautions.
   a. Persons entering the patient's room must adhere to strict hand-washing and masking procedures
   b. Persons who are ill must avoid any contact with the patient
4. Assess patient for signs of infection: Obtain blood, urine, sputum cultures if patient develops a fever.

F. Rejection
   1. Administer immunosuppression as per institution protocol
      a. Loading doses of cyclosporine or azathioprine are given preoperatively.
      b. A 500 mg–1000 mg of solumedrol bolus is given intraoperatively.
      c. Postoperatively a 3-drug maintenance regimen is started. Some centers will also administer induction therapy with a cytolytic agent for 1 week or until the cyclosporine levels are therapeutic.
   2. Follow trough cyclosporine or tacrolimus levels. Adjust dosing to maintain therapeutic levels.
   3. Assess for signs of rejection (see early postoperative complications). Administer augmented immunosuppression as per institution protocol.

G. Postoperative complications
   1. Primary graft failure: A severe form of pulmonary edema similar to an acute respiratory distress syndrome (ARDS) that occurs in about 15% of cases.
      a. Believed to reflect ischemia-reperfusion injury with surgical trauma and lymphatic disruption as contributing factors
      b. Diagnosed because the patient is hypoxemic and the CXR reveals generalized infiltrates within 72 hours of transplantation (other causes such as volume overload, pneumonia, rejection, occlusion of venous anastomosis and aspiration have been ruled out). Lung biopsies reveal a pattern of diffuse alveolar damage.
      c. Treatment is supportive—mostly mechanical ventilation.
      d. Additional supportive measures include: independent lung ventilation (for patients with single lung transplants), inhaled nitric oxide, Prostaglandin E1 infusion, and extracorporeal membrane oxygenation (ECMO).
      e. Mortality rate is approximately 60%.
      f. Patients who survive may have a long postoperative course but may achieve normal allograft function.
   2. Bleeding
      a. Patients with advanced lung disease frequently have dense pleural adhesions and hypertrophy of the bronchial circulation as a result of their underlying lung pathology. At the time of transplant, these

changes can require extensive dissection and lead to significant hemorrhage.

b. Patients who need cardiopulmonary bypass with Heparin anticoagulation are at even more risk of bleeding

c. If bleeding is severe, early surgical exploration is preferred over massive transfusion which may cause fluid overload in the lungs.

3. Airway complications

   a. In the past airway complications were common. Currently, these problems occur in less than 15% of patients because of improved surgical techniques and greater understanding of the contributions of immunosuppression to this problem.

   b. Types

      i. Complete dehiscence of the bronchial anastomosis requires immediate surgical correction or retransplantation.

      ii. Partial dehiscence: Treatment is more conservative with chest tube insertion to manage the associated pneumothorax and reduction of steroid therapy to foster healing.

   c. Anastomotic stenosis

      i. Most common airway complication.

      ii. Occurs several weeks to months after transplantation.

      iii. Symptoms include focal wheezing, recurrent lower respiratory tract infections, and suboptimal pulmonary function.

      iv. Narrowing may be caused by stricture, granulation tissue, or bronchomalacia.

      v. Can be corrected by laser removal of granulation tissue, placement of a stent, and/or balloon dilatation.

4. Infection

   a. The rate of infectious complications is higher in lung transplant recipients than in other solid organ transplant recipients. Interestingly, the lung is the only solid organ transplanted that is continually exposed to the external environment.

   b. The lung is the most frequent site of post-transplant infections.

5. Bacterial infection: Bacterial pneumonia is most common bacterial infection. It may occur as a result of several predisposing factors.

   a. Poor cough related to denervation and postoperative pain

   b. Poor lymphatic drainage

   c. Impaired mucociliary clearance as a result of diffuse ischemic injury to the bronchial mucosa and the airway anastomosis

   d. Narrowing of the bronchial anastomosis

   e. Transfer of microorganisms from the donor

   f. Harbored in the patient's sinuses, proximal airways, or native lung

   g. Immunosuppression

   h. Broad-spectrum antibiotics are used as prophylaxis in the perioperative period. In addition, if bronchial washings from the donor identify organisms, the recipient is treated accordingly.

i. Patients develop fever, new or increased infiltrates on chest X-ray, and a sputum culture identifying a new or predominant organism.

j. Treatment consists of a 2–4 week course of antibiotics specific to the culture results.

6. Viral infection

 a. In patients who are CMV positive or have a CMV positive donor lung, reactivation of CMV infection may occur in the postoperative period.

 b. For most patients, the reactivation is subclinical and presents as an asymptomatic viremia and/or shedding of the virus in the urine or respiratory tract. Other patients develop a mono-like illness with fever, malaise, liver enzyme elevation, and leukopenia. Organ specific manifestations include pneumonitis, colitis, gastritis, retinitis, and encephalitis.

 c. A quantitative CMV antigenemia assay shows the viral load and can reflect the effectiveness of therapy.

 d. Ganciclovir is used to treat CMV pneumonia or significant extrapulmonary disease.

 e. Some transplant centers use Ganciclovir prophylactically in CMV positive recipients or donors. Other centers match CMV negative patients with CMV negative donor lungs prophylactically

7. Fungal infection

 a. Both Candida and Aspergillus may cause invasive pneumonia and disseminated infection in transplant recipients.

 b. Candida infection usually arises from the donor trachea.

 c. Candida is treated with fluconazole therapy.

 d. Aspergillus infection typically develops as an ulcerative tracheobronchitis involving the anastomosis and large airways. Usually, the symptoms are subtle and not noticed until the infection has disseminated. The delay in diagnosis results in a high mortality.

 e. Aspergillus usually responds to oral itraconazole therapy. In more serious cases intravenous or inhaled Amphotericin B is used

8. Acute rejection

 a. Typically occurs in the first 3 months after transplant.

 b. Caused by the recipient's cellular immune response against the graft's HLA antigens.

 c. This complex response involves T lymphocytes creating perivascular and interstitial infiltrates.

 d. Graded in terms of severity from Grade 1 (minimal acute rejection) to Grade 4 (severe acute rejection).

 e. Signs/symptoms include low-grade fever, malaise, exercise desaturation or mild hypoxemia, decline in PFTs (restrictive pattern), and mild infiltrates and new or increased pleural effusion on chest X-ray.

 f. The diagnosis can be confirmed by transbronchial biopsy demonstrating perivascular lymphocytic infiltrate.

g. Initial treatment is solumedrol (0.5 mg–1 gm/day) for 3 days.

h. For persistent or recurrent rejection, adjusting the immunosuppressive regimen and/or courses of anti-lymphocytic therapy are used.

9. Cardiac arrhythmias
    a. Very common in the early postoperative period because of the direct involvement of the atria and pericardium in the surgery.
    b. Atrial arrythmias (particularly atrial fibrillation) are the most frequent types.
    c. Most arrythmias respond to drugs (such as digoxin, procanamide, and amiodarone) and resolve over time.
    d. Usually patients are treated for 3 months and then attempts are made to wean the antiarrhythmics off.

10. Diaphragm injury
    a. Incidence and course of the problem are not well documented.
    b. Occurs when the phrenic nerve is injured during dissection.
    c. Patients undergoing bilateral lung transplants or those with significant pleural adhesions are more at risk.
    d. The extent of diaphragm injury may vary from paresis (partial loss of function) to paralysis (complete loss of function).
    e. Diaphragm injury should be suspected in any patient who is not weaning well without an obvious reason.
    f. Unilateral diaphragmatic paralysis is evident on an inspiratory chest X-ray. The injured side will be elevated.
    g. Bilateral diaphragmatic paralysis may be present in a patient with paradoxical abdominal movement during spontaneous breathing.
    h. A "sniff" maneuver under fluoroscopy can confirm diagnosis.
    i. Affected patients may be hypercapnic and have reduced lung volumes. Treatment involves supporting the patient with either BiPAP or mechanical ventilation. Over time some patients will recover diaphragm function.

11. GI complications: Nausea is the most common GI problem. Some patients also develop bloating, anorexia, and vomiting.
    a. Usually occurs when the patient is beginning to take immunosuppressive medications orally.
    b. Some of the nausea may be caused by delayed gastric emptying or gastroparesis which occurs from some medications such as cyclosporine, steroids, and antibiotics.
    c. Unreliable gastric function might result in erratic absorption of drugs including immunosuppression medications.
    d. Treatment for this complication involves drugs to increase GI motility (metoclopramide, cisapride, domperidone).
    e. If symptoms are persistent or severe, consideration may be given to switching to another immunosuppressive agent or placement of a jejunal feeding tube to bypass the stomach

    f. In most cases, this problem tends to improve over time and usually the motility agents can be discontinued.

    g. Other GI complications include upper GI (severe gastritis or ulceration occurs in 10%–20%) and lower GI (diverticulitis, bowel obstruction, lymphoma of the gut, and lower GI bleeding).

  12. Other early postoperative complications that are less common include: chest wall complications, torsion of the lung allograft, seizures, pleural effusion, hyperacute rejection.

VIII. Long-term postoperative issues

  A. Posttransplant lymphoproliferative disorder (PTLD): A B-cell proliferative disorder that may result in limited polyclonal hyperplasia or in uncontrolled growth (lymphoma).

    1. Associated with the Epstein Barr virus, although its exact role in tumor development is unclear.

    2. Incidence is 6%–9% and usually occurs within the first year.

    3. Patients may present with incidental nodules or an unexplained infiltrate on chest X-ray. They report vague symptoms: low-grade fever, weight loss, fatigue, or nonspecific GI complaints.

    4. Presentations may vary from a nodule slowly increasing in size over a period of several months to a nodule that grows aggressively and disseminates rapidly.

    5. The optimal treatment is not well known. Because this disorder is believed to result in part by immunosuppression, a reduction in the immunosuppressive therapy is appropriate. Unfortunately, with a reduction in immunosuppression comes a higher risk of chronic rejection of the lung allograft.

    6. Mortality from PTLD is approximately 30%–60%.

  B. Chronic rejection

    1. Occurs 6 months or later with increasing incidence over time.

    2. The mechanism of chronic rejection is not well understood. It is theorized that the cumulative effect of several insults may play a role in development of this complication. These insults include recurrent episodes of acute rejection, chronic arterial insufficiency and progressive graft ischemia, and continual subclinical host-immune response against the graft.

    3. In the transplanted lung, chronic rejection is manifested as obliterative bronchiolitis (OB), which is an inflammatory process involving the small airways leading to progressive scarring and obliteration of the airway lumen.

    4. Affects approximately 40% of long-term survivors.

    5. Acute rejection within the first 6 months of transplant is an important risk factor for OB onset and progression.

    6. Clinical presentation is characterized by the insidious development of dyspnea and nonproductive cough. Patients may also develop recurrent episodes of purulent tracheobronchitis

7. The key diagnostic features (known as Bronchiolitis Obliterans Syndrome) are PFTs which show a 20% fall in FEV_1 from previous post-transplant baseline and the development of an obstructive pattern.
8. Chest X-ray is normal or significant only for hyperinflation.
9. High resolution CT scan may show evidence of bronchiectasis and mosaic pattern (due to areas of attenuated perfusion and to air trapping).
10. Transbronchial biopsy may not confirm the diagnosis because of the patchy distribution of OB in the lung.
11. Diagnosis is established on the basis of clinical presentation and evidence of progressive airflow obstruction on the PFTs.
12. Treatment consists of increasing the patient's immunosuppression. High dose steroids or cytolytic therapy may be used.
13. Unfortunately, OB is not very responsive to therapy and chronic rejection remains a common mortality.
14. For those patients who may be candidates for retransplantation, the outcomes are lower than the initial transplant with 45% one-year survival.

C. Infection
   1. Leading cause of early and late morbidity and mortality
      a. Bacterial infection
         i. *Pseudomonas aeruginosa*, a gram-negative bacterium is the most common isolate. Other common pathogens include: coagulase positive and coagulase negative *Staphylococcus* (including methicillin-resistant *Staphylococcus*). Patients with chronic rejection typically have *Pseudomonas* organisms colonize their lower airways. They develop recurrent episodes of infection as a patient with bronchiectasis.
        ii. Treatment is specific to organisms identified from cultures.
      b. Viral infection (refer to early postoperative complications): Other less common viruses include: herpes simplex (HSV), adenovirus, respiratory syncytial virus (RSV)
      c. Fungal infection (refer to early postoperative complications)

D. Medication side effects
   1. Cyclosporine (Sandimmune, Neoral)
      a. Renal insufficiency/renal failure → may contribute to electrolyte imbalances, systemic hypertension, fluid retention/edema, chronic anemia
      b. Gastroparesis/ gastric atony → anorexia, nausea, vomiting
      c. Systemic hypertension
      d. Electrolyte imbalances: hyperkalemia, hypomagnesemia
      e. Tremor
      f. Headache, subtle loss of concentration, seizures (2%–6% of patients), peripheral neuralgias/neuropathies, encephalopathy
      g. Osteoporosis
      h. Gingival hyperplasia
      i. Hypertrichosis

2. Tacrolimus (FK506)
   a. Renal insufficiency/renal failure
   b. Systemic hypertension
   c. Hyperglycemia
   d. Tremor
   e. Headache
3. Azathioprine (Imuran)
   a. Bone marrow suppression → leukopenia, anemia, thrombocyto-penia
   b. Pancreatitis
   c. Hepatotoxicity
4. Mycophenolate mofetil (Cellcept)
   a. Diarrhea
   b. Dyspepsia
   c. Leukopenia
   d. Anemia
5. Prednisone
   a. GI ulcers and bleeding
   b. Myopathy involving respiratory and peripheral muscles
   c. Osteoporosis → spontaneous fractures of vertebrae, ribs, etc.
   d. Mood disturbances (depression, mania, euphoria), delirium, psy-chotic reactions
   e. Fluid retention
   f. Hyperlipidemia
   g. Hyperglycemia
   h. Dermal atrophy (thinning of the skin) → bruising, poor wound healing
   i. Redistribution of subcutaneous fat (moon facies, obesity, Dowa-ger's hump, etc.)
   j. Cataracts

E. Managing medication side effects
   1. Perform bloodwork at least monthly for the first 3–6 months to recog-nize complications early.
   2. When changes are made in the cyclosporine or tacrolimus dose, the level should be rechecked in a few days to confirm if it is therapeu-tic.
   3. Follow blood pressure readings closely and treat hypertension aggres-sively. Calcium channel blockers are preferred (although these may affect blood levels of immunosuppressive agents).
   4. Educate patients to care for themselves and monitor for complica-tions.
      a. Reporting problems tolerating medications
      b. Recording their own BP, weight, temperature, spirometry readings
      c. Calling transplant coordinator with abnormal readings.
      d. Teach patients to eat a healthy and balanced diet. (Avoid high salt, high fat foods.)

e. Patients must be taught to avoid contact with other people who are or may be ill. They must learn to perform routine handwashing as a way to protect themselves from getting infections.

f. Patients should be encouraged to exercise regularly. They should be instructed on the health benefits of physical activity.

g. Notify transplant coordinator for any health issues, questions or concerns regarding how they feel or about the medical regimen (i.e., new symptoms, generalized "not feeling well," etc.).

h. Teach patients not to take any new medications without discussing first with the transplant coordinator. (Many drugs affect the immunosuppressive medications and can potentially cause serious effects.)

i. Avoid excessive sun exposure. Use sunscreens and light clothing for protection.

5. Identify patients with osteopenia (or osteoporosis) preoperatively with a baseline Dexa scan or radiograph. Begin aggressive therapy with calcium supplementation, estrogen replacement therapy, Calcitonin-salmon nasal spray (Miacalcin), alendronate (Fosamax) or raloxifene (Evista). Monitor effects of therapy on a routine basis.

6. Treat hyperlipidemia with HMG-CoA reductase inhibitors.

7. For patients with a family history of cancer, they should have screening procedures performed every 6–12 months.

8. All patients should have their skin checked at least annually for cancer.

F. Malignancy

1. Solid organ recipients have an increased incidence of cancer. According to the Cincinnati Transplant Registry, lymphomas, skin and lip carcinomas, perineal carcinomas, cervical cancer, and Kaposi's sarcoma are the most common.

2. Patients should be involved in routine screening procedures.

IX. Outcomes/statistics

A. Single lung transplants are most frequently performed for emphysema while bilateral lung transplants are most frequently performed for cystic fibrosis

B. The lung transplant actuarial survival for one, five, and seven years are 70%, 45%, and 32% respectively.

C. There is no significant difference in actuarial survival between single and bilateral lung transplants, with patient half-life of 3.6 years and 4.5 years respectively.

D. Patients over 55 years of age at the time of transplant had a significantly lower survival rate than younger patients.

E. Lung retransplantation survival rates are 45% for one year and 31% for three years.

F. The most common causes of death in patients less than one year after lung transplantation include nonspecific graft failure and infection. For patients one year or more following lung transplantation, the most common cause of death is bronchiolitis obliterans.

X. Future goals

    A. Increase the donor supply to meet the demand

        1. Xenotransplantation

            a. Involves the use of tissue from an animal donor.

            b. This option is not currently feasible because of preformed human antibodies against the animal tissue.

            c. Research is focused on genetically engineering animals, such as pigs.

    B. Management of chronic rejection to improve long-term survival

        1. Need to develop drugs that halt chronic rejection effectively

        2. Need to develop drugs with less toxic side effects

        3. Promotion of immune tolerance: Involves the infusion of donor bone marrow cells at the time of lung transplantation into the recipient as a method of transferring stem cells to foster the recipient to accept the alloantigens.

WEB SITE

A guide to lung transplantation: http://www.chestnet.org

SUGGESTED READINGS

American Thoracic Society. (1998). International guidelines for the selection of lung transplant candidates. *American Journal of Respiratory and Critical Care Medicine, 158,* 335–339.

Arcasoy, S. M., & Kotloff, R. M. (1999). Medical progress: Lung transplantation. *The New England Journal of Medicine, 340*(14), 1081–1091.

Barr, M. L., Schenkel, R. G., Cohn, R. G., Barbers, R. G., Fuller, C. B., Hagen, J. A., et al. (1998). Recipient and donor outcomes in living related and unrelated lobar transplantation. *Transplant Proceedings, 30,* 2261–2263.

Christie, J. D., Bavaria, J. E., Palevsky, H. I., Litzky, L., Blumenthal, N. P., Kaiser, L. R., et al. (1998). Primary graft failure following lung transplantation. *Chest, 114,* 51–60.

Collins, J., Kuhlman, J. E., & Love, R. B. (1998). Acute, life-threatening complications of lung transplantation. *RadioGraphics, 18,* 21–43.

de Hoyos, A., & Maurer, J. (1992). Complications following lung transplantation. *Seminars in Thoracic and Cardiovascular Surgery, 4,* 132–146.

Dorling, A., Riesbeck, K., Warrens, A., & Lechler, R. (1997). Clinical xenotransplantation of solid organs. *Lancet, 349,* 867–871.

Dusmet, M., Winton, T. L., Kesten, S., & Maurer, J. (1996). Previous intrapleural procedures do not adversely affect lung transplantation. *Journal of Heart and Lung Transplantation, 15,* 249–254.

Heng, D., Sharples, L. D., McNeil, K., Stewart, S., Wreghitt, T., & Wallwork, J. (1998). Bronchiolitis obliterans syndrome: Incidence, natural history, prognosis and risk factors. *Journal of Heart and Lung Transplantation, 17,* 1255–1263.

Hosenpud, J. D., Bennett, L. E., Berkeley, B. M., Fiol, B., Boucek, M. M., & Novick, R. J. (1998). The registry of the international society for heart and lung transplantation: 15th official report—1998. *Journal of Heart and Lung Transplantation, 17,* 656–668.

Maurer, J. M. (1996). Medical complications following lung transplantation. *Seminars in Respiratory and Critical Care Medicine, 17*(2), 173–185.

Maurer, J. R., Tullis, D. E., Grossman, R. F., Vellend, H., Winton, T. L., & Patterson, G. A. (1992). Infectious complications following isolated lung transplantation. *Chest, 101,* 1056–1059.

O'Donnell, M., & Parmeter, K. L. (1996). Transplant medications. *Critical Care Nursing Clinics of North America, 8*(3), 253–271.

Pham, S. M., Mitruka, S. N., Youm, Y., Li, S., Kawaharada, N., Yousem, S. A., Colson, Y. L., et al. (1999). Mixed hematopoietic chimerism induces donor-specific tolerance for lung allografts in rodents. *American Journal of Respiratory and Critical Care Medicine, 159,* 199–205.

Pigula, F. A., Griffith, B. P., Zenati, M. A., Dauber, J. H., Yousem, S. A., & Keenan, R. J. (1997). Lung transplantation for respiratory failure resulting from systemic disease. *Annals of Thoracic Surgery, 64,* 1630–1634.

Rao, A. S., Fontes, P., Iyengar, A., Shapiro, F., Dodson, F., & Corry, R. (1997). Augmentation of chimerism with perioperative donor bone marrow infusion in organ transplant recipients: A 44 month follow-up. *Transplant Proceedings, 29,* 1184–1185.

St. John, R. E. (1998). End-stage pulmonary conditions eligible for lung transplantation. In J. G. Alspach (Ed.), *American Association for Critical Care Nurses: Core curriculum for critical care nursing* (pp. 125–128). Philadelphia: W. B. Saunders.

Susanto, I., Peters, J. I., Levine, S. M., Sako, E. Y., Anzueto, A., & Bryan, C. L. (1998). Use of balloon-expandable metallic stents in the management of bronchial stenosis and bronchomalacia after lung transplantation. *Chest, 114,* 1330–1335.

Starnes, V. A., Barr, M. L., Schenkel, F. A., Horn, M. V., Cohen, R. G., Hagen, J. A., et al. (1997). Experience with living-donor lobar transplantation for indications other then cystic fibrosis. *The Journal of Thoracic and Cardiovascular Surgery, 114,* 917–922.

Tager, A. M., & Ginns, L. C. (1996). Complications of lung transplantation. *Critical Care Nursing Clinics of North America, 8*(3), 273–292.

Trulock, E. P. (1997). Lung transplantation. *American Journal of Respiratory and Critical Care Medicine, 155,* 789–818.

Yousem, S. A., Berry, G., & Cagle, P. T. (1996). Revision of the 1990 working formulation for the classification of pulmonary allograft rejection: Lung rejection study group. *Journal of Heart and Lung Transplantation, 15,* 1–15.

Pulmonary Rehabilitation

Bonnie Fahy, Paula Meek, and Janet Reardon

INTRODUCTION

1. Pulmonary rehabilitation is a standard of care for patients with chronic respiratory disease.
2. Patients with the diagnosis of Chronic Obstructive Pulmonary Disease (COPD) are not the only patients that can benefit from pulmonary rehabilitation services.
3. A comprehensive pulmonary rehabilitation program includes both education and exercise training.

Pulmonary rehabilitation is considered to be the standard of care for most patients with chronic respiratory disease. This chapter outlines all aspects of pulmonary rehabilitation from referral to outcome assessment.

I. Definition of pulmonary rehabilitation
Pulmonary rehabilitation is defined by the American Thoracic Society (ATS) as "a multidisciplinary program of care for patients with chronic respiratory impairment that is individually tailored and designed to optimize physical and social performance and autonomy" (American Thoracic Society [ATS], 1999a, p. 1668).
II. Benefits to patients with chronic respiratory disease (American College of Chest Physicians [ACCP]/American Association of Cardiovascular and Pulmonary Rehabilitation [AACVPR], 1997; Global Initiative for Chronic Obstructive Pulmonary Disease [GOLD], 2003).
A. Increased exercise tolerance
B. Decreased dyspnea
C. Improved health-related quality of life

III. Benefits to health care providers and payers
   A. Decrease in healthcare provider utilization
   B. Decrease in dollars spent for acute exacerbation and long-term care
IV. Appropriate referrals
   A. Any patient with symptoms from their lung disease is a potential candidate for pulmonary rehabilitation.
      1. Referral to pulmonary rehabilitation is appropriate for patients with COPD who: despite receiving optimal medical care continue to be dyspneic; are restricted in their functional ability to perform activities of daily living; experience a reduction in quality of life; or have had several hospital admissions or emergency room visits per year.
         a. Common ICD-9 codes used when referring patients to pulmonary rehabilitation.

i.	491.2–491.9	Chronic Bronchitis
ii.	492.8	Emphysema
iii.	493	Persistent Asthma
iv.	494	Bronchiectasis
v.	496	Chronic Airway Obstruction
vi.	515	Post-inflammatory Pulmonary Fibrosis
vii.	518.1	Interstitial Lung Disease
viii.	518.5	History of ARDS

      2. Relying only on a decreased FEV_1 as a sole referral criterion is inappropriate since symptoms have a better correlation with functional ability than pulmonary function measurements (Mahler & Harver, 1990).
      3. Disability and handicap are more appropriate indicators for need of referral to pulmonary rehabilitation than impairment as determined by pulmonary function testing (ATS, 1999a).
      4. The recommendation to refer patients with interstitial pulmonary fibrosis and other non-COPD indications including cystic fibrosis, lung cancer, post-polio syndrome, and selected neuromuscular diseases to pulmonary rehabilitation has been published by the ATS (ATS, 1999a, 2000).
      5. The American Association of Cardiovascular and Pulmonary Rehabilitation (AACVPR) expands the potential referral base beyond COPD and interstitial lung disease to include additional restrictive lung diseases (AACVPR, 1998).
      6. Because of the individualization of pulmonary rehabilitation services to patient specific needs, the referral of pediatric patients, pregnant patients, and the elderly to pulmonary rehabilitation programs may be appropriate.
V. Inappropriate referrals
   A. Patients not appropriate for referral to pulmonary rehabilitation are those patients that would be unable to participate in the exercise and/or education or for whom the physical activity could be detrimental to their health.
      1. Oftentimes a patient with a recent cardiac event and concomitant pulmonary disease is entered into cardiac rehabilitation until stable and then may enter a modified pulmonary rehabilitation program.

2. Patients with emotional/psychiatric disorders should be treated and stabilized before entry into the program.

3. Allowing smokers into pulmonary rehabilitation remains controversial. Most pulmonary rehabilitation programs accept smokers into their programs with the provision that they are currently enrolled in a smoking cessation program. The positive reinforcement they receive from staff and other patients who have successfully quit often help in achieving a successful outcome.

VI. Components of pulmonary rehabilitation

A. Initial assessment includes an evaluation of the patient's medical history with emphasis on their respiratory disease including nutritional status, current knowledge base, the impact of dyspnea on their level of functioning, their health-related quality of life, and their ability to exercise and oxygenate. The time and interest of the interviewer is the cornerstone on which the essential *trust* relationship between interviewer and patient is built.

1. The patient's rendition of their medical history as described to the interviewer can expose many insights that have never been discussed with another healthcare provider (AACVPR, 1998).

2. The patient's knowledge of their lung disease and strategies to cope with their symptoms are evaluated (AACVPR, 1998).

3. The impact of dyspnea on activities of daily livings prior to attending pulmonary rehabilitation and the effectiveness of rehabilitation interventions is measured. The UCSD Shortness of Breath Questionnaire (UCSD-SOBQ) or the Baseline and Transitional Dyspnea Index are two of the useful tools for this purpose (ATS, 1999b; Eakin, Resnikoff, Prewitt, Ries, & Kaplan, 1998).

4. Use of validated measures to evaluate pulmonary rehabilitation's impact on quality of life (QOL) are commonly used.

   a. The Medical Outcomes Study Short Form (SF-36 or SF-12) is a general health–related quality of life tool widely used in the United States for many populations. It can be used pre- and post-rehabilitation, includes a physical dimension and a psychosocial dimension, is self-administered, and takes about 16 minutes to complete (QualityMetric, 2000; Stewart, Hays, & Ware, 1988).

   b. The Chronic Respiratory Disease Questionnaire (CRQ) is more widely used internationally than the SF-36 and has the advantage, as the name implies, of being specifically designed for patients with a chronic respiratory disease. It measures the impact of dyspnea, in addition to fatigue, emotional function, and the feeling of mastery over the disease (Guyatt, Berman, Townsend, Pugsley, & Chambers, 1987).

   c. The St. George's Respiratory Disease Questionnaire (SGRQ) is also a popular and widely used tool. It contains 76 items, is self-administered, and has three categories: respiratory symptoms, activities limited by breathlessness, and emotional impact of breathlessness. The three domains can be calculated separately or aggregated to get a total score. A clinically significant difference (pre- to post-intervention) has been established at 4 points (Jones, Quirk & Baveystock, 1992).

    d. Refer to the ATS Web site at www.thoracic.org for more extensive information on QOL evaluation tools.

5. Analysis of the patient's ability to exercise and oxygenate is imperative prior to initiating exercise training.

    a. The information gleaned from an initial exercise study is used to determine an appropriate exercise prescription and to assess improvement when repeated at program completion.

    b. The type of exercise testing performed depends on the outcomes desired and the individual being tested.

        i. A symptom-limited treadmill or cycle graded exercise test (GXT), as performed on a cardiac patient, may not be an appropriate form of exercise testing in a patient with chronic lung disease. The intensity of this testing, in light of a pulmonary patient's physical deconditioning and dyspnea, may produce data that does not reflect their true exercise ability (Noseda, Carpiaux, Prigogine, & Schmerber, 1989).

        ii. Since most pulmonary rehabilitation programs promote increased *exercise endurance,* testing the patient at high intensities for short periods may also not be the best method to reflect improvements in exercise tolerance at program completion.

        iii. The measurements of expired gases and arterial blood gases are also not required to develop an exercise prescription.

        iv. In the majority of patients with chronic lung disease, a simple 6-minute or 12-minute walk test performed by walking in a level hallway while monitoring pulse oximetry is all that is needed prior to initiating exercise training (Larson et al., 1996; McGavin, Gupta, & McHardy, 1976; Steele, 1996).

        v. Measurement of dyspnea and rating of perceived exertion, using a Borg or visual analog scale (Gift, 1989; Skinner, Hutsler, Bergsteinnova, & Buskirk, 1973), before, during, and after exercise should be obtained with pre-program exercise testing for comparison with post-program values.

        vi. A protocol for performing a timed distance walk test can be found in AACVPR's *Guidelines for Pulmonary Rehabilitation Programs* (1998).

        vii. Knowing the MET level and duration the patient exercised, combined with an understanding of MET levels on various types of exercise equipment, an initial exercise prescription can be developed (AACVPR, 1998).

B. Exercise training

1. Exercise training is the area of pulmonary rehabilitation research that has received the most attention. The improvement in exercise

tolerance after attending pulmonary rehabilitation is well documented (ACCP/AACVPR, 1997; GOLD, 2003).

2. An exercise prescription is based on the principles of mode, intensity, duration, and frequency.

   a. Common modes of exercise are treadmill and stationary bicycle for lower extremity endurance training, supported arm ergometry for upper extremity endurance, unsupported weight training for upper extremity strength training, and weight training for lower extremity strength. A period of warm-up stretching/flexibility exercises and a cool-down period at the conclusion of the exercise session must accompany the endurance and strength building exercises.

   b. The use of ventilatory muscle training (VMT) in pulmonary rehabilitation remains controversial. The scientific evidence, as reviewed by the American College of Chest Physicians (ACCP) and the AACVPR, does not lend itself to result in the recommendation of including VMT as an essential component of pulmonary rehabilitation (ACCP/AACVPR, 1997).

   c. Determining appropriate intensity of exercise in the development of an exercise prescription utilizes the data obtained from the walk test and incorporates information from the initial assessment regarding level of activity prior to the program (most patients entering a pulmonary rehabilitation program have been relatively sedentary).

      i. Because of the level of deconditioning and disabling dyspnea in these patients, recommendations in the literature to exercise pulmonary rehabilitation patients at high intensities (60%–80% of their maximal workload) may be unrealistic, at least initially.

      ii. Initiating an exercise prescription that uses a MET level for each exercise that does not exceed the MET level determined during the submaximal walk test is usually appropriate.

      iii. With exercise endurance being a goal of pulmonary rehabilitation, the intensity of a specific exercise is increased only after the desired duration of exercise is attained.

      iv. Interval training, consisting of 1–3 minutes of high-intensity exercise during a regular exercise session, may be an option for those who cannot tolerate sustained high intensity training (Schols et al., 1996).

   d. The duration of each mode of exercise is determined from the data of the walk test for lower extremities and the patient's current ability to perform activities of daily living with their upper extremities, as identified during the initial assessment.

      i. The duration should not be such that the patient is exhausted at the end of exercise, never to return to pulmonary rehabilitation again.

      ii. Documentation of the need for rest periods during the walk test will be a baseline for the duration of each exercise.

      iii. Duration of the entire pulmonary rehabilitation program recommended to have a minimum duration of 2 months (GOLD, 2003).

Program duration is restricted mainly by insurance coverage limitations. Refer to your Local Medical Review Policy (LMRP) from your Fiscal Intermediary (FI) for local Medicare guidelines.

    iv. Since training effects are maintained for only as long as the exercise is continued, generally a strong recommendation is made that the patient continue in a maintenance exercise program or a home exercise program at the conclusion of a formal pulmonary rehabilitation program (Coyle et al., 1984; Coyle, Martin, Bloomfield, Lowry, & Holloszy, 1985).

  e. The frequency of exercising in pulmonary rehabilitation programs is often dictated by the availability of the pulmonary rehabilitation facility.

    i. Many pulmonary rehabilitation programs share staff and space with cardiac rehabilitation programs, without combining patient populations. With cardiac rehabilitation traditionally on Mondays, Wednesdays, and Fridays, pulmonary rehabilitation is usually 2 days a week, Tuesday and Thursday.

    ii. To gain the most benefit from an exercise program, the pulmonary rehabilitation patient is encouraged to exercise 30 to 90 minutes a minimum of 3 days a week and a maximum of 5 days a week.

  f. Factors responsible for variability in exercise improvement can include

    i. Age, FEV_1, disease severity

    ii. Frequency, intensity, and duration of exercise

    iii. Adherence with exercise prescription

C. Education including psychosocial/behavioral intervention

  1. The contribution of education including psychosocial/behavioral interventions to the outcomes of pulmonary rehabilitation is poorly represented in the literature.

  2. Despite this lack of documentation, expert opinion supports the inclusion of education and psychosocial/behavioral interventions as essential components in a comprehensive pulmonary rehabilitation program (ACCP/AACVPR, 1997; GOLD, 2003).

  3. The educational components included in a pulmonary rehabilitation program are individualized to the patient's needs as determined during the initial assessment interview and through ongoing patient-staff interactions.

  4. The goal of the educational component of a pulmonary rehabilitation program is for patients and significant other(s) to have a better understanding of their lung disease, improve adherence to therapies, and to put the patient in control of their lung disease rather than their lung disease controlling them. This is accomplished by educating the patient about their disease, therapies, and self-management skills. Specific examples of instructional content can be found in the texts by Morris and Hodgkin (1996) and by Ries and colleagues (1996).

a. Including the instruction of pursed lip and diaphragmatic breathing in a pulmonary rehabilitation curriculum receives mixed reviews in the literature.

    i. Research has shown that diaphragmatic breathing can increase work of breathing (Gosselink, Wagenaar, Sargeant, Rijswijk, & Decramer, 1995), but many patients state that pursed-lip and diaphragmatic breathing are the most beneficial information gained from attending pulmonary rehabilitation.

    ii. By instructing all patients in breathing techniques, those patients that find a lessening of dyspnea with their use will have a decrease in symptomatology.

    iii. The theme of utilizing breathing techniques to "remain in-control" is woven throughout all educational sessions.

b. Many patients have an incomplete/incorrect understanding of how the lung functions normally as an organ for gas exchange and what is actually wrong with their lungs.

    i. Pulmonary rehabilitation is an excellent venue for this instruction, with all treatment strategies then related to the pathophysiology.

    ii. Having a better understanding of their lung disease demystifies the fact that "sick lungs don't show" and patients state that with increased understanding that they feel a greater sense of control.

c. Instruction in the proper use of medications, including oxygen.

    i. When the patient's understanding of the rationale for the use of the medication is increased, medication compliance usually improves.

    ii. Patients should be instructed in the use of metered dose inhalers (MDI) with a spacer/chamber and dry powder inhalers (DPI), with return demonstration required at frequent intervals since deterioration in optimal technique occurs over time. Most patients are pleased when they discover that using an MDI with a spacer/chamber is as efficient as a small volume nebulizer, with much less bother.

    iii. The importance of oxygen use for the treatment of hypoxemia and not for dyspnea control alone is an often-misunderstood concept. Compliance will improve with a discussion of the indications for supplemental oxygen, a demonstration of its efficacy using an oximeter during activity and at rest, along with a recommendation of an oxygen delivery system that best meets the patient's needs.

    iv. Many ambulatory patients continue to receive supplemental oxygen from an oxygen concentrator and heavy E-tanks even though much more portable systems are available. More portable systems may be more costly and reimbursement may be an issue that can be addressed.

   d. Instruction in bronchial hygiene techniques.
      i. Not all patients enrolled in pulmonary rehabilitation will require instruction in bronchial hygiene techniques as intensive as postural drainage, percussion, and vibration or the use of a positive expiratory pressure device.
      ii. However, all patients can benefit from instruction in coughing techniques.
      iii. The importance of airway clearance can be related to the pathophysiology of the patient's chronic lung disease and individualized to their needs.
      iv. Clinical practice guidelines developed by the American Association of Respiratory Care (AARC) for bronchial hygiene techniques can be found on the AARC Web page (American Association of Respiratory Care, 2004).
   e. The importance of exercise and the concept of training reversibility, "use it or lose it."
      i. Maintenance exercise, either offered at the rehabilitation facility or self-monitored, must be encouraged after formal program completion.
   f. Energy conservation and work simplification techniques.
      i. Applying breathing techniques to daily activities, including exhaling as you exert, is important for inclusion in a comprehensive pulmonary rehabilitation program.
      ii. The goal is to have patients incorporate energy conservation and work simplification techniques, including the use of adaptive equipment, into their daily routine so that they have the ability to do more with less shortness of breath.
   g. General nutrition guidelines.
      i. At this time many misconceptions and current fads can be discussed.
      ii. If specific needs are identified and not resolved in the group setting, refer to dietitian/nutritionist for individual counseling. Needs for weight loss or weight gain that require individualized attention are common reasons for additional counseling.
      iii. Common problems such as weight gain from steroids, emotional air swallowing, and bloating, as well as need for increased caloric intake are addressed.
   h. Prevention and control of respiratory infections/irritant avoidance
      i. Discussion of signs and symptoms of a respiratory infection and the need to seek treatment immediately is often described as self-assessment and symptom management.
      ii. Hand washing before and after using exercise equipment is a launching point for further discussions on infection control.
      iii. In addition to counseling on the importance of avoiding outdoor air pollution, both primary and secondary smoking must be addressed.

i. Indications for calling the health care provider
   i. Effective communication with the health care provider is taught by instructing the pulmonary rehabilitation patient what information is important and how to best describe the symptoms.
j. Leisure, travel, and sexuality
   i. "Just because you have lung disease does not mean you have to stay at home and wait until you die" is the message of this session.
   ii. With the diagnosis of chronic lung disease often comes the notion of an inability to have fun and depression follows.
   iii. Pulmonary rehabilitation can explain to the patient how to have supplemental oxygen available on a cruise, airplane, train, or bus (www.breathineasy.com; Gorby, 2005) and that travel is possible.
   iv. The discussion of sexuality is usually reserved until one of the later educational sessions. This allows familiarity among the classmates so the mention of the topic alone is not dyspnea producing. An easy way to broach this subject is to equate sex with exercise. It is best to use your bronchodilator before exercise; if secretions are a problem, perform bronchial hygiene prior to exercise; if you use oxygen during exercise, use it during sex; and, avoid exercises where you have to support yourself using your arms (Hahn, 1989; Stockdale-Woolley, 1983).
k. Coping with chronic lung disease and end-of-life planning
   i. Patients are allowed to ventilate their frustrations most any time during the program but this session specifically focuses on their reaction to their disease and the effect of their reaction on others. Stress that depression and anxiety are common problems and are significantly under-treated (Yohannes, Baldwin, & Connolly, 2003). Openly discuss the former "stigma" associated with depression and encourage them to inquire about treatment options with their physician.
   ii. Pulmonary rehabilitation patients feel that rehabilitation is an appropriate setting for the discussion of advance directives (Heffner, Fahy, Hilling, & Barbieri, 1996). This discussion is not about what specific measures the patient requests; that should be a patient-physician discussion. Rather, this is a time to explain how a living will differs from a durable power of attorney for health care, to discuss treatment alternatives including hospice care, and to stress the importance of the patient-physician discussion.
   iii. Blank forms, often available from your state Hospital Association, for a living will and a durable power of attorney for health care are provided to the patient for their perusal prior to meeting with their physician.
l. Panic control
   i. Being short of breath can be very panic evoking. Therefore, if attending pulmonary rehabilitation reduces shortness of breath,

panic should also be reduced and in most cases it is. This session applies the breathing strategies to panic control.

D. Outcome assessment

1. Outcome assessment is required to quantify individual patient improvement after pulmonary rehabilitation and to quantify the effectiveness of the program as a whole.

2. The extent of measurement and the tools used will depend on the purpose of measurement, program goals, financial and staff resources, and level of clinician expertise.

3. All testing completed at the initial assessment should be repeated at program completion and evaluated.

4. Six, 12, and 24 month re-evaluation of outcomes would help to further determine long-term benefits of Pulmonary Rehabilitation if resources permit.

5. The absence of resources to aid in formal statistical analysis is not an acceptable excuse for not evaluating outcomes.

6. Simple differences in pre- and post-program values or analysis of trends are important to demonstrate.

7. Three major areas of measurement are recommended: Exercise ability, Dyspnea (overall and exertional), and Health-related Quality of Life.

8. Communicating with colleges or universities in the area may result in a relationship where your data is analyzed and interpreted by graduate students, fellows, or as a part of a large study.

9. A current listing of outcome measures and their availability are listed on the AACVPR Web site (AACVPR, 2004).

10. One mechanism available to evaluate the comprehensiveness of an existing program is to refer to the standards for pulmonary rehabilitation programs that are outlined in the requirements for AACVPR Pulmonary Rehabilitation Program Certification (AACVPR, 2004).

   a. This certification process is an attempt to insure that pulmonary rehabilitation programs are comprehensive and individualized, with measurable outcomes.

WEB SITES

American Association of Cardiovascular and Pulmonary Rehabilitation: http://www.aacvpr.org

American Association of Respiratory Care: http://www.aarc.org

American Lung Association: http://www.lungusa.org

American Thoracic Society: http://www.thoracic.org

Breathin' Easy Travel Guide: http://www.breathineasy.com

Global Initiative for Chronic Obstructive Lung Disease: http://www.goldcopd.com

The Pulmonary Education and Research Foundation (PERF): http://www.perf2ndwind.org

REFERENCES

American Association of Cardiovascular and Pulmonary Rehabilitation. (1998). *AACVPR guidelines for pulmonary rehabilitation programs* (2nd ed.). Champaign, IL: Human Kinetics.

American Association of Cardiovascular and Pulmonary Rehabilitation. (2004). Home page. Retrieved March 29, 2004, from http://www.aacvpr.org

American Association of Respiratory Care. (2004). Clinical Practice Guidelines. Retrieved March 29, 2004, from http://www.aarc.org

American College of Chest Physicians & American Association of Cardiovascular and Pulmonary Rehabilitation. (1997). Pulmonary Rehabilitation Guidelines Panel. Pulmonary rehabilitation: joint ACCP/AACVPR evidence-based guidelines. *Chest, 112,* 1363–1396.

American Thoracic Society. (1999a). ATS statement: pulmonary rehabilitation-1999. *American Journal of Respiratory and Critical Care Medicine, 159,* 1666–1682.

American Thoracic Society. (1999b). Dyspnea: Mechanisms, assessment, and management—a consensus statement. *American Journal of Critical Care and Pulmonary Medicine, 159,* 321–340.

American Thoracic Society. (2000). Joint statement of ATS and European Respiratory Society: idiopathic pulmonary fibrosis: Diagnosis and treatment. *American Journal of Respiratory and Critical Care Medicine, 161,* 658.

Coyle, E. F., Martin, W. H., Sinacore, D. R., Joyner, M. J., Hagberg, J. M., & Holloszy, J. O. (1984). Time course of loss of adaptations after stopping prolonged intense endurance training. *Journal of Applied Physiology, 57,* 1857–1864.

Coyle, E. F., Martin, W. H., Bloomfield, S. A., Lowry, O. H., & Holloszy, J. O. (1985). Effects of detraining on responses to submaximal exercise. *Journal of Applied Physiology, 59,* 853–859.

Eakin, E. G., Resnikoff, P. M., Prewitt, L. M., Ries, A. L., & Kaplin, R. M. (1998). Validation of a new dyspnea measure. *Chest, 113,* 619–624.

Gift, A. (1989). Visual analogue scales: Measurement of subjective phenomena. *Nursing Research, 38,* 286–288.

Global Initiative for Chronic Obstructive Pulmonary Disease. (2003). Workshop Report. Retrieved March 29, 2004, from http://www.goldcopd.com

Gorby, J. D. (2005). *Breathin easy travel guide: A guide for travelers with pulmonary disabilities.* Napa, CA: Author.

Gosselink, R., Wagenaar, R., Sargeant, A., Rijswijk, H., & Decramer, M. (1995). Diaphragmatic breathing reduces efficiency of breathing in chronic obstructive pulmonary disease. *American Journal of Respiratory and Critical Care Medicine, 151,* 1136–1142.

Guyatt, G., Berman, L., Townsend, M., Pugsley, S., & Chambers, L. (1987). A measure of quality of life for clinical trials in chronic lung disease. *Thorax, 42,* 773–778.

Hahn, K. (1989). Sexuality and COPD. *Rehabilitation Nursing, 14,* 191–195.

Heffner, J., Fahy, B., Hilling, L., & Barbieri, C. (1996). Attitudes regarding advance directives among patients in pulmonary rehabilitation. *American Journal of Respiratory and Critical Care Medicine, 154,* 1735–1740.

Jones, P. W., Quirk, F. H., & Baveystock, C. M. (1992). A self-complete measure of health status for chronic airflow limitation: The St. George's respiratory questionnaire. *American Journal of Respiratory and Critical Care Medicine, 145*, 1321–1327.

Larson, J. L., Covey, M. K., Vitalo, C. A., Alex, C. G., Patel, M., & Kim, M. J. (1996). Reliability and validity of the 12-minute distance walk in patients with chronic obstructive pulmonary disease. *Nursing Research, 45*, 203–210.

Mahler, D. A., & Harver, A. (1990). Clinical measurement of dyspnea. In D. A. Mahler (Ed.), *Dyspnea* (pp. 75–100). Mount Kisco, NY: Futera.

McGavin, C. R., Gupta, S. P., & McHardy, G. J. R. (1976). Twelve-minute walking test for assessing disability in chronic bronchitis. *British Medical Journal, 1*, 822–823.

Morris, K., & Hodgkin, J. (1996). *Pulmonary rehabilitation administration and patient education manual.* Gaithersburg, MD: Aspen.

Noseda, A., Carpiaux, J. P., Prigogine, T., & Schmerber, J. (1989). Lung function, maximum and submaximum exercise testing in COPD patients: Reproducibility over a long interval. *Lung, 167*, 247–257.

QualityMetric, Inc. (2001). SF-12 & SF-36 Health Surveys. Retrieved March 29, 2004, from http://www.qualitymetric.com

Schols, A. M., Coppoolse, J. R., Akkermans, M., Janssen, P., Mostert, P. R., & Wouters, E. F. M. (1996). Physiological effects of interval versus endurance training in patients with severe COPD [abstract]. *American Journal of Respiratory and Critical Care Medicine, 153*, A127.

Skinner, J., Hutsler, R., Bergsteinnova, V., & Buskirk, E. (1973). The validity and reliability of a rating scale of perceived exertion. *Medical Science and Sports, 5*, 94–96.

Steele, B. (1996). Timed walking tests of exercise capacity in chronic cardiopulmonary illness. *Journal of Cardiopulmonary Rehabilitation, 16*, 25–33.

Stewart, A., Hays, R., & Ware, J. J. (1988). The MOS short-form general health survey: Reliability and validity in a patient population. *Medical Care, 26*, 724–735.

Stockdale-Woolley, R. (1983). Sexual Dysfunction and COPD: Problems and management. *Nurse Practitioner, 8*, 16–17, 20.

Yohannes, A. M., Baldwin, R. C., & Connolly, M. J. (2003). Prevalence of sub-threshold depression in elderly patients with chronic obstructive pulmonary disease. *International Journal of Geriatric Psychiatry, 18*, 412–416.

SUGGESTED READINGS

Borg, G. (1988). *Borg's perceived exertion and pain scales.* Champaign, IL: Human Kinetics.

Cherniack, N., Altose, A., & Homma, I. (1998). *Rehabilitation of the patient with respiratory disease.* New York: McGraw-Hill.

Respiratory Nursing Society. (1994). *Standards and scope of respiratory nursing practice.* Washington, DC: American Nurses Publishing.

Ries, A. L., Moser, K. M., Myers, R., Limberg, T. M., Bullock, P. J., & Sassi-Dambron, D. E. (1996). *Shortness of breath: A guide to better living and breathing* (5th ed.). St. Louis: Mosby.

Self-Care Management Strategies

40

Cindy Kane

INTRODUCTION

I. Promotion of respiratory health
   A. Assessment of functional status: Balance of energy demands with supply
      1. The balance of energy resources and demands is determined by functional status.
      2. Functional status is characterized by one's ability to provide for the necessities of life.
         a. Basic self-care needs met
         b. Usual role fulfillment
         c. Maintenance of health and well-being.
      3. Foci includes activities of daily living, mental health, personal growth activities, social activities, work, and spiritual dimensions. Patient-identified goals should be set.
      4. Four dimensions of functional status
         a. Capacity
         b. Performance
         c. Reserve
         d. Capacity utilization
      5. Full capacity for performance is only partially activated at any one time, leaving functional reserve. This involves physical and mental components, value placed by the patient.
      6. Functional status of persons with chronic pulmonary disease is often severely limited.
         a. Pulmonary causes are among the top 15 listed as main cause of activity limitations.

b. Pulmonary function is not a key predictor of functional status.

c. Pulmonary function negatively affects dyspnea, exercise capacity, and desaturation.

d. Poor endurance/exercise capacity worsens dyspnea, mood, and functional performance.

e. Depression and anxiety negatively affect functional status.

f. Younger persons with emphysema report difficulty with self-care activities more often but report that connectedness activities (i.e., playing with children) are more important.

B. Nursing interventions in promotion of energy reserve

1. Strategies that are valued by each individual are important.

2. Those with increasing number of co-morbid conditions often report a much greater decrease in functional performance.

3. Functional status may be enhanced by energy conservation methods.

4. Take frequent rest periods, space daily living activities, especially upper-body utilization which uses respiratory muscles for functional activities.

5. Prioritize activities, allowing for most important to be done first, with rest periods.

6. Acceptance of assistance, allowing family to perform non-essential self-care skills.

7. Use quick-relief inhaled bronchodilators prior to activities as needed.

8. Pace activities, using controlled breathing techniques with all activities.

C. Dyspnea and self-care management

1. Dyspnea is multifactorial with neurologic, muscle fiber, chest wall, chemoreceptor, and mechanoreceptor feedback.

2. Patients with chronic lung disease often have higher levels of anxiety and depression, which may be causative or reactive to dyspnea.

D. Assessment of dyspnea

1. Measurement of dyspnea is a subjective assessment, which uses the patient as his or her own control. Methods such as the Borg scale, Visual Analogue Scale (VAS), St. George Respiratory Questionnaire, Chronic Respiratory Disease Questionnaire, Pulmonary Functional Status, and Functional Performance Inventory are variations of simple numbered dyspnea scales to functional-related questions of dyspnea and performance (see chapter 39 "Pulmonary Rehabilitation").

E. Nursing intervention of dyspnea

1. Dyspnea is of multisystem origin; therefore, treatment requires multiple approaches.

2. Optimization of air exchange using pursed lip and diaphragmatic breathing may provide relief for those with air trapping (Emphysema).

3. More intensive management with Pulmonary Rehabilitation provision of exercise and education; inspiratory muscle training, and nutritional support allow for patient investment in longer-term improvement (see chapter 39 "Pulmonary Rehabilitation").

4. Management of stressors and co-morbid issues such as nutrition, pain, anxiety, and depression is an important contributor. Regular relaxation therapy such as music, progressive muscle relaxation, or massage may decrease the overwhelming loads of fatigue, dyspnea, and anxiety. However, alternative methods such as acupuncture are currently unproven.

5. Patients with lung cancer may be dyspneic from cachexia and increased work of breathing. Nutritional support may relieve some dyspnea during treatment such as chemotherapy and/or radiation.

6. Non-invasive ventilatory support or surgical interventions are other options in very severe lung disease.

F. Fatigue

1. Fatigue is closely linked with dyspnea and increased work of breathing, and may augment complaints of dyspnea. Fatigue has been shown to correlate with FEV1, exercise tolerance, depression, and overall quality of life.

2. Cognitive components of fatigue, such as decreased motivation and mental fatigue have not been shown to correlate with physical components of quality of life. Depression is correlated with higher fatigue.

3. Fatigue interferes with ability to perform functional activities, independently from dyspnea.

G. Nursing intervention of fatigue

1. Patients with chronic lung disease often develop adaptive mechanisms for fatigue quite easily.

2. Stress reduction prevents general loss of control.

3. Problem-focused coping skills include
   a. Energy conservation
   b. Utilization of focused active energy
   c. Restoration of energy

4. Emotion-focused coping includes
   a. Positive thinking
   b. Accepting physical limitations
   c. Distracting oneself
   d. Normalizing current status

5. Other management strategies include
   a. Moderate exercise
   b. Nutritional supports/supplementation
   c. Adequate sleep
   d. Social support systems, faith/belief communities

H. Immunizations

1. Influenza vaccinations are recommended for those over age 65, with chronic health conditions, such as COPD, asthma, and other chronic pulmonary disorders. The vaccine is generally available early October, for use through the flu season (November–March). The influenza vaccine will generally protect 6–12 months.

2. In non-vaccinated elderly, hospitalization rates double during flu season.
3. Influenza vaccination is associated with fewer outpatient visits.
4. Pneumococcal vaccinations are recommended as above, with coverage lasting approximately 5–7 years.

I. Nutrition
1. 19%–60% of those with COPD have been classified as malnourished, due to increased resting energy expenditure.
2. Weight loss occurs due to hypermetabolism, cost of infections, work of breathing, and decreased caloric intake.
3. The results of weight loss include decreased immune system functioning, decreased muscle endurance, increased functional impairment, and decreased surfactant production.
4. Prolonged use of steroids contributes to muscle catabolism.

J. Nutritional assessments should include
1. History and physical exam
2. Body weight comparative to ideal body weight; height
3. Skinfold exam, muscle mass, inspiratory muscle testing, handgrip strength
4. Creatine height index

K. Nursing intervention in altered nutritional status in chronic lung disease
1. Acute management should meet caloric needs.
2. In home settings, nutritional repletion can occur at a goal of 0.25–0.5 lbs/day.
3. Start with isotonic (1 cal/cc), at ratios of 50% carbohydrate, 20% protein, and 30% fat.
4. Support should be individualized, with focus on meeting nutritional and comfort goals.

II. Peak flow meter and asthma action plans
A. Asthma patient education and self-management are essential for optimal patient outcomes.
B. Peak expiratory flow (PEF, PF) measures bronchial hyperreactivity, as a response to inflammatory changes of the airways.
C. PF is the largest expiratory flow achieved with maximal effort from maximal inspiration, usually within the first 100 ml of exhalation. PF is less sensitive than spirometric measures. Normal range is age and height dependant, generally 380–700 ml.
D. PF is recommended to be obtained daily in the A.M. by those with moderate-persistent to severe asthma. Diurnal variation and A.M. dip (changes of 15%–20%) are signs of worsening asthma.
E. PF-best may be obtained after approximately 2 weeks of inhaled steroid initiation.
F. Symptom assessment is less sensitive to airway changes, up to 60% of asthmatic patients will have no correlation between PF and symptom description. Consistency of measure is more important than actual number accuracy. The best of three efforts is used.

G. Young children may not accurately be able to use PF, assessment of technique is crucial.

H. Regular use of PF has been shown to decrease ER visits and hospitalization; and to improve quality of life.

I. Aged patients may have decreased nocturnal awareness of symptoms and show higher PF variability.

J. Asthma Action Plan: All patients with asthma need an Asthma Action Plan.

    a. Written guideline outlining levels of care in asthma management

    b. Typical plans include three levels of care

        i. Stable, asymptomatic, little PF variability: use regular controller medicines.

        ii. Symptomatic, 20%–50% variability in PF: use inhaled/oral rescue meds.

        iii. Severe, 50% airflow compromise: emergent evaluation and treatment.

III. Oxygen treatment and home respiratory care modalities

Indications for oxygen: $PaO_2 < 55$ mm Hg or $SaO_2 < 88\%$ during rest, activity, or sleep.

A. Contributive indications include cor pulmonale with PaO_2 55–59 mm Hg or SaO_2 89% with P-pulmonale on EKG; and evidence of congestive heart failure (CHF).

B. Oxygen therapy has been shown to increase life expectancy, decrease cor pulmonale, enhance cardiac function, improve exercise performance, improve neuropsychological functioning, and reduce hospitalization rates.

C. Oxygen should be assessed and prescribed at certain flow rates for rest, exertion, sleep, and altitude if applicable. Nocturnal desaturation may occur without daytime hypoxemia. Many patients self-adjust wearing time, oxygen is most beneficial if worn greater than 17 hours per day. Portable units are most helpful for those with exertional oxygen needs.

D. Short-term use criteria

    1. Management of hypoxemia, maintaining normal oxygenation.

    2. With CO_2 retainers, increase gradually, assessing CO_2 levels frequently. Other methods of ventilation (invasive and or non-invasive) may be needed in this group of patients if hypoxemia and hypercarbia worsen.

E. Long-term use criteria

    1. Evaluate oxygen need at rest, exercise, and sleep.

    2. Post-hospital initiation of oxygen needs re-evaluation at 2 weeks, and 1–2 months to follow, as 30%–45% of patients will normalize oxygenation.

    3. Many patients with COPD (25%–45%) have evidence for nocturnal desaturation and should have night-time oxygen monitoring, via oximetry, or they may need polysomnography.

    4. Daily living activities use both upper and lower body muscles, and may require careful assessment; often not evaluated with traditional exercise testing.

5. Thorough patient education regarding the rationale, safety, and utilization of oxygen systems is important to prevent injury and improve adherence.

6. Commitment to wearing oxygen appropriately may be built by addressing issues of social isolation, depression, and anxiety.

F. Oxygen delivery

   1. Oxygen concentrators are non-mobile electrical units, which use sieve beds to concentrate oxygen molecules from room air. Flows may be up to 12 LPM, but generally range 4–6 LPM. A back-up supply of oxygen is necessary in case of equipment malfunction or electrical power outage. This is the most cost-effective method.

   2. Compressed gas cylinders are available in several different sizes, with some portable units weighing 3–5 lbs, although time duration of flow is less for these sizes. Standard "E" tanks generally last 6–8 hours but weigh 17 lbs.

   3. Liquid oxygen is frozen to compress storage and is refillable from a reservoir in the home. It holds more oxygen for longer portability, although it loses small amounts of volume due to evaporation leakage. Liquid oxygen systems are a higher cost to the supplier due to service costs.

   4. All oxygen systems deliver gaseous oxygen at the point of delivery (usually nasal cannula), whether the storage is concentrator, gas, or liquid.

   5. Demand flow systems deliver a pulse of oxygen during early inspiration, to minimize dead space O_2 flow as during exhalation. This decreases the total amount of oxygen used, however, some patients with severe COPD may not tolerate the amount of O_2 available during inspiration only, and may desaturate with activity. This bears careful evaluation by oximetry.

   6. Transtracheal oxygen catheters deliver oxygen directly to a small catheter inserted into the cervical trachea. The catheter may be inserted as a simple outpatients procedure. Patients need careful follow-up for assessment of infection, mucous balls, and for self-care education needs. This procedure hides the entry point for the oxygen and decreases O_2 flow needs due to direct delivery into the lower airway. Disadvantages include cost, increased need for site management, risk of local infection, and mucous balls at the catheter tip.

IV. Indications for nebulized medications

A. Inhaled medications are often preferable to oral or parenteral routes because delivery gives direct benefits with limited systemic side effects.

B. Typical nebulized medications include bronchodilators, inhaled steroids, mucolytics, and antibiotics.

C. Nebulized medications may be given when (a) metered dose versions are not available; or (b) nebulization is considered more effective. In adults, if the vital capacity is less than one and a half times the predicted tidal volume of 7 ml/Kg; or breath-hold is less than 4 seconds. Those with hand strength or decreased vision issues may not be able to use inhalers. Nebulizers may be more effective in young children who cannot appropriately perform inhaler with spacer steps. Nebulization creates airborne liquid particulates that are inhaled through the mouthpiece.

D. Activity limitation may occur due to the frequency of electric Nebulizers, battery options may be available but reimbursement often is an issue. Patients also need to be taught care of the machine.

V. Airway clearance

    A. Indications: Airway clearance techniques are recommended when coughing > 30 cc mucous per day. Patients with cystic fibrosis, bronchiectasis. Bronchitis, pneumonia or those with weak cough are examples of those who benefit from regular airway clearance.

    B. Methods

        1. Cough and deep breathing: perform a deep inspiration to vital capacity, followed by rapid exhalation (cough). Incidence of atelectasis and pneumonia in post-surgical patients, the elderly, and those with limited respiratory strength is decreased.

        2. Chest physiotherapy: CPT uses cupped hands or vibrator with rapid clapping over the lung fields to loosen mucous. Patients must lie with head lower than hips for 2–5 minutes in 4–6 positions. CPT is best done after bronchodilator use. Those with chest pain, fractures, pneumothorax, osteoporosis, or are intolerant to positioning are not good candidates.

        3. Mechanical exhalation vibratory devices
        The Flutter and Acapella are examples of two devices that cause endobronchial oscillations, thus loosening mucous. These devices are as effective, if not better than, CPT.

        4. PEP therapy: the PEP valve uses exhalation against a mouthpiece resistor to loosen mucous.

        5. Thairapy vest: This inflatable vest offers high frequency air compression/vibration. This system can be used independently, but cost is a consideration.

VI. Self-care strategies: Artificial airways—tracheostomy

    A. Indications for tracheostomy management

        1. Airway protection

        2. Secretion management

        3. Prevention of airway obstruction

    B. Patient care instructions

        1. Suction—perform as needed to remove secretions. In-hospital guidelines vary; home care includes clean technique. Suction catheters are cleaned with soapy water with water and vinegar rinse. Children's suctioning should not be performed deeply or greater than 5 seconds. Hyper-oxygenating with ambu bag is recommended.

        2. Change tracheostomy tubes monthly, per manufacturer recommendations; children's may be changed weekly or up to every 6 months.

        3. Site care should be performed per individual hospital guideline, generally every shift. Daily cleaning in home settings is acceptable. Disposable inner cannulas should not be re-used.

4. Complications of tracheostomies include
   a. Infection: Report purulent secretions to the health care provider, including amount and viscosity.
   b. Bleeding: Inspect the stoma for granulation tissue and report. Sudden bleeding of large amounts necessitates application of pressure and emergent help.
   c. Loss of airway patency: This is seen in difficulty suctioning, replacing the tracheostomy tube or loss of airflow volumes. Tracheal wall malacia/weakening may occur secondary to cuff pressure. Granulation tissue may partially occlude the end of the tube, or mucous plugging may obstruct the airway. These all need to be reported.

5. Communication
   a. Communication limitation causes withdrawal, depression, and limits the patient's ability to participate in their own care.
   b. Speech therapy should be consulted early in the tracheostomy process.
   c. Communication may be enhanced by writing tablets, computer boards, and in-line speaking valves.

Quality of Life and Functional Ability Issues

Georgia L. Narsavage

INTRODUCTION

This chapter examines quality of life (QoL) as a subjective determination of satisfaction with life experienced by an individual or family living with respiratory disorders. Problems associated with QoL in individuals with respiratory disorders are described and the role of social support, cost constraints, and ethical dilemmas are examined. The clinician is assisted to consider educational and support needs of patients and caregivers in living with respiratory disorders.

- Limitations in functional ability and QoL changes are commonly seen in people with respiratory disorders.
- Psychological issues such as control, self-esteem, and so forth, arise when there is little or no power to affect illness, when there is forced dependence on caregiver or health care team, and/or when life has lost meaning and value.
- Sociocultural issues such as social support, family impact, cultural interpretation of illness, spirituality, and economic status impact QoL.
- Assessment of social support includes support resources available and willingness to use them.
- Financial burdens impact QoL; may be expense of illness care or inability to work.
- Ethical considerations include continuation and adherence to treatment; examine in light of medical benefit to the patient, as well as patient and family's perception of positive effects of treatment vs. impact on QoL.
- Assessment of patient/family's strengths and weaknesses, self-esteem, understanding of respiratory disease and treatment, congruence of perceptions of the patient's functional ability, expectations of independence, external

strengths and needs, and the availability and knowledge of community and financial resources are warranted.

■ Assessment of QoL should consider
  ■ Who will be assessed
  ■ Physical location of the assessment (home vs. clinic, etc.)
  ■ Characteristics of the assessment tool and method of administration
    ■ General: useful in comparing and contrasting across populations and diseases
    ■ Disease specific: focus on areas affected, or that affect QoL, in specific conditions; useful when evaluating treatment effects
  ■ Focus of the assessment
  ■ Who will perform the assessment
  ■ Resources available for analysis

I. Quality of life (QoL), health-related quality of life (HQoL), and functional ability

These three terms have been used interchangeably in the literature. An understanding of their differences can organize clearer assessment and interventions in caring for individuals with respiratory disorders. QoL is a subjective determination of satisfaction experienced by an individual or family living with respiratory disorders. HQoL is characterized by level of satisfaction with factors that have been affected by a respiratory disorder or its treatment or can be affected by health care providers and systems. Functional ability refers to the degree to which individuals with respiratory disorders are limited in engaging in physical and psychosocial activities. Limitations in functional ability may affect an individual's HQoL (Leidy & Traver, 1995).

A. QoL defined

Definitions reflect that QoL is multi-dimensional and subjective and can only be determined by the individual and family involved. Their perception of satisfaction with life in areas they consider important will include both positive and negative characteristics. In respiratory disorders their QoL appraisal often reflects their satisfaction with their functional level compared to what they think would be an ideal or possible level of functioning. QoL is unique to the situation, person, and family (Parse, 1994).

B. HQoL defined

HQoL includes psychological and sociocultural indicators related to the patient and family as well as traditional physiological clinical indicators. These distinct areas are influenced by patients' experiences, as well as health beliefs, functional expectations, and health-related perceptions. Functional impairments (physical, emotional, and social) are important components of HQoL for individuals with respiratory disorders and their families because they affect daily living. In determining HQoL, identifying areas that can be affected by health care providers and systems is useful in planning care (Juniper, 1997; Testa & Simonson, 1996).

Useful Web site: http://www.atsqol.org/key.html

C. Functional ability defined

Functional ability not only includes the extent to which the patient and family are able to continue functioning in activities of daily living (ADLs), such as self-care, and Instrumental Activities of Daily Living (IADLs) but also their level of independence in completing developmental and situational tasks and their ability to meet bio-psychosocial and spiritual needs. Functional ability also relates to assessment of self-esteem (Lubkin, 2002; Cohen & De Back, 1999). Examples of ADLs include bathing, dressing, ambulation, and stair climbing. Examples of IADLs include shopping, meal preparation, child care, and use of public transportation systems.

II. Problems associated with QoL and functional ability

A. Physical issues

1. Patients with respiratory disorders may have limitations in self-care when oxygen desaturation or dyspnea makes activities increasingly difficult or impossible to complete. Changes in functional ability necessitate attention to potential changes in perceived QoL.

2. The distress of physical symptoms also affects psychological and sociocultural issues as activities outside the home are limited and self-esteem decreases. Visible indicators of disability such as oxygen use may also be perceived as negative and affect QoL.

B. Psychological issues

1. Self-esteem: As respiratory illness affects multiple areas, negative feelings about oneself or one's capabilities may be directly or indirectly expressed. Issues arise when there is little or no power to affect the illness, when there is forced dependence on the caregiver or health care team, or when life has lost meaning and value (Sparks & Taylor, 1998).

2. Control: One method to promote functioning is to increase the individual's perception of control, such as in helping control dyspnea through activity limitation or knowing which medications to take in an acute asthma attack. However this can become an issue when little or no control is possible; the physiological effects of respiratory illness may not be controllable (Narsavage, 1997).

3. Psychological distress: Psychological distress has been shown to impact QoL. Changing psychological distress factors, such as addressing anxiety and depressive symptoms can have an impact on QoL (Andenaes, Kalfoss, & Wahl, 2004).

C. Sociocultural issues

1. Social support affects how meaning is attributed to the respiratory illness and how coping strategies are used when stress is encountered. The availability of social support may increase motivation to adapt to situations such as being driven versus walking long distances when change is not possible, and helps maintain self-esteem and a positive mood. Assessment of social support includes not only what is available but also use or willingness to use such support (Lubkin, 2002).

2. Family impact can be observed when the family serves as caregiver and advocate by interacting, protecting, assisting, controlling, and changing situations related to the respiratory illness. Additional issues arise when they refuse or are unable to act, such as not monitoring physiological status because of distance, or not providing medications or care because of cost (Marshall, 1990; Musil, Morris, Warner, & Saeid, 2003).

3. Cultural interpretation of illness: The social meaning of respiratory illness varies. Health beliefs such as the acceptability and use of alternative treatments (e.g., relaxation therapy versus medications for dyspnea), and functional expectations such as cooking for oneself versus having meals provided by others has been viewed differently by gender and ethnicity. Cultural issues arise when the caregiver or health care provider does not acknowledge differences that are real and significant to the individual and family, such as the need to have the family "take care of" the ill person rather than promote independence (Warner, 1999).

4. Spirituality viewed as the meaning and purpose of one's life becomes an issue when the caregiver ascribes a different attribution to a respiratory disorder or its consequences (Taylor, Jones, & Burns, 2002).

5. Economic status: The family's economic needs remain, and strain can increase by additional expenses related to unemployment and treatment; many medications that control and treat respiratory disorders are expensive.

III. Role of social support, cost constraints, and ethical dilemmas

A. Social support

1. There have been multiple roles suggested for the contribution of social support to QoL. Social support has been shown to improve or help prevent problems by affecting the interpretation of the illness and the mood of the patient, providing a coping method, motivating the individual toward recovery or self-care, and providing for patients tangible needs, especially assistance in ADLs.

2. The availability of social support should not be assumed to indicate that there is positive support or that support is being used appropriately. Health-related QoL measures, administered to patients with lung disease and their support people can provide direction for supportive care and appropriate nursing interventions (Low & Gutman, 2003).

3. For many years, researchers have noted gender differences in forming and using networks of social support. Women are often the ones who provide support to children, friends, and relatives. If low levels of support are provided to women, because of perceptions of male gender superiority for example, demoralization and depression may result. Women with chronic obstructive pulmonary disease, usually diagnosed after they are 50 years of age, are at high risk for decreased social support.

4. *The Outcomes Mandate: Case Management in Health Care Today* emphasizes the necessity of identifying and maximizing the use of social support in promoting cost-effective positive patient outcomes (Cohen & De Back, 1999).

B. Cost constraints

1. QoL is affected when illness creates a financial burden on individuals and their families, not only directly through the expense of illness care but also indirectly through loss of the patient's ability or care provider's opportunity to work. Respiratory disease that limits functional ability has been a major cause of disability in the United States.

2. Financial resources and health insurance provide access to health care and protection from poor health but many individuals and families have little or no health insurance, thus limiting access to care and increasing out-of-pocket expenses to the point where even basic care is beyond the limits of many—decreasing QoL (Philipp & Black, 2002). Additionally chronic respiratory disease involves costs for long periods of time, such that insurance limits may be reached (and reimbursement ended) as care needs increase.

C. Ethical dilemmas

1. Ethical QoL issues focus on dilemmas related to an individual's right of self-determination, the principle of beneficence (doing good without harm), and the sanctity of life versus the QoL (see chapter 45). Whether individuals with severe respiratory disease who determine that their QoL is poor (such as being immobile and on a respirator) should be allowed to have therapy withdrawn.

2. Adherence or lack of adherence to treatment must be examined not only in light of the medical benefit to the patient but also the patient and family's perception that the "good" effects, such as a longer life, are or are not outweighed by a negative impact on QoL (Dean, 1990).

IV. Educational and support needs of patient and caregiver/family

A. Patient

1. Areas to assess for educational needs relative to QoL include internal strengths and needs, level of self-esteem, understanding of the respiratory disease and treatment, perception of functional ability, and expectations of independence (Hymovich & Hagopian, 1992).

2. Research on chronic illness suggests that the expressed need for disease specific information ranks second to a need for social support and the key to effective group support is the relationships formed among participants (Narsavage, Romeo, Lawless, & Nagy, 1999).

3. A support group can provide for multiple needs of those with chronic illness from regular exercise to group discussions of spirituality and philosophical views of life. Even when physical concerns can be treated and resolved, psychosocial and spiritual areas remained significant issues (Wyatt & Friedman, 1996).

B. Caregiver/family
1. Areas to assess for educational needs of the caregiver, family relative to QoL include their strengths and needs, level of self-esteem, understanding of the respiratory disease and treatment, congruence of perceptions of the patient's functional ability, and expectations of independence. Additionally external strengths and needs, as well as availability and knowledge of access to community and financial resources should be considered (Hymovich & Hagopian, 1992). The "Caregiver Quality of Life Cystic Fibrosis (CQOLCF) Scale" is one example of a disease-specific measure that can be used as an assessment tool (Boling, Macrina, & Clancy, 2003).
2. Research suggests that respiratory patients and their caregivers can have enhanced coping and confidence for living through assistance with learning needs, supportive education, and increased familiarity with disease facts and figures (Grahn & Danielson, 1996).
3. Anticipatory guidance, including teaching about the effects of respiratory illness on both mental and physical states, should be combined with education on skills needed to provide care, stress reduction, coping strategies and available resources (Sparks & Taylor, 1998).

C. Providing education and support
1. Once the assessment is completed, patients and families can be taught various techniques to improve QoL. Relaxation techniques and stress management programs can all be used with patients and families living with respiratory disease. The caregiver may need relaxation and stress management as much or more than the patient. Selection of a specific intervention can be accessed through multiple Web sites and will not be repeated here.
2. Keeping a diary of symptoms, treatments, and reactions can assist the patient, family and respiratory nurse specialist to identify what works and what is ineffective. Discussion of the diary record can be a useful communication tool in identifying areas of importance when the focus is on improving QoL (Narsavage, 1997).
3. Additional resources such as physical therapy, nutrition, occupational therapy, skilled home care nursing, personal care attendants, and community support groups such as "Easy Breathers" may be of value and referrals should be considered.
4. Treatment and intervention components may need to focus on improving nutritional status, exercise, and developing understanding and skills to use medications and oxygen therapy. These areas are usual components of pulmonary rehabilitation programs. Researchers have consistently demonstrated that pulmonary rehabilitation has positively affected QoL, although the improvement is often not long-lasting.
5. Alternative and complementary therapy may be useful for patients with respiratory problems. The effect of acupuncture and acupressure, for example, have allowed patients with chronic respiratory disease

to experience clinically significant improvements in QoL (Maa et al., 2003).

V. Evaluation of QoL and functional ability

   A. Issues in development of QoL instruments

      1. One major issue in selection of an instrument is their multiplicity—there are hundreds of generic and disease-specific measures of different aspects of QoL. This can be noted in the American Thoracic Society (ATS) Web site and multiple articles on measures of QoL for patients with respiratory disease.

      2. Acknowledgment that QoL is a valid outcome measure in clinical trials was hindered by the conceptual vagueness of QoL, questionable validity and reliability of the measures, the use of inappropriate research methods, and weak statistical findings (Fallowfield, 1996).

      3. There is a need for normative data in QoL, HQoL, and functional ability measures so that findings can be compared across populations and specific diseases (McHorney, 1997).

   B. Issues in selection of instruments and techniques

      1. Measures and methods used to assess QoL are different for providers, patients, families, caregivers, etc. Other factors that should be considered are where the evaluation will be completed (e.g., clinic, hospital, home), characteristics of the questionnaire and method of administration (e.g., short or long form, self-report or interview, clinic or hospital survey, telephone or mail survey), the focus of the evaluation (e.g., quality improvement, program development, research), who is to collect the data, and what resources are available for analysis (Testa & Simonson, 1996).

      2. In measuring QoL and HQoL for patients with respiratory disorders, we are more interested in the clinical significance of findings than a statistically significant difference. This involves both the patient and the provider's interpretation of significance. Clinically meaningful improvement has been defined as "the smallest difference in score in the domain of interest which patients perceive as beneficial and which would mandate, in the absence of troublesome side-effects and excessive cost, a change in the patient's management" (Juniper, Guyatt, Willan, & Griffith, 1994, p. 81).

      3. Instruments for use in patients with adult asthma may have small changes because of the intermittent nature of the disease, but there may be an impact that is clinically significant. It may be more appropriate to use general instruments to provide comparison with a "healthy" population when examining the impact of adult asthma on QoL.

      4. Because functional performance depends on the capacity or potential for performance, instruments must be selected that measure what has been defined as functional ability (Leidy & Traver, 1995).

      5. Because the development of many functional ability instruments are not related to a conceptual framework, it is important to ask whether

the measure is conceptually consistent with its intended application, that is, are we interested in limitations in functional ability or actual performance, in QoL or HQoL, level of dyspnea, or the impact of dyspnea on HQoL (Weaver, Narsavage, & Guilfoyle, 1998).

6. Selection of disease-specific instruments such as the St. George's Respiratory Questionnaire, the Pulmonary Functional Status Scale, the Pulmonary Functional Status and Dyspnea Questionnaire, the Asthma Quality of Life Questionnaire, or a general measure such as the Quality of Well-being Scale or the SF36 should be related to the goals of the assessment. General measures are useful in comparing and contrasting across populations and diseases. Disease-specific measures focus on areas that usually are affected or affect QoL in specific conditions, such as ADLs and dyspnea in pulmonary disease. Disease-specific tools may be more sensitive to changes and are useful when evaluating treatment effects. A combination of global and disease-specific measures may be beneficial but the burden on the patient may be greater than desired.

C. Sources of instruments on the Internet

1. An Index of QoL and HQoL Instruments is available on the ATS "Quality of Life Resource" Web site at http://www.atsqol.org/qinst.asp. This Web site provides information about measures that have been used in evaluating QoL and functioning of patients with respiratory disorders. It also has definitions of key QoL concepts and explains terminology such as validity and reliability. Specific diseases with recommendations for measures include adult and pediatric asthma, COPD, cystic fibrosis (CF), critical care patients, lung cancer, rhinosinusitis, sarcoidosis, sleep-disordered breathing, pulmonary hypertension, and smoking tobacco addiction. Detailed information about the QoL and functional assessment tools is available on the Web sites is not repeated here. The frequency of updates makes this a very informative site.

2. "Quality of life questionnaires that work" can be found at the Medical Outcomes Trust Web site at http://www.outcomes-trust.org:80/healthplan.html

3. Functional ability measures as well as QoL measures can be accessed through the "Quality of Life Assessment in Medicine: Internet Resource" links to both multiple global and disease-specific measure, as well as major organizations and research groups. It can be found at http://www.qlmed.org/url.html. Most of the links provide not only the instrument but also a reference or link to the reliability and validity of the tool. For example the Childhood Asthma Questionnaire http://www.psy.uwa.edu.au/user/davina/caq.html provides reports for children in specific age groups (4–7, 8–11, and 12–16).

4. Many of the measures that are widely used have developed their own Web sites. An example may be found on the RAND site for MOS shortforms (SF-36) accessible at http://www.sf-36.com/tools. This site offers not only the questionnaire—which is public domain—but also

methods for administering, reliability and validity, information that is available on its use, and references.

5. The HQoL section of the National Center for Chronic Disease Prevention and Health Promotion (CDC) Web site provides methods and measures for different populations. One example is the Healthy (and unhealthy) Days Measure that can be used to compare QoL in multiple diseases. It can be found at http://www.cdc/gov/nccdphp/hrqol/index.html.

6. The World Health Organization has published instruments designed to measure QoL cross-culturally. These may be downloaded and printed in PDF format for the WHO Web site at http://www.who.int/mental_health/Publication_Pages/Pubs_General.html.

D. Additional issues in QoL evaluation

1. QoL and HQoL are not the same for all ages and diseases. It is preferable to select an instrument that has been validated on the population (children versus adults, men and women, asthma versus COPD) that is being studied or treated. If data are not available on the ability of the selected questionnaire to measure the QoL impact of the specific disease, the clinician should ask a group of patients with the disease to review the questions for appropriateness. Other respiratory nurse specialists can also provide their expert opinion to support content validity.

2. If a new measure is being used the clinician should trial it with a small group of patients who can be expected to change after treatment (e.g., pre-inhaler prescription for newly diagnosed COPD). By having the patients (and families) complete the tool before the change as well as after treatment, the clinician is more likely to be able to identify an impact.

3. Because QoL and HQoL are perceived, it is important that evaluation methods include self-appraisal, in which the client and family answer the questions (Bopp & Lubkin, 2002).

4. Evaluation of teaching and use of educational and support resources may be obtained by examining medical records for clinical status evidence, however declining clinical status does not in and of itself constitute poor QoL.

5. Evaluation of QoL remains a social rather than a medical judgment. The patient and family are the ultimate judges of their QoL.

6. A holistic concept of QoL includes social, psychological, and spiritual well-being that extends beyond ADLs and disease categories. Despite respiratory illness and functional limitations, people can find meaning, value, and the motivation to persist in the face of a disruptive condition. Those who report having a high QoL are reported to have an understanding of their condition, take control, conserve energy, seek balance, search for resources to better manage their lives, engage in social networks, and remain connected, while providing emotional support to others (Albrecht & Devlieger, 1999).

E. Pediatric considerations
   1. Children may begin to realistically conceptualize and process the meaning for respiratory illness at 11 to 12 years of age. Therefore, logical reasoning regarding medical decision making often cannot occur before the teenage years. Yet children, even at young ages, should be informed of their choices in a developmentally appropriate manner and assent (indicating some understanding and agreement with treatment) should be obtained.
   2. Ethical dilemmas or conflicts can occur if the developing child's moral views of the respiratory illness and death differ from those held by parents or adults. It may be necessary to formalize the consideration of such ethical issues by an Ethics Board of Review.
   3. Other pediatric issues include surrogacy to determine the authority, responsibility, and competence of parents to promote the best interests of their dependent children. QoL discussion must reflect the potential life of the infant or young child and the normal nurturing dependence of the child upon his family (Hays, 1991).

F. Pregnancy considerations
   1. Studies suggest that using medications during pregnancy (e.g., inhaled beta-agonist bronchodilators) to attain an optimal QoL and control of asthma is justified—especially in the one-third of women for whom asthma worsens with pregnancy (Schatz, 2001). Alternative therapies such as Sahaja yoga have also been beneficial as measured by the Asthma-related QoL in the area of improved mood (Manocha, Marks, Kenchington, Peters, & Salome, 2002).
   2. In pregnancies complicated by diabetes, reducing complications and improving QoL can promote healthy infant and family functioning and reduce long-term complications (Samson, 1992).
   3. QoL in adults with CF demonstrated different patterns in men and women. The decision to become pregnant and the ability to bring a pregnancy to term have correlated with improved QoL for women. Looking after the home, social life, hobbies, and holiday responsibilities were less in women with CF when compared with women who had minor non-acute conditions (Congleton, Hodson, & Duncan-Skingle, 1996).

WEB SITES

http://www.nih.gov—This Web site provides links to the National Heart Lung and Blood Institute as well as Alternative Medicine and http://www.clinicaltrials.gov. The search engine on this site can help clinicians to identify which measures of QoL are currently being used in research with particular diseases.

http://www.cdc.gov—This site links to disease specific data and local health departments for information about demographics and characteristics on disease populations

http://www.ncqa.org—Although not specific to QoL, this site can be useful in identifying what insurers are rating. It links to a related site, http://www. healthgrades.com, which has information on clinics and nursing homes.

Medical center Web sites such as http://www.mayoclinic.com and http://www. oncolink.com (University of Pennsylvania) can provide information about disease management, guidelines, and clinical trials that are incorporating QoL measures.

REFERENCES

Albrecht, G. L., & Devlieger, P. J. (1999). The disability paradox: High quality of life against all odds. *Social Science and Medicine, 48,* 977–988.

Andenaes, R., Kalfoss, M. H., & Wahl, A. (2004). Psychological distress and quality of life in hospitalized patients with chronic obstructive pulmonary disease. *Journal of Advanced Nursing, 46,* 523–530.

Boling, W., Macrina, D. M., & Clancy, J. P. (2003). The Caregiver Quality of Life Cystic Fibrosis (CQOLCF) scale: Modification and validation of an instrument to measure quality of life in cystic fibrosis family caregivers. *Quality of Life Research, 12,* 1119–1126.

Bopp, A., & Lubkin, I. (2002). Teaching. In I. M. Lubkin (Ed.), *Chronic illness: Impact and interventions* (pp. 343–362). Boston: Jones & Bartlett Publishers.

Cohen, E. L., & De Back, V. (1999). *The outcomes mandate.* Philadelphia: Mosby.

Congleton, J., Hodson, M. E., & Duncan-Skingle, F. (1996). Quality of Life in adults with cystic fibrosis. *Thorax, 51,* 936–940.

Dean, H. E. (1990). Political and ethical implications of using quality of life as an outcome measure. *Seminars in Oncology Nursing, 6,* 303–308.

Fallowfield, L. (1996). Quality of quality-of-life data. *Lancet, 348,* 421–422.

Grahn, G., & Danielson, M. (1996). Coping with the cancer experience. II. Evaluating an education and support program for cancer patients and their significant others. *European Journal of Cancer Care, 5,* 182–187.

Hays, R. (1991). Health care ethics and pediatric rehabilitation. *Physical Medicine and Rehabilitation Clinics of North America, 2,* 743–763.

Hymovich, D. P., & Hagopian, G. A. (1992). *Chronic illness in children and adults.* Philadelphia: W. B. Saunders.

Juniper, E. F. (1997). Quality of life in adults and children with asthma and rhinitis. *Allergy, 52,* 971–977.

Juniper, E. F., Guyatt, G. H., Willan, A., & Griffith, L. E. (1994). Determining a minimal important change in a disease-specific quality of life questionnaire. *Journal of Clinical Epidemiology, 47,* 81–87.

Leidy, N. K., & Traver, G. A. (1995). Psychophysiologic factors contributing to functional performance in people with COPD: Are there gender differences? *Research in Nursing and Health, 18,* 535–546.

Low, G., & Gutman, G. (2003). Couples' ratings of chronic obstructive pulmonary disease patients' quality of life. *Clinical Nursing Research, 2,* 28–48.

Lubkin, I. M. (2002). *Chronic illness: Impact and interventions* (5th ed.). Boston: Jones & Bartlett Publishers.

Maa, S. H., Sun, M. F., Hsu, K. H., Hung, T. J., Chen, H. C., Yu, C. T., et al. (2003). Effect of acupuncture or acupressure on quality of life of patients with chronic obstructive asthma: A pilot study. *Journal of Alternative & Complementary Medicine, 9,* 659–670.

Manocha, R., Marks, G. B., Kenchington, P., Peters, D., & Salome, C. M. (2002). Sahaja yoga in the management of moderate to severe asthma: A randomised controlled trial. *Thorax, 57,* 110–115.

Marshall, P. S. (1990). Cultural influences on perceived quality of life. *Seminars in Oncology Nursing, 6,* 278–284.

McHorney, C. A. (1997). Generic health measurement: Past accomplishments and a measurement paradigm for the 21st century. *Annals of Internal Medicine, 127,* 743–750.

Musil, C. M., Morris, D. L., Warner, C. D., & Saeid, H. (2003). Issues in caregivers stress and providers support. *Research on Aging, 25*(5), 505–526.

Narsavage, G. L. (1997). Promoting function in clients with chronic lung disease by increasing their perception of control. *Holistic Nursing Practice, 12*(1), 17–26.

Narsavage, G. L., Romeo, E., Lawless, P., & Nagy, E. (1999). Adaptation to stress: Meeting cancer patients needs. *The European Respiratory Journal, 14,* 70S.

Parse, R. (1994). Quality of life: Sciencing and living the art of human becoming. *Nursing Science Quarterly, 7,* 16–21.

Philipp, T., & Black, L. (2002). Financial impact. In I. M. Lubkin (Ed.), *Chronic illness: Impact and interventions* (pp. 501–527). Boston: Jones & Bartlett Publishers.

Samson, L. F. (1992). Infants of diabetic mothers: Current perspectives. *Journal of Perinatal and Neonatal Nursing, 6,* 61–70.

Schatz, M. (2001). The safety of inhaled beta-agonist bronchodilators during pregnancy. In GINA Workshop Report. Retrieved February 8, 2002, from http://www.getasthmahelp.org

Sparks, S. M., & Taylor, C. M. (1998). *Nursing diagnosis reference manual* (4th ed.). Springhouse, PA: Springhouse Corporation.

Taylor, E. J., Jones, P., & Burns, M. (2002). Quality of life. In I. M. Lubkin (Ed.), *Chronic illness: Impact and interventions* (pp. 207–226). Boston: Jones & Bartlett Publishers.

Testa, M. A., & Simonson, D. C. (1996). Assessment of quality-of-life outcomes. *New England Journal of Medicine, 334,* 835–840.

Warner, R. (1999). The emics and etics of quality of life assessment. *Social Psychiatry and Psychiatric Epidemiology, 34,* 117–121.

Weaver, T. E., Narsavage, G. L., & Guilfoyle, M. J. (1998). The Development and Psychometric Analysis of the Pulmonary Functional Status Scale (PFSS): An Instrument to Assess Functional Status in Pulmonary Disease. *Journal of Cardiopulmonary Rehabilitation, 18*(2), 105–111.

Wyatt, G., & Friedman, L. L. (1996). Long-term female cancer survivors: Quality of life issues and clinical implications. *Cancer Nursing, 19,* 1–7.

Legal and Ethical Issues

Resource Utilization

42

Donna Smaha

INTRODUCTION

An appreciation of costs, reimbursement issues, and impact of lung disease on society should enhance the clinician's approach to health care. This chapter will attempt to speak to some of the key points surrounding the broad topic of resource utilization. It will address epidemiology, costs of disease and associated health care, technological impact, and approaches to optimizing utilization of resources while maintaining focus on patient-centered care.

I. Costs and resource utilization of pulmonary disease
   To evaluate resource utilization in health care, it is important to understand the epidemiology of specific disease states, resource requirements, and availability and access to those resources. As well as serving other purposes, biostatistical data offers an objective profile of burden of disease and the financial impact on society.
   A. Terminology used in statistical reporting (Thomas, 1997)
      1. Prevalence—the actual number of cases of a disease present in a specified population at a given time
      2. Incidence—the frequency of occurrence of any condition over a period of time in relation to the population in which it occurs
      3. Morbidity rates—"the number of cases per year of certain diseases in relation to the population in which they occur" (Thomas, 1997, p. 163). They can be expressed per 100, 1,000, 10,000, or 100,000 of all living persons with the disease.
      4. Mortality rates—"the number of deaths in a specified population, usually expressed per 100,000 population, over a given period, usually one year" (Thomas, 1997, p. 163).

5. Resource utilization can be expressed in terms of direct and indirect costs (American Lung Association [ALA], 1996b).
    a. Direct costs include hospital care, emergency care, outpatient and ambulatory care services, physician and professional health care services, drugs, durable medical equipment, nursing home and other extended care, such as hospice and rehabilitation services
    b. Indirect costs
        i. Indirect morbidity costs reflect lost days at work, either from personal illness or that of a child or other family member, resulting in the loss of earnings
        ii. Indirect mortality costs reflect lost future earnings by those who died from the given disease
B. Acute and chronic respiratory disorders rank among the highest in prevalence, incidence, morbidity and mortality, and resource utilization of all diseases in the United States. Ranking of lung disease in the United States between 1979 and 1997 were reported by the Epidemiology and Statistics Unit of the American Lung Association (1999b). Unless otherwise indicated, data and date ranges apply to all Section B statistics. Table 42.1 summarizes some of this data
    1. Lung cancer is the leading cause of cancer mortality in both men and women in the United States, surpassing breast cancer for women in 1987 (ALA, 1999f).
        a. 171,500 estimated new cases in 1998 or 14% of all cancer diagnoses, of which >80% are non-small cell lung cancer (NSCLC); 76% of those cases are diagnosed at Stage III or IV; close to 50% of all new cases are not eligible for surgery because of late stage at diagnosis.
        b. The surveillance, epidemiology and end results (SEER) program of the National Cancer Institute reports there has been a 10.9% increase in incidence from 1989 to 1995 (ALA, 1999).
        c. The most significant cause of lung cancer is smoking. Approximately 90% of all lung cancer patients are smokers or former smokers. Incidence risk is directly proportional to smoker pack-years. Two-pack-per-day smokers have 15–25 times greater risk of lung cancer than those who have never smoked. Five-year survival rates for diagnosed lung cancer is just over 10% (Department of Health and Human Services [DHHS], 1998).
        d. Lung cancer caused an estimated 161,000 deaths in 1998, accounting for 28% of all cancer deaths.
        e. 80%–90% of all lung cancer patients also have COPD (Wilson, 1997).
        f. Respiratory cancers lead in total costs of lung diseases at $27.9 billion in 1998, with direct costs of $3.5 billion and indirect costs of $24.3 billion (ALA, 1999b).
    2. Chronic obstructive pulmonary disease (COPD) is a general category of lung disease characterized by coughing, chronic sputum production, and dyspnea. Chronic bronchitis, emphysema, bronchiectasis,

| Table 42.1 | Statistical Data for Common Lung Diseases in the United States | | | |

Disease	Deaths	Prevalence	Prevalence Rates	Mortality Rates
Lung Cancer	161,000 (1998)	171,500 (1998)	N/A	N/A
COPD	103,595 (1997)	16.4 million (1995)		Up 41% (1979–97)
Emphysema	N/A	1.9 million (1998)	Down 30% (1982–95)	N/A
Bronchitis	N/A	14.5 million (1995)	Up 64% (1982–95)	N/A
Asthma	3500 (1997)	15 million (1997)	Up 63% (1980–94) Up 160% <4yrs old (1980–94)	Up 55% (1979–97)
Pneumonia/ influenza	86,448 (1997)	Pneumonia 108 million episodes (1995)	N/A	Up 15.2% (1979–97) 99% were pneumonia in 1997
Tuberculosis	N/A		Up 20% (1985–92)	
Sleep Disorders	N/A	40 million (1999)	N/A	

N/A: not applicable or not available.

and sometimes asthma and cystic fibrosis are included in this group (Seidel, Ball, Dains, & Benedict, 2003). The American Thoracic Society defines COPD as "a disease state characterized by the presence of airflow obstruction due to chronic bronchitis or emphysema . . . [which] is generally progressive, [and] may be accompanied by airway hyperactivity" (American Thoracic Society [ATS], 1995, pg. 11). In this section, COPD will refer to chronic bronchitis and emphysema.

a. Together, these two diseases rank fourth among the leading causes of death in the United States, and fifth in the world.

b. Approximately 16.4 million Americans were affected in 1995.

c. In 1997, COPD mortality increased by almost 41% from 1979, accounting for 103,595 deaths; the overall age-adjusted death rates for all causes decreased 17% during this same period (ALA, 1999b).

d. Of the major disease groups, only COPD continues to increase in mortality rates (Doherty, Mandel, & Haggerty, 2000).

e. COPD is second only to heart disease as a cause of disability in adults younger than 65 years of age (McCance & Huether, 2002).

591

f. From 1979–1981, there were 169 million days of restricted activity in this population, for an average of 2 months per year per person. "COPD is the third most frequent medical diagnosis (after congestive heart failure and stroke) for patients receiving home care" (ATS, 1995, p. S78).

g. "The most expensive 10% of Medicare beneficiaries with COPD (account) for nearly half of total expenditures for this population" (Grasso, Weller, Shaffer, Diette, & Anderson, 1998, p. 134).

h. Although emphysema and chronic bronchitis are commonly considered together as COPD, and occur simultaneously in a large number of cases, the following data illustrates the difference in incidence and prevalence of emphysema and chronic bronchitis (ALA, 2000).

    i. Emphysema data between 1982 and 1995

    ii. 30% *decrease* in prevalence rate, a significant decline

    iii. 1.9 million cases in 1995, of which 93% were >45 years

    iv. Significantly higher prevalence rates in whites over blacks

    v. 44% of persons with emphysema report limitations in activities of daily living

i. Chronic bronchitis data between 1982 and 1995

    i. Ninth in prevalence of chronic conditions

    ii. 8% increase in reported incidence

    iii. 64% increase in reported prevalence

    iv. A statistically significant increase in prevalence rate of 27% occurred in females between 1983 and 1995

    v. 14.5 million cases in 1995, an increase from 7.7 million in 1982

C. Asthma

Asthma incidence and mortality has increased globally over the last few decades and has become a major health problem for persons of all ages (National Institutes of Health, 1995). It is an obstructive lung disease that is chronic in nature. However, because of its primary characteristics of inflammation and *reversibility* of airflow obstruction, in recent years it has been considered separately from COPD (ATS, 1995; Maltais & Bourbeau, 1995). Asthma is defined by the National Asthma Education and Prevention Program (NAEPP) Expert Panel Report 2 as "a chronic inflammatory disorder of the airways in which many cells and cellular elements play a role, in particular, mast cells, eosinophils, T-lymphocytes, neutrophils, and epithelial cells [which] in susceptible individuals . . . causes recurrent episodes of wheezing, breathlessness, chest tightness, and cough, particularly at night and in the early morning" (National Asthma and Education Prevention Program [NAEPP], 1997, p. 3).

1. Asthma currently affects approximately 15 million Americans (NAEPP, 1997).

2. Its overall prevalence increased 63.2% from 1980 to 1994, and in children under the age of four, 160% (ALA, 1999a).

3. The age-adjusted death rate increased 55.6%, from 0.9 per 100,000 in 1979 to 1.4 per 100,000 in 1997 (ALA, 1999a).
4. Pediatric considerations
    a. Asthma is the most common chronic disorder in children and adolescents under the age of 18, about 5 million, of which 1.3 million are under the age of 5 years (American Academy of Allergy, Asthma, & Immunology [AAAAI], 1999).
    b. Children under 18 years of age account for over 33% of the medically underserved (AAAAI, 1999).
    c. The highest increase in prevalence has been in the 18–44 year age group, an increase of 86.8% (AAAAI, 1999)!
    d. Hospitalization discharge rates increased 6.7% from 1988 to 1997 (ALA, 1999); the National Hospital Discharge Survey of 1994 reported 164,000 hospitalizations for children under age 15 (AAAAI, 1999).
    e. >44% of asthma patients discharged in 1997 were <15 years of age; only 22% of the general population is in that age group (AAAAI, 1999).
5. Sly (2000) reported hopeful news in the *Annals of Allergy, Asthma and Immunology*: Asthma deaths decreased for the year 1997. Annual economic costs (in 1998 dollars) total $11.2 billion (ALA, 1999a); "20% of patients with asthma account for 80% of the costs of the disease due to high utilization of urgent care services"(AAAAI, 1999). In a comparative study of 1.4 million covered lives in corporate health care plans, there was a significantly higher utilization of resources in asthmatic versus non-asthmatic patients, accounting for double the number of resources used and 2–3 times higher amounts paid by health care plans for the asthmatic population, an average of $3,243 versus $1,502 per patient (Nelson, Oritz, Fitterman, & Markson, 1998).
    a. Direct costs $7.5 billion; inpatient hospitalizations account for $3.2 billion of that total (ALA, 1999a)
    b. Indirect costs $3.8 billion; lost *school* days represent the largest portion in reduced productivity of $1 billion; 100 million days of restricted activity for adults and children combined (NAEPP, 1997), including 10 million missed school days annually, an average of greater than three times that of children without asthma (AAAAI, 1999).
D. Pneumonia, influenza, and acute respiratory illness are significant contributors to morbidity, mortality, and health care costs in the United States (ALA, 1999c). The American Lung Association reported the following data through the Epidemiology and Statistics Unit in November 1999.
    1. Pneumonia and influenza together were the sixth leading cause of death.
        a. 86,448 deaths in 1997 alone; 90% of all deaths occur in those over 65 years of age
        b. The fifth leading cause of death for people over 65 years of age

2. The mortality rate for those of the age of 65 has increased 15.2%, and over 99% of 1997 cases were from pneumonia.

3. Combined with other acute respiratory illnesses such as the common cold and acute bronchitis, they are substantial contributors to lost days at work and school.

4. In 1995, acute respiratory illness ranked first (85.2 per 100 persons) as causes of sick days.

    a. Lost days at school (191.7 episodes per 100 children) and lost days at work (107.8 per 100 employed)

    b. An estimated 223 million respiratory conditions reported of which influenza accounted for 108 million episodes and the common cold, 60.5 million episodes

5. Immunization

    a. Administration of annual flu vaccines and once or twice in a life-time Pneumococcal Polysaccharide Vaccine (PPV) improves health outcomes, reduces hospitalization and death rates, and reduces health care costs (Nichol, 1999).

    b. Vaccination rates for influenza and pneumonia vary by state.

    c. Recommendations are that all persons aged 65 and over, as well as younger patients meeting specific criteria, receive the PPV, which can be administered any time of year; yet the Centers for Disease Control estimates that only 40% of all Medicare beneficiaries have *ever* received the PPV.

6. Costs of pneumonia and the flu in 1998 were $22.9 billion.

    a. Direct costs totaled $17.5 billion.

    b. Indirect costs totaled $5.4 billion.

7. A significant increase in influenza deaths of epidemic proportions, exceeding 40,000 deaths compared to an average annual 20,000 deaths, has occurred in 4 of the past 5 years. Twenty percent to 40% of the population are affected each year and hospitalizations now exceed 300,000 annually (Blaiss, 1999).

E. Tuberculosis (TB) is an airborne infection caused by *Mycobacterium tuberculosis*, an acid-fast bacillus usually affecting the lungs but that may invade other organs and tissues (McCance & Huether, 2002).

1. TB is the leading cause of death from a single infectious agent worldwide.

2. By the year 2020, global estimates predict: 1 billion people will become infected, 200 million will become ill, 70 million will die (ALA, 1999d).

3. Prevalence rates in the United States declined steadily until a surge increasing the number of cases by 20% were reported between 1985 and 1992 (ALA, 1999d).

4. This mounting trend can be attributed in large part to the acquired immune deficiency syndrome (AIDS) epidemic, as well as to the increasing number of drug-resistant strains (McCance & Huether,

2002). However, the years between 1992 and 1998 showed a 31% overall decline.

5. Total costs $1.054 billion
   a. Direct costs: $703.1 million
   b. Indirect costs: $351 million

6. To address the rise in cases during the late 1980s and early 1990s, the government supported prevention programs for HIV-infected persons, TB screenings, and preventive therapy for high-risk patients. Screening programs will be necessary to address the high rate of TB in immigrants and refugees (ALA, 1999d).

F. The total cost of lung disease as estimated by the National Heart, Lung and Blood Institute (NHLBI) in 1999 was $127.2 billion, of which $88.1 billion was attributed to direct costs and $39.1 to indirect costs (ALA, 1999b). A breakdown of figures for 1998 are shown below (see Table 42.2).

G. Sleep disorders (Siegel, 1999)
   1. 40 million Americans are affected by chronic sleep disorders.
   2. 20–30 million have periodic sleep-related problems.
   3. 95% of all people with sleep disorders are undiagnosed.
   4. About 30% of motor vehicle accidents occur from drivers falling asleep at the wheel.
   5. Accidents in the workplace are caused by sleep-deprived workers with impaired concentration and psychomotor skills.
   6. Direct costs are estimated at $15.9 million per year, indirect costs at $50–$100 billion.
   7. "Less than 4 or more than 9 hours' sleep (per night) is associated with higher mortality than is the average 8 hours" (Brown, 1999, p. 52).

| Table 42.2 | Estimates of Direct and Indirect Costs of Lung Disease, 1998 (Dollars Expressed in Billions) |

Condition (ICD-9-CM)	Total Costs	Direct Costs	Indirect Mortality	Costs Morbidity	Total Indirect
COPD (490–92,494,496)	26.0	13.6	6.0	6.4	12.4
Asthma (493)	11.3	7.5	2.4	1.4	3.8
Pneumonia/Influenza	22.9	17.5	5.4	–	5.4
Tuberculosis (010–165)	1.054	0.703	–	–	0.351
Respiratory Cancer (160–165)	27.9	3.5	20.8	3.5	24.3
Lung Disease Total	**89.1**	**42.8**	**34.6**	**11.3**	**46.3**

From: American Lung Association, Epidemiology & Statistics Unit. (1999, November). Trends in chronic bronchitis and emphysema. *Morbidity and Mortality.*

8. Treatment of sleep disorders such as obstructive sleep apnea may be covered by some insurance, but many are not, or only partial service and/or equipment is covered (Eisenberg, 1999).

II. Reimbursement issues and managed care

A. Managed care began as a result of ever-increasing health care costs in the 1980s and has developed into a complicated mix of traditional and so-called managed insurance plans, both in the private and public sectors. Economic recession and inflation, bureaucratic organizational structures of health care institutions (Blancett & Dominick, 1995), and unregulated payment of fee-for-service by insurance companies led to an unprecedented escalation of health care spending. Spending grew from 4% of the gross national product in the 1950s to an alarming 12% by 1990 (CBS Healthwatch, 2000). Industry, government, and the public have clamored for reform, which has come in numerous strategic forms and continues to be debated.

1. Alain Enthoven, an economist from Stanford University, became a major player in economic health care reform. His goal to convert providers into economic units in order to develop competition, thereby promoting cost controls in health care delivery, is referred to as *managed competition* (Bodenheimer & Grumbach, 1995; Fox, 1993).

2. Another strategy used to control costs is patient cost sharing through out-of-pocket expenses for a share of insurance premiums, deductibles, co-payments, and non-covered services. The amount of these out-of-pocket expenses varies widely by type of plan (Bodenheimer & Grumbach, 1995).

3. Utilization management (UM) is one other major cost containment strategy whereby physicians and other providers are monitored for amount and cost of services provided with the threat of denial of payment for services if not pre-authorized. UM has been used by Medicare and Medicaid for quite some time and is performed by the entity at financial risk, whether it be the health care institution, the insurance company, or private physician (Bodenheimer & Grumbach, 1995).

4. Types of health coverage: Private sector

   a. Traditional reimbursement—Fee-for-service and/or indemnity plan, which usually covers most treatments and illnesses but may not cover preventive care, requires a deductible out-of-pocket expense prior to any payment, holds patients responsible for filing insurance claims, and allows choice of providers without limitation (CBS Healthwatch, 2000).

   b. Preferred Provider Organization (PPO)—Networks of providers who provide price discounts for contracted services, limits choice but allows out-of-network choice, which requires a higher co-pay or deductible, does not require primary care physician (Edelman & Mandle, 1994), and usually covers pre-existing conditions (CBS Healthwatch, 2000).

    c. Health maintenance organization (HMO)—"Proto-typical managed care model [which] provides health care in return for a preset, prepaid amount of money on a per member per month basis" (Edelman & Mandle, 1994, p. 26), limits access to providers, and which covers pre-existing conditions; can be divided into Individual Practice Associations (IPA) and Group or Staff Model HMOs like Kaiser-Permanente.

    d. Capitation—Not a health plan but a form of payment based on membership rather than services delivered, as in an HMO, with the added restriction of each physician or practice providing care for a given number of "lives" for a flat annual fee with the objective of containing costs through health promotion and disease prevention, or preventive services (Edelman & Mandle, 1994); a shortfall in managed care, financial incentives to health care providers often promote acute, episodic care rather than continuity of care (AAAAI, 1999).

5. Types of health coverage: Public sector

    a. Medicare—The Federal insurance program established as an amendment to the Social Security Act in 1966 funding health care for persons aged 65 and older, amended in 1973 to include those under age 65, who are totally and permanently disabled who qualify for Social Security, to receive benefits for 2 years, and those in end-stage renal failure requiring hemodialysis or a kidney transplant. For inpatient hospitalizations, Medicare makes payment based on a Diagnosis Related Group (DRG) system, whereby the facility is paid according to the diagnosis rather than cost. This system incentives hospitals to be efficient. Medicare beneficiaries do have the benefit of choice of providers and service agencies (Edelman & Mandle, 1994). A major shortfall in the Medicare program is the lack of prescription drug coverage, a strategic political and economic issue during the 2000 Presidential election campaign.

    b. Medicaid—jointly managed federal and state government assistance program begun in 1967 as an amendment to the Social Security Act to provide funding for basic health services of those too poor to pay and who receive either welfare, Aid to Families with Dependent Children, Supplemental Security Income, Old Age Assistance, Aid to the Blind, or Aid to Totally and Permanently Disabled; additional eligibility and services vary by state (Edelman & Mandle, 1994). Generally, Medicaid only allows for 16 hospital days per year and pays for many prescription drugs. But like Medicare beneficiaries, Medicaid patients have a choice of providers.

    c. Uninsured—Approximately one-third of Americans are uninsured and rely primarily on urgent care services for their health care, also the most expensive and inefficient means of care (Chande, Krug, & Warm, 1996; Edelman & Mandle, 1994). Recent immigrants and their families account for about 25% of the nation's uninsured, half of whom live at or below the poverty level. If passed by Congress, restoring Medicaid and federal Children's Health Insurance Benefits (CHIPS) to immigrant children and pregnant women is estimated to cost $1.6 billion over the next 10 years (Zwillich, 2000).

B. Balanced Budget Act of 1997—As described in an economics brief by the Health Care Advisory Board, "The Balanced Budget Act [BBA] of 1997 was the most significant legislation for health care finance in at least a decade. After implementation began in 1998, hospitals and health systems began reporting—almost immediately—devastating declines in financial performance, with the blame for the downturn assigned almost exclusively to the BBA" (1999, p. v). Average hospital incomes dropped over 30% in 1998, two-thirds of which is estimated to be attributable to the BBA. Despite the fact that the BBA far surpassed original projections in the first year resulting in the current budget surplus, little relief is in sight for appreciable restoration of funding.

1. The BBA can be summarized into six major changes/reforms to be implemented over a 5-year period from 1998–2002 (Health Care Advisory Board, 1999).

a. Slowdown in inpatient price increases—payment rate to hospitals for inpatient admissions were initially frozen with gradual increases over 5 years to market rate minus 1.1 points

b. Early transfer penalties—minimum length of stay required in order to receive full payment for a hospital admission on 10 specified DRGs when transferred to either a skilled nursing facility or home with home health in 1999, increasing to 25 DRGs in 2000, and possibly all by 2001.

c. Skilled Nursing Facility (SNF) Prospective Payment System (PPS)–progressing from a blended formula of historic and national costs paying a set amount by diagnosis, similar to hospital DRGs, to payment based on national rates regardless of provider costs by 2002

d. Home Health prospective payment—15% across-the-board cut in payments in 2000 progressing toward full PPS in 2002

e. Outpatient payment modification—implementation of outpatient PPS in August, 2000 called Ambulatory Payment Classification (APCs; DHHS, 1998); patient co-pays were frozen

f. Teaching, DSH (disproportionate share) cutbacks—9% reduction in indirect medical education (IME) payments and 1% in DSH in 1998, with additional deductions for a total of 28.5% for IME and 5% for DSH by 2002

2. Estimated impact on pulmonary DRGs related to SNF discharges—using a 300-bed community hospital as an example, an increased inpatient length of stay secondary to new transfer rules could be a $375,000 loss in 1 year (Health Care Advisory Board, 1999).

3. Fear of loss of insurance coverage for a pre-existing condition due to the diagnosis of a chronic illness often prevents people from seeking

care until very ill. By that time, costs are higher for urgent care. Illustrating this point is the large number of asthmatic children who are often treated for multiple upper respiratory infections, rather than receiving a diagnosis of asthma and subsequently, appropriate treatment (AAAAI, 1999).

C. One other issue to be considered in a discussion of cost and resource utilization is individual patient quality of life goals. For example, the use of liquid oxygen versus the E-cylinder versus the H-tank, each of which has pros and cons to consider. Patients and their health care providers must balance cost issues with compliance and quality of life issues.

III. Impact of technology

A. Technology has exploded in almost every domain of modern life and is especially apparent in the medical field. However, rapidly expanding technology also translates into increases in health care costs. Examples of newer technologies related to respiratory care are whole body positron-emission tomography (PET) for the improved rate of detection of metastases in non-small cell lung cancer (Pieterman et al., 2000), photodynamic therapy (PDT), low-dose spiral computed tomography (CT) with the promise of dramatically increasing the early detection of lung cancer and ultimately lengthen survival (Henschke et al., 1999), lung transplantation and lung surfactants, to name a few.

B. Diagnostic studies account for approximately 20% of health care expenditures in the United States (Tierney, McPhee, & Papadakis, 1996), signifying the importance of establishing criteria for use of screening procedures, including properties of useful diagnostic tests and the impact on treatment, survival, and quality of life.

C. Implications for prolongation of care for severely and incurably ill— shortages of available funds for expensive technology, the projected nursing shortage over the next 20 years, and ethical considerations of autonomy, distributive justice, beneficence, maleficence should give us pause to re-think issues of futile care.

D. Reimbursement issues and the separation of the socioeconomic classes poses ethical problems as well. Americans have come to expect the best and latest in technology, even when not proven as a standard of care. The mentality has become one of "do everything" possible regardless of cost, even though few could afford the high-tech and high-cost procedures, such as lung transplantation, without insurance coverage. Medicare and some Medicaid programs pay for medically necessary organ transplants, but the uninsured have virtually no access (Bodenheimer & Grumbach, 1995). Some private insurance will also pay but many procedures will not be covered until research proves outcomes to be beneficial *and* cost-effective enough to be established as the standard of care.

IV. Strategies to improve effective utilization of resources

We have reviewed strategies used by payors in an effort to decrease costs. However, the public, as well as the healthcare industry, must also be prudent in the utilization of resources while maintaining or improving health outcomes.

A. The American Academy of Allergy, Asthma & Immunology included suggestions for improving resource utilization for asthmatic children in their 1999 guide (p. 137), many of which can be applied to health care in general.

1. Promote best practice guideline to clinicians and the public alike by respected community experts.

2. Encourage public and private funding for implementing and researching preventive care programs that are specifically targeted to at-risk groups.

3. Allocate funds for education.

4. Identify the most expensive users of care and develop systems to provide effective and cost-efficient care.

5. Consider ways to make transportation to clinic appointments possible for those in need (e.g., cab, bus, train, bus vouchers).

B. Smoking cessation—In general, cigarette smoking is the foremost cause of preventable morbidity and mortality in the United States. It accounted for 434,000 deaths and over 1.1 million years of potential life lost in 1993 alone. It is responsible for $100 billion in health care costs and lost productivity, 1 in every 5 deaths (ALA, 1999e) and untold suffering. Smoking cessation is the single most important lifestyle change a person can make.

1. Smoking cessation contributes to reversal of chronic bronchitis and improved pulmonary function (Tierney et al., 1996).

2. After 10–20 years of smoking cessation, lung cancer rates approach the rates of lifelong non-smokers (DHHS, 1991).

3. A Danish study by Dr. Kirsten Wisborg and colleagues of almost 25,000 live births over a 7-year period revealed women who smoked had more than three times the risk of losing a child to Sudden Infant Death Syndrome (SIDS) and that smoking cessation could potentially reduce mortality by up to 40% (Reuters Medical News, 2000).

4. There is no current standard for reimbursement of smoking cessation, though some corporations have had the foresight to incorporate a variety of services into their Health and Wellness disease management programs. Studies are currently being conducted to assess the effectiveness of smoking cessation aids in conjunction with education support programs.

5. The American Lung Association (1999e) advocates tobacco excise taxes, enforcement of youth access laws, restriction of smoking in public places, and restriction of tobacco advertising and promotion to reduce smoking prevalence and aid in cessation efforts.

C. Health promotion and disease prevention, the historical nursing model, can have significant impact on cost and quality of life. Vaccination is a simple intervention that significantly improves health outcomes while reducing health care costs.

1. Although annual flu severity is unpredictable, influenza vaccination is efficacious 70%–90% of the time in general. In the frail elderly, it is

less effective at prevention but is useful in reducing the complications of illness and death. At the current rate of illness and cost per case, an estimated $50 per patient episode could be saved (Blaiss, 1999).

2. The pneumococcal vaccine is less recognized by the general population and is even more underutilized than the flu vaccine. Although Medicare has paid for PPV since 1981, the Centers for Disease Control and Prevention estimates only 40% of Medicare patients have ever received it. The Health Care Financing Administration (HCFA) began an initiative through hospitals, then outpatient services, to screen Medicare beneficiaries for vaccination status in an effort to increase the rate of administration (Alabama Quality Assurance Foundation, 1999).

D. Pulmonary rehabilitation goals are to alleviate symptoms and optimize independent function. For patients with chronic lung disease, primarily COPD, the impact of a pulmonary rehab program following evidence-based guidelines is statistically and clinically significant. It is appropriate for any patient with stable pulmonary disease. Recommendations are based on evidence grades of A, B, and C, with A being the highest grade for established scientific evidence (American College of Chest Physicians [ACCP]/American Association of Cardiovascular and Pulmonary Rehabilitation [AACPR], 1997). Albeit rehab does not reverse or improve airflow obstruction (Maltais & Bourbeau, 1995), it does have multiple benefits

1. Impact on dyspnea—strength of evidence A; Pulmonary rehabilitation improves the symptoms of dyspnea in patients with COPD.
2. Impact on exercise tolerance—strength of evidence A; lower extremity exercise training improves exercise tolerance and ambulation.
3. Impact on quality of life—strength of evidence B; improvement in health-related quality of life (QOL) outcomes have been shown in comprehensive pulmonary rehab programs but further studies are required to measure disease-specific QOL.
4. Impact of health care utilization—strength of evidence B; the majority of studies evaluating resource utilization relating to pulmonary rehab have been non-randomized or observational. However, these have demonstrated a trend toward a decrease in the total number of hospital admissions as well as length of stay "in the years following completion of a comprehensive pulmonary rehab program compared to the year preceding rehabilitation" (Reuters Medical News, 2000).
5. Impact on mortality—strength of evidence C; there is no consistent evidence to support this conclusion; age and baseline FEV1 are the best predictors of mortality.

V. Implications for the clinician

As previously stated, having an understanding of costs, reimbursement issues, and impact of lung disease on society improves the clinician's approach to health care. For example, knowing that asthma education and utilization of self-management strategies decreases the number of asthma exacerbations, emergency visits, and mortality rates provides motivation for implementation of time-consuming education activities, such as peak flow monitoring and written Action Plans. Similarly, administration of the pneumococcal vaccine in high-risk patients decreases the incidence of pneumococcal pneumonia, and thereby reduces mortality rates, as well as the expense, pain and suffering of illness and hospitalization.

WEB SITES

http://www.medscape.com/pulmonarymedicine
http://www.lungusa.org
http://www.ginasthma.com
http://www.healthypeople.gov/
http://www.cdc.gov/nchs/products/pubs/pubd/hp2k/hp2k.htm

REFERENCES

Alabama Quality Assurance Foundation. (1999). Although underutilized, immunizations enhance care. *Quality Perspective*. Retrieved from http://www.aafp.org

American Academy of Allergy, Asthma & Immunology. (1999). *Pediatric asthma: Promoting best practice*. Milwaukee, WI: Author.

American College of Chest Physicians/American Association of Cardiovascular and Pulmonary Rehabilitation Pulmonary Rehabilitation Guidelines Panel. (1997). Pulmonary rehabilitation: Joint ACCP/AACVPR evidence-based guidelines. *Journal of Cardiopulmonary Rehabilitation, 17*, 371–405.

American Lung Association. (1999). *Estimated prevalence and incidence of lung disease by lung association territory*. Retrieved from http://www.lungusa. org/data/lae_00/EstPrev2pdf

American Lung Association, Epidemiology and Statistics Unit. (1999a). *Trends in asthma morbidity and mortality*. Retrieved from http://www.lungusa.org/data/asthma/asthma_700.pdf

American Lung Association, Epidemiology and Statistics Unit. (1999b). *Trends in chronic bronchitis and emphysema: Morbidity and mortality*. Retrieved from http://www.lungusa.org/data/copd/copd1.pdf

American Lung Association, Epidemiology and Statistics Unit. (1999c). *Trends in morbidity and mortality: Pneumonia, influenza and acute respiratory conditions*. Retrieved from http://www.lungusa.org/pi/pi_1.pdf

American Lung Association, Epidemiology and Statistics Unit. (1999d). *Trends in tuberculosis morbidity and mortality*. Retrieved from http://www.lungusa. org/data/tb/part1.pdf

American Lung Association, Epidemiology and Statistics Unit. (1999e). *Trends in cigarette smoking*. Retrieved from http://www.lungusa.org/data/smoke/smoke_1.pdf

American Lung Association, Epidemiology and Statistics Unit. (1999f). *Trends in lung cancer morbidity and mortality.*. Retrieved from http://www.lungusa.org/lc/lc_1.pdf

American Lung Association. (2000). *What is emphysema?* Retrieved from http://www.lungusa.org/diseases/lungemphysem.html

American Thoracic Society. (1995). Definitions, epidemiology, pathophysiology, diagnosis and staging. *American Journal of Respiratory and Critical Care Medicine, 152,* S78.

Blaiss, M. S. (1999). Influenza prevention and treatment: New options. *1999 American College of Allergy, Asthma & Immunology Annual Meeting.* Retrieved from www.medscape.com/medscape/cno/1999/ACAAI/Sory.cfm?story_id=879

Blancett, S. S., & Dominick, L. F., (Eds.). (1995). Changing paradigms: The impetus to reengineer health care. In *Reengineering nursing and health care: The handbook for organizationl transformation.* Gaithersburg, MD: Aspen Publishers.

Bodenheimer, T. S., & Grumbach, K. (1995). *Understanding health policy: A clinical approach* (1st ed.). Norwalk, CT: Appleton & Lange.

Brown, D. B. (1999). Managing sleep disorders. *Clinician Reviews, 9, 10,* 51–69.

CBS Healthwatch. 2000 Medscape, Inc. *Mastering managed care.* Retrieved from http://cbshealthwatch.medscape.com/medscape/p/G_library/article.asp

Chande, V. T., Krug, S. E., & Warm, E. F. (1996). Pediatric emergency department utilization habits: A consumer survey. *Pediatric Emergency Care, 12*(1), 27–30.

Doherty, D., Mandel, M., & Haggerty, M. (Eds.) (2000). Report from "Update on the management of COPD," presented at the annual meeting of the American College of Chest Physicians. *COPD: The Journal of Management, 1*(1), 16–19.

Edelman, C. L., & Mandle, C. L. (1994). *Health promotion throughout the lifespan* (3rd ed.). St. Louis, MO: Mosby-Year Book.

Eisenberg, L. D. (1999). Insurance coding for the diagnosis and treatment of obstructive sleep disorders. *Ear, Nose & Throat Journal, 78*(11), 858–860.

Fox, J. C. (1993). The role of nursing in public policy reform. *Journal of Psychosocial Nursing and Mental Health Service, 31*(8), 9–12.

Grasso, M. E., Weller, W. E., Shaffer, T. J., Diette, G. B., & Anderson, G. F. (1998). Capitation, managed care, and chronic obstructive pulmonary disease. *American Journal of Respiratory and Critical Care Medicine, 158*(1), 133–138.

Health Care Advisory Board. (1999). *Medicare Payment Reform: Executive Briefing on Health System Financial Performance under the Balanced Budget Act of 1997.* Washington, DC: The Advisory Board Company.

Henschke, C. I., McCauley, D. I., Yankelevitz, D. F., Naidich, D. P., McGuinness, G., Miettinen, O. S., et al. (1999). Early lung cancer action project: Overall design and findings from baseline screening. *The Lancet, 354,* 99–105.

Maltais, F., & Bourbeau, J. (1995). Medical management of emphysema. *Chest Surgery Clinics of North America, 5*(4), 673–689.

McCance, K. L., & Huether, S. E. (Eds.). (2002). Alterations of pulmonary function. *Pathophysiology: The Biologic Basis for Disease in Adults and Children* (4th ed., pp. 1158–1200). St. Louis: Mosby.

National Asthma and Education Prevention Program. (1997). *Expert Panel Report 2: Guidelines for the diagnosis and management of asthma.* National Institutes of Health, National Heart, Lung, and Blood Institute, Publication No. 97–4501.

National Heart, Lung, and Blood Institute/World Health Organization. (1995, January). Workshop Report. *Global Initiative for Asthma: Global Strategy for Asthma Management and Prevention.* National Institutes of Health, National Heart, Lung, and Blood Institute, Publication No. 95–3659.

Nelsen, L. M., Oritz, E., Fitterman, L. K., & Markson, L. E. (1998). *Evaluation of resource utilization among asthmatic and nonasthmatic patient populations.* Retrieved from http://www.ahsr.org/1998/abstracts/nelsen.htm

Nichol, K. L. (1999). Health and economic benefits of influenza and pneumococcal vaccinations in elderly patients. *Immunizing Adults Against Influenza and Pneumonia. Post Graduate Medicine: A Special Report.* Retrieved from www.postgradmed.com

Pieterman, R. M., van Putten, J. W. G., Meuzelaar, J. J., Mooyaart, E. L., Vaalburg, W., Koeter, G. H., et al. (2000). Preoperative staging of non-small cell lung cancer with positron-emission tomography. *The New England Journal of Medicine, 343,* 254–261.

Reuters Medical News. (2000). Link between smoking and SIDS confirmed in prospective study. Retrieved from http://respiratorycare.medscape.com/reuters/prof/2000/08/08.25/2000825clin002.html

Seidel, H. M., Ball, J. W., Dains, J. E., & Benedict, G. W. (Eds.). (2003). Chest and lungs. *Mosby's guide to physical examination* (5th ed., pp. 356–413). St. Louis: Mosby.

Siegel, C. (1999). Airway obstruction and sleep disorders: More common than you thought. *1999 American College of Allergy, Asthma & Immunology Annual Meeting, Day 1—November 12, 1999.* Retrieved from http://www.medscape.com/Medscape/cno/1999/ACAAI/Story.cfm?story_id=880

Sly, R. M. (2000). Decreases in asthma mortality in the United States (Abstract). *Annals of Allergy, Asthma and Immunology, 85*(2), 121–127.

Thomas, C. L. (Ed.). (1997). *Taber's Cyclopedic Medical Dictionary* (18th ed.). Philadelphia: F. A. Davis.

Tierney, L. M., McPhee, S. J., & Papadakis, M. A. (1996). Diagnostic testing & medical decision making. In S. J. MePhee, M. A. Papadakis, & L. M. Tireney (Eds.), *Current medical diagnosis & treatment* (35th ed., pp. 26–35). Stamford, CN: Appleton & Lange.

U.S. Department of Health and Human Services, Public Health Service. (1991). *Healthy People 2000: National Health Promotion and Disease Prevention Objectives.* Washington, DC: U.S. Government Printing Office.

U.S. Department of Health and Human Services (1998). Health Care Financing Administration, Office of Inspector General. Medicare Program; Prospective Payment System for Hospital Outpatient Services; Proposed Rules. *Federal Register, 63*(173), 47561.

Wilson, D. J. (1997). Pulmonary rehabilitation exercise program for high-risk thoracic surgical patients. *Chest Surgery Clinics of North America, 7*(4), 697–706.

Zwillich, T. (2000). Immigration curbs recommended to reduce number of uninsured. Reuters Medical News, August 3, 2000. Retrieved from http://respiratorycare.medscape.com/reuters/prof/2000/08/08.03/20000803plcy002.html

SUGGESTED READINGS

Landis, S. H., Murray, T., Bolden, S., & Wingo, P. A. (1998). Cancer statistics 1998. *Cancer Journal for Clinicians, 48,* 6–29.

Landis, S. H., Murray, T., Bolden, S., & Wingo, P. A. (1999). Cancer statistics 1999. *Cancer Journal for Clinicians, 49,* 8–31.

Patient Advocacy

43

Anne H. Boyle and Dianne L. Locke

INTRODUCTION

Patient advocacy is a key part of the nurse's role in caring for vulnerable persons with pulmonary disease and their families. While there are barriers to the nurse's fulfilling this role, both the American Nurses Association and the Respiratory Nursing Society strongly endorse advocacy as a significant part of nursing practice. One area in which nurses often find themselves advocating on behalf of the patient and family is in the area of advance directives.

1. An advocate is one who acts as an instrument on behalf of a vulnerable individual.
2. The professional role mandates advocacy.
3. Advance directives include both living wills and Durable Powers of Attorney for Health Care.

I. What it means to advocate
   A. Definition—acting as an instrument on behalf of the vulnerable individual as needed
   B. Historical perspective
      1. Health care providers have long struggled with decisions about appropriate care, especially in critically and/or chronically ill individuals.
      2. Physician held complete control over plan of care.
      3. Society is recognizing individual's having a right to control own fate.
      4. Managed care has severely limited physician time with patients.
      5. Non-physician professionals have successfully demonstrated skills and unique contributions to multidisciplinary teams.
      6. Physician may no longer be "team captain."
      7. Interdisciplinary care is now the norm and often expected by consumers.

C. Barriers to advocacy
  1. System
     a. Administrative structures that inhibit full interdisciplinary participation
     b. Policies and procedures that interfere with professional practice
        i. Who can talk to the MD
        ii. Who can make referrals, etc.
     c. Fear of reprisal for advocacy behavior (Hewitt, 2002)
  2. Interpersonal
     a. "Doctor-nurse game" style of communication (Stein, 1967)
        i. Classic article by Stein describing game between physicians and nurses based on male-female power relationships
        ii. Physician asks for and gets advice in way that makes it possible to retain pretense of omnipotence
        iii. Nurse "makes suggestions" to doctor in a way that allows him to think course of action was his idea
     b. Passive-aggressive behaviors by patient, family, or clinicians
     c. Unwillingness or insecurity in assuming professional role
     d. Older and less educated individuals defer to physician
     e. Opportunities for misunderstanding and disagreement
        i. Physician to physician
        ii. Physician to nurse and other team members
        iii. Nurse to other health care team members, including physician
        iv. Staff to patient and family
     f. Inadequate communication skills: Staff lack assertiveness skills
     g. Inadequate communication skills: Patients and families communicate information to the MD that is different from the information given the other caregivers
        i. "I'm fine" when severe pain is the reality
        ii. "The doctor's so busy, I didn't want to bother ..."
     h. Inadequate communication skills: Patients and families often need coaxing to be entirely forthright about certain situations (e.g., financial issues)
     i. Failure to appreciate the skills and contributions of the various health care team members
  3. Physiologic (See chapter 45 "End-of-Life Issues")
     a. Often difficult to determine when time to "care" vs. "cure"
     b. Often subjective with only a few physiologic parameters to guide decision process
  4. Legal: fear of tort claim or other disciplinary action for acting on behalf of the patient
  5. Patient preferences may be fluid as patient or agent for care may change goals or desires on a day to day basis making it difficult to discern the plan of care

D. Professional role and mandates regarding advocacy
  1. Statements from American Nurses Association (ANA) Code of Ethics (American Nurses Association [ANA], 2001)
    a. The nurse's primary commitment is to the patient, whether an individual, family, group, or community.
    b. The nurse promotes, advocates for, and strives to protect the health, safety, and rights of the patient.
  2. Position Statements from ANA
    a. The nurse's role in advocacy is critical to ongoing implementation of the Patient Self-Determination Act (ANA, 1996).
    b. It is the responsibility of nurses to facilitate informed decision making for patients making choices (ANA, 1996).
  3. Standards and statement on the scope of Respiratory Nursing Society. (Dean-Barr et al., 1994) (See Table 43.1)
  4. Legal precedents have affirmed advocacy role for nurses (Davidson & Degner, 1998)
  5. Patient Bill of Rights and Responsibilities
E. Arenas of advocacy (Liaschenko, 1995)
  1. Physical
    a. Secure competent care for physical needs
      i. Assessment of status
      ii. Symptom management
      iii. Reduction of restraint use
    b. System navigation
      i. Information regarding resources and availability of resources (Hellwig, Yam, & DiGiulio, 2003)
      ii. Referrals, as needed
    c. Accurate reporting of symptoms, signs, or patient/family concerns and re-reporting as needed to secure appropriate care or response
    d. Environmental assessment and modification
  2. Psychological
    a. Support information seeking by patient and family
    b. Interpret and explain complex language and procedures
    c. Assure informed decision making and consent by providing complete information regarding options and approaches
    d. Actively encourage asking of questions—assist in their formulation
    e. Supportive presence, as needed
  3. Integrity of self
    a. Ascertain patient's desires regarding therapies and treatment
    b. Assess patient's *desired* level of participation as not all want to exert control or self-manage
    c. Assist with clarification of values and goals
    d. Promote use of identified values and goals in decision making
    e. Refrain from imposing own values and goals upon patient and family

Table 43.1

Standard V

The respiratory nurse's decisions and actions on behalf of clients are determined in an ethical manner.

Measurement Criteria

1. The nurse's practice is guided by the Code for Nurses.
2. The nurse maintains client confidentiality.
3. The nurse acts as a client advocate.
4. The nurse promotes the provision of information and discussion regarding the respiratory client's right to an advance directive.
5. The nurse ascertains the respiratory client's desires regarding ventilatory support.
6. The nurse delivers care in a non-judgmental and non-discriminatory manner that is sensitive to client diversity.
7. The nurse delivers care in a manner that preserves and protects client autonomy, dignity and rights.
8. The nurse seeks available resources to help formulate ethical decisions.
9. The nurse participates in decision making regarding allocation of scarce resources.

From *Standards and Statement on the Scope of Respiratory Nursing Practice,* (1994), p. 17.

F. Effective approaches for advocacy enhancement
   1. "As members of a multidisciplinary health team, nurses have a moral and ethical responsibility to ensure that their patients have the ability and capacity to make treatment decisions, and medical information they have been given concerning treatment options" (Davidson & Degner, 1999, p. 131).
   2. Assertiveness and communication skills education
   3. Interdisciplinary team meetings
   4. Organizational structure that empowers staff while encouraging openness to critical review (Hart, Yates, Clinton, & Windsor, 1998)
      a. Group problem solving.
      b. Groups characterized by collegial or collaborative relationships, defined by Aroskar (1998, p. 313) as "working together with mutual respect for the contributions and accountabilities of each profession to the shared goal of quality patient care."
   5. Health care system structure that enhances patient autonomy
   6. Education of staff, consumers, and the public
   7. Ethics committee consults initiated by any interested party without reprisal
II. Values and beliefs
   A. Influence upon decision making
      1. Self-concept and self-identity

       2. Personal values regarding life quality, pain and suffering, independence, life and death, and economics have profound impact

       3. Awareness of cultural influences (Seifert, 2002), family dynamics and previous experiences with health care enable staff to understand and accept patient/agent decisions; respect for patient/agent decision making does not imply agreement

  B. Staff vs. patient

       1. Patient autonomy is foremost concept.

       2. Staff role is to support patient in decision making by providing correct and complete information and encouraging open dialogue.

       3. Nurse may decide to remove self from setting if activities and practices violate personal value system by seeking employment in another setting or requesting removal from case.

  C. Conflict resolution

       1. Must refrain from paternalistic approach that imposes own values and goals upon the patient

       2. Active advocacy on behalf of patient within parameters of known patient preferences

       3. Ethics committee consultation as needed to assist in conflict resolution

III. Advance directives (Scanlon, 2003)

  A. Historical perspective

       1. Patient Self-Determination Act 1990 mandated that health care systems that receive federal funds must inform patients of their rights to participate in determining the goals and directions of their care.

       2. The Study to Understand Prognoses and Preferences for Outcomes and Risks of Treatment (SUPPORT) found that advance directives were largely ignored (SUPPORT Investigators, 1995).

       3. Subsequent studies indicate that a Durable Power of Attorney for Health Care is significantly associated with do not resuscitate (DNR) orders and comfort care plans (Ramsey, 2001).

  B. Purpose: to provide direction in the case of terminal or irreversible illness, when the patient can no longer speak for him/herself

       1. Can be done by any competent adult.

       2. Guidelines for those under 18 vary among states.

       3. Can be changed either verbally or in writing and any subsequent changes take precedence over previous wishes as long as the patient can speak for self.

       4. Generally requires two physicians to determine that this status has been reached.

  C. Types

       1. Living will: directives to physicians about treatments that individual would or would not want to prolong life (Ramsey, 2001)

          a. Has legal status that varies from state to state.

          b. Does not allow for designation of agent—someone to speak legally for patient in event of coma, altered mental status, etc.

c. If individual is pregnant, living will is invalid if physician aware of pregnancy.

2. Durable power of attorney for health care (Ramsey, 2001)
   a. Legal document that enables patient to designate the individual(s) to speak on his/her behalf in event of incapacity to do so
      i. Applies *only* to health care issues
      ii. Is not related to financial or business or other personal power of attorney
   b. Person who has been appointed by patient is called proxy, surrogate, or health care agent
   c. Agent has been informed by patient about wishes and values regarding health care in the event of terminal or irreversible illness and is to convey those wishes to the health care team
   d. Written, signed, and witnessed
   e. Preferred over living will
      i. Communicates individual's values and may be used for health care decisions, not just life-sustaining treatment (Ramsey, 2001)
      ii. Has legal standing and decreases conflict in determining plan of care since patient has already determined it
      iii. Increases awareness of health care team of individual's right to autonomy
      iv. Increases lay population awareness of issues regarding self-determination

3. Nurse's role (Briggs & Colvin, 2002; Sheehan & Schirm, 2003)
   a. Determine existence of document.
      i. Obtain copy for medical record.
      ii. Be aware of contents.
      iii. Ascertain with patient/family as to current accuracy.
      iv. Ensure that all members of health team aware of and use document in planning care.
   b. If none exists, explore with patient and family advisability of initiating and using advance directive.
      i. Work in conjunction with physician
      ii. Consult social work and pastoral care, as needed
      iii. Role model by having own advance directive in place
      iv. Participate in family and community to enhance knowledge and development of advance directives
   c. Communicate to physician any changes verbalized by the individual.
   d. Initiate appropriate action if advance directive appears to be violated or ignored.
      i. "Nurses, because of their insights into patients' preferences and their role as patient advocates, have a legitimate role in monitoring compliance of treatment with patient's preferences as expressed in advanced directives" (Johns, 1996, p. 152).

ii. Court actions have upheld individual right to autonomy vs. paternalistic control by medical team.

iii. Interdisciplinary team meeting.

iv. Ethics committee consult.

v. Reporting via chain of command.

e. Thorough documentation of any conversations, questions, or requests made by patient or agent regarding care.

i. Courts view oral advance directives favorably.

ii. When made by competent individuals, courts have considered these statements when making decisions to terminate life-prolonging treatments (Ramsey, 2001).

f. Mentor and role model for other health care professionals in the practice of patient advocacy.

g. Participate on relevant committees and organizational structures.

h. Recognize the moral and ethical conflicts that influence individual decision making and approach these discussions with respect.

WEB SITES

Alpha 1 Association: http://www.alpha1.org
American Lung Association: http://www.lungusa.org
American Nurses Association: http://www.nursingworld.org/
Asthma and Allergy Foundation of America: http://www.aafa.org
Asthma and Allergy Network Mothers of Asthmatics: http://www.aanma.org
Center for Patient Advocacy: http://www.patientadvocacy.com
Cystic Fibrosis Foundation: http://www.cff.org/
Efforts: Emphysema Foundation for our Right to Survive: http://www.emphysema.net
The National Emphysema Foundation: http://www.emphysemafoundation.org
Initiative for Chronic Obstructive Pulmonary Disease: www.goldcopd.org
Pulmonary Fibrosis Foundation: http://www.pulmonaryfibrosis.org/
Pulmonary Hypertension Association: http://www.phassociation.org/
Second Wind Lung Transplant Association: http://www.2ndwind.org/

REFERENCES

American Nurses Association. (1996). *Position statements on the nurse's role in end-of-life decisions*. Washington, DC: American Nurses Association.

American Nurses Association. (2001). *Code of ethics for nurses with interpretive statements*. Washington, DC: American Nurses Association.

Aroskar, M. A. (1998). Ethical working relationships in patient care: Challenges and possibilities. *Nursing Clinics of North America, 33*(2), 313–324.

Briggs, L., & Colvin, E. (2002). The nurse's role in end-of-life decision-making for patients and families. *Geriatric Nursing, 23*(6), 302–310.

Davison, B. J., & Degner, L. F. (1998). Promoting patient decision-making in life and death situations. *Seminars in Oncology Nursing, 14*(2), 129–136.

Dean-Barr, S. L., Gieger-Bronsky, M., Gift, A., & Hagarty, E. (Eds.). (1994). *Standards and statement on the scope of respiratory nursing practice/American Nurses Association.* Washington, DC: American Nurses publishing.

Hart, G., Yates, P., Clinton, M., & Windsor, C. (1998). Mediating conflict and control: Practice challenges for nurses working in palliative care. *International Journal of Nursing Studies, 35*(5), 252–258.

Hellwig, S. D., Yam, M., & DiGiulio, M. (2003). Nurse case managers' perceptions of advocacy: A phenomenological inquiry. *Lippincott's Case Management, 8*(2), 53–65.

Hewitt, J. (2002). A critical review of the arguments debating the role of the nurse advocate. *Journal of Advanced Nursing, 37*(5), 439–445.

Johns, J. (1996). Advanced directives and opportunities for nurses. *Image, 28*(2), 149–153.

Liaschenko, J. (1995). Ethics in the work of acting for patients. *Advances in Nursing Science, 18*(2), 1–12.

Ramsey, G. C. (2001). Legal aspects of palliative care. In B. R. Ferrell & N. Coyle (Eds.), *Textbook of palliative nursing* (pp. 180–216). New York: Oxford University Press.

Scanlon, C. (2003). Ethical concerns in end-of-life care. *American Journal of Nursing, 103*(1), 48–55.

Seifert, P. (2002). Ethics in perioperative practice: Commitment to the patient. *AORN Journal, 76*(1), 153–154, 156–160.

Sheehan, D. K., & Schirm, V. (2003). End-of-life care of older adults. *American Journal of Nursing, 103*(11), 48–58.

Stein, L. L. (1967). The doctor-nurse game. *Archives of General Psychiatry, 16,* 699–703.

SUPPORT Principal Investigators. (1995). A controlled trial to improve care for seriously ill hospitalized patients. *Journal of the American Medical Association, 274*(20), 1591–1958.

Ethical Dilemmas

44

Sue Galanes

INTRODUCTION

This chapter will address ethical theory, ethical principles, ethical rules, and virtues in professional roles.

The primary ethical principles are: autonomy, beneficence, nonmaleficence, futility, and justice. Ethical rules of veracity, privacy, confidentiality, and fidelity, as well as the virtues compassion, discernment, trustworthiness, and integrity support the ethical principles.

I. Ethical theory: Both traditional and contemporary theories provide structure for needed discussion. This discussion may lead to choices for action or nonaction. They are not meant as absolute solutions (Beauchamp & Childress, 1994; Mappes & DeGrazia, 1996; Veatch, 1997).

    A. Utilitarianism (consequence-based theory): Accepts the principle of utility. Consequentialism-based theory holds that actions are right or wrong according to the balance of their good and bad consequences. This principle asserts that we should always produce the maximal balance of positive value over disvalue (or the least possible disvalue, if only undesirable results can be achieved). The greatest good should be assessed in terms of the total intrinsic value produced by an action. It concerns outcome, or the consequences of the action. Found in the writings of Jeremy Bentham (1748–1832) and John Stuart Mill (1806–1873).

    B. Kantianism (obligation-based theory): Also called deontological (a theory that some features of actions other than or in addition to consequences make the actions right or wrong). This theory is called Kantian from the ethical thought of Immanuel Kant (1724–1804), who shaped many of its formulations. Kantian thought is that morality is grounded in pure reason, not in tradition, intuition, conscience, emotion, or attitudes such as sympathy. Human beings are creatures with power to resist desire and the capacity to act by rational considerations. Moral obligation depends on the rule that determines the individual's will. An action possesses moral worth only if performed by an agent with a good will and morally valid reason. One must not act only in accordance with but for the sake of obligation, that a person's motive for acting must come from recognition of what is morally required. It concerns obligation or duty.

C. Character ethics (virtue-based theory): Emphasizes that the agents who perform actions make choices. A morally good person is more likely than others to understand what should be done and more likely to act on moral ideals. This is a person with ingrained motivation and desire to perform right actions (not a rule follower, but a moral model). This questions which action is right, best, or obligatory when addressing the ethical principles and corresponding virtues.

D. Liberal individualism (rights-based theory): A right is a justified claim validated by moral principles and rules. It consists of the concept that in a democratic society the individual is protected and allowed to pursue personal projects. Statements of rights provide protection of life, liberty, expression, and property. They protect against oppression, unequal treatment, intolerance, and arbitrary invasion of privacy.

E. Communitarianism (community-based theory): This theory is based on ethics being derived from communal values, the common good, social goals, traditional practices and cooperative virtues.

F. Ethics of care (relationship-based accounts): An emphasis on traits valued in intimate personal relationships, such as sympathy, compassion, fidelity, discernment, and love. Caring refers to the emotional commitment and willingness to act on behalf of persons with whom one has a significant relationship. Two constructive themes are present: mutual interdependence and emotional response.

G. Casuistry (case-based reasoning): Moral belief and knowledge evolve incrementally through reflection on cases in which a consensus is formed. This consensus is then extended to new cases by analogy.

H. Convergency of theories: In moral reasoning we often blend principles, rules, rights, virtues, passions, analogies, and interpretations of the above theories.

II. Ethical principles

A. Autonomy: self-determination, individual choice; freedom of will.
1. Essential conditions to autonomy
   a. Liberty: independence from controlling influences
   b. Capacity for intentional action
2. Traits of the autonomous person include the capacity of self-governance such as, understanding, reasoning, deliberating, and independent choice.
3. Competence in decision making is closely connected to questions about the validity of consent: questions about if the subject is psycho-

logically or legally capable of adequate decision making (American Thoracic Society [ATS], 1991; Beauchamp & Childress, 1994).

   a. A patient has decision making capacity when a patient has

      i. The ability to comprehend information relevant to the decision at hand.

      ii. The ability to deliberate in accordance with his or her own values and goals.

      iii. The ability to communicate with caregivers.

   b. In complex cases, psychiatric consultations should be sought when the state of competence cannot be clearly identified.

   c. If a patient lacks decision-making capacity, respecting autonomy means that an appropriate surrogate should make decisions based upon

      i. The patient's explicit directions, or

      ii. If there are none; knowledge of the patient's preferences and values, or

      iii. If sufficient knowledge is not available, on the basis of how a reasonable person in the patient's circumstances would choose.

4. Informed consent: One can give an informed consent to an intervention if one is competent to act, receives a thorough disclosure, comprehends the disclosure, acts voluntarily, and consents to the intervention (ATS, 1991).

5. If the patient is capable of participating in the discussion, it is imperative to respect his or her autonomy, even if the family is in disagreement with the patient's decision.

   a. The patient's consent to involve the family in the discussion should be obtained.

   b. Under conditions of severe disagreement, the health care provider may choose to repeat conversations with the patient in the presence of the family, so that they may witness for themselves the patient's decision (McGee, Weinacker, & Raffin, 2000).

B. Beneficence: The biomedical ethical principle is the principle to do good; to benefit the patient; and to promote the patients well-being. Fundamentally this means the health care provider attempts to preserve the patient's life. The obligation to promote the patient's good involves identifying the benefits and burdens of the treatment from the patient's perspective.

1. Paternalism: Conflicts between beneficence and autonomy. An intentional overriding of one person's known preference or actions by another person, where the person who overrides justifies the action, with the goal of benefiting or avoiding harm to the person whose will is overridden (Beauchamp & Childress, 1994).

C. Nonmaleficence: The ethical principle that means to do no harm.

1. Moral rules that support nonmaleficence (Beauchamp & Childress, 1994):

   a. Do not kill.

   b. Do not cause pain or suffering to others.

        c. Do not incapacitate others.

        d. Do not cause offense to others.

        e. Do not deprive others of the goods of life.

    2. Life-sustaining treatment is not obligatory if its burdens outweigh its benefits to the patient (Gilligan & Raffin, 1996).

        a. Life-sustaining treatment sometimes violates patient's interests. Such as, pain can be so severe and physical restraints so burdensome that they outweigh the anticipated benefit of a brief prolongation of life. In this case treatment would be inhumane or cruel and in violation of the principle of nonmaleficence.

  D. Futility: A futile action is one that cannot achieve the goals of the action (Ethics Committee of the Society of Critical Care Medicine, 1997). The likelihood of failure may be predictable; it may be immediately obvious or may become apparent only after many failed attempts. The intended physiologic effect cannot be produced. Claims of futility involve the prediction and evaluation of outcomes, which are usually probable rather than certain (Schneiderman, Jecker, & Jonsen, 1990; Youngner, 1996).

    1. The right to refuse treatment does not imply a right to demand treatment (Emmanuel, 1988). If health professionals cannot provide medical benefits, no obligation exists to follow patient or surrogate demands for interventions (Luce, 1995; Ethics Committee of SCCM, 1997; ATS, 1991).

    2. Futility should be distinguished from hopelessness (Schneiderman, Jecker, & Jonsen, 1990). Hope and hopelessness have more relation to desire, faith, and denial. Hope may replace reasonable expectation. As the chance for success decreases, hope may actually increase. Hope is what human beings summon up to seek a miracle against overwhelming odds.

    3. A fact of life is that life has an ending (Richmond, 1994).

  E. Justice: Supports the fair allocation of medical resources. This pertains both to the individual's access to an adequate level of health care, and to the distribution of available health care resources. The terms *fairness*, what is deserved, and *entitlement* are used to explain justice. Justice places ethical limits on the patient's liberty to demand scarce medical resources as well.

III. Ethical rules

  A. Veracity: Truthfulness; to deal honestly with patients and colleagues. Virtues of candor and truthfulness are among the most widely praised character traits of health professionals in contemporary biomedical ethics (Beauchamp & Childress, 1994).

  B. Privacy: Respect for privacy. Shielding information from others and protecting an area of individual freedom without interference. It is a right to limit physical or informational accessibility to others.

  C. Confidentiality: Involves rules of privacy and safeguarding patient confidences. It is present when one person discloses information to another and the person to whom the information is disclosed pledges not to divulge the information without the confider's permission.

    D. Fidelity: The faithfulness of one human being to another. A disposition to be true to one's word. The health care relationship is founded on trust and confidence resulting in professional loyalty.

IV. Virtues in professional roles (Beauchamp & Childress, 1994)

    A. Compassion: The moral sentiment of caring; an attitude of active regard for another persons welfare, with sympathy and tenderness.

    B. Discernment: Practical wisdom; the ability to make judgments and reach decisions without being influenced by outside fears or personal attachments.

    C. Trustworthiness: A confident belief in and reliance upon the ability and moral character of another person.

    D. Integrity: An individual's core beliefs about himself; soundness, reliability, wholeness, and integration of moral character; fidelity in adherence to moral norms.

V. Conclusion

Complex situations abound in health care, and use of ethical principles, ethical rules, and virtues in professional roles can assist the health caregiver, the patient, and significant others to achieve intentional chosen outcomes on the patient's behalf.

REFERENCES

American Thoracic Society (ATS). (1991). Withholding and withdrawing life-sustaining therapy. *American Review of Respiratory Diseases, 144,* 726–731.

Beauchamp, T., & Childress, J. (1994). *Principles of biomedical ethics.* Oxford: Oxford University Press.

Emanuel, E. (1988). A review of the ethical and legal aspects of terminating medical care. *The American Journal of Medicine, 84,* 291–301.

Ethics Committee of the Society of Critical Care Medicine. (1997). Consensus Statement of the Society of Critical Care Medicine's Ethics Committee regarding futile and other possible inadvisable treatments. *Critical Care Medicine, 25,* 887–891.

Gilligan, T., & Raffin, T. A. (1996). Rapid withdrawal of life support. *Chest, 108,* 1047–1048.

Luce, J. (1995). Physicians do not have a responsibility to provide futile or unreasonable care if a patient of family insists. *Critical Care Medicine, 23,* 760–766.

Mappes, T., & DeGrazia, D. (1996). *Biomedical ethics.* New York: McGraw-Hill.

Mc Gee, D. C., Weinacker, A. B., & Raffin, T. A. (2000). Withdrawing life support from the critically ill. *Chest, 118,* 1238–1239.

Richmond, K. (1994). A time to die. *The Journal of Pastoral Care, 48,* 407–409.

Schneiderman, L., Jecker, N., & Jonsen, A. (1990). Medical futility: Its meaning and ethical implications. *Annals of Internal Medicine, 112,* 949–954.

Veatch, R. (1997). *Medical ethics.* Sudbury, MA: Jones and Bartlett Publishers.
Youngner, S. (1996). Medical futility. *Critical Care Clinics, 12,* 165–178.

SUGGESTED READINGS

ACCP/SCCM Consensus Panel. (1990). Ethical and moral guidelines for the initiating, continuation, and withdrawal of intensive care. *Chest, 97,* 949–958.
Campbell, M. (1995). Interpretation of an ambiguous advance directive. *Dimensions of Critical Care Nursing, 14,* 226–232.
Curtis, J., & Hudson, L. (1994). Emergent assessment and management of acute
respiratory failure in COPD. *Clinics in Chest Medicine, 15,* 481–500.
Heffner, J., Fahy, B., & Barbieri, C. (1996). Advance directive education during
pulmonary rehabilitation. *Chest, 109,* 373–379.

End-of-Life Issues

45

Anne H. Boyle and Dianne L. Locke

INTRODUCTION

Palliative care is directed primarily toward symptom management and improving quality of life. Patients with advanced pulmonary disease often experience unpleasant symptoms, such as severe dyspnea, at the end of life. Respiratory nurses interacting with patients and families across the care continuum must be advocates for adequate symptom relief and an appropriate focus on palliation. In critical care units, terminal weaning is a process that must be managed well with the goal of allowing the patient to terminate mechanical ventilation with maximum comfort.

1. Dyspnea is a distressing symptom experienced by many patients at the end of life.
2. Palliative care is patient and family centered and directed toward managing symptoms and improving quality of life.
3. Hospice care is only one aspect of palliative care. It has been underused by patients with advanced respiratory disease because of difficulty in determining prognosis.
4. Focus on palliation often begins too late to be effective.

I. Palliative care
   A. Definition—active and compassionate care directed toward symptom management and improving quality of life for the patient whose disease does not respond to curative treatment; not all palliative care patients are nearing the end of life (Ferrell & Coyle, 2002)
   B. Goals identified by World Health Organization (Johnston & Abraham, 1995)
      1. Affirms life and regards dying as a normal process
      2. Provides relief from pain and other distressing symptoms

3. Integrates psychological and spiritual aspects of patient care
4. Offers support system to help patients live as actively as possible
5. Offers support system to help family cope during patient's illness and their own bereavement

C. Principles of palliative care (Last Acts, 1997)
   1. An approach that is foremost patient-centered
   2. Encourages family involvement
   3. Identifies and honors preferences of patient and family
   4. Assists patients in establishing goals of care
   5. Strives to meet patients' preferences
   6. Encourages advance care planning
   7. Recognizes potential for conflict among stakeholders
   8. Appreciates that dying is a critical period in life of patient and responds aggressively to suffering
   9. Places high priority on physical comfort and functional capacity
   10. Provides holistic support to patient and family
   11. Alleviates isolation
   12. Assists with issues of life review, life completion, and life closure
   13. Extends support to family in their bereavement
   14. Utilizes strengths of interdisciplinary resources
   15. Acknowledges and addresses caregiver concerns
   16. Builds systems and mechanisms of support

D. Recommended competencies for end-of-life nursing care (American Association of Colleges of Nursing [AACN], 1997)
   1. Recognize dynamic changes in population demographics, health care economics, and service delivery that necessitate improved professional preparation for end-of-life care
   2. Promote the provision of comfort care to the dying as an active, desirable, and important skill, and an integral component of nursing care
   3. Communicate effectively and compassionately with the patient, family, and health care team members about end-of-life issues
   4. Recognize one's own attitudes, feelings, values, and expectations about death and the individual, cultural, and spiritual diversity existing in these beliefs and customs
   5. Demonstrate respect for patient's views and wishes during end-of-life care
   6. Collaborate with interdisciplinary team members while implementing the nursing role in end-of-life care
   7. Use scientifically based standardized tools to assess symptoms (e.g., pain, dyspnea [breathlessness], constipation, anxiety, fatigue, nausea/vomiting, and altered cognition) experienced by patients at the end of life
   8. Use data from symptom assessment to plan and intervene in symptom management using state-of-the-art traditional and complementary approaches
   9. Evaluate the impact of traditional, complementary, and technological therapies on patient-centered outcomes

10. Assess and treat multiple dimensions, including physical, psychological, social, and spiritual needs, to improve quality at the end of life

11. Assist the patient, family, colleagues, and one's self to cope with suffering, grief, loss, and bereavement in end-of-life care

12. Apply legal and ethical principles in the analysis of complex issues in end-of-life care, recognizing the influence of personal values, professional codes, and patient preferences

13. Identify barriers and facilitators to patients' and caregivers' effective use of resources

14. Demonstrate skill at implementing a plan for improved end-of-life care within a dynamic and complex health care delivery system

15. Apply knowledge gained from palliative care research to end-of-life education and care

E. Current health care system as reflected by recent studies
   1. Results of SUPPORT study (1995)
      a. Study to Understand Prognoses and Preferences for Outcomes and Risks of Treatment—study of seriously ill, hospitalized patients
      b. Goal: to improve five outcomes of care at the end of life
         i. Patient-physician agreement on CPR preferences
         ii. Incidence and timing of DNR orders
         iii. Days in ICU, in coma, or on ventilator before death
         iv. Pain
         v. Hospital resource use
      c. Study intervention, designed to improve outcomes, had no effect
      d. Findings: most end-of-life care is "routine" and not necessarily based on patient/family wishes
   2. Institute of Medicine study (Field & Cassel, 1997)
      a. Concluded that there were serious problems in end-of-life care
      b. Made recommendations for policymakers aimed at improving care and addressing deficiencies in the health care system

F. When to focus on palliation—how do providers know when it's time?
   1. Illness trajectory for pulmonary disease
      a. Characterized by uncertainty
      b. Ambiguous dying trajectory (Pattison, 1984)
      c. Patients with advanced lung disease tend to live for variable lengths of time in a "continuous state of poor health punctuated by exacerbations" (Fox et al., 1999, p. 1644)
      d. Although there are many types of advanced pulmonary disease, end-stage events limited to a few frequent pathways (Herbst, 1996)
         i. Respiratory failure (hypoxemia and/or hypercapnea)
         ii. Congestive heart failure
         iii. Infection
   2. Goals of care
      a. While most care in chronic lung diseases is palliative, dilemma facing clinicians is determining when to focus on palliation.

623

    b. Multiple goals may apply at the same time, and goals may also change over time, with a gradual shift of focus to palliative care.

    c. Initially, goals may focus more on attempts at cure and prolongation of life.

    d. Relief of suffering should be pursued at same time as life prolongation, providing early access to symptom management and supportive care; palliative care can begin at time of diagnosis.

G. Prognostic Indicators: Determination of prognosis in persons with advanced lung disease complex and challenging (van Gunten & Twaddle, 1996)

  1. Impaired functional ability (van Gunten & Twaddle, 1996)

    a. Indicated by declining ability to perform activities of daily living

    b. Greater the functional impairment, more advanced the illness

    c. Karnovsky Performance Status Scale a useful assessment tool; scores range in 10-point increments from 0 (death) to 100 (fully functional); patient with advanced disease and score of 50 or less has increased risk of dying in next 6 months

  2. Impaired nutritional status (van Gunten & Twaddle, 1996)

    a. Unintentional weight loss of more than 10% over a 6-month time period

    b. Serum albumin less than 2.5 g/dL

    c. Body weight < 90% of ideal body weight

  3. Advanced age and FEV_1 less than 30% predicted (Hodgkin, 1990) for patients with COPD

    a. Prospective study of 985 patients with COPD found above two factors somewhat predictive.

    b. These patients had marked increase in mortality, but there was significant variability.

  4. Other markers of decline in COPD

    a. Cor pulmonale

    b. Rate of decline in FEV_1 > 40 ml/yr

    c. Failure of therapy

    d. Prior episodes of respiratory failure

  5. BODE index proposed by Celli et al. (2004) for COPD patients includes body-mass index, FEV_1 % predicted, dyspnea score, and distance walked in 6 minutes

H. Management of dyspnea: Use of opioids (see chapter 10 "Dyspnea") Morphine is the most common (see Table 45.1) and standard treatment for relief of dyspnea near death.

  1. Site of action opioid receptors located in CNS

  2. Stimulation of μ-1 receptors provides analgesia

  3. Hypothesized mode of action in dyspnea

    a. Stimulate μ-2 receptors, which alters perception of breathlessness and decreases ventilatory response to changes in blood gases (Weatherill, 1995)

    b. Reduce pulmonary edema through venodilation and resultant decrease in preload

4. Routes of administration
   a. Choose least invasive, most effective route (Kazanowski, 2001)
   b. Oral preferred as patient tolerates
   c. Sublingual may be used
      i. Although not intended for this route, may be used if patient unable to swallow
      ii. Use liquid or crush and dissolve pills and place under tongue or against buccal mucosa—most is actually swallowed and not absorbed through mucosa (Kazanowski, 2001)
   d. Intravenous
      i. May be used for rapid onset of action and in terminal weaning situations
      ii. Patient-controlled analgesia (PCA) appropriate if patient able to use
   e. Subcutaneous
   f. Nebulized
      i. Effects possibly related to delivery of rapid air flow into nasopharynx (Farncombe & Chater, 1994)
      ii. Anecdotal evidence supports this method, but research results conflicting
   g. Rectal
5. Principles of dose selection
   a. No ceiling effect
   b. Titrate to patient response
   c. When used to manage breathlessness, pharmacologic tolerance not a clinically significant problem
   d. Oral
      i. Appropriate starting dose morphine 5–10 mg every 4 hours as needed, if patient opioid-naïve (Coyne, Lyne, & Watson, 2002)
      ii. Those already on opioids for pain will need to have breakthrough dose of morphine increased by 50% to relieve dyspnea (Kazanowski, 2001)
      iii. Use of long-acting preparations
   e. Intravenous
      i. Regimen reported by Cohen et al. (1991) for terminal dyspnea: morphine 1–2 mg every 5–10 minutes until relief obtained, then continuous IV infusion with hourly dose equal to 50% of cumulative bolus dose
      ii. Mean dose of morphine for dyspnea relief 5.6 mg/hr whereas for pain relief 20 mg/hr
   f. Nebulized
      i. Initial doses of morphine range from 5 to 20 mg (Picella, 1997)
      ii. Fentanyl also used—preferred by some practitioners because of concern regarding nebulized sulfates causing irritation
   g. Rectal dose generally same as oral

6. Side effects (SEs)
   a. Constipation
      i. Opioids decrease G-I motility, thus promoting fluid absorption in colon
      ii. Start patients on bowel regimen—easier to prevent than treat
      iii. Only SE to which patients do not develop tolerance
   b. Nausea
      i. Vomiting center, located in medulla, coordinates stimuli from various areas, including chemoreceptor trigger zone, pharynx and G-I tract, cerebral cortex, vestibular system, and intracranial pressure receptors (Rousseau, 1996)
      ii. Usually multifactorial in dying patients; occurs during initiation of opioids and becomes less of a problem as tolerance develops—usually within days
      iii. Treatment with anti-emetics until nausea resolves (see Table 45.1)
      iv. Comfort measures (e.g., foods at room temperatures, if desired; limiting sights, sounds, smells; providing fresh air)
I. Management of dyspnea: Other methods
   1. Benzodiazepines (see Table 45.1)—more commonly used than phenothiazines (potential for extrapyramidal side effects)
   2. Other drug treatments, such as, bronchodilators; steroids; diuretics, especially furosemide (Lasix); antibiotics; mucolytics; oxygen as appropriate; must consider potential side effects and interactions of any treatments and possibility of increasing suffering (see chapter 35 "Respiratory Pharmacology")
   4. Bedside fan
      a. Stimulates trigeminal nerve receptors
      b. Alters perception of breathlessness
      c. Place at low speed and direct at face
   5. Air conditioned room
   6. Position for comfort as selected by patient able to do so
   7. Energy conservation measures
   8. Focused breathing; pursed-lip breathing for COPD patients
      a. Inhale through nose and use diaphragm
      b. Exhale slowly through pursed lips
      c. Relaxation techniques work better after patient has gained some control through focused breathing
   9. Assessment of dyspnea relief (Campbell, 1996)
      a. Patient report, using valid and reliable dyspnea assessment tool (American Thoracic Society [ATS], 1999)
      b. In non-verbal patient, assess for decrease in tachycardia, tachypnea, restlessness, and accessory muscle use
J. Fear and anxiety
   1. As much a part of suffering as pain and dyspnea
   2. Anticipatory
      a. Patients fear dying alone with unremitting suffering

| Table 45.1 | Medications Most Commonly Used in Palliative Care of Respiratory Patients |

Drug	Route	Usual Dose	Comments
Opioids for Severe Dyspnea			
morphine	po, sublingual (SL)	2.5–10 mg q 4 hr	rarely require doses in excess of 15–20 mg q 4 hr to control dyspnea
	IV	1–2 mg q 5–10 minutes until relief obtained, then continuous infusion with hourly dose equal to 50% of cumulative bolus dose	for urgent situations or when oral route not available
	nebulized	5–20 mg in 2 ml NS	
	per rectum	same as oral dose	
oxycodone	po, SL	5–10 mg q 4 hr	
hydromorphone (Dilaudid)	po, SL	0.5–2.0 mg q 4 hr	
fentanyl	nebulized	25 mcg in 2 ml NS	
Anxiolytics—Benzodiazepines			
alprazolam (Xanax)	po	0.25–0.5 mg bid–tid	
lorazepam (Ativan)	po, SL	0.5–2.0 mg q 1 hr prn until settled, then q 4–6 hr	
	IV	0.5–2.0 mg q 1 hr prn until settled, then q 4–6 hr	longer acting than midazolam
diazepam (Valium)	po	2–10 mg q 6–8 hr	long half life
	per rectum	5–10 mg q 8–12 hr	
clonazepam (Klonopin)	po	0.25–3 mg q 8–12 hr	long half life
midazolam (Versed)	IV	0.5 mg q 15 min until settled, then by continuous infusion; 2–5 mg/hr	short half-life and more pronounced amnesiac effect (Campbell, 1996)
Agitation			
haloperidol (Haldol)	po	0.5–5 mg q 4–6 hr	also anti-emetic
	IV	0.5–5 mg q 6 hr	titrate to pt response; monitor for extrapyramidal effects
Ativan, Benadryl, & Haldol (ABH)	per rectum	1 suppository q 8 hr prn	used for severe nausea & vomiting or if patient is very agitated

(continued)

Table 45.1	Medications Most Commonly Used in Palliative Care of Respiratory Patients (*continued*)		
Drug	**Route**	**Usual Dose**	**Comments**
Anti-Emetics			
metoclopramide (Reglan)	po	5–20 mg po q 6 hr	most commonly used prokinetic agent
	IV	5–10 IV q 6 hr	extrapyramidal side effects possible
promethazine (Phenergan)	po	25 mg q 4–6 hr	more commonly used in acute care setting
	IV	12.5–25 mg q 4–6 hr	
	per rectum	25 mg q 4–6 hr	
prochlorperazine (Compazine)	po	10–20 mg q 6 hr	
	IV	5–10 mg q 6 hr	
	per rectum	25 mg q 8–12 hr	
hydroxyzine (Vistaril)	po	25 mg q 4–6 hr	
Secretion Management			
hyoscyamine (Levsin)	po/SL	0.125–.25 mg q 6 hr prn	anticholinergic; used to manage "death rattle"
scopolamine	SC	0.1–0.4 mg q 4 hr	Anticholinergic
scopolamine (Transderm-Scop)	transdermal	1–3 patches q 72 hr	patch contains 1.5 mg; releases 1 mg in 3 days

    b. "I've been told that strangulation is the worst death there is" (Wise, Schiavone, & Sitts, 1988, p. 143)

3. Fear of loss of control, loss of dignity, and loss of relationships
4. Assure patient of appropriate symptom management and that health care team will not abandon them
5. Use of benzodiazepines (See Table 45.1)
    a. Relieve anxiety and agitation
    b. Also useful for dyspnea with careful management of symptomatic response (ATS, 1999)
6. Relaxation techniques
7. Guided imagery
8. Spiritual needs
    a. Aspects of spirituality important contributors to quality of life (Kemp, 1999)
    b. Religious beliefs and practices are helpful coping strategies for many patients in dealing with fear and anxiety
    c. Spiritual assessment—FICA (Puchalski, Larson, & Post, 2000)

i. Faith or beliefs

ii. Importance and influence

iii. Community—"Are you part of a spiritual or religious community?"

iv. Address—"How would you like me to address these issues?"

K. Depression

1. Presence of refractory depression related to increased mortality

a. Loss of "will to live" may be independent predictor of mortality (van Gunten & Twaddle, 1996, p. 150)

b. Help patient to find meaning (Davies & Oberle, 1990)

i. Help patient make sense of illness and prognosis

ii. Offer hope

iii. Facilitate reflection—reminiscence and life review

iv. Refer for counseling, as appropriate

2. Use of anti-depressants

a. Selective serotonin uptake inhibitors (SSRIs) more rapid therapeutic effect than tricyclics

b. SSRIs: sertraline (Zoloft); fluoxetine (Prozac); paroxetine (Paxil)

c. Methylphenidate (Ritalin) can be used for up to 6 weeks; has more immediate effects, and can be used while other drug achieving therapeutic effects

L. Complementary therapies

1. Acupressure

2. Acupuncture

3. Therapeutic touch

4. Aromatherapy (use carefully—some patients may not be able to tolerate smells)

5. Music therapy

a. Use headphones

b. String music particularly relaxing

6. Humor therapy

M. Ethical issues in palliative care

1. Relevant ethical principles

a. Autonomy

i. Respect for persons and their inherent dignity and worth is the most fundamental ethical principle for nursing (American Nurses Association [ANA], 2001); included is a respect for individual autonomy

ii. Individuals have the liberty to determine their own actions according to plans they have chosen (Fry, 1996)

iii. Loss of control common fear of terminally ill patients

b. Beneficence (benefits)

i. Commonly defined as doing good

ii. Palliation of symptoms

iii. Relief of suffering

iv. Improving quality of life

     c. Non-maleficence (no harm)
        i. Commonly defined as doing no harm
        ii. Unwarranted fear of violating this principle by causing respiratory depression leads to unnecessary withholding of comfort measures and resultant patient suffering
     d. Justice
        i. Equal treatment of equals and those who are unequal are treated differently according to needs (Fry, 1996)
        ii. Distribute palliative care according to need

2. Application of principles in palliative care
     a. Double effect—balancing principles of beneficence and non-maleficence—requires four conditions (Weatherill, 1995)
        i. Desired effect of action not evil in itself, although action may have harmful effects
        ii. Only the good effect is intended
        iii. Harmful effect is not used to achieve good effect
        iv. Benefit of action is proportionate to harmful effect
     b. Futility
        i. Unlikely to be of particular benefit for a patient.
        ii. Futile interventions often increase pain and discomfort—violating principle of non-maleficence.
        iii. Provision of care felt to be futile by practitioners invariably results in conflict and can compromise efforts to provide psychosocial support to patient and family (Fins, 2000).
     c. Principles applied by nurse not from a detached position, but from one of involvement and connection with patient and family

3. Duties owed by nurse to patient and family
     a. Fidelity
        i. Faithful to one's commitments—keeping promises, maintaining confidentiality, and caring (Fry, 1996)
        ii. Promise to prevent and relieve suffering
        iii. Promise not to abandon patient and family
     b. Veracity
        i. Obligation to tell the truth
        ii. Individuals have the right to be told the truth about their diagnosis and prognosis
        iii. Studies of terminally ill persons have shown that they want to be told the truth about their condition (Fry, 1996)

N. Communication in palliative care
1. Basic listening skills
     a. Create the right setting
     b. Ensure privacy and time
     c. Sit and face patient
     d. Use touch, as appropriate
2. Specific communication skills related to palliative care
     a. Give permission for patient to talk about concerns

b. May introduce in a general way—"Many people in your situation think about dying. Is that something you are thinking about?"
c. Explore what patient is expecting or hoping for
d. Translate medical information into terms patient can understand
e. Repeatedly explain end-of-life treatment options
f. Use reflective, empathic statements, for example, "This must be very frightening for you"
g. Recognize cultural and ethnic influences on communication (Griffie, Nelson-Marten, & Muchka, 2004)
h. Facilitate patient-family communication (Griffie et al., 2004)
  i. Identify family decision makers
  ii. Ask "how are things going?" and explore
  iii. Recognize that patient's and family members' information needs may be different
  iv. Interpret behaviors and help family members to see each other's points of view (Davies & Oberle, 1990)
3. Communicating with family during bereavement process
a. Normalize grief for survivors; let them know that responses like inability to concentrate are normal (Egan & Arnold, 2003)
b. Active listening
c. Open-ended statements or acknowledgement of feelings
4. Communicating with other professionals (see chapter 43 "Patient Advocacy")
O. Special considerations for pediatric patients (Coyle & Layman-Goldstein, 2001)
1. Child and family are unit of care.
2. Parents and caregivers must be incorporated into the therapeutic alliance, which also includes child and health care providers.
3. Pharmacologic symptom management principles are similar to those for adults, except starting doses are determined by weight.
4. Death of a child particularly difficult—seen as out of the ordinary.
II. Role of hospice
A. Historical development of hospice (Ferrell & Coyle, 2002)
1. From same root word as hospitality; in early Western civilization, the word described place of shelter or rest for weary or sick travelers.
2. First applied to care of dying patients in modern times at St. Christopher's Hospice in London, England, by Dame Cicely Saunders in 1967.
3. First hospice program in United States began in 1974; today over 3,000 programs.
4. Federal funding through Medicare since 1982 when hospice benefit established to pay for hospice services for Medicare beneficiaries.
B. What is hospice?
1. One aspect of palliative care for those in terminal phase of illness
a. Interdisciplinary, team approach
b. Focus on care, not cure—treats person, not disease

   c. Patient and family are unit of care (Von Gunten & Twaddle, 1996)

   d. Death expected—not hastened or prolonged (Von Gunten & Twaddle, 1996)

   e. Relief of suffering, palliation of symptoms, and enhancing quality of life are primary goals (Von Gunten & Twaddle, 1996)

  2. Variety of settings; philosophy of care, not a setting

   a. Home—90% of hospice patient time spent in a personal residence (Egan & Labyak, 2001)

   b. Hospitals

   c. Long-term care facilities

   d. Freestanding inpatient facilities

  3. Requirements for hospice

   a. Certification by patient's attending physician and hospice medical director that patient's life expectancy is 6 months or less

   b. Informed consent

   c. One or more persons (family or friend/significant other) who will assist with care

   d. DNR order

 C. Financial aspects of hospice

  1. Coverage provided by various third-party payers

   a. Medicare nationally

   b. Medicaid in most states

   c. Most private insurers, including HMOs and managed care organizations

  2. Hospices also rely on grants and community support

  3. Services covered by Medicare (Department of Health and Human Services [DHHS], 2003)

   a. Physicians' services and nursing care

   b. Medical supplies and equipment

   c. Drugs for pain relief, symptom control

   d. Short-term acute inpatient care, including respite

   e. Home health aide and homemaker services

   f. Physical, occupational, and speech therapy

   g. Social services

   h. Dietary counseling

   i. Bereavement counseling

  4. Medicare beneficiaries enrolled for specified periods of time, known as "election periods" (DHHS, 2003)

   a. Two initial 90-day election periods

   b. Following initial election periods, may be enrolled for unlimited number of 60-day periods

 D. Advanced lung disease patients as candidates for hospice

  1. Patient's physician and hospice medical director certify that patient is terminally ill with 6 months or less to live

  2. Determination difficult with end-stage pulmonary disease—cancer most common cause of death among hospice patients

III. Terminal weaning
 A. Withdrawal of mechanical ventilation without belief that patient will maintain respiration
 B. Decision to terminate
  1. Ethical issues
   a. Principle of autonomy guides decision making
    i. Right to refuse treatment, even when death may be the consequence
    ii. Patient's values/beliefs should guide decisions (Scanlon, 1998)
    iii. "Nurse ascertains the respiratory client's desires regarding use of ventilatory support" a stated standard of performance for respiratory nurse (Respiratory Nursing Society, 1994, p. 17)
    iv. American Nurses Association Code of Ethics states that nurse's primary commitment is to patient (ANA, 2001)
   b. Beneficence and non-maleficence
    i. Withdrawing futile treatments supports both principles (McGee, Weinacker, & Raffin, 2000)
    ii. Goal of withdrawing treatments to remove those no longer providing comfort to patient (Rubenfeld, 2000)
    iii. Palliation of any resulting symptoms
   c. Justice
    i. Allocation of scarce resources
    ii. Costly interventions, like mechanical ventilation, should be used only in those situations in which patient is likely to benefit (Shekleton et al., 1994)
  2. Importance of advance care planning and frank discussions between providers, patients, and families
   a. Discussions with patient and family prior to event requiring intubation and mechanical ventilation ideal, but generally does not occur (Pfeifer, Mitchell, & Chamberlain, 2003; SUPPORT, 1995)
   b. Physicians less likely to discuss advance directives and resuscitation issues with COPD patients than with patients who have cancer or AIDS, despite similar prognoses (Von Gunten & Twaddle, 1996)
   c. Percent predicted FEV_1 not helpful in determining patient readiness to discuss end-of-life issues (Pfeifer et al., 2003)
   d. Involvement of ethics team or ethics committee, as necessary
  3. Decisions to withdraw most often made by family members in consultation with health team members (Brody, Campbell, Faber-Langendoen, & Ogle, 1997)
 C. Process
  1. Adequate sedation and analgesia should be provided before withdrawal of mechanical ventilatory support (Rubenfeld, 2000)
   a. Sole purpose to relieve symptoms associated with process
   b. Before removal from life support, patients should be completely comfortable

      c. Titrate medications until objective signs of discomfort have been eliminated

      d. Current guidelines recommend combination of morphine or similar drug with a benzodiazepine (Rubenfeld, 2000)

  2. All electronic alarms and monitors should be removed (Rubenfeld, 2000)

      a. Purpose of monitoring during withdrawal of support is to provide comfort and detect time of death, which can be accomplished without electronic monitoring.

      b. Since lifesaving role of critical care units so closely linked to monitoring devices, removal of alarms is a clear indication that goals of care have changed (Rubenfeld, 2000).

      c. Assess whether transfer to floor or move to a private room is necessary, with the primary goal of providing support and comfort for patient and family; transfer may be disruptive for family, especially if there are established relationships with unit staff.

  3. Gradual decrease in ventilator rate, PEEP, oxygen levels, or tidal volumes

      a. May first reduce ventilator rate to rate of spontaneous breathing

      b. Then gradually decrease oxygen concentration to room-air level

      c. Re-assess patient comfort after each ventilator change

  4. May leave endotracheal tube in place or extubate

      a. Extubation appears to be used less frequently (one survey found used exclusively by only 13% of critical care physicians but at least occasionally by 67%).

      b. Advocates of each method cite patient comfort and family's perceptions as factors in choice (Brody et al., 1997).

      c. Few data to determine best practice regarding airway management.

D. Nurse's role

  1. Increased role in collaborative decision making

      a. Open communication

      b. Participation of family crucial; patient generally unable to participate (<5% of the time)

  2. Preservation of own integrity (Davies & Oberle, 1990)

      a. Periodic self-reflection

      b. Valuing of own worth

      c. Acknowledging and accepting own grief reaction

      d. Awesome sense of responsibility felt by care providers during terminal weaning (Shekleton et al., 1994)

  3. Primary role as patient and family advocate

      a. Use palliative care principles throughout process with relief of symptoms and maintenance of patient comfort as top priorities

      b. Family preparation and support

        i. Education of family regarding what to expect (Haisfield-Wolfe, 1996)

    ii. A set time to begin withdrawal should be agreed upon (Shekleton et al., 1994)

    iii. Allow to remain with patient, as desired

WEB SITES

American Academy of Hospice and Palliative Medicine: http://www.aahpm.org

American College of Surgeons: http://www.facs.org/palliativecare

American Hospice Foundation: http://www.americanhospice.org

American Nurses Association (position statements on end-of-life issues): http://www.nursingworld.org/mainmenucategories/

Barbara Ziegler Palliative Care Education Program—Memorial Sloan-Kettering Cancer Center: http://www.mskcc.org/mskcc/html/2607.cfm

Before I Die—PBS Online: http://www.wnet.org/bid/index.html

Center for Advanced Illness Coordinated Care: Pocket Guide: http://www.coordinatedcare.net

Center to Advance Palliative Care: http://www.capc.org/

Crossing the Creek: A Practical Guide to Understanding Dying Process: http://crossingthecreek.com

Dying Well: http://www.dyingwell.org/

End-of-Life Nursing Education Consortium (ELNEC) Project: http://www.aacn.nche.edu/elnec/

End of Life/Palliative Education Resource Center (EPERC): http://www.eperc.mcw.edu/

Growth House, Inc.: http://www.growthhouse.org/

Hospice and Palliative Nurses Association: http://www.hpna.org/

Hospice Foundation of America: http://www.hospicefoundation.org/

Innovations in End-of-Life Care—online journal: http://www2.edc.org/lastacts

International Association for Hospice & Palliative Care: http://www.hospicecare.com/

Medical College of Wisconsin Palliative Medicine Program: http://www.mcw.edu/pallmed/

Medline Plus—End of Life Issues—National Library of Medicine: http://www.nlm.nih.gov/medlineplus/endoflifeissues.html#specificconditionsaspe

National Hospice and Palliative Care Organization: http://www.nhpco.org/templates/1/homepage.cfm

On Our Own Terms: Moyers on Dying: http://www.pbs.org/wnet/onourownterms/

Promoting Excellence in End-of-Life Care: http://www.promotingexcellence.org

REFERENCES

American Association of Colleges of Nursing. (1997). *Peaceful death: Recommended competencies and curricular guidelines for end-of-life nursing care.* Retrieved February 27, 2004, from http://www.aacn.nche.edu/Publications/deathfin.htm

American Nurses Association. (2001). *Code of Ethics for Nurses with Interpretive Statements.* Washington, DC: ANA Publications.

American Thoracic Society. (1999). Dyspnea—Mechanisms, assessment, and management. *American Journal of Respiratory and Critical Care Medicine, 159*(1), 321–340.

Brody, H., Campbell, M. L., Faber-Langendoen, K., & Ogle, K. S. (1997). Withdrawing intensive life-sustaining treatment—Recommendations for compassionate clinical management. *New England Journal of Medicine, 336*(9), 652–657.

Campbell, M. L. (1996). Managing terminal dyspnea: Caring for the patient who refuses intubation or ventilation. *Dimensions of Critical Care Nursing, 15*(1), 4–15.

Celli, B. R., Cote, C. G., Marin, J. M., Casanova, C., Montes de Oca, M., Mendez, R. A., et al. (2004). The body-mass index, airflow obstruction, dyspnea, and exercise capacity index in chronic obstructive pulmonary disease. *NEJM, 350*(10), 1005–1012.

Cohen, M. H., Anderson, A. J., Krasnow, S. H., Spagnolo, S. V., Citron, M. L., Payne, M., et al. (1991). Continuous intravenous infusion of morphine for severe dyspnea. *Southern Medical Journal, 84*(2), 229–234.

Coyle, N., & Layman-Goldstein, M. (2001). Pain assessment and management in palliative care. In M. L. Matzo & D. W. Sherman (Eds.), *Palliative care nursing: Quality care at the end of life* (pp. 362–486). New York: Springer Publishing.

Coyne, P., Lyne, M., & Watson, A. (2002). Symptom management in people with AIDS. *American Journal of Nursing, 102*(9), 48–56.

Davies, B., & Oberle, K. (1990). Dimensions of the supportive role of the nurse in palliative care. *Oncology Nursing Forum, 17*(1), 87–94.

Department of Health and Human Services, Centers for Medicare and Medicaid Services. (2003). *Medicare Hospice Benefits*—Publication No. CMS 02154. Baltimore: Author.

Egan, K. A., & Arnold, R. L. (2003). Grief and bereavement care. *American Journal of Nursing, 103*(9), 42–52.

Egan, K. A., & Labyak, M. J. (2001). Hospice care: A model for quality end-of-life care. In B. R. Ferrell & N. Coyle (Eds.), *Textbook of palliative nursing* (pp. 7–26). New York: Oxford University Press.

Farncombe, M., & Chater, S. (1994). Clinical application of nebulized opioids for treatment of dyspnea in patients with malignant disease. *Supportive Care in Cancer, 2*, 184–187.

Ferrell, B., & Coyle, N. (2002). An overview of palliative nursing care. *American Journal of Nursing, 102*(5), 26–31.

Field, M. J., & Cassel, C. K. (Eds.) (1997). *Approaching death: Improving care at the end of life. Report of the Institute of Medicine Task Force on End of Life Care.* Washington, DC: National Academy of Sciences. Retrieved February 27, 2004, from http://www.nap.edu/readingroom/books/approaching/

Fins, J. J. (2000). Principles in palliative care: An overview. *Respiratory Care, 45*(11), 1320–1330.

Fox, E., Landrum-McNiff, K., Zhong, Z., Dawson, N. V., Wu, A. W., & Lynn, J., for the SUPPORT investigators. (1999). Evaluation of prognostic criteria for determining hospice eligibility in patients with advanced lung, heart, or liver disease. *JAMA, 282,*(17), 1638–1645.

Fry, S. (1996). Ethical dimensions of nursing and health care. In J. L. Creasia & B. Parker (Eds.), *Conceptual foundations of professional nursing care* (2nd ed., pp. 260–284). St. Louis: Mosby.

Griffie, J., Nelson-Marten, P., & Muchka, S. (2004). Acknowledging the "elephant": Communication in palliative care. *American Journal of Nursing, 104*(1), 48–57.

Haisfield-Wolfe, M. E. (1996). End-of-life care: Evolution of nurse's role. *Oncology Nursing Forum, 23*(6), 931–935.

Herbst, L. H. (1996). Prognosis in advanced pulmonary disease. *Journal of Palliative Care, 12*(2), 54–56.

Hodgkin, J. E. (1990). Prognosis in chronic obstructive pulmonary disease. *Clinics in Chest Medicine, 11,* 5555–5569.

Johnston, G., & Abraham, C. (1995). The WHO objectives for palliative care: Are we achieving them? *Palliative Medicine, 9,* 123–137.

Kazanowski, M. K. (2001). Symptom management in palliative care. In M. L. Matzo & D. W. Sherman (Eds.), *Palliative care nursing: Quality care at the end of life* (pp. 327–361). New York: Springer Publishing.

Kemp, C. (1999). *Terminal illness: A guide to nursing care* (2nd ed.). Philadelphia: Lippincott.

Last Acts. (1997). *Precepts of palliative care.* Electronic Newsletter of the Last Acts Campaign. Princeton, NJ: Robert Wood Johnson Foundation. Retrieved February 28, 2004, from http://www.rwjf.org/index

McGee, D. C., Weinacker, A. B., & Raffin, T. A. (2000). The patient's response to medical futility. *Archives of Internal Medicine, 160*(11), 1565–1566.

Pattison, E. M. (1984). Chronic lung disease. In H. B. Roback (Ed.), *Helping patients and their families cope with medical problems* (pp. 190–215). San Francisco: Jossey-Bass.

Pfeifer, M. P., Mitchell, C. K., & Chamberlain, L. (2003). The value of disease severity in predicting patient readiness to address end-of-life issues. *Archives of Internal Medicine, 163*(5), 609–612.

Picella, D. V. (1997). Palliative care for the patient with end stage respiratory illness. *Perspectives in Respiratory Nursing, 8*(4), 1, 4, 6, 8–10.

Puchalski, C. M., Larson, D. B., & Post, S. G. (2000). Physicians and patient spirituality. *Annals of Internal Medicine, 133*(9), 748–749.

Respiratory Nursing Society/American Nurses Association. (1994). *Standards and statement on the scope of respiratory nursing practice.* Washington, DC: ANA.

Rousseau, P. (1996). Nonpain symptom management in terminal care. *Clinics in Geriatric Medicine, 12*(2), 313–327.

Rubenfeld, G. D. (2000). Withdrawing life-sustaining treatment in the intensive care unit. *Respiratory Care, 45*(11), 1399–1410.

Scanlon, C. (1998). Unraveling ethical issues in palliative care. *Seminars in Oncology Nursing, 14*(2), 137–144.

Shekleton, M. E., Burns, S. M., Clochesy, J. M., Goodnough-Hanneman, S. K., Ingersoll, G. L., & Knebel, A. R. (1994). Terminal weaning from mechanical ventilation: A review. *AACN Clinical Issues, 5*(4), 523–533.

SUPPORT Principal Investigators. (1995). A controlled trial to improve care for seriously ill hospitalized patients. *Journal of the American Medical Association, 274*(20), 1591–1958.

Von Gunten, C. F., & Twaddle, M. L. (1996). Terminal care for noncancer patients. *Clinics in Geriatric Medicine, 12*(2), 349–358.

Weatherill, G. G. (1995). Pharmacologic symptom control during the withdrawal of life support: Lessons in palliative care. *AACN Clinical Issues, 61*(2), 344–351.

Wise, T. N., Schiavone, A. A., & Sitts, T. M. (1988). The depressed patient with chronic obstructive pulmonary disease. *General Hospital Psychiatry, 10*(2), 142–147.

SUGGESTED READING

Dean-Baar, S. L., Geiger-Bronsky, M., Gift, A., & Hagarty, E. (1994). *Standards and statement on the scope of respiratory nursing practice: American Nurses Association.* Washington, DC: American Nurses Publishing.

Index

AACN. *See* American Association of Critical Care Nurses (AACN)

Abnormal values, clinical implications
  arterial blood gases, 84–85
  complete blood count (CBC) with differential, 91
  end tidal CO_2, 76–77
  immunoglobulins, 94
  magnetic resonance imaging (MRI), 80
  pulmonary function test (PFT), 78
  pulse oximetry, 76
  spontaneous respiratory parameters, 79

Active breathing, 30

Activity-exercise pattern, 62

Adenocarcinoma, 277

Adherence, of patients, 102–103

Adolescent issues
  cystic fibrosis, 207–208, 214, 217, 221, 224
  education, 101–102
  impaired sleep, 124, 125, 127
  marijuana use, 422
  respiratory muscle weakness, 335
  respiratory system growth, 46
  tobacco avoidance programs, 6–7

Adult issues, cystic fibrosis
  dating/marriage, 209
  education/career planning, 208–209
  pregnancy, 209
  reproductive decisions, 209

Adult learning theory (Knowles), 98

Adult obstructive sleep apnea. *See* Obstructive sleep apnea

Advance directives
  historical perspective, 611
  nurses role, 612–613
  purpose, 611
  types
    durable power of attorney, 612
    living will, 611–612

Advocacy. *See* Patient advocacy

Airway resistance (R_{aw}), 31

Alveolar hypoventilation
  causes, 53–54
  definition, 52–53
  physiologic features, 53
  treatment, 54

American Association of Critical Care Nurses (AACN), 12–13

American Lung Association (ALA), 3

American Nurses Association, 4

American Thoracic Society (ATS), 3, 12

Amyotrophic lateral sclerosis
  assessment, 328
  defined, 327
  etiology, 327
  incidence/clinical manifestations, 327–328
  life span considerations, 328
  pathophysiology, 327
  therapeutic modalities, 328–331

Anatomy/physiology of respiratory system
  basic structures, 28–29
  breathing mechanics, 29–32
  fetal/neonatal development, 43–49
  functional anatomy, 32–36
    lower airway, 33–36
    upper airway, 32–33
  functions, 27–28
  gas exchange, 37–43
  vascular supply, 36–37

Anti-inflammatory medication
  leukotriene modifiers, 487
  mast cell stabilizer, 487–488

Anti-inflammatory medication (*continued*)
  side effects, 223
  steroids
    inhaled/intranasal, 486
    oral, 485–486
Antibiotics
  bronchiectasis, 233, 237, 239
  considerations, 493–495
  cystic fibrosis, 222–223
  emphysema/bronchitis, 170
  laryngotracheobronchitis, 468
  newborn respiratory disorders, 438
  sinusitis, 181
  upper respiratory tract infection, 193, 195,
    198–199
Anxiety
  assessment, 138–139
  cultural considerations, 138
  definition, 135–136
  etiology, 136–137
  home care considerations, 140
  incidence, 137
  life span considerations, 138
  pathophysiology, 137
  theories, 137
  therapeutic modalities, 139–140
Arterial blood gases (ABGs), 169, 219, 455, 456, 540
  clinical indications/abnormal values, 84–85
  complications, 85
  contraindications, 85
  indications, 84
  nursing implications, 84
  procedure, 84
  purpose, 84
Arterial hypertension, 396–397
Aspergillosis, 259
Assessment. *See also* Pediatric assessment
  aging related normal findings, 66–70
  amyotrophic lateral sclerosis, 328
  anxiety, 138–139
  asthma, 178–180
  bronchiectasis, 234–237
  bronchopulmonary dysphasia, 440–441
  cocaine/marijuana use, 424
  COPD, 167–169
  cor pulmonale, 368–371
  cystic fibrosis, 215–221
  depression, 145–146
  dyspnea, 113–116
  epiglottitis, 467–468
  functional health patterns, 62–63
  Guillain-Barré Syndrome, 333
  history, 61–62
  impaired sleep, 128–129
  influenza, 190–191
  interstitial lung disease, 246–248
  Kaposi's Sarcoma (KS), 386
  key tips, 70
  lung cancers, 280–281

meconium aspiration syndrome, 437–438
mononucleosis, infectious, 196–197
multiple sclerosis, 326
muscular dystrophy, 335
myasthenia gravis, 338
objective data, 63–65
obstructive sleep apnea, 312–313
otitis media, 198
patient educational needs, 97–98
persistent cough, 154, 156–157
pharyngitis, 193
Pneumocystis pneumonia (PCP), 383
pneumonias, 264–265
pulmonary hypertension, 400–405
pulmonary rehabilitation, 557–558, 564
pulmonary thromboembolism, 296–301
respiratory distress syndrome (newborns),
  434–435
respiratory failure, 358–359
respiratory syncytial virus (RSV), 454
spinal cord injury, 343–344
tobacco use, 423–424
upper respiratory infections (URI), 188–189
Asthma
  assessment, 178–180
  complications/sequelae, 178
  definitions, 175
  dyspnea, 110
  etiology, 175–176
  home care considerations, 183
  interventions, 182–184
  life span considerations, 177
  pathophysiology, 176
  pharmacotherapy, 180
  prevalence, 176–177
  research, highlights/directions, 14
  self-management behaviors, 99
  therapeutic modalities, 180–182
  web sites, 184
ATS. *See* American Thoracic Society (ATS)
Auscultation, respiratory assessment, 65
  pediatric assessment, 73

Bacterial pneumonia, 256–259
Barriers, to patient education, 100–101
Bilateral sequential lung transplantation, 542
Bipolar disorder, 141, 142. *See also* Depression
Blood filter, systemic, 28
Blood reservoir, 28
Breathing
  act of
    central nervous system, neural pathways, 319
    motor control/functional level disruption,
     319–323
    respiratory muscles, 317–319
  control of
    chemical, 31
    mechanical, 31
    neural, 31

mechanics of
  breathing control, 31
  lung volumes, 31–32
  mechanical properties, 30–31
  patterns, 29–30
  respiratory muscles, 30
Bronchiectasis
  assessment, 234–237
  complications/sequelae, 234
  definition, 231
  etiology, 231–232
  home care considerations, 239–240
  incidence/prevalence, 233
  life span considerations, 233–234
  pathophysiology, 232–233
  surgical interventions, 239
  therapeutic modalities, 237–239
Bronchioalveolar carcinoma (BAC), 277
Bronchiolitis
  assessment, 448–449
  complications/sequelae, 448
  definition, 447
  etiology, 447
  home care considerations, 451
  incidence, 448
  interventions/outcomes, 450–451
  pathophysiology, 447–448
  therapeutic modalities, 449
  web sites, 451
Bronchitis, chronic
  definition, 166
  etiology, 166
  incidence, 167
  pathophysiology, 166–167
Bronchodilators
  anticholinergics
    long-acting, 483–484
    short-acting, 483
  beta-adrenergic
    long-acting, 476, 482–483
    short-acting, 475–476
  methylxanthine derivatives, 484–485
  side effects, 476, 482, 483, 484–485
Bronchopulmonary dysphasia
  assessment, 440–441
  complications/sequelae, 440
  definition, 439
  etiology, 439
  home care considerations, 443–444
  incidence, 440
  interventions/outcomes, 442
  pathophysiology, 439–440
  therapeutic modalities, 441–442
  web sites, 444
Bronchoscopy procedure, 93, 157, 211, 236, 239
  complications, 87
  definition/purpose, 86
  indications, 87
  nursing implications, 87

  precautions, 87
  procedure, 86–87

Caregiver considerations
  cystic fibrosis, 226
  dyspnea, 118
  evaluation reports, 104
  impaired sleep, 118, 131
  newborn respiratory disorders, 443
  persistent cough, 160–161
  QoL/functional ability issues, 580
  treatment decisions, 101
Centers for Disease Control (CDC), 6–8, 594, 601
Chemotherapy
  Kaposi's Sarcoma, 386–387
  lung cancers, 277–278, 281, 284–287
  side effects, 111, 192, 569
Chest X-ray reading/interpretation, 81–83
  clinical indications, 81
  clinical indications/abnormal findings, 82–83
  normal findings, 81–82
  patient preparation, 81
  purpose, 81
  setting, 81
Chest X-ray, digital imaging (noninvasive), 84
  clinical indications, 84
  clinical indications/abnormal findings, 84
  normal values, 84
  patient preparation, 84
  purpose, 84
  setting, 84
Chlamydiae pneumonia, 259
Chronic obstructive pulmonary disease
    (COPD), 6.
  assessment, 167–169
  complications/sequelae, 167
  dyspnea, 110
  home care considerations, 171
  incidence, 167
  life span considerations, 167
  pharmacotherapy, 170
  research directions, 14–15
  stages, based on global initiative, 169
  therapeutic modalities, 170–171
  web sites, 171
  See also Bronchitis, chronic; Emphysema
Chronic thrombotic/embolic disease, 398–399
Clark, E. G., 9
Clinical indications
  chest X-rays, 81, 84
  computerized tomography (CT), 80
  end tidal CO_2, 76
  magnetic resonance imaging (MRI), 80
  polysomnogram/nocturnal desaturation
    study, 79
  pulmonary function test (PFT), 77
  pulse oximetry, 75
  spontaneous respiratory parameters, 78
  sputum diagnostics, 93

Clinical manifestations
  amyotrophic lateral sclerosis, 327
  anxiety, 138
  croup, 465
  cystic fibrosis, 204
  depression, 144
  epiglottitis, 467
  Guillain-Barré Syndrome, 332
  muscular dystrophy, 334–335
  myasthenia gravis, 337
  respiratory muscle weakness, 325–326
  spinal cord injury, 341–342
Clinical nurse specialist (CNS), 3
Cocaine use
  assessment, 424
  incidence, 422
  life span considerations, 422–423
  mechanism of action, 419
  pathophysiology, 420–421
  therapeutic modalities, 426–427
Cognitive-perceptual pattern, 62
Communitarianism (community-based theory),
    616
Community-acquired pneumonia, 255–256, 262
Compensatory mechanisms, hypoxia, 57–58
Complementary therapies, palliative care, 629
Complete blood count (CBC) with differential,
    91–92
  clinical implications/abnormal values, 91
  complications, 91
  indications, 91
  normal values, 91
  nursing implications, 91
  precautions, 91
  procedure, 91
  purpose, 91
Complications/sequelae
  arterial blood gases, 85
  asthma, 154, 178
  bronchiectasis, 234
  bronchopulmonary dysphasia, 440
  bronchoscopy, 87
  COPD, 167
  coughing, 154
  cystic fibrosis, 210–215
  dyspnea, 113
  immunoglobulins, 94
  impaired sleep, 127–128
  influenza, 190
  interstitial lung disease, 246
  Kaposi's Sarcoma (KS), 385
  lung biopsy, 88
  lung cancers, 278–280
  lung transplantation, 545–549
  meconium aspiration syndrome, 437
  mediastinoscopy, 90
  mononucleosis, infectious, 196
  multiple sclerosis, 326
  muscular dystrophy, 335

myasthenia gravis, 337–338
obstructive sleep apnea, 312
persistent cough, 154–155
pharyngitis, 192–193
Pneumocystis pneumonia (PCP), 382–383
pneumonias, 263
pulmonary angiography, 86
pulmonary hypertension, 400
pulmonary thromboembolism, 296
respiratory distress syndrome (newborns), 434
skin tests, 95
spinal cord injury, 342–343
sputum diagnostics, 93
thoracentesis, 89
thoracoscopy, 90
tobacco use, 423
tracheostomy, 528–530
upper respiratory infections, 188
ventilation perfusion scan, 86
Computerized tomography (CT), 80–81
  clinical indications, 80
  clinical indications/abnormal findings, 81
  normal values, 80
  patient preparation, 80
  purpose, 80
  settings, 80
Congestive heart failure (CHF), 48
  anxiety, 136, 139
  cor pulmonale, 440
  depression, 142
  dyspnea, 111
  impaired sleep disorder, 124
Contraindications
  arterial blood gases, 85
  lung biopsy, 88
Coping-stress tolerance pattern, 63
Cor pulmonale
  assessment, 368–371
  definitions, 363–364
  etiology, 364
  home care considerations, 375
  pathophysiology, 364–368
  therapeutic modalities, 371–375
  web sites, 375–376
Cough. *See* Persistent cough
Cough preparations
  antitussives, 489–490
  expectorants, 490
Croup
  assessment, 465–466
  clinical manifestations, 465
  definition, 459
  etiology, 459
  pathophysiology, 459–462
  therapeutic modalities, 462–465
Cultural considerations
  anxiety, 138
  cystic fibrosis, 210
  depression, 144–145

dyspnea, 113
impaired sleep, 127
persistent cough, 154
Cyclothymic disorder. *See* Depression
Cystic fibrosis
assessment, 215–221
complications, 210–215
cultural considerations, 210
definition, 203
etiology, 203–204
home/continuity of care, 225–226
incidence, 207
life span considerations, 207–210
pathophysiology, 204–207
pharmacotherapy, 222–224
research directions, 15
risk factors, 204
surgical interventions, 213, 221, 224–225
therapeutic modalities, 221–225
web sites, 226

Depression
assessment, 145–146
cultural considerations, 144–145
definition, 141–142
etiology, 142–143
home care considerations, 148
incidence, 143–144
interventions/outcomes, 147–148
life span considerations, 144
theories, 143
therapeutic modalities, 146–147
Diagnostic studies
invasive
arterial blood gases, 84–85
bronchoscopy, 86–87
CBC with differential, 91–93
immunoglobulins, 93–94
lung biopsy, 87–88
mediastinoscopy, 89–90
pulmonary angiography, 86
skin tests, 94–95
thoracentesis, 88–89
thoracoscopy, 90–91
ventilation perfusion scan, 85–86
noninvasive
chest X-ray reading/interpretation, 81–83
chest X-ray, digital imaging, 84
computerized tomography (CT), 80–81
end tidal CO_2, 76–77
magnetic resonance imaging, 80
polysomnogram/nocturnal desaturation
study, 79–80
pulmonary function test (PFT), 77–78
pulse oximetry, 75–76
spontaneous respiratory parameters, 78–79
Diagnostic testing
adult obstructive sleep apnea, 313
asthma, 179–180

bronchiectasis, 235
bronchiolitis, 449
COPD, 169
cor pulmonale, 369
coughing, 157
croup, 466
cystic fibrosis, 218
depression, 146
dyspnea, 114
emphysema/chronic bronchitis, 169
epiglottitis, 467–468
HIV, 383, 386
impaired sleep, 129
infectious mononucleosis, 197
influenza, 191
interstitial lung disease, 248
lung cancers, 280
newborn respiratory disorders, 434–435, 438,
441
otitis media, 198
pharyngitis, 193, 195
pneumonia, 264
pulmonary hypertension, 402, 403
pulmonary thromboembolism, 297, 298–301
respiratory muscle weakness, 326, 328, 333,
335, 338, 344
sinusitis, 195
tobacco use, 424
upper respiratory infections, 189, 191, 193,
197, 198
Diffusion defect
causes, 54
definition, 54
physiologic features, 54
treatment, 54
Drugs. *See* Pharmacotherapy
Durable power of attorney, 612
Dyspnea
assessment, 113–116
complications, 113
cultural considerations, 113
dimensions, 110
etiology, 109–110
home care considerations, 118
incidence/prevalence, 112
life span considerations, 112
management/palliative care, 112
pathophysiology, 110–113
physiologic mechanisms
attention/judgment, 110
neuro-chemical, 110
neuro-mechanical, 109–110
psychosocial factors, 110
related diseases/disorders, 110–112 (*See also
individual diseases/disorders*)
research directions, 15
risk factors, 110–113
therapeutic modalities, 116–118
Dysthymia. *See* Depression

Education of patients
  adherence, 102–103
  adults/cystic fibrosis, 208–209
  asthma, 99, 182–183
  barriers, 100–101
  determination of need, 97–98
  influential factors, 101–102
  interventions, 98–100
    evaluation of, 104–105
  teaching and learning formats, 100
  upper respiratory infections (URI), 189
Elderly issues
  anxiety, 138
  asthma, 178
  depression, 144, 145, 147
  dyspnea, 112
  impaired sleep, 127
  influenza, 190
  interstitial lung disease, 246
  otitis media, 198
  Pneumocystis pneumonia (PCP), 382
  pneumonias, 263
  pulmonary hypertension, 399–400
  tobacco use, 423
  tobacco/substance abuse, 423
  upper respiratory infections, 188
Elimination pattern, 62
Emphysema
  definition, 165
  etiology, 165–166
  pathophysiology, 166
End tidal CO_2
  clinical indications, 76
  clinical indications/abnormal values, 76–77
  normal values, 76
  patient preparation, 76
  purpose, 76
  setting, 76
End-of-life issues
  decision making/research directions, 14
  hospice, role of, 631–632
  palliative care
    communication, 630–631
    complementary therapies, 629
    current system, 623
    definition, 621
    depression, 629
    dyspnea management, 112, 624–626
    ethical issues, 629–630
    fear and anxiety, 626, 628–629
    focus determination, 623–624
    pediatric considerations, 631
    principles, 622
    prognostic indicators, 624
    recommended competencies, 622–623
    WHO goals, 621–622
  terminal weaning, 633–635
  web sites, 635

Epiglottitis
  assessment, 467–468
  clinical presentation, 467
  definition, 466
  etiology, 466
  pathophysiology, 466–467
  scoring system, 469
  therapeutic modalities, 468–469
  web sites, 469
Erythrocytosis, 51, 58
Ethical dilemmas
  principles
    autonomy, 616–617
    beneficence, 617
    futility, 618
    justice, 618
    nonmaleficence, 617–618
  rules
    confidentiality, 618–619
    fidelity, 619
    privacy, 618
    veracity, 618
  theories
    causality, 616
    character ethics (virtue-based theory), 616
    communitarianism, 616
    convergence of theories, 616
    ethics of care (relationship-based accounts), 616
    Kantianism (obligation-based theory), 615–616
    liberal individualism (rights-based theory), 616
    utilitarianism (consequence-based theory), 615
  virtues in professional roles, 619
Etiology
  amyotrophic lateral sclerosis, 327
  anxiety, 137
  bronchiectasis, 231–232
  bronchitis, chronic, 166
  bronchopulmonary dysphasia, 439
  cor pulmonale, 364
  cystic fibrosis, 203–204
  depression, 142–143
  dyspnea, 109–110
  emphysema, 165–166
  epiglottitis, 466
  Guillain-Barré Syndrome, 331
  impaired sleep, 124–125, 125–126
  influenza, 189–190
  interstitial lung disease, 243–244
  Kaposi's Sarcoma (KS), 384
  meconium aspiration syndrome, 437
  mononucleosis, infectious, 196
  multiple sclerosis, 325
  muscular dystrophy, 334
  myasthenia gravis, 337
  obstructive sleep apnea, 311

otitis media, 197
persistent cough, 153
pharyngitis, 192
Pneumocystis pneumonia (PCP), 381
pneumonias, 255–256
pulmonary hypertension, 393–394
pulmonary thromboembolism, 291–293
respiratory distress syndrome (newborns), 433
respiratory failure
  hypercapnic respiratory failure, 356
  hypoxemic respiratory failure, 355–356
spinal cord injury, 340
Evaluation, of patient education, 104–105
Expiration, muscles, 30
Extrinsic hypoxia, 51–52

Fear
  anxiety, 136, 140
  cystic fibrosis, 207, 209, 211
  dyspnea, 111–112, 114
  impaired sleep disorder, 125, 128
Fetal/neonatal development, 43–49
Fluid exchange, lungs, 28
Functional ability.
  associated problems, 577
    physical issues, 577
    psychological issues, 577
    sociocultural issues, 577–578
  definition, 577
  See also Quality of life (QoL) issues
Functional anatomy of respiratory system
  lower airway, 33–36 (*See also* Lower airway)
  upper airway, 32–33 (*See also* Upper airway)
Functions of respiratory system
  blood reservoir, 28
  fluid exchange, 28
  gas exchange, 27–28
  metabolic function of lungs, 28
  systemic blood filter, 28
  ventilation, 28

Gas exchange
  A-a gradient, 38–39
  carbon dioxide transport, 41
  cellular respiration, 27–28
  diffusion, 38
  external respiration, 27
  internal respiration, 27
  oxygenation principles, 39–41
  pressure gradients, 38
  ventilation and perfusion (V/Q), 41–43
Generalized anxiety disorder. *See* Anxiety
Guillain-Barré Syndrome
  assessment, 333
  definition, 331
  etiology, 331
  home care considerations, 334
  incidence/clinical manifestations, 332
  life span considerations, 332–333

pathophysiology, 331
therapeutic modalities, 333–334

Health patterns (functional), respiratory
    assessment, 62–63
Health-related quality of life (HQoL), 576
    See also Quality of life (QoL) issues
Heart-lung transplantation, 542–543
History, respiratory assessment, 61–62
    functional health patterns, 62
    pediatric assessment, 71–72
    subjective data, 61–62
Home care considerations
    anxiety, 140
    asthma, 183
    bronchiectasis, 239–240
    bronchopulmonary dysphasia, 443–444
    COPD, 171
    cor pulmonale, 375
    cystic fibrosis, 225–226
    depression, 148
    dyspnea, 118
    Guillain-Barré Syndrome, 334
    high-tech research directions, 14
    impaired sleep, 131
    interstitial lung disease, 251
    Kaposi's Sarcoma (KS), 387
    lung cancers, 286–287
    mechanical ventilation, 521–522
    multiple sclerosis, 327
    muscular dystrophy, 336
    myasthenia gravis, 339
    newborn respiratory disorders, 443–444
    obstructive sleep apnea, 313–314
    otitis media, 199
    oxygen treatment, 571–572
    persistent cough, 160–161
    Pneumocystis pneumonia (PCP), 384
    pneumonias, 267
    pulmonary hypertension, 412–413
    pulmonary thromboembolism, 307–308
    respiratory failure, 360
    respiratory syncytial virus (RSV), 457
    spinal cord injury, 347
    tobacco use, 427
Hospital-acquired pneumonia, 255, 260–261
Human immunodeficiency virus (HIV),
    complications
    definitions, 379
    incidence, 380
    Kaposi's Sarcoma (KS) (*See* Kaposi's Sarcoma
      [KS])
    life span considerations, 380
    Pneumocystis pneumonia (PCP) (*See*
      Pneumocystis pneumonia [PCP])
Hypercapnia, 48, 51, 52, 55, 69–70
    causes, 353
    clinical assessment, 358–359
    croup, 461

Hypercapnia (*continued*)
  definition, 51
  depression, 146
  dyspnea, 110
  lung transplantation, 544
  mechanical ventilation, 497, 498
  newborn respiratory disorders, 440, 441
  respiratory distress syndrome, 436
  respiratory failure, 354, 357
Hyperventilation, 354, 356
  croup, 464–465
  diagnostic studies, 76, 84
  hypoxia, 57
  mechanical ventilation, 519
  respiratory syncytial virus, 456
Hypoxemia, 54–56
  bronchiectasis, 233, 234
  causes, 52
  croup, 462
  cystic fibrosis, 225
  definition, 51
  diagnostic studies, 93
  dyspnea, 110, 114
  interstitial lung disease, 246, 248, 250
  lung transplantation, 544
  pulmonary thromboembolism, 293, 296
  respiratory assessment, 69–70
  respiratory failure, 353, 354–358
  respiratory syncytial virus, 454
Hypoxia
  causes
    alveolar hypoventilation, 52–54
    diffusion defects, 54
    extrinsic, 51–52
    oxygen, inadequate transport/delivery,
      56–57
    V/Q mismatch, 54–56
  compensatory mechanisms
    cardiac output, 57–58
    erythrocytosis, 58
    hyperventilation, 57
    oxyhemoglobin curve shift, 58
  definition, 51

Immunoglobulins, 93–94
  clinical indications/abnormal values, 94
  complications, 94
  indications, 94
  normal values, 94
  nursing implications, 94
  precautions, 94
  procedure, 93
  purpose, 93
Impaired sleep
  assessment, 128–129
  complications/sequelae, 127–128
  cultural considerations, 127
  definition, 123–124
  etiology, 124–125

  home care considerations, 131
  incidence, 125
  interventions/outcomes, 130–132
  life span considerations, 125–127
  pathophysiology, 125
  risk factors, 125
  therapeutic modalities, 129–130
Incidence
  amyotrophic lateral sclerosis, 327–328
  anxiety, 137
  bronchiectasis, 233
  bronchitis, chronic, 167
  bronchopulmonary dysphasia, 440
  cocaine, 422
  COPD, 167
  cystic fibrosis, 207
  depression, 143–144
  dyspnea, 112
  Guillain-Barré Syndrome, 332
  impaired sleep, 125
  influenza, 190
  interstitial lung disease, 245–246
  Kaposi's Sarcoma (KS), 385
  lung cancers, 276–277
  marijuana, 421–422
  meconium aspiration syndrome, 437
  mononucleosis, infectious, 196
  muscular dystrophy, 334–335
  myasthenia gravis, 337
  obstructive sleep apnea, 312
  otitis media, 197
  persistent cough, 154
  pharyngitis, 192
  Pneumocystis pneumonia (PCP), 381–382
  pneumonias, 261–262
  pulmonary hypertension, 395–396
  pulmonary thromboembolism, 294
  respiratory distress syndrome (newborns), 434
  spinal cord injury, 341–342
  upper respiratory infections (URI), 188
Influenza
  complications/sequelae, 190
  definition, 189
  definition/etiology, 189–190
  life span considerations, 190
  pathophysiology, 190
  resource utilization, 593–594
  therapeutic modalities, 191
  vaccines/immunizations, 490–491
Insomnia
  anxiety, 136
  as side effect
    amantadine, 495
    anti-inflammatories, 485
    nasal decongestants, 488
    smoking cessation, 492
  depression, 141, 144, 145, 146, 147
  impaired sleep, 124, 125, 129, 130
  therapeutic modalities, 130

Inspection, respiratory assessment, 63–64
  pediatric assessment, 72–73
Inspiration, muscles, 30
Instrument development, research directions, 16–17
Interstitial lung disease
  assessment, 246–248
  complications/sequelae, 246
  definition, 243
  elderly issues, 246
  etiology, 243–245
  home care considerations, 251
  incidence, 245–246
  interventions/outcomes, 249–251
  life span considerations, 246
  pathophysiology, 244–245
  pediatric issues, 246
  pharmacotherapy, 249
  pregnancy issues, 246
  therapeutic modalities, 248–249
  web sites, 251
Interventions. *See also* Pharmacotherapy
  anxiety, 139–140
  asthma, 182–184
  bronchiectasis, 239
  bronchopulmonary dysphasia, 442
  depression, 147–148
  energy reserve promotion, 568
  futile interventions, 630
  impaired sleep, 130–132
  interstitial lung disease, 249–251
  mechanical ventilation, 497, 500, 507, 508–517, 520
  meconium aspiration syndrome, 438–439
  obstructive sleep apnea, 313
  patient education, 98–100
  persistent cough, 160
  pneumonias, 265–267
  pulmonary hypertension, 411–412
  respiratory distress syndrome (newborns), 435–436
  respiratory syncytial virus, 455–456
  respiratory syncytial virus (RSV), 455–457
Invasive diagnostic studies. *See under* Diagnostic studies
Involuntary (passive) smoking, 8

Janson-Bjerklie, Susan, 97–105
Joint Commission of Accreditation of Hospital Organizations (JCAHO), 16

Kantianism (obligation-based theory), 615–616
Kaposi's Sarcoma (KS)
  assessment, 386
  complications/sequelae, 385
  definition, 384
  etiology, 384
  home care considerations, 387
  incidence, 385

  pathophysiology, 385
  therapeutic modalities, 386–387
  transmission, 384–385
  web sites, 387–388
Knowles, Malcolm, 98

Lareau, Suzanne C. 3–4
Large cell carcinoma, 277–278
Larson, Janet, 3–4
Larynx, 33
Leavell, H. R., 9
Legionnaire's disease, 259
Leukotriene modifiers, 487
Liberal individualism (rights-based theory), 616
Life span considerations.
  amyotrophic lateral sclerosis, 328
  anxiety, 138
  asthma, 177
  bronchiectasis, 233–234
  COPD, 167
  cystic fibrosis, 207–210
  depression, 144
  dyspnea, 112
  Guillain-Barré Syndrome, 332–333
  impaired sleep, 125–127
  influenza, 190
  interstitial lung disease, 246
  mononucleosis, infectious, 196
  multiple sclerosis, 326
  muscular dystrophy, 335
  myasthenia gravis, 337
  obstructive sleep apnea, 312
  otitis media, 198
  pharyngitis, 192
  Pneumocystis pneumonia (PCP), 382
  pneumonias, 262–263
  pulmonary hypertension, 399–400
  pulmonary thromboembolism, 295–296
  spinal cord injury, 342
  upper respiratory infections (URI), 188
  See also Adolescent issues; Elderly issues; Pediatric issues; Pregnancy issues
Life trajectory changes (of respiratory system)
  aging, normal changes, 47–49
  childhood periods
    adolescence, 46
    infancy, 44–45
    preschool, 45
    school age, 45–46
    toddler, 45
  fetal circulation, 43
  neonatal, 43–44
  pregnancy, 46–47
Living wills, 611–612
Lobar transplantation (from living donor), 543
Long-term mechanical ventilation (LTMV), 13, 14
Lower airway, 33–36
  acinar, 35–36
  conducting airway tissue, 34

Lower airway (*continued*)
  major airways
    bronchi (lobar/segmental), 34
    bronchi (main stem), 34
    bronchi (subsegmental), 34
    bronchioles, terminal, 34
    carina (cartilage), 34
    trachea, 33–34
  tracheobronchial surface lining, 35
LTMV. *See* Long-term mechanical ventilation
    (LTMV)
Lung biopsy, 249, 294, 383, 386, 404
  complications, 88
  contraindications, 88
  definition/purpose, 87
  indications, 88
  nursing implications, 88
  procedure, 87–88
Lung cancers.
  assessment, 280–281
  causes, 275–276
  chemotherapy, 277–278, 281, 284–287
  complications/sequelae, 278–280
  definition, 275
  home care considerations, 286–287
  incidence, 276–277
  pathophysiology, 277, 278
  research directions, 15
  risk factors, 275–276
  stage grouping/TNM subsets, 283
  staging, 90, 280, 281–283
  TNM descriptors, 282
  treatment methods, 283–286
  web sites, 287–288
  See also Non-bronchiogenic carcinomas; Non-
    small cell lung cancer (NSCLC); Oat cell
    carcinoma; Small-cell lung cancer
Lung infections, 3
Lung transplantation
  allocation issues, 542
  diagnostic studies, 540–541
  goals for future, 553
  historical perspective, 537
  operative considerations
    bilateral sequential transplantation, 542
    heath-lung transplantation, 542–543
    lobar transplantation (from living donor), 543
    single lung transplantation, 542
  outcomes/statistics, 552–553
  patient selection
    amenable diseases, 538–540
    contraindications, 540
    general considerations, 537–538
  postoperative issues, long-term
    chronic rejection, 549–550
    infection, 550
    malignancy, 552
    medication side effects, 550–552
    PTLD, 549

  postoperative management
    complications, 545–549
    fluids/electrolytes, 544
    hemodynamic management, 543
    infections, 544–545
    pain management, 544
    pulmonary management, 543–544
    rejection, 545
  preoperative considerations, 541–542
  research directions, 15
Lungs
  mechanical properties, 30–31
  metabolic functions, 28
  structure, 29
  volumes, 31–32

Magnetic resonance imaging (MRI), 80
Major depressive disorder. *See* Depression
Managed care
  Balanced Budget Act (1997), 598–599
  historical background, 596
  private sector coverage types, 596–597
  public sector coverage types, 596–597
Marijuana use
  assessment, 424
  incidence, 421–422
  life span considerations, 422–423
  mechanism of action, 418–419
  pathophysiology, 420
  therapeutic modalities, 426–427
Mast cell stabilizer, 487–488
Mechanical ventilation
  discontinuation of support, 519–520
  long-term/home care considerations, 521–522
  modes and function, 502–507
    classification of ventilators, 502
    common settings, 506–507
  noninvasive techniques
    negative pressure support, 498–499
    noninvasive postural pressure ventilation
      (NPPV) support, 499–501
    postural devices, 499
  problem management, 507–519
  weaning guidelines, 520–521
  web sites, 522
Meconium aspiration syndrome
  assessment, 437–438
  complications/sequelae, 437
  definition, 436–437
  etiology, 437
  incidence, 437
  interventions/outcomes, 438–439
  pathophysiology, 437
  therapeutic modalities, 438
Mediastinoscopy, 89–90, 280
  abnormal findings, 89
  complications, 90
  definition/purpose, 89
  indications, 89

nursing implications, 90
precautions, 90
procedure, 89
Mediastinum, 28–29
Medications. *See* Pharmacology;
Pharmacotherapy
Minitracheostomy
approach, 530–531
definition, 530
indications, 530
pre-/postoperative considerations, 531
Mononucleosis, infectious
assessment, 196–197
complications/sequelae, 196
definition, 196
etiology, 196
incidence, 196
life span considerations, 196
pathophysiology, 196
therapeutic modalities, 197
Mood disorders, 141–142. *See also* Anxiety;
Depression
Multiple sclerosis, 323–327
assessment, 326
clinical manifestations, 325–326
complications/sequelae, 326
definition, 325
etiology, 325
home care considerations, 327
life span considerations, 326
pathophysiology, 325
therapeutic modalities, 326–327
Muscles, of respiratory system, 30
Muscular dystrophy
assessment, 335
complications/sequelae, 335
definition, 334
etiology, 334
home care considerations, 336
incidence/clinical manifestations, 334–335
lifespan considerations, 335
pathophysiology, 334
therapeutic modalities, 335–336
Myasthenia gravis
assessment, 338
complications/sequelae, 337–338
definition, 336–337
etiology, 337
home care considerations, 339
incidence/clinical manifestations, 337
lifespan considerations, 337
pathophysiology, 337
therapeutic modalities, 338–339

Narcolepsy, therapeutic modalities, 130
National Asthma Education and Prevention
Program (NAEPP), 592
National Institute of Nursing Research (NINR),
12

National Tuberculosis & Respiratory Disease
Association (NTRDA), 3
National Tuberculosis Association (NTA), 3
Neuromuscular diseases
amyotrophic lateral sclerosis, 327–331
Guillain-Barré Syndrome, 331–334
multiple sclerosis, 323–327
muscular dystrophy, 334–336
myasthenia gravis, 336–339
spinal cord injury, 339–347
Newborn respiratory disorders
bronchopulmonary dysphasia, 439–442
home care considerations, 443–444
meconium aspiration syndrome, 436–439
respiratory distress syndrome, 433–436
web sites, 444
NINR. *See* National Institute of Nursing
Research (NINR)
Nocturnal desaturation study, 79–80
Non-bronchiogenic carcinomas, 278
Non-small cell lung cancer (NSCLC), 277, 278,
284–285
Noninvasive diagnostic studies. *See under*
Diagnostic studies
Nose, 32
Nursing implications
arterial blood gases, 84
bronchoscopy, 87
immunoglobulins, 94
lung biopsy, 88
mediastinoscopy, 90
skin tests, 95
sputum diagnostics, 93
thoracentesis, 89
thoracoscopy, 90
ventilation perfusion scan, 85–86
Nutritional-metabolic pattern, 62

Oat cell carcinoma, 278
Obesity
dyspnea, 111
hypercapnia, 52
lung transplantation, 551
mechanical ventilation, 498, 519
respiratory failure, 353, 356, 357, 359
sleep apnea, 311, 312
Objective data, respiratory assessment
auscultation, 65
inspection, 63–64
palpation, 64
percussion, 64–65
physical exam/vital signs, 63
Obsessive-compulsive disorder, 136
See also Anxiety
Obstructive lung diseases, 3
Obstructive sleep apnea
assessment, 312–313
complications/sequelae, 312
definition, 311

Obstructive sleep apnea (*continued*)
  etiology, 311
  home care considerations, 313–314
  incidence, 312
  interventions, 313
  life span considerations, 312
  pathophysiology, 311–312
  research directions, 15
  risk factors, 311
  therapeutic modalities, 129–130, 313
Oral cavity, 32–33
ORYX initiative, 16
Otitis media
  assessment, 198
  definition, 197
  etiology, 197
  home care considerations, 199
  incidence, 197
  life span considerations, 198
  pathophysiology, 197
  therapeutic modalities, 198–199
  web sites, 199–200
Outcome and Assessment Information Set
    (OASIS), 16
Outcomes
  anxiety, 139–140
  bronchopulmonary dysphasia, 442
  depression, 147–148
  impaired sleep, 130–132
  interstitial lung disease, 249–251
  meconium aspiration syndrome, 438–439
  persistent cough, 160
  pneumonias, 265–267
  pulmonary hypertension, 411–412
  pulmonary thromboembolism, 307
  respiratory distress syndrome (newborns),
    435–436
  respiratory syncytial virus (RSV), 455–457
Oxygen delivery systems, research
    directions, 14
Oxygen, inadequate transport/delivery
  causes, 56–57
  definition, 56
  physiologic features, 56
  treatment, 57

Palliative care
  communication, 630–631
  complementary therapies, 629
  current system, 623
  definition, 621
  depression, 629
  dyspnea management, 112, 624–626
  ethical issues, 629–630
  fear and anxiety, 626, 628–629
  focus determination, 623–624
  pediatric considerations, 631
  principles, 622
  prognostic indicators, 624

  recommended competencies, 622–623
  WHO goals, 621–622
Palpation, respiratory assessment, 64
  pediatric assessment, 73
Panic disorder, 135–136
  See also Anxiety
Passive (involuntary) smoking, 8
Pathophysiology
  amyotrophic lateral sclerosis, 327
  anxiety, 137
  asthma, 176
  bronchiectasis, 232–233
  bronchitis, chronic, 166–167
  bronchopulmonary dysphasia, 439–440
  cocaine, 420–421
  cor pulmonale, 364–368
  cystic fibrosis, 204–207
  depression, 143
  dyspnea, 110–113
  emphysema, 166
  epiglottitis, 466–467
  Guillain-Barré Syndrome, 331
  impaired sleep, 125
  influenza, 190
  interstitial lung disease, 244–245
  Kaposi's Sarcoma (KS), 385
  lung cancers, 277–278
  marijuana, 420
  meconium aspiration syndrome, 437
  mononucleosis, infectious, 196
  multiple sclerosis, 325
  muscular dystrophy, 334
  myasthenia gravis, 337
  obstructive sleep apnea, 311–312
  otitis media, 197
  persistent cough, 153–154
  Pneumocystis pneumonia (PCP), 381
  pneumonias, 256–261
  pulmonary hypertension, 394–395
  pulmonary thromboembolism, 293
  respiratory distress syndrome (newborns),
    433–434
  respiratory failure
    hypercapnic respiratory failure, 356
    hypoxemic respiratory failure, 355–356
  respiratory syncytial virus (RSV), 454
  spinal cord injury, 340–341
  tobacco, 419–420
  upper respiratory infections (URI), 188
Patient advocacy
  advance directives, 611–613
  arenas, 609
  barriers to, 608
  definition, 607
  enhancement approaches, 610
  historical perspective, 607
  professional role/mandates regarding, 609
  values/beliefs, 610–611
  web sites, 613

Patient preparation
  chest X-ray, digital imaging, 84
  chest X-rays, 81
  computerized tomography (CT), 80
  end tidal CO_2, 76
  magnetic resonance imaging (MRI), 80
  polysomnogram/nocturnal desaturation
      study, 79–80
  pulmonary function test (PFT), 77
  pulse oximetry, 76
  spontaneous respiratory parameters, 78
Patient selection, lung transplantation, 538–540
Patterns of breathing, 29–30
Peak flow meter, asthma action plans, 570–571
Pediatric assessment
  age-specific findings, 73–74
  auscultation, 73
  history, 71–72
  inspection, 72–73
  key tips, 74
  palpation, 73
  percussion, 73
  pneumonias, 262
  quality of life (QoL), 584
Pediatric issues
  anxiety, 137
  asthma, 177, 181, 422, 593
  common cold, 188
  cystic fibrosis, 207
  depression, 144
  dyspnea, 112
  end-of-life/palliative care, 631
  HIV/AIDS, 380
  impaired sleep, 125–127
  influenza, 190
  interstitial lung disease, 246
  otitis media, 198
  Pneumocystis pneumonia (PCP), 382
  pulmonary hypertension, 399
  substance abuse/tobacco, 422
  tobacco use, 422
Percussion, respiratory assessment, 64–65, 73
Performance improvement (PI)
  definition/purpose, 16
  system samples, 16–17
  team leaders, hints for, 17
  See also ORYX initiative
Persistent cough
  assessment, 154, 156–157
  complications, 154
  cultural considerations, 154–155
  definitions, 151–152
  etiology, 153
  home care considerations, 160–161
  incidence, 154
  interventions/outcomes, 160
  pathophysiology, 153–154
  risk factors, 153
  therapeutic modalities, 157–159

Pharmacology
  anti-inflammatories
    leukotriene modifiers, 487
    mast cell stabilizer, 487–488
    steroids, inhaled/intranasal, 486
    steroids, oral, 485–486
  antibiotics
    classifications, 493
    considerations, 493–495
  bronchodilators
    anticholinergics, long-acting, 483–484
    anticholinergics, short-acting, 483
    beta-adrenergic, long-acting, 476,
        482–483
    beta-adrenergic, short-acting, 475–476
    methylxanthine derivatives, 484–485
  cough preparations
    antitussives, 489–490
    expectorants, 490
  nebulized medications, 572–573
  smoking cessation
    nicotine replacement, 492
    non-nicotine, 492–493
  upper respiratory medications
    antihistamines, 488–489
    nasal decongestants, 488
  vaccines/immunizations
    influenza, 490–491
    pneumonia, 491–492
Pharmacotherapy
  amyotrophic lateral sclerosis, 330
  anxiety, 139
  asthma, 180
  bronchiectasis, 237–238
  COPD, 170
  cor pulmonale, 373–375
  cystic fibrosis, 222–224
  depression, 147
  dyspnea, 116
  impaired sleep, 130
  influenza, 191
  interstitial lung disease, 249
  muscular dystrophy, 336
  myasthenia gravis, 338–339
  persistent cough, 158–159
  pulmonary thromboembolism, 301–304
  respiratory muscle weakness, 330, 333, 336
  sinusitis, 195–196
Pharyngitis
  assessment, 193
  complications/sequelae, 192–193
  definition, 192
  etiology, 192
  incidence, 192
  life span considerations, 192
  therapeutic modalities, 193–194
Phobic disorder, 136. *See also* Anxiety
Physiology of respiratory system. *See* Anatomy/
    physiology of respiratory system

Pneumocystis pneumonia (PCP)
  assessment, 383
  complications/sequelae, 382–383
  definition, 380
  diagnosis, 383
  etiology, 381
  home care considerations, 384
  incidence, 381–382
  life span considerations, 382
  pathophysiology, 381
  therapeutic modalities, 384
  transmission, 381
Pneumonias
  assessment, 264–265
  complications/sequelae, 263
  definition, 253–254
  etiology, 255–256
  home care considerations, 267
  incidence, 261–262
  interventions/outcomes, 265–267
  life span considerations, 262–263
  pathophysiology, 256–261
  resource utilization, 593–594
  risk factors
    gastric colonization, 259
    hospital-acquired pneumonia, 260–261
    oropharyngeal colonization, 258
  therapeutic modalities, 265
  vaccines/immunizations, 491–492
  web sites, 267–268
  See also Bacterial pneumonia; Chlamydiae
    pneumonia; Community-acquired
    pneumonia; Hospital-acquired
    pneumonia; Pneumocystis pneumonia
    (PCP)
Polysomnogram/nocturnal desaturation study,
    79–80
  clinical indications, 79
  patient preparation, 79–80
  purpose, 79
  setting, 79
Post-traumatic stress disorder (PTSD), 136
  See also Anxiety
Practice Resource Network (AACN), 12–13
Pregnancy issues
  asthma, 177
  cystic fibrosis, 203, 209–210
  dyspnea, 112
  first-third trimester changes, 46–47
  impaired sleep, 127
  influenza, 190, 491
  interstitial lung disease, 246
  otitis media, 198
  Pneumocystis pneumonia (PCP), 382
  pneumonia, 491
  pneumonias, 263
  pulmonary hypertension, 399
  quality of life (QoL), 584
  tobacco/substance abuse, 7, 422–423
  upper respiratory infections, 188

Private sector coverage types, 596–597
Procedures
  arterial blood gases (ABGs), 84, 169, 219, 455,
    456, 540
  bronchoscopy, 86–87, 93, 157, 211, 236, 239
  immunoglobulins, 93
  lung biopsy, 87–88, 249, 294, 383, 386, 404
  mediastinoscopy, 89, 280
  pulmonary angiography, 86, 295
  skin tests, 49, 72, 94–95, 211, 489, 541
  sputum diagnostics, 92
  thoracentesis, 88, 281
  ventilation perfusion scan, 85, 295, 299, 403
Promotion of respiratory health
  prevention programs
    primary, secondary, tertiary, 5–6
    tobacco avoidance, 6–8
Psychological disorders. *See* Anxiety; Depression
Public sector coverage types, 596–597
Pulmonary angiography, 86, 295
  abnormal findings, 86
  complications, 86
  indications, 86
  nursing implications, 86
  precautions, 86
  procedure, 86
  purpose, 86
Pulmonary function test (PFT)
  clinical indications, 77
  clinical indications/abnormal values, 78
  normal values, 77–78
  patient preparation, 77
  purpose, 77
  setting, 77
Pulmonary hypertension
  assessment, 400–405
  classification/types
    arterial hypertension, 396–397
    chronic thrombotic/embolic disease,
     398–399
    pulmonary vasculature, 399
    respiratory system/hypoxemia, 398
    venous hypertension, 398
  complications/sequelae, 400
  definition, 393
  etiology, 393–394
  home care considerations, 412–413
  incidence, 395–396
  interventions/outcomes, 411–412
  life span considerations, 399–400
  pathophysiology, 394–395
  therapeutic modalities, 405–411
  web sites, 413
Pulmonary rehabilitation (PR)
  benefits
    to patients, 555
    to providers/payers, 556
  components
    assessment, initial, 557–558
    assessment, outcome, 564

education, 560–564
    exercise training, 558–560
definition, 555
referrals
    appropriate, 556
    inappropriate, 556–557
research directions, 15
web sites, 564
Pulmonary thromboembolism
assessment, 296–301
classifications/types, 294–295
complications/sequelae, 296
definition, 291
etiology, 291–293
home care considerations, 307–308
incidence, 294
life span considerations, 295–296
outcomes, 307
pathophysiology, 293
pharmacotherapy, 301–304
surgical interventions, 304–306
therapeutic modalities
    pharmacotherapy, 301–304
    surgical interventions, 304–306
Pulmonary vasculature, 399
Pulse oximetry
clinical implications/abnormal values, 76
clinical indications, 75
normal values, 76
patient preparation, 76
purpose, 75
setting, 76

Quality of life (QoL) issues
associated problems
    physical issues, 577
    psychological issues, 577
    sociocultural issues, 577–578
cost constraints, 579
definition, 576
educational needs
    caregiver/family, 580
    patients, 579–580
    support for, 580–581
ethical dilemmas, 579
evaluation of
    additional issues, 583
    development of QoL instruments, 581
    instruments/techniques, 581–582
    Internet sources of instruments, 582–583
pediatric considerations, 584
pregnancy considerations, 584
social support, role of, 578–579
web sites, 584–585
Quiet breathing, 29

Radiation therapy, 285–286
Reimbursement issues/managed care
Balanced Budget Act (1997), 598–599
historical background, 596

private sector coverage types, 596–597
public sector coverage types, 596–597
Research Priorities in Respiratory Nursing
    (ATS Nursing Assembly), 12
Research Work Group (AACN), 12
Research, highlights/directions, 11–17
acute care therapeutic strategies
    critical care, 13–14
    end-of-life decision making, 14
    high-tech home care, 14
    oxygen delivery systems, 14
    weaning from LTMV, 13
chronic therapeutic strategies
    asthma, 14
    COPD, 14–15
    cystic fibrosis, 15
    dyspnea, 15
    lung cancer, 15
    lung transplantation, 15
    pulmonary rehabilitation (PR), 15
    sleep apnea, 15
disease prevention/health promotion
    postoperative pulmonary complications
        (PPC), 13
    tobacco use, 13
health delivery, 15–17
priorities, 11–13
    AACN, 12–13
    ATS, 12
    NINR, 12
Resource utilization
asthma, 592–593
implication for clinicians, 601–602
lung disease costs, 595
pneumonia/influenza, 593–594
ranking of lung diseases, 590–592
reimbursement issues/managed care
    Balanced Budget Act (1997), 598–599
    historical background, 596
    private sector coverage types, 596–597
    public sector coverage types, 596–597
sleep disorders, 595–596
statistical reporting terminology, 589–590
strategies for improvement, 599–601
technology, impact of, 599
tuberculosis (TB), 594–595
web sites, 602
Respiratory distress syndrome (RDS/newborns)
assessment, 434–435
complications/sequelae, 434
definition, 433
etiology, 433
incidence, 434
interventions/outcomes, 435–436
pathophysiology, 433–434
therapeutic modalities, 435
Respiratory failure
assessment, 358–359
definitions, 354–355
home care considerations, 360

Respiratory failure (*continued*)
  pathophysiology/etiology
    hypercapnic respiratory failure, 356
    hypoxemic respiratory failure, 355–356
  therapeutic modalities, 359–360
  web sites, 360
Respiratory medicine/healthcare
  associated specializations, 3
  historical background, 3
  interdisciplinary approach, 4
  settings for, 8–9
Respiratory muscle weakness
  breathing, act of, 317–323
  diagnostic testing, 326, 328, 333, 335,
    338, 344
  neuromuscular diseases
    amyotrophic lateral sclerosis, 327–331
    Guillain-Barré Syndrome, 331–334
    multiple sclerosis, 323–327
    muscular dystrophy, 334–336
    myasthenia gravis, 336–339
    spinal cord injury, 339–347
  pharmacotherapy, 330, 333, 336
Respiratory nursing
  historical background, 3–4
  strategy promotion by, 4
Respiratory Nursing Society (RNS), 4
Respiratory parameters, spontaneous, 78–79
Respiratory syncytial virus (RSV)
  assessment, 454
  epidemiology, 453
  home care considerations, 457
  interventions/outcomes, 455–457
  pathophysiology, 454
  therapeutic modalities, 454–455
Respiratory system
  breathing mechanisms, 29–32
  function of, 27–28
  structures, basic, 28–29
Risk factors
  anxiety, 136
  bronchiolitis, 447
  community-acquired pneumonia, 262
  cystic fibrosis, 204
  depression, 142–143
  dyspnea, 110–113
  gastric colonization, 259
  hospital-acquired pneumonia, 260–261
  impaired sleep, 125
  lung cancer
    biological, 276
    lifestyle, 275
    occupational, 275–276
  lung cancers, 275–276
  mechanical ventilation, 501
  meconium aspiration syndrome, 436
  obstructive sleep apnea, 311
  oropharyngeal colonization, 258
  persistent cough, 153

  pneumonias
    gastric colonization, 259
    hospital-acquired pneumonia,
     260–261
    oropharyngeal colonization, 258
  respiratory distress syndrome, 433
  tobacco use, 6
Role-relationship pattern, 63

Schuyler, Linda, 5–9
Self-care management strategies
  airway clearance, 573
  artificial airways/tracheostomy,
    573–574
  asthma, 99
    peak flow meter, 570–571
  dyspnea, 568–569
  energy reserve interventions, 568
  fatigue, 569
  functional status assessment, 567–568
  immunizations, 569–570
  nebulized medications, 572–573
  nutrition, 570
  oxygen treatment/home modalities,
    571–572
Sequelae. *See* Complications/sequelae
Sexually-reproductive pattern, 63
Side effects
  anti-inflammatories, 223
  antibiotics, 493–494
  antihistamines, 489
  antitussives, 490
  anxiety medication, 139
  benzodiazepines, 626
  bronchodilators, 476, 482, 483, 484–485
  calcium channel blockers, 372
  cor pulmonale medication, 373–374
  corticosteroids, 180, 249, 441
  cytotoxic medications, 249
  expectorants, 490
  leukotriene modifiers, 487
  lung transplantation medication, 550–551
  mast cell stabilizer, 488
  muscular dystrophy medication, 336
  myasthenia gravis medication, 338, 339
  nasal decongestants, 488
  opioids, 626
  pulmonary hypertension medication,
    405–409
  radiation therapy, 287
  smoking cessation, nicotine/non-nicotine,
    492–493
  SSRIs, 147
  steroids, inhaled/oral, 485–487
  vaccines
    influenza, 491
    pneumonia, 492
Single lung transplantation, 542
Sinuses, paranasal, 32

Sinusitis
assessment, 195
complications/sequelae, 195
definition, 194
etiology, 194
incidence, 195
life span considerations, 195
pathophysiology, 194–195
therapeutic modalities, 195–196
Skin testing, 49, 72, 211, 489, 541
complications, 95
indications, 95
nursing implications, 95
precautions, 95
procedure, 94–95
purpose, 94
Sleep apnea. *See* Obstructive sleep apnea
Sleep-rest pattern, 62
Small-cell lung cancer (NSCLC)
chemotherapy, 285
pathophysiology, 278
radiation therapy, 285–286
Smoking cessation
nicotine replacement, 492
non-nicotine, 492–493
See also Tobacco avoidance programs
Spinal cord injury
assessment, 343–344
complications/sequelae, 342–343
definition, 339–340
etiology, 340
home care considerations, 347
incidence/clinical manifestations, 341–342
life span considerations, 342
pathophysiology, 340–341
therapeutic modalities, 344–347
Spontaneous respiratory parameters, 78–79
clinical indications, 78
clinical indications/abnormal values, 79
normal values, 78–79
patient preparation, 78
purpose, 78
setting, 78
Sputum diagnostics, 92–93
clinical indications/abnormal findings, 93
complications, 93
indications, 92–93
normal values of sputum, 93
nursing implications, 93
precautions, 93
procedure, 92
purpose, 92
Squamous cell carcinoma, 277
Staging, lung cancers, 90, 280, 281–283
Standards of Care (American Nurses Association), 4
Sternum, 28
Structures of respiratory system, 28–29
See also Thorax
Systemic blood filter, 28

Therapeutic modalities
alveolar hypoventilation, 54
amyotrophic lateral sclerosis, 328–331
anxiety, 139–140
asthma, 180–182
bronchiectasis, 237–239
bronchopulmonary dysphasia, 441–442
cocaine use, 426–427
COPD, 170–171
cor pulmonale, 371–375
cystic fibrosis, 221–225
depression, 146–147
diffusion defect, 54
dyspnea, 116–118
epiglottitis, 468–469
Guillain-Barré Syndrome, 333–334
hypoxia, extrinsic, 52
impaired sleep, 129–130
influenza, 191
interstitial lung disease, 248–249
Kaposi's Sarcoma (KS), 386–387
lung cancers, 283–286
marijuana use, 426–427
meconium aspiration syndrome, 438
mononucleosis, infectious, 197
multiple sclerosis, 326–327
muscular dystrophy, 335–336
myasthenia gravis, 338–339
obstructive sleep apnea, 129–130, 313
otitis media, 198–199
oxygen, inadequate transport/delivery, 57
persistent cough, 157–159
pharyngitis, 193–194
Pneumocystis pneumonia (PCP), 384
pneumonias, 265
pulmonary hypertension, 405–411
pulmonary thromboembolism, 301–307
respiratory distress syndrome (newborns), 435
respiratory failure, 359–360
respiratory syncytial virus (RSV), 454–455
sinusitis, 195–196
spinal cord injury, 344–347
tobacco use, 424–426
upper respiratory infections (URI), 189
V/Q mismatch, 56
Thoracentesis, 88–89, 281
abnormal findings, 89
complications, 89
definition/purpose, 88
indications, 88
nursing implications, 89
precautions, 89
procedure, 88
Thoracoscopy, 90–91
abnormal findings, 90
complications, 90
indications, 90
nursing implications, 90
precautions, 91

Thoracoscopy (*continued*)
  procedure, 90
  purpose, 90
Thorax
  lungs, 29
  mediastinum, 28–29
  rib cage, 28
  sternum, 28
Tobacco avoidance programs
  adolescents, 6–7
  involuntary smoking, 8
  women, 7–8
Tobacco use
  assessment, 423–424
  complications/sequelae, 423
  definition, 417
  etiology, 417
  home care considerations, 427
  incidence, 421
  life span considerations, 422–423
  mechanism of action, 418
  pathophysiology, 419–420
  research programs, 13
  smoking cessation programs
    nicotine replacement, 492
    non-nicotine, 492–493
  therapeutic modalities, 424–426
  web sites, 427
Tracheostomy
  approach, 525–526
  complications, 528–530
  definition, 525
  indications, 525
  minitracheostomy, 530–531
  pre-/postoperative considerations, 526
  preoperative considerations, 526
  self-care management strategies, 573–574
  troubleshooting
    abnormal bleeding, 526–527
    infection, 528
    obstructed airway, 527
    subcutaneous emphysema, 528
    tube dislodgment, 527–528
  tube types, 531–534
Transtracheal oxygen delivery (TTOD), 14
Treatment. *See* Pharmacology;
    Therapeutic modalities
Tube types, tracheostomy
  cuffed, 532
  cuffless, 532
  double-lumen, 531–532
  fenestrated trachea, 532
  Passy Muir valve, 533
  single cannula, 532
  tracheostomy button/plug, 533
  uncuffed single lumen, 532
Tuberculosis (TB)
  antibiotics, 493
  historical background, 3

HIV association, 379
lung cancer association, 280
persistent cough, 153, 157
resource utilization, 594–595
skin test reliability, 49
sputum diagnosis, 92
thoracentesis association, 88–89, 91

Upper airway, 32–33
  larynx, 33
  nose, 32
  oral cavity, 32–33
  pharynx, 33
  sinuses, paranasal, 32
Upper respiratory infections (URI)
  assessment, 188–189
  complications, 188
  definition, 187
  etiology, 187–188
  incidence, 188
  life span considerations, 188
  pathophysiology, 188
  therapeutic modalities, 189
Upper respiratory medications
  antihistamines, 488–489
  nasal decongestants, 488
Utilitarianism (consequence-based theory), 615

V/Q mismatch. *See* Ventilation and perfusion
    (V/Q) mismatch
Vaccines/immunizations
  influenza, 490–491
  pneumonia, 491–492
Value-belief pattern, 63
Vascular supply, of respiratory system
  bronchial circulation, 37
  lymphatic circulation, 37
  metabolic activity, 37
  pulmonary circulation, 36–37
Ventilation and perfusion (V/Q), 41–43
Ventilation and perfusion (V/Q) mismatch,
    42–43
  causes, 55–56
  definition, 54–55
  physiologic features, 55
  treatment, 56
Ventilation perfusion scan, 295, 299, 403
  clinical indications/abnormal scan, 85
  complications, 86
  definition/purpose, 85
  indications, 85
  nursing implications, 85–86
  precautions, 86
  procedure, 85

Weaning issues
  mechanical ventilation guidelines, 520–521
  research, highlights/directions, 13
  terminal weaning, 633–635

Weaver, Terri E., 124–132
Web sites
    bronchopulmonary dysphasia, 444
    COPD, 171
    cor pulmonale, 375–376
    cystic fibrosis, 226
    end-of-life issues, 635
    epiglottitis, 469
    impaired sleep, 132
    interstitial lung disease, 251
    Kaposi's Sarcoma (KS), 387–388

lung cancers, 287–288
mechanical ventilation, 522
newborn respiratory disorders, 444
otitis media, 199–200
patient advocacy, 613
pneumonias, 267–2268
pulmonary hypertension, 413
quality of life (QoL) issues,
    584–585
respiratory failure, 360
tobacco use, 427